# Epidermal Growth Factors and Cytokines

## CLINICAL DERMATOLOGY

*Series Editor*

**ALAN R. SHALITA, M.D.**

*Professor and Chairman*
*Department of Dermatology*
*State University of New York*
*Health Science Center at Brooklyn*
*Brooklyn, New York*

1. Cutaneous Investigation in Health and Disease: Noninvasive Methods and Instrumentation, *edited by Jean-Luc Lévêque*
2. Irritant Contact Dermatitis, *edited by Edward M. Jackson and Ronald Goldner*
3. Fundamentals of Dermatology: A Study Guide, *Franklin S. Glickman and Alan R. Shalita*
4. Aging Skin: Properties and Functional Changes, *edited by Jean-Luc Lévêque and Pierre G. Agache*
5. Retinoids: Progress in Research and Clinical Applications, *edited by Maria A. Livrea and Lester Packer*
6. Clinical Photomedicine, *edited by Henry W. Lim and Nicholas A. Soter*
7. Cutaneous Antifungal Agents: Selected Compounds in Clinical Practice and Development, *edited by John W. Rippon and Robert A. Fromtling*
8. Oxidative Stress in Dermatology, *edited by Jürgen Fuchs and Lester Packer*
9. Connective Tissue Diseases of the Skin, *edited by Charles M. Lapière and Thomas Krieg*
10. Epidermal Growth Factors and Cytokines, *edited by Thomas A. Luger and Thomas Schwarz*

*ADDITIONAL VOLUMES IN PREPARATION*

# Epidermal Growth Factors and Cytokines

edited by

**Thomas A. Luger**
**Thomas Schwarz**

*Ludwig Boltzmann Institute for Cell Biology*
*and Immunobiology of the Skin*
*University of Münster*
*Münster, Germany*

Marcel Dekker, Inc. New York • Basel • Hong Kong

**Library of Congress Cataloging-in-Publication Data**

Epidermal growth factors and cytokines / edited by Thomas A. Luger, Thomas Schwarz.
p. cm.
Includes bibliographical references and index.
ISBN 0-8247-9102-9 (alk. paper)
1. Cytokines. 2. Growth factors. 3. Epidermal growth factor.
4. Epidermis--Molecular aspects. I. Luger, Thomas A.
II. Schwarz, Thomas.
[DNLM: 1. Epidermal Growth Factor–Urogastrone--physiology.
2. Cytokines--physiology. W1 CL69L v. 10 1994 / WK 170 E64 1994]
QR185.8.C95E63 1994
612.7'9--dc20
DNLM/DLC
for Library of Congress 93-27742
CIP

The publisher offers discounts on this book when ordered in bulk quantities. For more information, write to Special Sales/Professional Marketing at the address below.

This book is printed on acid-free paper.



Marcel Dekker, Inc.
270 Madison Avenue, New York, New York 10016

Current printing (last digit):
10 9 8 7 6 5 4 3 2 1

PRINTED IN THE UNITED STATES OF AMERICA

# Series Introduction

During the past decade there has been a vast explosion in new information relating to the art and science of dermatology as well as fundamental cutaneous biology. Furthermore, this information is no longer of interest only to the small but growing specialty of dermatology. Scientists from a wide variety of disciplines have come to recognize both the importance of skin in fundamental biological processes and the broad implications of understanding the pathogenesis of skin disease. As a result there is now a multidisciplinary and world-wide interest in the progress of dermatology.

With these factors in mind, we have undertaken a new series of books specifically oriented to dermatology. The series will be purposely broad in focus and will range from pure basic science to practical, applied clinical dermatology. Thus, while there will be something for everyone, all editions in the series should ultimately prove to be valuable additions to the dermatologist's library.

*Epidermal Growth Factors and Cytokines*, edited by Drs. Thomas A. Luger and Thomas Schwarz, is an outstanding example of the type of scholarly and practical book we hope will be the hallmark of this series. The editors have assembled a group of authors who are internationally known for their expertise. They have put together a work on cytokines and other epidermal growth factors that will be a most valued addition to the libraries of the clinical practitioner as well as of great use to residents, fellows, and other students of skin biology.

I sincerely hope that you will enjoy reading these books as much as I have enjoyed planning them with the authors and editors of this series.

*Alan R. Shalita*
SUNY Downstate Medical Center
Brooklyn, New York

# Foreword

For many years, keratinocytes, the major subpopulation of epidermal cells, were thought to function primarily in the manufacture of keratins and other structural proteins. It is only within the past 10 years that an explosion of new information has indicated that keratinocytes, as well as other epidermal cells, are a rich source of cytokines and other growth factors. Cytokines are hormone-like peptides that are extremely potent at very low concentrations and generally act on cells near where they are produced (in a paracrine manner) or on the cells that produce them (in an autocrine manner). Thus, cytokine molecules produced by epidermal cells may exert their activity on cells within the epidermis, or the dermis, or at distant sites (such as hormones produced by endocrine glands).

This new information has opened new vistas in the study of skin biology, pathophysiology of skin disease, and potential therapeutic interventions. The ready accessibility of skin for study and the recent availability of recombinant cytokines in sufficient quantities to test in various diseases make skin an attractive model system in which to study the activities of cytokines in health and disease.

The editors of this book, Thomas Luger and Thomas Schwarz, have contributed greatly to our knowledge regarding identification and function of epidermis-derived cytokines. They have assembled a noteworthy group of authors who have also generated significant information and enthusiasm about cytokines—both as important epidermis-derived regulatory molecules and as effector molecules in inflammatory and neoplastic disease. The discussions regarding physical and chemical modulation of cytokine production as well as therapeutic interventions based on this entirely new scientific discipline provide exciting prospects for the future study and use of epidermis-derived cytokines and growth factors.

*Stephen I. Katz, M.D., Ph.D.*
*Dermatology Branch*
*National Cancer Institute*
*Bethesda, Maryland*

# Preface

Research on cytokines and growth factors has become one of the most rapidly advancing and expanding fields in medicine and bioscience. Almost two decades after the description of the first cytokines, we are dealing with dozens of these mediators, which are of importance for almost any biological process. With the increasing number of cytokines and growth factors, however, the subject has become gradually more complicated and difficult to survey. There is also evidence for a strong network of interacting cytokines and growth factors and we are just beginning to understand this communication. In addition, it has been established for almost a decade that the skin not only is a target for cytokines but can also function as a source for these mediators. Nowadays it is known that a variety of cytokines and growth factors are produced within the epidermis and that these mediators are involved in the modulation of inflammatory and immunological cutaneous reactions.

In spite of the availability of numerous books dealing with cytokines and growth factors, none of these is dedicated to the skin. In making epidermal cytokines and growth factors the subject of this book, it has been our aim to examine a selection of cytokines and growth factors that are produced by the epidermis or influence this organ. We have been fortunate in having a number of experts contribute to this book and are very grateful to them for their considerable efforts. Although most chapters deal with cytokines and growth factors produced within the skin, it was necessary to include also "non-epidermal" cytokines, such as lymphocyte-activating cytokines, to reflect the importance of the interaction of cytokines and growth factors within the cytokine network. Rather, we hope that this book will contribute to these efforts by furthering understanding of physiological and pathological reactions in general within the skin.

We have not attempted to demonstrate how cytokines are related specifically to particular skin diseases since, in order to address these issues sufficiently, much more information needs to be obtained.

The stimulating environment at the Dermatology Units of the University of Vienna, where both of us worked for more than a decade, was a prerequisite for us to be able to edit this book. In addition, we are gratified to find that this stimulating atmosphere has continued since our move to the University of Münster. Finally, we are grateful to Marie Luise Hülsmann and Monika Orschel for their excellent secretarial assistance. The editorial assistance of Barbara Dunleavy and Tammerly Booth of Marcel Dekker, Inc., was also of major importance.

*Thomas A. Luger*
*Thomas Schwarz*

# Contents

# Contributors

**Günther R. Adolf, Ph.D.** Head, Department of Cell Biology, Bender & Co. GmbH, Vienna, Austria

**John C. Ansel, M.D.** Associate Professor, Dermatology Service, Veterans Affairs Medical Center, and Department of Dermatology, Oregon Health Sciences University, Portland, Oregon

**Cheryl A. Armstrong, M.D.** Assistant Professor of Dermatology, Dermatology Service, Veterans Affairs Medical Center, and Department of Dermatology, Oregon Health Sciences University, Portland, Oregon

**Detlef Becker, M.D.** Department of Dermatology, University of Mainz, Mainz, Germany

**Enno Christophers, M.D.** Professor, Department of Dermatology, University of Kiel, Kiel, Germany

**Michael J. Cork, B.Sc., Ph.D., M.R.C.P.** Section of Dermatology, University Department of Medicine and Pharmacology, University of Sheffield and Royal Hallamshire Hospital, Sheffield, S. York, England

**Beate M. Czarnetzki, M.D.** Full Professor and Director, Department of Dermatology, Rudolf Virchow Clinics, Free University, Berlin, Germany

**Gordon W. Duff, M.A., Ph.D., F.R.C.P.** Professor of Molecular Medicine, Section of Molecular Medicine, University of Sheffield and Royal Hallamshire Hospital, Sheffield, S. York, England

**Beate Eckes, Ph.D.** Department of Dermatology, University of Cologne, Cologne, Germany

**James T. Elder, M.D., Ph.D.** Departments of Dermatology and Radiation Oncology (Cancer Biology), University of Michigan, Ann Arbor, Michigan

**Alexander H. Enk, M.D.*** Dermatology Branch, National Cancer Institute, National Institutes of Health, Bethesda, Maryland

**Sergij Goerdt, M.D.** Institute of Experimental Dermatology, University of Münster, Münster, Germany

**Matthias Grell, Ph.D.** Institute for Cell Biology and Immunology, University of Stuttgart, Stuttgart, Germany

**Hans-Hermann Hagemeier, M.D.** Institute of Experimental Dermatology, University of Münster, Münster, Germany

**Ruth Halaban, Ph.D.** Senior Research Scientist, Department of Dermatology, Yale University School of Medicine, New Haven, Connecticut

**Charles E. Hart, Ph.D.** Senior Scientist, Department of Protein Chemistry, ZymoGenetics Inc., Seattle, Washington

**Conrad Hauser, M.D.** Associate Professor of Dermatology, Department of Dermatology, Hôpital Cantonal Universitaire, Geneva, Switzerland

**Christine Heufler, Ph.D.** Department of Dermatology, University of Innsbruck, Innsbruck, Austria

**Eckhart Kämpgen, M.D.**† Department of Dermatology, University of Innsbruck, Innsbruck, Austria

**Tadamitsu Kishimoto, M.D., Ph.D.** Professor and Chairman, Department of Medicine III, Osaka University Medical School, Osaka, Japan

**Jürgen Knop, M.D., Ph.D.** Professor, Department of Dermatology, University of Mainz, Mainz, Germany

**Franz Koch, Ph.D.** Department of Dermatology, University of Innsbruck, Innsbruck, Austria

**Thomas Krieg, M.D.** Professor and Chairman, Department of Dermatology, University of Cologne, Cologne, Germany

**Current affiliation*: Professor, Department of Dermatology, University of Mainz, Mainz, Germany

†*Current affiliation*: Department of Dermatology, University of Würzburg, Würzburg, Germany

**Jean Krutmann, M.D.** Associate Professor, Head, Photodermatology Section, Department of Dermatology, University of Freiburg, Freiburg, Germany

**Thomas S. Kupper, M.D.** Thomas B. Fitzpatrick Associate Professor of Dermatology, Harvard Medical School, and Director of Research, Division of Dermatology, Department of Medicine, Brigham & Women's Hospital, Boston, Massachusetts

**Thomas A. Luger, M.D.** Director and Chairman, Department of Dermatology, Ludwig Boltzmann Institute for Cell Biology and Immunobiology of the Skin, University of Münster, Münster, Germany

**Cornelia Mauch, M.D., Ph.D.** Division of Cytokines and Wound Healing, Department of Dermatology, University of Cologne, Cologne, Germany

**Gisela Moellmann, Ph.D.** Associate Research Scientist, Department of Dermatology, Yale University School of Medicine, New Haven, Connecticut

**Annelie Möller, M.D.** Scientific Assistant, Department of Dermatology, Rudolf Virchow Clinics, Free University, Berlin, Germany

**Kai M. Müller, M.Sc.** Department of Dermatology, Hôpital Cantonal Universitaire, Geneva, Switzerland

**Takashi Oono, M.D.** Department of Dermatology, University of Cologne, Cologne, Germany

**Sidney Pestka, M.D.** Professor and Chairman, Department of Molecular Genetics and Microbiology, Robert Wood Johnson Medical School, University of Medicine & Dentistry of New Jersey, Piscataway, New Jersey

**Martin Röcken, M.D.*** National Institute of Allergy and Infectious Diseases, National Institutes of Health, Bethesda, Maryland

**Nikolaus Romani, Ph.D.** Associate Professor, Department of Dermatology, University of Innsbruck, Innsbruck, Austria

**Peter Scheurich, Ph.D.** Professor, Institute for Cell Biology and Immunology, University of Stuttgart, Stuttgart, Germany

**John W. Schrader** The Biomedical Research Centre, University of British Columbia, Vancouver, British Columbia, Canada

**Current affiliation*: Department of Dermatology, Ludwig-Maximilians-University Munich, Munich, Germany

**Jens-Michael Schröder, Ph.D.** Department of Dermatology, University of Kiel, Kiel, Germany

**Gerold Schuler, M.D.** Professor, Department of Dermatology, University of Innsbruck, Innsbruck, Austria

**Thomas Schwarz, M.D.** Professor of Dermatology and Head of the Division of Photobiology and Phototherapy, Department of Dermatology, Ludwig Boltzmann Institute for Cell Biology and Immunobiology of the Skin, University of Münster, Münster, Germany

**Pavel Smid, M.D.** Department of Dermatology, University of Kiel, Kiel, Germany

**Clemens Sorg, Ph.D.** Professor, Institute of Experimental Dermatology, University of Münster, Münster, Germany

**Michael Sticherling, M.D.** Department of Dermatology, University of Kiel, Kiel, Germany

**J. Wayne Streilein, M.D.** Professor and Chairman, Department of Microbiology and Immunology, University of Miami School of Medicine, Miami, Florida

**Gerda Topar, M.D.** Department of Dermatology, University of Innsbruck, Innsbruck, Austria

**Franz Trautinger, M.D.*** Department of Dermatology, Ludwig Boltzmann Institute for Cell Biology and Immunobiology of the Skin, University of Münster, Münster, Germany

**Agatha Urbanski** Department of Dermatology, Ludwig Boltzmann Institute for Cell Biology and Immunobiology of the Skin, University of Münster, Münster, Germany

**Sharon M. Wahl, Ph.D.** Chief, Cellular Immunology Section, National Institute of Dental Research, National Institutes of Health, Bethesda, Maryland

**Kazuyuki Yoshizaki, M.D., Ph.D.** Assistant Professor, Department of Medicine III, Osaka University Medical School, Osaka, Japan

**Current affiliation*: Department of Dermatology, University of Vienna, Vienna, Austria

# Epidermal Growth Factors and Cytokines

# Introduction: Immunobiology of the Skin

**J. Wayne Streilein**
*University of Miami School of Medicine*
*Miami, Florida*

The immune system, comprised chiefly of antigen-specific T and B lymphocytes, is a vertebrate adaptation that permits the host to recognize and respond to a startlingly diverse array of molecules expressed by environmental pathogens and antigens. Recognition of an antigen by cells of the immune system leads to the generation of effector responses that destroy, inactivate, or otherwise eliminate specific environmental threats carrying that antigen. Almost invariably, successful completion of the immune effector response involves the recruitment and participation of phylogenetically older nonspecific host defense mechanisms. Thus, the success with which a vertebrate organism can ward off pathogens requires a collaboration between adaptive immunity and inflammatory processes.

Among vertebrates, the immune system encounters potential pathogens/antigens usually (but not always) through one of the two major specialized interfaces that separate the host from the environment: the integument and the mucosa (alimentary, respiratory, and urogenital tracts). Although these interfaces are similar in overall design (each has a specialized barrier epithelium supported by a connective tissue stroma), they are vastly different in their anatomical, physiological, and molecular details. Moreover, the range of pathogens/antigens that pose a risk of violating the barrier surface of the integument is vastly different from that which confronts mucosal surfaces. It is no surprise, therefore, to learn that the immune system itself, and its specific effector responses, undergo tissue-specific specializations that allow for protection at the cutaneous and mucosal surfaces that is adequate, appropriate, and in many ways unique.

In a book dedicated to epidermal cytokines and growth factors, it is important to point out that the parenchymal cells that comprise the environmental interfaces—the epithelia of the skin and mucous membranes—play a major role in promoting and defining the unique characteristics of the immune response that provides the protective shields. In large measure, cytokines, secreted by the keratinocytes of skin, bind to receptors expressed on cells of the lymphoreticular system that occupy the cutaneous microenvironment and thereby modify the functional activities of these cells.

## I. SKIN-ASSOCIATED LYMPHOID TISSUES

It has been more than 15 years since it was first proposed that a portion of the lymphoid apparatus was dedicated primarily to providing immune protection for the skin [1]. The concept was fashioned after the formulation of gut-associated lymphoid tissues (GALT) in which it was believed that the lymphoid tissues associated with the gastrointestinal tract—tonsils, adenoids, appendix, Peyer's patches—were primarily responsible for handling and responding to antigenic information entering through mucosal surfaces [2]. In the case of skin, the associated lymphoid tissues were envisioned to be the lymph nodes that punctuate lymph drainage pathways from cutaneous surfaces. As in the concept of GALT, these skin-associated lymphoid tissues (SALT) contained T and B lymphocytes, some of which were believed to possess the unique capacity to bind to dermal vascular endothelium and thereby gain entrance preferentially into the cutaneous milieu. This belief was strengthened considerably by the knowledge that malignant T cells in cutaneous T-cell lymphomas display skin-seeking properties. Support for the idea that a skin-associated lymphoid tissue exists also came from the dramatic demonstrations that epidermal Langerhans cells function as potent antigen-presenting cells, thereby providing the epidermis with a capacity to capture, process, and present antigens that penetrate beyond the barrier of the stratum corneum [3].

There appear to be, therefore, two great tissue-specific specializations of the immune apparatus and response: one, mucosa-associated lymphoid tissues (MALT), focuses its activities on pathogens and antigens encountered through mucosal surfaces, while the other, SALT, is dedicated to responding to pathogens and antigens encountered through epidermal surfaces. As it is currently understood, SALT is comprised of (1) skin-seeking T (and B) lymphocytes, which have the responsibility of recognizing via surface receptors the antigens found within skin, (b) epidermal Langerhans cells and dermal dendritic cells/macrophages that capture antigens and prepare them for presentation to antigen-specific lymphocytes, (c) specialized dermal high-endothelial cells that can promote the migration of bloodborne lymphocytes into the cutaneous compartment, and (d) draining lymph nodes that provide an appropriate microenvironment in which naive and memory antigen-specific T and B lymphocytes can be primed and expanded to skin-derived antigens [4, 5]. Similar specializations of lymphoid tissues, lymphocytes, antigen-presenting cells, and microvasculature are found in MALT. Yet, MALT and SALT produce quite different immune effector responses, and evidence is considerable that the differences between these two systems are dictated by the unique parenchymal cells in which the responses are mediated. In the case of skin, keratinocytes directly and indirectly establish a unique microenvironment wherein the functions of lymphocytes, dendritic cells, and vascular endothelial cells are molded to the purpose of providing appropriate cutaneous immunity.

## A. SALT: Immune Surveillance

When the skin is at rest immunologically, i.e., when no cognate immune response is taking place, SALT is thought to provide a surveillance system designed to detect subliminal antigenic threats to the host's survival [6]. In this presumed "steady state," Langerhans cells reside in the suprabasilar epidermis, their dendrites insinuated between and around surrounding keratinocytes [3]. Deployed in this manner, Langerhans cells provide an extensive weblike surface for the entrapment of molecules in the extracellular space of the epidermis. Counterpart cells with antigen-processing and presentation capacity also reside in the dermis; however, their anatomical configuration and relationship to other dermal cells are not well understood [7]. In the aggregate, both the epidermis and dermis are equipped under resting conditions with specialized cells that can entrap and endocytose (or phagocytose) molecules and particles of potential interest to the immune system.

A small but steady stream of T (and B) lymphocytes exits continuously from the blood via the superficial dermal postcapillary venules. Circumstantial evidence indicates that some of the immigrant T cells move toward the epidermis, penetrate the basement membrane, and enter the extracellular space of the epidermis [8]. Evidence also suggests that T cells that find themselves within the epidermis can return to the dermis and, along with dermally located lymphocytes, pass with the flow of tissue fluid in lymph channels to the draining lymph node. T cells that follow this migration pathway typically express $\alpha\beta$ T-cell receptors for antigen and are thought to include naive cells—as well as memory cells—that have previously encountered and responded to skin-derived antigens. The surveillance function they subserve relates to conventional antigenic encounters.

In mice, a second population of epidermally located T cells exists in surprisingly large numbers [9]. These cells express $\gamma\delta$ T-cell receptors and populate the epidermis by proliferation after a "wave" of precursor cells reaches the skin during ontogeny [10]. These dendritic T cells do not participate in the recirculation pathways described for $\alpha\beta$ T cells. Although the immune functions of $\gamma\delta$ T cells in murine skin are unknown, highly speculative and provocative proposals have attempted to assign unique functional properties to these cells. Moreover, it is not clear that homologous populations of epidermal T cells bearing $\gamma\delta$ receptors exist in other species, including humans. Therefore, at this time it is difficult to know whether a conceptual framework of SALT should include $\gamma\delta$ T cells, and, if so, what role these intriguing cells should be assigned.

In resting skin, dermal endothelial cells do not appear to display surface ligands of the type that have been shown to promote lymphocyte migration through specialized and inflammatory endothelia. If this statement is true, then the T cells in skin that provide surveillance function must rely on constitutive processes such as diapedesis in order to enter the cutaneous environment. Much remains to be learned about the cytokines and/or cell-adhesion molecules that are responsible for the baseline flow of lymphocytes and antigen-presenting cell precursors to the skin, as well as about the non–antigen-dependent processes that govern their fate.

## B. SALT: Induction of Cutaneous Immunity

Introduction of antigen into the "resting" cutaneous environment causes sweeping changes among the cellular participants in SALT, the consequence of which is the development of cutaneous immunity. The experimental model system that has been most extensively studied is contact hypersensitivity (allergic contact dermatitis), and it is believed, but by no means proven, that the principles that have emerged from these studies will apply generically to antigens expressed by pathogens that invade the skin and to neoantigens displayed by malignant cells that arise within the skin. Epicutaneously applied antigens (highly reactive haptens, such as dinitrochlorobenzene) are able to form covalent bonds with proteins in the epidermal compartment and thereby create new antigenic determinants that include the hapten itself. The first component of SALT to encounter hapten-derivatized neoantigens is the epidermal Langerhans cells. Shortly after hapten has penetrated through the stratum corneum into the suprabasilar space, Langerhans cells are found to contain the hapten—either because the cell's own surface proteins have been derivatized or because derivatized proteins have been endocytosed [11]. Within a few hours, "veiled" cells bearing hapten appear in the dermal lymph channels [12]; these cells are presumed to represent Langerhans cells that have migrated across the dermal-epidermal junction. Shortly thereafter, hapten-bearing dendritic cells can be identified in the parafollicular areas of the draining lymph node [13, 14]. At this point, the cells are exceedingly immunogenic: small numbers of hapten-bearing $Ia^+$ dendritic cells from a draining lymph node can immunize naive, syngeneic recipients when injected subcutaneously. By 24–48 h after epicutaneous hapten painting, interfollicular dendritic cells in the draining node are found to be surrounded by activated and proliferating T cells [15]. At this time, the postcapillary venules of the deep cortex of the node are engorged with lymphocytes migrating from the blood, and shortly thereafter T cells that can mediate contact hypersensitivity are found—first locally (within the node) and then systemically. In the induction of contact hypersensitivity, hapten-specific CD4+ and CD8+ T cells that are generated within these nodes are distributed throughout the body.

## C. SALT: Expression of Cutaneous Immunity

Reexposure of a sensitized individual to hapten via an epicutaneous application evokes an intense local inflammatory response that is delayed in onset, and when fully formed, the inflammation involves both the epidermis and the dermis. It is not clear when or where the *initial* encounter between hapten and bloodborne, recirculating hapten-specific T cells takes place in contact hypersensitivity. Two different views have been advanced: in the first, which places the initial event within the epidermis, surface proteins associated with Langerhans cells, keratinocytes, and potentially other resident cells of the epidermis become derivatized by the epicutaneously applied hapten. As in initial sensitization, these derivatized proteins are taken up by Langerhans cells and presented on the surface to hapten-specific T cells that "happen" to be in the epidermis at the time (a surveillance function). An alternate possibility is that both Langerhans cells and keratinocytes are capable of presenting hapten-derivatized peptides to T cells in the epidermis. Upon recognition of hapten, T cells that "happen" to be passing through the epidermis release lymphokines (e.g., gamma-interferon, lymphotoxin) that promote inflammation by (a) permeating the local epidermis, inducing up-regulation of MHC molecules on epidermal cells, and therefore expanding the antigen-presenting substrate within this tissue space, and (b) diffusing into the dermis where activation of endothelial cells of the dermal postcapillary venules leads to dilatation, leakage of plasma products, and recruitment of circulating monocytes, lymphocytes, and other leukocytes that will contribute to specific and nonspecific amplification of the response. In the second view, which places the initial recognition of hapten by T cells in the dermis, hapten percolates through the epidermis into the dermis, derivatizing proteins promiscuously in the process. Among the cells that either express proteins to be derivatized or can take up derivatized proteins are the endothelial cells of the postcapillary venules. Hapten-specific T cells within the vascular tree are thus able to recognize antigen on the endothelial surface. In this view of the process, release of inflammatory lymphokines at this surface causes endothelial cells to undergo a functional transformation, which leads to dilatation, leakage of plasma proteins into the dermis, and, most important, recruitment of monocytes, T cells, and other leukocytes into the local site. As additional hapten-specific T cells enter the dermis, and after they migrate into the epidermis, they are confronted by a sea of hapten-derivatized proteins. Amplification then ensues as more and more cutaneous cells are endowed with the capacity to express class I and class II molecules, expanding the antigen-presenting stratum.

## II. CONCERNING THE CUTANEOUS MICROENVIRONMENT(S) CREATED BY KERATINOCYTES

The specializations of the immune system, of which SALT is an important expression, are dictated largely by the microenvironment in which immunity is carried out. This may seem axiomatic, but it is worth pointing out that the only unique components of SALT are the parenchymal cells of the skin. The immune cellular participants, lymphocytes, appear to arise during ontogeny as generic rather than skin-specific cells. Similarly, Langerhans cells arise from bone marrow–derived precursors and apparently adopt their intraepidermal functional program once they have invaded the site. The endothelial cells that line the dermal microvessels share a common ontogeny and functional properties with dermal endothelial of most (but not all) tissues of the body. The fact that these diverse cells collaborate in providing the skin with a relatively unique brand of immune protection reflects the extent to which they have come under the influence of the parenchymal cells of skin—keratinocytes.

Except among excitable tissues and among organs where gap junctions provide direct electrical and chemical means of intercellular communication, all other forms of cellular communication appear to be mediated by cytokines and receptors, by cell-adhesion molecules and their co-receptors, and by small molecular weight mediators (of inflammation). The skin is no exception; the extent to which keratinocytes can influence cells of the lymphoreticular apparatus and the microvasculature is the extent to which keratinocytes secrete cytokines and express cell surface molecules of interest. When the skin is at rest, immunologically speaking, keratinocytes are constitutively secreting only a few cytokines of potential relevance to the immune system: transforming growth factor-alpha (TGF-$\alpha$), interleukin 1$\alpha$ (IL-1$\alpha$), and (probably) transforming growth factor-beta (TGF-$\beta$) (see Chapter 16). It may be that keratinocytes also constitutively secrete alpha-interferon (IFN-$\alpha$)

and alpha-melanocyte stimulating hormone (MSH-$\alpha$). The numerous other cytokines that have been demonstrated to be secretory products of cultured and perturbed keratinocytes are *not* constitutively produced in resting skin: IL-1$\beta$, tumor necrosis factor alpha (TNF-$\alpha$), IL-6, IL-3, and granulocyte/macrophage colony-stimulating factor (GM-CSF) among others. Therefore, under "resting" conditions, Langerhans cell precursors that enter the epidermal compartment are confronted by a rather subtle microenvironment that is able to promote (or allow the natural endogenous expression of) the cells to adopt the "fresh" functional program. Migratory lymphocytes that enter this compartment also find little that would promote their activation potential. Similarly, the microenvironmental state of the dermis under "resting" conditions allows for the steady trickle of bloodborne granulocytes, lymphocytes, monocytes, etc. that regularly pass through the dermal endothelium by diapedesis.

The quiescence of resting skin is undoubtedly more apparent than real. Even so, the cutaneous microenvironment "at rest" is decidedly less provocative to cells of the immune system than when the skin is assaulted by a pathogen, a highly reactive hapten, or by ultraviolet radiation. The range of changes that can and do take place among perturbed keratinocytes, in terms of cytokine and cytokine receptor expression, display of cell-adhesion molecules, and production of mediators of inflammation, is enormous and clearly beyond the scope of this chapter, to say nothing of the expertise of the author. As subsequent chapters will reveal, the "perturbed" keratinocyte comes to resemble cultured keratinocytes in its ability to transcribe and produce a large array of cytokines and mediators that directly and indirectly affect keratinocytes and other nonepithelial cells that occupy the cutaneous space. Langerhans cells, lymphocytes, endothelial cells, fibroblasts, mast cells, dermal dendritic cells, and other temporary or permanent occupants of the skin have surface receptors that allow them to respond to keratinocyte-derived signals and in so doing to change the proliferative and differentiation status of the skin itself, impact on the dermal elements of the cardiovascular system, and (in the context of this chapter) alter the systemic and local immune response to cutaneous antigens.

In the last section of this chapter, three examples are selected and described in order to give a flavor of the molecular mechanisms by which keratinocytes can influence immunity in the skin. In so doing, the point is made that once keratinocytes begin to alter the properties of cells of the immune and vascular system, and destabilize thereby the "resting" microenvironment of skin, keratinocytes themselves can become the targets of activation products of the invading, nonparenchymal cells. Understanding of this complex set of actions and counteractions is incomplete and a fruitful area of current research.

## III. ALTERED CUTANEOUS MICROENVIRONMENTS AND THEIR CONSEQUENCES

The three examples selected for the following segment of this chapter represent research areas of particular interest to the author. In each case, keratinocytes play a major role in changing their microenvironment and, in so doing, alter the functional properties of the indigenous cells and the immune potential of the site.

### A. Corneal Epithelium, Langerhans Cells, and Cell-Mediated Immunity

Of all cutaneous surfaces of the body, the cornea is unique. At its attachment to the sclera, the limbus, Langerhans cells are densely packed within the suprabasilar space of the epithelium on the conjunctival side. However, on the corneal side, few Langerhans cells can be found, especially as one approaches the central cornea [17]. Since Langerhans cells are regarded as the critical antigen-presenting cells of skin, their absence from the central corneal epithelium is of considerable theoretical and practical interest. It has been known for some time that migration of limbal Langerhans cells into the central cornea can be induced by various stimuli, including (a) a suture of silk thread placed through the central cornea (epithelium and upper stroma), (b) application of a hapten, such as dinitrofluorobenzene (DNFB), to the corneal surface, (c) 1-$\mu$m plastic beads placed in extremely thin slits carved in the superficial central corneal epithelium, and (d) infection of the cornea with herpes simplex virus. Niederkorn and coworkers [18–20] have conducted an elegant series of experiments that reveal one molecular mediator responsible for migration of Langerhans cells into the cornea and indicate the important immunological consequences of bringing Langerhans cells into the cornea. This group of investigators has demonstrated that limbal Langerhans cells can be called into the central cornea simply by injecting IL-1 into the corneal stroma, indicating that Langerhans cell migration into and through the epithelium is likely to be cytokine dependent. Other cytokines may have similar effects, but that remains to be seen. It could be postulated that under "resting" conditions, little or no IL-1 activity exists in the central cornea, and therefore Langerhans cells fail to migrate in. Niederkorn et al.'s data strongly suggest that injury or trauma to central corneal epithelial cells induces the production and release of IL-1 and that, as a consequence, Langerhans cell movement into the central corneal epithelium is instigated.

Fortunately for the immunodermatologists who have conceptualized an important role for Langerhans cells in the epidermis, the (abnormal) presence of Langerhans cells in the central corneal epithelium has important immunological consequences. Using a model system in rats that contrasts immune responses to corneal allografts placed in orthotopic as opposed to heterotopic sites, Niederkorn et al. have demonstrated that, whereas orthotopic corneal allografts are usually accepted, rejection is greatly promoted if Langerhans cells are present in the graft epithelium [20]. Thus, the absence of Langerhans cells in cornea may be important in the extraordinary success of human corneal allografts. In addition, Niederkorn et al. have discovered that heterotopic corneal allografts containing Langerhans cells induce cell-mediated immunity comprised of both delayed hypersensitivity and cytotoxic T cells, whereas heterotopic normal corneal grafts (i.e., devoid of Langerhans cells) only engender cytotoxic T-cell activation. Recipients of these grafts fail to display alloantigen-specific delayed hypersensitivity. It has long been known that immunity that is selectively deficient in delayed hypersensitivity is the typical outcome when antigens are placed in the anterior chamber of the eye [18]. It has been suspected that the absence of Langerhans cells in the normal cornea may contribute to the unusual and deviant form of systemic immunity elicited by antigens injected into the anterior chamber. In support of this suspicion, Williamson et al. [21] and McLeish et al. [22] have independently verified that injections of antigen into the anterior chambers of eyes in which the corneal epithelium already contains Langerhans cells induce a conventional immune response, replete with vigorous antigen-specific delayed hypersensitivity.

In this example of an altered cutaneous microenvironment, corneal epithelial cells (the equivalents of epidermal keratinocytes) preside over a local microenvironment in which Langerhans cells are absent and in which immune responses are unusual and deficient in delayed hypersensitivity. The data imply that this microenvironment normally lacks IL-1 and that corneal epithelial cells—by their failure to secrete IL-1 constitutively—are responsible. In fairness, the morphological appearance of Langerhans cells at the limbus of a normal eye suggests that their absence from the central epithelium could be due to a factor that inhibits their migration into the cornea. Numerous inhibitory cytokines (TGF-$\beta$, MSH-$\alpha$, vasoactive intestinal peptide) have now been identified in the aqueous humor, the clear fluid that fills the anterior chamber and penetrates into the corneal stroma [23]. It remains to be seen whether the unique qualities of the central corneal microenvironment are dominated by a keratinocyte failure or by inhibitory influences derived from the internal components of the eye itself.

## B. Ultraviolet Light, TNF-$\alpha$, and Cutaneous Immunity

For more than a decade it has been known that acute low-dose radiation with ultraviolet B light (UVB) impairs the induction of contact hypersensitivity

(CH) to epicutaneously applied haptens, such as DNFB—at least in some inbred strains of mice [24] and in certain humans [25]. Recently, the genetic basis of the effects of UVB on CH induction has been elucidated in mice [26]. Polymorphic alleles at the *Lps* and *Tnfα* loci conspire to produce the phenotypes of UVB susceptibility (UVB-S) and UVB resistance (UVB-R). At the *Lps* locus, UVB-S mice possess an *Lps* allele that contributes to increased TNF-α production, primarily by stabilizing TNF-α mRNA. At the *Tnfα* locus, all UVB-R mice possess a unique *Tnfα* allele that is defined by a restriction fragment length polymorphism following DNA digestion with BamH1 (Streilein, unpublished observations). The precise reasons for the ability of this allele to confer UVB resistance remains to be determined, but it is reasonable to suspect a regulatory segment in the 5′-untranslated region that interferes with transcription of *Tnfα*. Even though the precise molecular basis of UVB-S and UVB-R is still unclear, the facts that (a) intradermally injected recombinant murine TNF-α can reproduce the effects of UVB radiation on induction of CH, and (b) these effects of UVB are abrogated by systemic anti–TNF-α antibody treatment strongly support the contention that TNF-α is the primary mediator of the deleterious effects of UVB and CH induction. Since a single exposure to UVB and a single injection of TNF-α produce comparable changes in local epidermal Langerhans cells, it is likely that TNF-α impairs CH induction by interfering with the ability of hapten-bearing Langerhans cells to carry to the draining lymph node the essential immunogenic signal that activates naive hapten-specific T cells.

The cellular source of TNF-α that mediates the effect of UVB on CH induction is a matter of considerable interest. Whereas intradermally-injected TNF-α produces changes in Langerhans cells within 5 min, UVB radiation achieves a similar effect only after 2 h [27]. The delay is thought to represent the time it takes for UVB radiation to induce up-regulation of transcription of the *Tnfα* gene within keratinocytes, where it is usually silent in “resting” skin. An alternative view is that the TNFα-containing granules of mast cells in the superficial dermal papillae (which receive approximately 5% of UVB radiation when the skin is exposed) may release TNF-α in response to radiation injury. A third possibility is that Langerhans cells themselves serve as the source of UVB-induced TNF-α. The first and third possibilities are the more compatible with the genetic basis of the effects of UVB on CH induction, and of these, we favor the first because cultured keratinocytes are known to secrete large amounts of TNF-α following exposure to UVB radiation in vitro.

This example highlights the role of keratinocytes in influencing immunity engendered by cutaneous antigens. According to the scenarios described earlier in this chapter, hapten painted on normal skin leads to sensitization when epidermal Langerhans cells take up hapten-derivatized proteins, carry them across the dermal-epidermal junction into the extracellular compartment of the dermis, and are then swept (as veiled cells) to the draining lymph node. Following UVB radiation, local release of TNF-$\alpha$ profoundly alters the functional properties of epidermal Langerhans cells. Their morphological appearance (round soma, lost dendrites) reflects the fact that the cells are virtually immobilized within the epidermal compartment. As a consequence hapten-bearing $Ia^+$ cells fail to arrive in sufficient numbers in the draining lymph node during the first 24 h after irradiation.

UVB-perturbed keratinocytes also appear to be responsible for the observation that UVB irradiation of mouse skin leads to the exaggerated expression of contact hypersensitivity [29]. This paradoxical result has been explored by Yoshikawa et al. [30] and found to be explainable, once again, as the consequence of intraepidermal release of TNF-$\alpha$. These investigators have found that injection of TNF-$\alpha$ into the pinnae of DNFB-immune mice prior to application of hapten leads to enhanced CH expression—approximately to the same degree as that induced by UVB radiation of the ears. Moreover, enhanced CH expression following UVB radiation is eliminated if the mice are treated systemically with neutralizing anti–TNF-$\alpha$ antibodies. It was first reported by Bergstresser et al. [31] that epicutaneous application of a hapten produces a significant reduction in local Langerhans cells, presumably because hapten-bearing cells in larger numbers are induced to migrate out of the epidermis. Preliminary evidence from our laboratory indicates that, although intradermal injection of TNF-$\alpha$ produces an almost immediate change in Langerhans cells, including a slight reduction in the number of Ia-bearing cells, subsequent application of hapten causes no further reduction in Ia-bearing cells. In fact, within 24 h, the density of Langerhans cells in epidermis injected with TNF-$\alpha$ and then exposed to hapten is slightly above normal. Moreover, expression of cell adhesion molecules, both on keratinocytes themselves and Langerhans cells, within UVB-treated epidermis is significantly up-regulated [32]. We interpret these results to mean that UVB, via TNF-$\alpha$ released from keratinocytes, immobilized Langerhans cells within the epidermis for a significant period of time. Consequently, although hapten-bearing cells are unable to deliver an immunogenic signal to the draining lymph node, the cells are retained in large numbers within the epidermis to serve as targets of hapten-specific T cells. Increased expression of cell-adhesion molecules on epidermal cells also serves to focus and retain migratory lymphocytes and other leukocytes that comprise the inflammatory response.

It is apparent that not all of the elements contributing to the effects of UVB radiation on the induction and expression of CH have been identified, nor have all the complicated cellular interactions been elucidated. However, even at this early time, experimental results clearly indicate that keratinocytes, through the release of cytokines and expression of cell-adhesion molecules, make a major impact on the manner in which the immune system detects and responds to antigens in the cutaneous environment.

## C. Psoriasis and the Functional Properties of Fresh and Cultured Langerhans Cells

In the previous example, keratinocytes responded to an environmental stimulus, UVB radiation, by assuming novel functional properties that drastically altered the epidermal, and presumably dermal, microenvironments. As a consequence, the ability of the immune system to recognize and respond to cutaneous antigens was greatly distorted. As the primary parenchymal cells of the skin, keratinocytes are responsible for dictating the specific nature of the microenvironment over which they preside. In the cutaneous setting, cells of the immune system (lymphocytes, Langerhans cells) resemble pawns in a game over which they exert no direct control. In the third example, represented by the common form of psoriasis, keratinocytes may not always dominate their environment. When the immune system invades the skin inappropriately, a novel microenvironment can be created, one that fundamentally distorts the functions of cutaneous cells resulting in a pathological state.

Within the past decade, in light of the remarkable ability of systemic treatment with the immunosuppressive drug cyclosporin A to ameliorate the cutaneous signs and symptoms of psoriasis, attention has been drawn to the possibility that the immune system may participate in the pathogenesis of this disease [33]. Theories have been advanced implicating (a) T-cell responses to cutaneous antigens, either exogenous (e.g., streptococcal antigens) or endogenous (autoantigens of keratinocytes, etc.), or (b) abnormalities in the dermal microvasculature through which immunoreactive cells enter the dermis and epidermis. Streilein has recently advanced the notion that psoriasis may be a disorder in which cytokines of the immune system act as driving forces to alter the cutaneous microenvironment in a fashion that leads to the psoriasis phenotype [34, 35].

Like most cells, keratinocytes, T lymphocytes, Langerhans cells, and dermal endothelial cells respond to environmental signals in order to carry out their genetic programs of proliferation, differentiation, and function. Even though their individual genetic programs are unique, the environmental signals to which these disparate cells respond are sometimes very similar. This simply underscores the fact that a relatively limited number of cytokines and receptors, as well as cell-adhesion molecules and other molecular mediators, are used over and again by different tissues in the body as the means by which signals are communicated. Keratinocytes, especially following activation or being placed in culture, become factories for the production of cytokines, such as IL-1, IL-3, IL-6, TNF-$\alpha$, GM-CSF, TGF-$\beta$, and others. In the previous two examples, production of these cytokines accounted, in part, for the influence keratinocytes exerted over the activities of Langerhans cells, lymphocytes, and vascular endothelium. Similarly, T lymphocytes also become cytokine factories when activated, secreting IL-3, GM-CSF, lymphotoxin, IFN-$\gamma$, etc. Production of lymphokines equips T cells with the potential to influence Langerhans cells, vascular endothelial cells, and even keratinocytes. It is the inherent redundancy of cytokine signals that makes it possible for lymphocytes to invade skin and to establish a novel microenvironment that subverts the normal functions of keratinocytes and fibroblasts. Such a situation, occurring during the course of expression of contact hypersensitivity, is not a long-term threat, because the response subsides as antigen is eliminated from the skin and keratinocytes can reestablish their hegemony. It is the thesis advanced here and elsewhere that in psoriasis T lymphocytes maintain a prolonged influence over the skin with long-term pathological consequences.

Demidem et al. have conducted a series of experiments examining the functional properties of fresh and cultured Langerhans cells obtained from normal skin in comparison with cells harvested from involved and uninvolved skin of patients with psoriasis [36–39]. As anticipated, fresh epidermal cells from normal human skin displayed functional properties similar to those described for freshly obtained murine Langerhans cells. They were unable to activate autologous T cells, but readily able to activate allogeneic T cells in the presence of TGF-$\beta$, but not in medium containing chloroquine. These properties were not shared with fresh cells obtained from psoriatic skin. Instead, fresh epidermal cells from involved and uninvolved psoriatic skin performed in vitro in a manner very similar to that of cultured normal epidermal cells. They were able to activate autologous T cells as well as allogeneic T cells, capacities that were enhanced in the presence of chloroquine but impaired when TGF-$\beta$ was present. Perhaps the most important aspect of these results is the discovery that cells harvested from uninvolved psoriatic skin already possessed the functional phenotype usually associated with cultured Langerhans cells. This indicates that abnormalities in Langerhans cells can precede the appearance of a psoriatic lesion and raises the possibility that this abnormality may contribute to the lesion's development.

A hypothesis that links the changes in Langerhans cells in psoriasis with the immunopathogenesis of the disease has been advanced [34, 35]. Briefly, it is proposed that a primary (perhaps the first) immune abnormality in psoriasis is the functional transformation of epidermal Langerhans cells from a "fresh" to a "cultured" phenotype. In the absence of antigenic stimuli, this transformation is silent, and the skin clinically appears to be "uninvolved." However, if the skin is assaulted with "antigen," the abnormal Langerhans cells display their capacity to present antigen in a highly immunogenic way, sufficient to activate unprimed T cells in situ. Activated T cells not only undergo replication, but they also secrete lymphokines, such as GM-CSF, IL-3, and IL-2. Under normal circumstances, this type of activation of unprimed T cells occurs in lymph nodes or spleen; however, when activation occurs extranodally—for example, in the skin—the lymphokines secreted by T cells permeate the local microenvironment. Langerhans cell function is particularly enhanced by GM—CSF, which means that further enhancement of their capacity to activate T cells can occur within an epidermis containing activated T cells; moreover, dermal dendritic cells and macrophages are also susceptible to this T-cell cytokine. T-cell–derived cytokines, released within the skin, have direct access to dermal endothelial cells. In fact, the transformation of dermal vessels in psoriasis into "high" endothelial cells that promote leukocyte emigration may reflect the consequences of intracutaneous T-cell activation [8]. Recruitment of additional T cells and leukocytes into this site of psoriasis-prone skin serves to amplify T-cell activation, leading to further increases in concentration of T-cell–derived lymphokines within the cutaneous microenvironment. Eventually, as this response becomes self-sustaining and the microenvironment becomes saturated with T-cell lymphokines, keratinocytes find themselves bathed in fluids that promote their proliferation and inhibit their differentiation. On the crest of this wave, the clinical lesion of psoriasis emerges.

Whether this scenario eventually proves to have any validity in the pathogenesis of psoriasis is less important than the value it has in suggesting novel experimental approaches to understanding the pathogenesis of immunopathogenic diseases of the skin. It may be that one reason cyclosporin A (CsA) is so effective in psoriasis is that it inhibits T-cell activation, not only by a direct action on T cells, but indirectly by suppressing the delivery of accessory signals to T cells from CsA-susceptible antigen-presenting cells located in the skin. Similarly, the idea that chloroquine is deleterious to psoriasis [40, 41] and may even precipitate new lesions seems to be related to the capacity of this drug to amplify the antigen-presenting potential of cells—cultured Langerhans cells and cells freshly obtained from psoriatic skin (uninvolved as well as involved) that already express considerable accessory cell function. Perhaps chloroquine's ability to exaggerate the accessory properties of antigen-presenting cells in uninvolved skin is sufficient to permit the local activation of T cells, culminating eventually in the appearance or exaggeration of psoriatic lesions.

## IV. SUMMARY

The specialization of the immune system represented by SALT is dictated ultimately by the intracutaneous microenvironment created primarily by keratinocytes. This microenvironment is comprised chiefly of the cytokines and other secretory products of so-called "resting" keratinocytes and is appropriate not only for the orderly proliferation and differentiation of keratinocytes, but also for ensuring that, on the one hand, induction of immunity to cutaneous antigens takes place in draining lymph nodes, rather than in the skin itself, whereas, on the other hand, expression of immunity occurs within the skin itself. Maintenance of a keratinocyte "sphere of influence" within the skin is essential to the integrity of the skin. When this influence is breached—e.g., following irradiation of the skin with UVB or when T cells invade the skin and establish their own novel microenvironment—cutaneous immunity is impaired and the physiological properties of skin itself are distorted. Much remains to be learned about the complexities of cellular communication in providing skin with its physiological functional properties. Progress in identifying the individual cytokines that influence the functions of indigenous and exogenous cells of the skin will eventually help us reach a suitable understanding.

## ACKNOWLEDGMENTS

This work was supported by USPHS Grant AI-22072 and American Cancer Society Grant PDT-383.

## REFERENCES


1. J. W. Streilein, *J. Invest. Dermatol. 71*, 167 (1978).
2. M. McWilliams, J. M. Philips-Quagliata, and M. E. Lamm, *J. Immunol. 115*, 54 (1975).
3. J. W. Streilein and P. R. Bergstresser, *Immunobiology 168*, 285 (1984).
4. J. W. Streilein, *J. Invest. Dermatol. 80*, 12S (1983).
5. J. W. Streilein, in *The Skin Immune System (SIS)*, (J. Bos, ed.), CRC Press, Inc., Boca Raton, Florida, 1990, p. 26.
6. F. M. Burnet, *Immunological Surveillance*, Pergamon Press, Oxford, 1970.
7. J. W. Streilein, *J. Invest. Dermatol. 93*, 443 (1989).
8. Y-H. Chin, V. Falanga, J. W. Streilein, and R. Sackstein, *J. Invest. Dermatol. 93*, 82S (1989).
9. P. R. Bergstresser, R. Tigelaar, and J. W. Streilein, *J. Invest. Dermatol. 85*, 85S (1985).
10. W. L. Havran, Y-H. Chien, and J. P. Allison, *Science 252*, 1430 (1991).
11. C. D. Bucana, J-M. Tang, K. Dunner, and M. L. Kripke, *J. Invest. Dermatol. 99*, 205 (1992).
12. D. J. McKeever, N. D. MacHugh, B. M. Goddeeris, E. Awino, and W. I. Morrison, *J. Immunol. 147*, 3703 (1991).
13. S. T. Macatonia, S. C. Knight, A. J. D. Edwards, S. Griffihs, and P. Fryer, *J. Exp. Med. 166*, 1654 (1987).

14. M. L. Kripke, C. G. Munn, A. Jeevan, J-M. Tang, and C. Bucana, *J. Immunol. 145*, 2833 (1990).
15. M. Cumberbatch, I. Illingworth, and I. Kimber, *Immunology 74*, 139 (1991).
16. A. Gottlieb, C. K. Chank, D. N. Posnett, B. Fanelli, and J. P. Tam, *J. Exp. Med. 167*, 670 (1988).
17. J. W. Streilein, G. B. Toews, and P. R. Bergstresser, *Nature 282*, 326 (1979).
18. J. Y. Niederkorn, *Adv. Immunol. 48*, 191 (1990).
19. J. Y. Niederkorn, J. S. Peeler, and J. Mellon, *Reg. Immunol. 2*, 83 (1989).
20. J. Ross, Y-G. He, M. Pidherney, J. Mellon, and J. Y. Niederkorn, *Transplantation 52*, 857 (1991).
21. J. S. P. Williamson, S. DiMarco, and J. W. Streilein, *Invest. Ophthalmol. Vis. Sci. 28*, 1527 (1987).
22. W. McLeish, P. Rubasamen, S. S. Atherton, and J. W. Streilein, *Reg. Immunol. 2*, 236 (1989).
23. J. W. Streilein, G. A. Wilbanks, A. Taylor, and S. Cousins, *Curr. Eve. Res. 11*, 41 (1992).
24. G. B. Toews, P. R. Bergstresser, and J. W. Streilein, *J. Immunol. 124*, 445 (1980).
25. T. Yoshikawa, V. Rae, W. Bruins-Slot, J-W. Van den Berg, J. R. Taylor, and J. W. Streilein, *J. Invest. Dermatol. 95*, 530 (1990).
26. T. Yoshikawa and J. W. Streilein, *Immunogenetics 32*, 398 (1990).
27. M. Vermeer and J. W. Streilein, *Photodermatol. Photoimmunol. & Photomed 7*, 258 (1990).
28. M. Bigby, R. Vargas, and M-D. Sy, *J. Immunol. 143*, 3867 (1989).
29. L. Polla, R. Margolis, C. Goulston, J. A. Parrish, and R. D. Granstein, *J. Invest. Dermatol. 86*, 13 (1986).
30. T. Yoshikawa, I. Kurimoto, and J. W. Streilein, *J. Invest. Dermatol. 96*, 625 (abstract) (1991).
31. P. R. Bergstresser, G. B. Toews, and J. W. Streilein, *J. Invest. Dermatol. 75*, 73 (1980).
32. D. A. Norris, B. Lyons, M. H. Middleton, J. J. Yohn, and M. Kashihara-Sawami, *J. Invest. Dermatol. 95*, 132 (1990).
33. C. Ellis, D. Gorsulowsky, T. Hamilton, J. Billings, M. Brown, J. Headington, K. Cooper, O. Baadsgaard, E. Duell, T. Annesley, J. Turcotte, and J. Voorhees, *JAMA 256*, 3110 (1986).
34. J. W. Streilein, *J. Invest. Dermatol. 95*, 20S (1990).
35. J. W. Streilein, S. F. Grammer, T. Yoshikawa, A. Demidem, and M. Vermeer, *Immunol. Rev. 117*, 159 (1990).
36. A. Demidem, J. R. Taylor, S. F. Grammer, and J. W. Streilein, *J. Invest. Dermatol. 96*, 401 (1991).
37. A. Demidem, J. R. Taylor, S. F. Grammer, and J. W. Streilein, *Reg. Immunol. 3*, 297 (1991).
38. A. Demidem, J. R. Taylor, S. F. Grammer, and J. W. Streilein, *J. Invest. Dermatol. 97*, 454 (1991).
39. A. Demidem, J. R. Taylor, S. F. Grammer, and J. W. Streilein, *J. Invest. Dermatol. 98*, 181 (1992).
40. H. Baker, *Br. J. Dermatol. 78*, 161 (1966).
41. G. A. Slagel and W. D. James, *J. Am. Acad. Dermatol. 12*, 857 (1983).

# I
# CYTOKINES

# 1
# Interleukin 1

**Michael J. Cork and Gordon W. Duff**
*University of Sheffield and*
*Royal Hallamshire Hospital*
*Sheffield, S. York, England*

## I. INTRODUCTION

There are two classes of interleukin 1 (IL-1) molecule, IL-1$\alpha$ and IL-1$\beta$, each encoded by a separate gene but seeming to act on common receptors. They are polypeptides involved in the regulation of immune and inflammatory responses. IL-1 belongs to a group of cytokines with overlapping biological properties, the others being TNF-$\alpha$ and IL-6. IL-1 is a primary macrophage-derived cytokine which stimulates the transcription of many other cytokines, and it is thought that production of IL-1, its receptors, and its inhibitors may be important in many inflammatory diseases such as psoriasis and rheumatoid arthritis.

## II. HISTORICAL PERSPECTIVE

Products of macrophages with activities now ascribed to IL-1 have been studied for many years under different names. A granulocyte pyrogen (GP) was initially described as a soluble protein released by activated peritoneal exudate cells which, when injected into animals or humans, produced fever (Bennett and Beeson 1953). This activity was further characterized as endogenous pyrogen (EP) (Atkins 1960).

A lymphocyte-activating factor (LAF) extracted from mouse peritoneal macrophages augmented the proliferation of lymphocytes in response to suboptimal doses of antigens or mitogens such as phytohemagglutinin (Gery and Waksman 1972). A similar substance isolated from keratinocytes by several groups was called epidermal thymocyte-activating factor (ETAF) (Luger et al. 1981, Sauder et al. 1982). Subsequent studies revealed that ETAF was a heterogeneous mixture of IL-1$\alpha$, IL-1$\beta$, and probably also TNF-$\alpha$ and IL-6 (Sauder et al. 1984b, Kupper 1990a).

Several other factors with similar properties and structures have been demonstrated: leukocyte endogenous mediator (LEM) (Merriman et al. 1977), mononuclear cell factor (MCF) (Krane et al. 1985), catabolin (Saklatvala et al. 1985), osteoclast-activating factor (OAF) (Dewhurst et al. 1985), hemopoietin-1 (HP-1) (Moore and Warren 1987), and B-cell–activating factor (BAF). At the International Lymphokine Workshop in 1979 it was proposed that the term interleukin 1 (IL-1) should replace GP, EP, LEM, LAF, OAF, HP-1, BAF, and others (Aarden et al. 1979).

## III. CELLS PRODUCING IL-1

Virtually all cells are capable of producing IL-1 or molecules with similar biological activity (Table 1). IL-1 is not only found in mammalian species but has also been demonstrated in some invertebrates where it may serve as an "all-purpose" proinflammatory cytokine (Beck and Habicht 1986). The cells of the mononuclear phagocyte lineage are a major source of IL-1, predominantly IL-1$\beta$ (March et al. 1985, Gray et al. 1986, di Giovine et al. 1991a). This is because mRNA for IL-1$\beta$ in lipopolysaccharide-activated monocytes constitutes approximately 5% of the total polyadenylated RNA species (March et al. 1985, Auron et al. 1987, Tocci et al. 1987) and monocytes can translocate IL-1 molecules rapidly across the plasma membrane (Hazuda et al. 1988).

The epidermis contains very high levels of IL-1, 100–1000 times greater than most normal tissues (Schmitt et al. 1986). Keratinocytes are the major source of IL-1 in the epidermis and, unlike monocytes, are able to produce it constitutively without deliberate stimulation (Kupper et al. 1986), although it is difficult to exclude inadvertant stimulation during cell processing (e.g., by bacterial endotoxin or UV light). Human keratinocytes produce both IL-1$\alpha$ and IL-1$\beta$, although IL-1$\alpha$ is the predominant secreted type (Kupper 1989, Romero et al. 1989, Camp et al. 1990a, Anittila et al. 1990). The keratinocyte, unlike other cells, produces biologically active IL-1$\alpha$ but cannot convert the inactive pro–IL-1$\beta$ (precursor) into active IL-1$\beta$ because it lacks the monocyte IL-1 convertase enzyme (Mizutani et al. 1989). Keratinocyte IL-1 predominantly remains in a cell-associated fraction either bound to the cell membrane or in the cytoplasm (Goldminz et al. 1987, Kupper et al. 1987, Blanton et al. 1989), although high concentrations of biologically inactive IL-1$\beta$ have been demonstrated in basal keratinocytes (Didierjean et al. 1989).

**Table 1** Cells Producing IL-1

| |
|---|
| Monocytes |
| Blood (Gery et al. 1983) |
| Placenta (Flynn et al. 1982) |
| Macrophages |
| Alveolar macrophages (Simon et al. 1981) |
| Kupffer cells (Dinarello et al. 1968) |
| Synovial cells (Wood et al. 1985, di Giovine et al. 1987) |
| Peritoneal macrophages (Murphy et al. 1980) |
| Lymphocytes |
| $CD4^+$ helper T cells (Tartakovsky et al. 1986) |
| B cells (Matsushima et al. 1985a,b) |
| NK cells (Scala et al. 1984) |
| Epidermal/Dermal |
| Keratinocytes (Luger et al. 1982) |
| Langerhans cells (Sauder et al. 1984a) |
| Vascular Cells |
| Smooth muscle cells (Libby et al. 1986) |
| Endothelial cells (Wagner et al. 1985) |
| CNS Cells |
| Astrocytes (Fontana et al. 1982) |
| Microglia (Giulian et al. 1985) |
| Glioma cells (Fontana et al. 1984) |
| Miscellaneous |
| Dendritic cells (Duff et al. 1985) |
| Kidney mesangial cells (Lovett et al. 1983) |
| Neutrophils (Goto et al. 1984) |
| Fibroblasts (Iribe et al. 1983) |
| Chondrocytes (Ollivierre et al. 1986) |
| Corneal epithelium (Grabner et al. 1982) |
| Liver (Tovey et al. 1988) |
| Spleen (Tovey et al. 1988) |
| Thymic epithelium (Le et al. 1987b) |
| Noradrenergic neural cells (Schultzberg et al. 1989) |

Dermal fibroblasts and smooth muscle cells contain mostly pro–IL-1$\beta$, but they are unable to process this to the active form (Elias et al. 1989, Mizutani et al. 1991). Following trauma or infection, inflammatory cells may release serine proteases, which could cleave the pro–IL-1$\beta$ to its active form.

The differentiation of keratinocytes in vitro can be influenced by the concentration of calcium in the culture medium (Ansel et al. 1988a,b). Undifferentiated keratinocytes produce large amounts of IL-1, but with differentiation the production of IL-1 ceases. Terminal differentiation of the keratinocytes is then associated with release of IL-1 into the medium (Ansel et al. 1988a,b, 1990a,b). This is analogous to the situation in vivo, where IL-1 is normally produced in situ and, if the epidermis is not perturbed, is subsequently lost by the normal desquamation of the stratum corneum. This sequestration of IL-1 inside keratinocytes is a powerful protective mechanism against trauma and other stimuli, which by releasing a large preformed pool of IL-1 can trigger a rapid inflammatory response.

## IV. INDUCTION OF IL-1 PRODUCTION AND RELEASE

Monocyte or macrophage IL-1 production in vitro is very sensitive to bacterial lipopolysaccharide (LPS) (Duff and Atkins 1982, Loppnow 1986). The ubiquitous contamination of in vitro systems by LPS makes interpretation of studies of IL-1 induction by other stimuli difficult to interpret (di Giovine and Duff 1990). Numerous other stimuli are capable of inducing IL-1 production (Figs. 1 and 2).

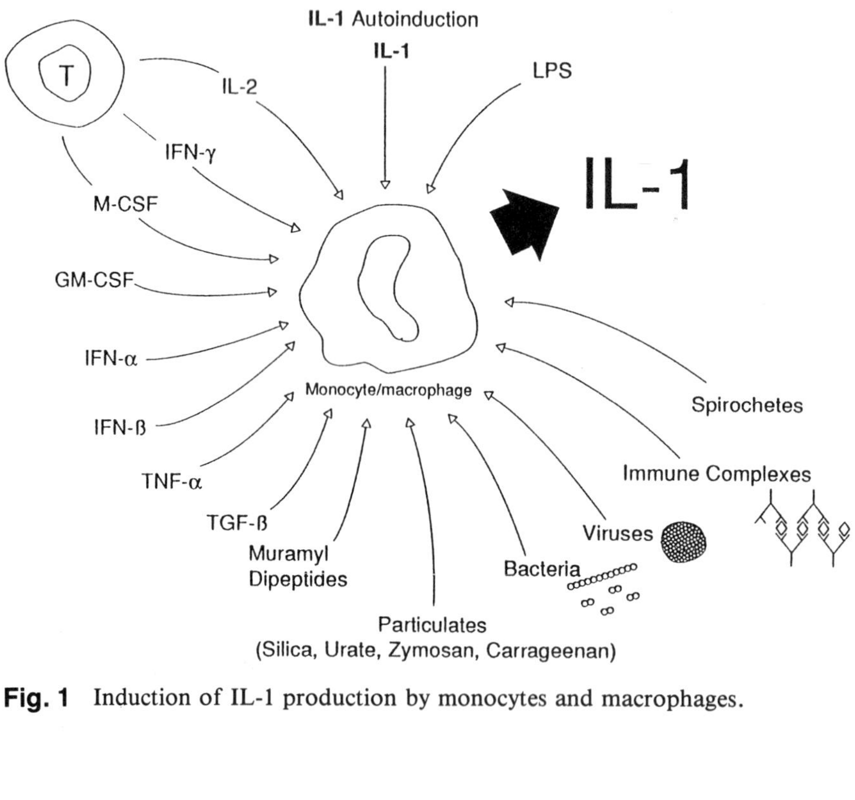


**Fig. 1** Induction of IL-1 production by monocytes and macrophages.

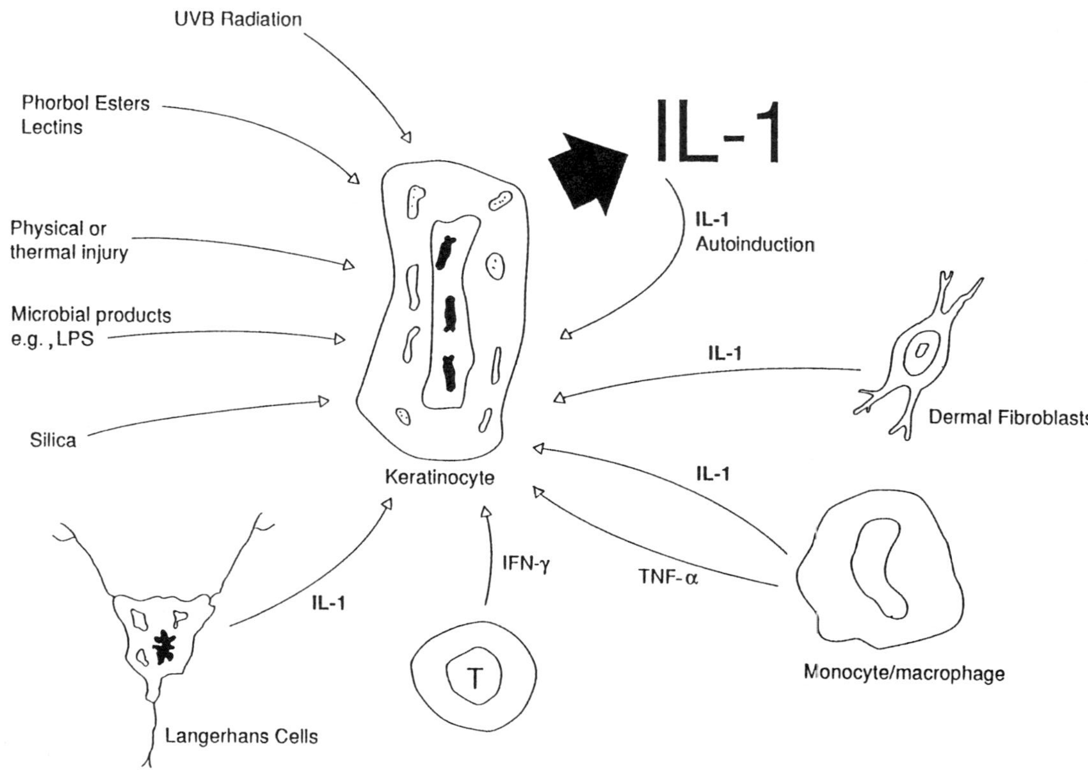


**Fig. 2** Stimuli inducing IL-1 production by keratinocytes.

In addition to the many exogenous and endogenous agents that stimulate IL-1 production, IL-1 itself can stimulate its own production in vascular smooth muscle (Warner et al. 1987a), endothelial cells (Warner et al. 1987b), blood mononuclear cells (Dinarello et al. 1987), and keratinocytes (Ristow 1987). The production of prostaglandin $E_2$ ($PGE_2$) by macrophages and connective tissue cells is enhanced by IL-1, but $PGE_2$ inhibits the production of IL-1 by these cells (Knudsden et al. 1986, Kunkel et al. 1986). In certain circumstances IFN-$\gamma$ may also inhibit IL-1 autocrine production but by a $PGE_2$-independent mechanism (Ghezzi and Dinarello 1988).

Manson et al. (1989) demonstrated that exposure of human mononuclear cells to recombinant IL-1$\alpha$ or IL-1$\beta$ at high or low concentrations stimulated their production of IL-1. In contrast, intermediate concentrations of added recombinant IL-1 failed to stimulate mononuclear cell IL-1 production and inhibited the low level of background IL-1 production. This was independent of $PGE_2$ production and the presence of IFN-$\gamma$. Thus it appears that IL-1 can both up- and down-regulate its own production depending on its concentration, providing another potential homeostatic or pathogenic mechanism.

## V. BIOCHEMISTRY

The two forms of IL-1 are initially translated as 31 kd precursors (pro IL-1), and these are cleaved by proteases from the carboxy-terminal portion to produce 17 kd mature IL-1 (Beuscher et al. 1988, Kobayashi et al. 1988, Bursten et al. 1988). Mature IL-1$\alpha$, IL-1$\beta$, and pro–IL-1$\alpha$ are biologically active, while pro–IL-1$\beta$ has very little activity (Jobling et al. 1988). Active IL-1$\alpha$ weighs 17.5 kd and contains 159 amino acids, IL-1$\beta$ weighs 17.3 kd and contains 153 amino acids (Young et al. 1988, Boraschi et al. 1988). Studies of site-specific mutagenesis have ascribed different biological functions to particular amino acid sequences (Priestle et al. 1989), but there is no general consensus in this area.

It is not clear how IL-1, which lacks a hydrophobic leader sequence, is transported out of the cell, but this may happen via lysosomal vesicles (Bakouche et al. 1987). Evidence for a release pathway other than the classical endoplasmic reticulum/Golgi system has been reported (Rubartelli et al. 1990). In human mononuclear cells, pro–IL-1$\alpha$ remains in a predominantly cell-associated form, while pro and active IL-1$\beta$ are released into the supernatant (Hazuda et al. 1988). IL-1$\alpha$ may therefore have a role as a membrane-bound cytokine stimulating lymphocytes by direct cell-cell interactions, while IL-1$\beta$ exerts predominantly paracrine and distant effects after release from the cell. This is consistent with the predominance of IL-1$\alpha$ in keratinocytes (Romero et al. 1989) and IL-1$\beta$ in monocytes (Auron et al. 1987).

## VI. GENE EXPRESSION

In humans, the two IL-1 genes are on the long arm of chromosome 2 (Auron and Webb 1984, Lomedico et al. 1984, March et al. 1985), and each gene contains 7 exons coding for IL-1 mRNA (Webb et al. 1986), with similar exon/intron boundaries (Telford et al. 1987). Each gene contains a 7-nucleotide repetitive motif at its 3′ end, which is shared by other endotoxin-induced cytokines (Shaw and Kamen 1986). These sequences may code for mRNA instability, which is counteracted by endotoxin (Caput et al. 1986). The human IL-1$\alpha$ gene is 10.5 kb (Clark et al. 1986, Webb et al. 1986, Bensi et al. 1987) and the IL-1$\beta$ gene is 7.8 kb (Furutani et al. 1986, Lafarge et al. 1989, Dinarello 1991). Although IL-1$\alpha$ and IL-1$\beta$ bind to the same receptor, there is only 25% amino acid homology, suggesting that some regions may contain minimal structural information for receptor interactions (Casagli et al. 1989). IL-1$\alpha$ and IL-1$\beta$ are both highly conserved between species (Takacs et al. 1988).

Each gene contains potential binding sites for the glucocorticoid receptor, which may explain the effects of glucocorticoids on the transcription of IL-1 genes (Clark et al. 1988). This receptor belongs to the superfamily of transacting transcriptional regulatory factors, which includes thyroid, retinoic acid, and vitamin D receptors (Lazare 1991). In vitro, dexamethasone blocks transcription and reduces the half-life of IL-1$\beta$ mRNA (Knudsden et al. 1987, Lee et al. 1988). Dexamethasone also reduces serum levels of IL-1 in vivo (Staruch and Wood 1985).

Relatively little has been published on promoter mechanisms and *cis*-acting elements in 5′-flanking DNA (Clark et al. 1988). Intron 6 of the IL-1$\alpha$ gene contains a 46-base-pair variable tandem repeat (Furutani et al. 1986), which could act as a transcriptional enhancer or suppressor. Each repeat contains the recognition sequence for the SP1 transcription factor, a viral enhancer element, and a complementary sequence of the glucocorticoid receptor binding site. This potential glucocorticoid response element may be important because, as noted above, corticosteroids inhibit the production of IL-1 (Dillard and Bodel 1980, Lew et al. 1988). Recent results indicate that there is considerable length polymorphism within intro 6 of the IL-1$\alpha$ gene that can be accounted for by variable numbers of the 46 base pair repeats (up to 19) (Bailly and Duff 1992). A polymorphism has also been demonstrated in the 5′ region of the IL-1$\beta$ gene (di Giovine et al. 1992). This polymorphism is in a region that could influence transcription.

## VII. MEMBRANE IL-1

Surface recognition events are thought by some to be crucial to the activation of T cells and other immune cells (Patarroyo et al. 1990). The presentation of IL-1 at the cell surface may facilitate these events when cells are in close contact in tissues such as the epidermis. Membrane IL-1 has been proposed on a large number of activated cells including monocytes (Hurme 1987), lymphocytes (Kurt-Jones et al. 1985), dendritic cells, fibroblasts (Le et al. 1987a), and endothelial cells (Kurt-Jones et al. 1987). Several groups have proposed that IL-1$\alpha$ is the only cell surface–bound form, while soluble IL-1 is composed of both IL-1$\alpha$ and IL-1$\beta$ (Schmidt and Tocci 1990). This is an area of some continuing disagreement.

## VIII. IL-1 RECEPTORS

The initial studies of IL-1 binding demonstrated a single receptor (IL-1R) that bound IL-1$\alpha$ and IL-1$\beta$ (Dower et al. 1985). IL-1 receptors have been demonstrated on many cell types including T cells, B cells, fibroblasts, keratinocytes, and endothelial cells (Schmidt and Tocci 1990). Subsequently, receptors of 30, 68, 80, 105, and 220 kd were demonstrated (Bird and Saklatvala 1986, Resch et al. 1986, Bird et al. 1987, Kroggel et al. 1988). It has emerged that there are two distinct classes of IL-1 receptor. The IL-1 receptor type 1 (IL-1R1) is an 80 kd glycoprotein that has been cloned from mouse and human cells and is found on T cells, fibroblasts, keratinocytes, endothelial cells, synovial lining cells, chondrocytes, and hepatocytes (Sims et al. 1988). The type 1 receptor belongs to the immunoglobulin superfamily and has an extracellular domain with disulfide intrachain bonds. There is a transmembrane portion and a cytosolic region, which is phosphorylated after binding of IL-1 (Gallis et al. 1989) and is thought to be important in signal transduction.

The multiple glycosylation sites on the type 1 receptor may determine its binding affinities and specificities. The binding of IL-1$\alpha$ or IL-1$\beta$ may be determined by the pattern of nitrogen and oxygen glycosylation (Mancilla et al. 1989). After IL-1 has bound to the type 1 IL-1R, it is internalized and is apparently not degraded, as it seems to be detectable in the nucleus several hours after binding (Mizel et al. 1987, Qwarnstrom et al. 1988, Curtis et al. 1990).

The second type of IL-1 receptor (IL-1R2) has a molecular weight of 68 kd and is found on B-cell lineages, neutrophils, and bone marrow cells (Matsushima et al. 1986a, Horuk et al. 1987, Horuk and McCubrey 1989). It is also a member of the immunoglobulin superfamily, and there is 28% homology between the extracellular portions of the type 1 and 2 receptors (Dower et al. 1990). The main structural difference between the two receptors is the shorter cytoplasmic domain in the IL-1R2, which may explain differences in signal transduction (Dower et al. 1990).

The two IL-1 receptors differ in their binding affinities, signal transduction, and cell surface expression (Solari 1990, Solari et al. 1990). Transformed

T cells and fibroblasts express IL-1R1 but produce little IL-1, while B cells and neutrophils express type 2 receptors. An IL-1R1 has been demonstrated on monocytes (Sims et al. 1988), but other studies have failed to demonstrate it on murine macrophages (Uhl et al. 1989). Many cell lines express both types of IL-1 receptors. IL-1 bound to IL-1R1 is rapidly internalized, whereas that bound to the IL-1R2 remains at the cell surface and is then shed and degraded (Matsushima et al. 1986b, Horuk et al. 1987).

IL-1$\alpha$ and IL-1$\beta$ can induce markedly different biological responses on the same cell (Bird et al. 1987, Gottschall et al. 1989). Blocking antibody studies to distinct regions on the IL-1 receptors indicate that IL-1$\alpha$ and IL-1$\beta$ bind to different regions on the same receptor. IL-1$\alpha$ may bind preferentially to IL-1R1 and IL-1$\beta$ to IL-1R2 (Uehara et al. 1987, Scapigliati et al. 1989, Clark et al. 1990).

IL-1 stimulates biological responses at very low levels of receptor occupancy. In chinese hamster ovary (CHO) cells transfected with the murine IL-1 receptor, binding studies have revealed that occupation of as few as 3–7 receptors per cell can elicit a biological response (Curtis et al. 1989). Several groups have reported a discrepancy between the biological effects of IL-1 and its binding affinities, suggesting that the actions of IL-1 may not always be mediated by a classical receptor pathway (Rosoff et al. 1988, Dinarello et al. 1989).

The distribution of IL-1 receptors on cultured dermal fibroblasts has been studied using radiolabeled IL-1$\beta$. Most of the receptors were localized to focal adhesions where intercellular processes and extracellular matrix are in apposition (Qwarnstrom et al. 1988). This observation is relevant to the effects of IL-1 on cell–extracellular matrix interactions.

IL-1 stimulates the production of platelet-derived growth factor (PDGF) from fibroblasts (Raines et al. 1989) (Fig. 3), which then act as a fibroblast mitogen (Schmidt et al. 1982). PDGF also seems to cause a significant increase in IL-1 receptor expression on fibroblasts (Bonin et al. 1988, Dower et al. 1990). PDGF is released by endothelial cells when blood vessels are damaged and by up-regulating IL-1 receptors may mediate part of the response to trauma.

Keratinocytes express high affinity receptors for IL-1 (Kupper et al. 1988a, Blanton et al. 1989). In normal epidermis only a few IL-1 receptors are expressed, but this is increased in response to UVB radiation and trauma (Kupper et al. 1989). IL-1 receptors can also be induced on keratinocytes by T-cell–derived IFN-$\gamma$ and phorbol esters (Kupper et al. 1988b) (Fig. 2). Studies with IL-1R-transfected CHO cells indicate that the number of IL-1 receptors occupied rather than the ratio of occupied to unoccupied receptors is crucial to cell activation (Curtis et al. 1989). The inducibility of IL-1 receptor expression on keratinocytes in the presence of static levels of IL-1

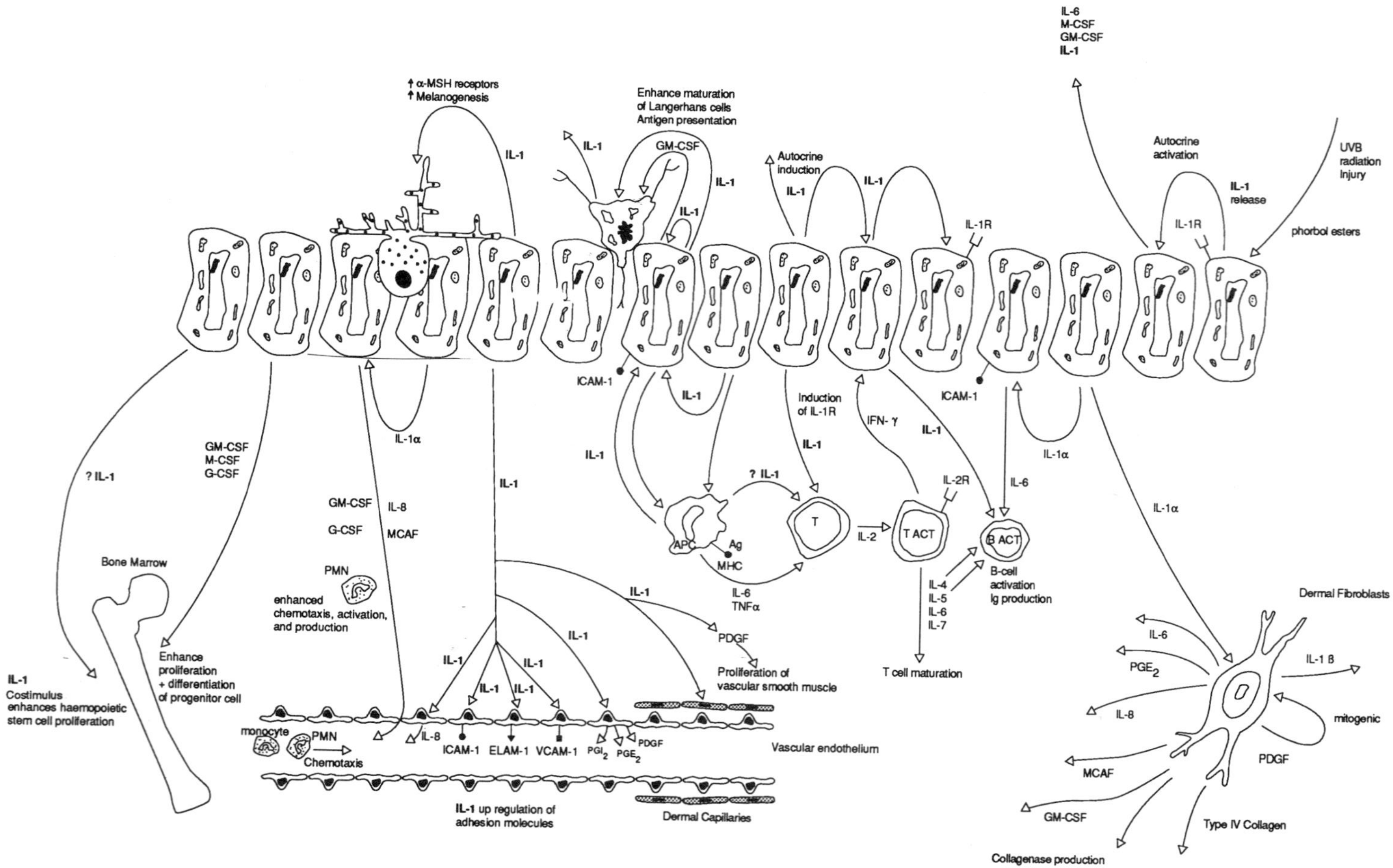


**Fig. 3** Multiple actions of IL-1 derived from keratinocytes in the epidermis and dermis.

may be very important for the regulation of immune and inflammatory responses in the skin (Kupper 1990a,b).

## IX. INHIBITORS OF IL-1

Proinflammatory cytokines are designed to combat infection and promote wound healing, but if their actions are not controlled they can cause extensive tissue damage and the death of the host. Not surprisingly, many inhibitors of IL-1 have been demonstrated (Table 2). Two groups of inhibitors appear to be central to the physiological control of the actions of IL-1 and other cytokines (Gehr et al. 1992).

### A. Type 1 IL-1 Inhibitors

Type 1 inhibitor proteins are structural homologs of a cytokine that competes with it for binding to its receptor, e.g., the IL-1 receptor antagonist (IL-1ra) (Mazzei et al. 1990). Binding of the IL-1ra to the IL-1 receptor does not produce detectable cell activation and so acts as a competitive inhibitor (Hannum et al. 1990, Dripps et al. 1991). The cDNA sequence for the IL-1ra has been cloned from human monocytes and codes for a 17 kd protein (Carter et al. 1990, Eisenberg et al. 1990, Hannum et al. 1990). It has a 19% amino acid homology to IL-1$\alpha$ and 26% homology to IL-1$\beta$ (Carter et al. 1990). Genomic cloning shows that the gene contains 4 exons, which code for the secreted form of IL-1ra (Lennard et al. 1992). By in situ fluorescence hybridization the gene was demonstrated on the long arm of chromosome 2 at 2q13-14.1 (Lennard et al. 1992). This is the same region to which the IL-1$\alpha$ and IL-1$\beta$ genes have been mapped, and this organization may have a regulatory function.

Recombinant human IL-1ra blocks the binding of IL-1$\alpha$ and IL-1$\beta$ to both IL-1R1 and IL-1R2 in humans (Hannum et al., 1990, Granowitz et al. 1991), but it did not find to a murine B-cell IL-1R2, presumably due to species variation of the IL-1ra (Hannum et al. 1990, Carter et al. 1990, Granowitz et al. 1992). Although IL-1 and IL-1ra bind to IL-1 receptors with equal affinity (Arend and Coll 1991, Dripps et al. 1991), target cells require only 1–2% receptor occupancy with IL-1 to produce a biological response. The IL-1ra must therefore be present in 10–100 times excess over IL-1 in order to block cell stimulation (Arend et al. 1990).

*Epidermal IL-1 Receptor Antagonist*

The cDNA for a specific epithelial form of the IL-1ra has been cloned from lysates of keratinocytes (Haskill et al. 1991). This keratinocyte IL-1ra appears to be predominantly intracellular (icIL-1ra) and is almost identical to

**Table 2** Reported Inhibitors of IL-1

| |
|---|
| Naturally Occurring Nonspecific Inhibitors |
| Lipoproteins (Rosenstreich et al. 1988) |
| alpha-2 Macroglobulin (Borth and Luger 1989) |
| Uromodulin (Muchmore and Decker 1986) |
| Specific Polypeptide Inhibitors |
| Serum from endotoxin injected patients (Dinarello et al. 1981) |
| Urine from febrile patients (Liao et al. 1984) |
| Plasma posthemodialysis (Shaldon et al. 1987) |
| Urine patients monocytic leukemia (Seckinger et al. 1987) |
| Monocytes adhering to IgG-coated surfaces (Arend et al. 1989) |
| 52–66 kd Inhibitors |
| Human myelomonocytic cell line (Barack et al. 1986) |
| Macrophage cell line P388D (Isono et al. 1989) |
| Viral-Infected Cells |
| HIV (Locksley et al. 1988) |
| CMV (Rodgers et al. 1985) |
| EBV (Lotz et al. 1986) |
| Syncitial virus (Roberts et al. 1986) |
| Other Cytokines |
| IFN-$\gamma$ (Browning et al. 1987) |
| TGF-$\beta$ (Wahl et al. 1988) |
| IL-4 (Hurme et al. 1988) |
| IL-10 (Zlotnik and Moore 1991) |
| Type 1 IL-1 Receptor Inhibitors |
| IL-1 receptor antagonist (Dayoff et al. 1983, Balavoine et al. 1986, Barack et al. 1986, Seckinger et al. 1987, Arend et al. 1989, Dayer et al. 1989, Isono et al. 1989, Carter et al. 1990, Eisenberg et al. 1990, Hannum et al. 1990, Mazzei et al. 1990) |
| Antibodies to IL-1Rt1 (Chizzonite et al. 1989, Lewis et al. 1990) |
| Type 2 IL-1 Receptor Inhibitors |
| Soluble IL-1R proteins (Fanslow et al. 1990, Symons et al. 1990, 1991, Symons and Duff 1990) |
| Other Inhibitors |
| $PGE_2$ (Knudsden et al. 1986) |
| alpha-MSH (Deeter et al. 1988, Hiltz et al. 1989, Hiltz et al. 1990) |
| Methyl ester muramyl dipeptide (Cady et al. 1989) |
| ACTH |
| Glucocorticoids (Knudsden et al. 1987) |
| Inhibitors of protein kinase C and calmodulin-dependent kinase (Kovacs et al. 1988) |
| Metalloendopeptidase 24.11 (Pierart et al. 1988) |

the mature extracellular form of IL-1ra produced by monocytes, termed secretory IL-1ra (sIL-1ra). The icIL-1ra has an additional 7 amino acids at its $NH_2$ terminus and is in a 17 kd nonglycosylated form. The sIL-1ra possesses a 25-residue leader sequence and is in a 22–25 kd glycosylated form (Haskill et al. 1991). These structural differences may explain the failure of secretion of the keratinocyte intracellular IL-1ra, but despite this variation their receptor binding affinity is identical (Arend and Coll 1991, Dripps et al. 1991). This structural variation is probably due to a different first exon for keratinocyte icIL-1ra arising from alternative splicing of mRNA (Bigler et al. 1992).

Cultured keratinocytes produce icIL-1ra, and production is significantly enhanced in medium containing high concentrations of calcium, which promotes their differentiation (Bigler et al. 1992). This is analogous to the increased production of sIL-1ra as monocytes mature into macrophages in vitro (Janson et al. 1992). Immunofluorescence studies indicate a band of IL-1ra immediately below the stratum corneum in normal epidermis (Bigler et al. 1992).

Keratinocyte icIL-1ra may be important in the control of inflammation triggered by IL-1$\alpha$ released from dead or damaged keratinocytes and those primed to release IL-1 by other mechanisms (e.g., IFN-$\gamma$). Dysregulation of the production and release of icIL-1ra could contribute to loss of IL-1 homeostasis and the development of inflammatory dermatosis.

#### *IL-1 Receptor Antagonist Genetic Polymorphism*

A trialleic variable-length polymorphism has been detected within intron 2 of the IL-1ra gene (Steinkasserer et al. 1991). Two further alleles have subsequently been demonstrated, and it appears that the length variation is due to variable numbers of an 86 bp repeat. Pedigree analysis confirms that these alleles follow mendelian segregation (Tarlow et al. 1992). The significance of such polymorphisms in cytokine and related genes requires further study.

#### *Antibodies to IL-1*

Antibodies to the IL-1R1 on murine cells block the effects of IL-1 in vivo and in vitro (Chizzonite et al. 1989, Lewis et al. 1990). Mice injected with IL-1 intraperitoneally develop peritonitis, a neutrophil infiltrate, and raised IL-6 levels. Pretreatment of these mice with an antibody to IL-1R1 prevents these changes (Chizzonite et al. 1989).

### B. Type 2 IL-1 Inhibitors

These IL-1 inhibitors, components of the cell membrane–associated IL-1 receptor, are cleaved from it and shed into the circulation where they bind to IL-1 (Symons et al. 1990, Dinarello 1991, Gehr et al. 1992). A soluble protein that binds IL-1$\beta$ (sIL-1R) selectively has been isolated from normal human serum, human synovial inflammatory exudates, culture supernatants from human peripheral blood mononuclear cells, and a keratinocyte cell line (Eastgate et al. 1990, Symons et al. 1990, 1991, J. A. Symons personal communication).

This inhibitor is also released by a human B-cell line, and its release is increased by treatment with dexamethasone (Symons et al. 1990), which also increases the expression of IL-1R2 on these cells (Akahoshi et al. 1988, Scapigliati et al. 1989). Release of this IL-1$\beta$-binding protein (sIL-1R) was inhibited by aprotinin, a serine protease inhibitor. It therefore appears that this soluble IL-1 inhibitor could be produced by the action of serine proteases on the 60 kd IL-1 receptor (IL-1R2) (Symons and Duff 1990).

Purification of the sIL-1R from a Raji cell line revealed a 47 kd protein that specifically bound IL-1$\beta$ with an affinity kd of 2.7 nm (Symons et al. 1991). The sIL-1R may function as a specific regulator of the actions of IL-1$\beta$ in vivo. This is analogous to the soluble IL-2 receptor (sIL-2R), which may also inhibit the action of IL-2 (Symons et al. 1988, Symons and Duff, 1991). The production of the sIL-1R by keratinocytes may therefore provide another mechanism for control of the actions of IL-1 in the skin (Symons et al. 1992).

## X. SIGNAL TRANSDUCTION

The observation that very few IL-1 receptors need to be occupied to elicit a biological response (Curtis et al. 1989) implies that a potent amplification mechanism exists during signal transduction. There is no clear consensus concerning the form of IL-1 signal transduction and putative second messengers that lead to a cellular response (Mizel 1990, O'Neil et al. 1990).

### A. Calcium Homeostasis

In many in vitro systems cytosolic calcium fluxes have been shown to be important second messengers for cell growth (Hesketh et al. 1983). Several groups have been unable to demonstrate an increase in intracellular calcium following IL-1 stimulation of T-cell lines (Abraham et al. 1987, Mukaida et al. 1987, Didier et al. 1988, Freedman et al. 1988, Rosoff et al. 1988) and neutrophils (Georgilis et al. 1987). However IL-1 inhibition of mesangial cell growth in vitro is associated with an inhibition of extracellular calcium entry into the cytosol (Ikeda et al. 1991). The glucose-induced uptake of calcium into the islets of Langerhans is also inhibited by IL-1 (Wolf et al. 1989), but IL-1 induces an increase in cytosolic calcium in dermal fibroblasts (Bouchelouche et al. 1988).

## B. Kinases

There is a dichotomy of results in this area. Some indicate a protein kinase A (PKA)-dependent second messenger (Mizel 1990), while others demonstrate a kinase that is neither PKA nor protein kinase C (PKC) (O'Neil et al. 1990, Stylianou et al. 1991, Guesdon et al. 1991). A rise in cAMP production following IL-1 stimulation has been reported in several cell types including human synovial cells, human and murine fibroblast cell lines, and murine T cells (Bomsztyk et al. 1989, Chizzonite et al. 1989). Analogs of cAMP and forskolin mimic several actions of IL-1, inducing T-cell proliferation in the presence of suboptimal levels of PKA (Mizel 1990). If IL-1–responsive cells are transfected with an expression plasmid containing a cDNA encoding a specific inhibitor of PKA, this abrogates IL-1–induced stimulation of gene transcription (Mizel 1990).

In contrast, other groups have not demonstrated increased levels of cAMP or diacylglycerol (DAG) in cells responding to IL-1 (Carroll 1986, Didier et al. 1988). Prostaglandin $E_2$ ($PGE_2$), which elevates levels of cAMP, does not mimic the action of IL-1, and in T cells $PGE_2$ inhibits IL-2 production (Rappaport and Dodge 1982).

Cytokines can alter gene expression by activating or inducing transcription factors such as NF-$\kappa$B and AP-1 complex, which regulate specific genes (Lenardo and Baltimore 1989). Following the binding of IL-1 to its receptor, NF-$\kappa$B (Osborn et al. 1989) and the AP-1–dependent gene transcription occur (Muegge et al. 1989, Espel et al. 1990). This is probably via a protein kinase. The demonstration that activation of NF-$\kappa$B can be produced by cAMP analogs and forskolin suggested a PKA mechanism (Shirakawa and Mizel 1989, Shirakawa et al. 1989b). In contrast, a specific activation of NF-$\kappa$B via the type 1 IL-1 receptor was not mediated by PKA or PKC (Stylianou et al. 1991).

A cytoplasmic inhibitor of NF-$\kappa$B, I$\kappa$B complexes with NF-$\kappa$B and inhibits its binding to DNA. This complex can be dissociated by treatment with PKC or PKA, facilitating translocation of NF-$\kappa$B to the nucleus (Baeuerle and Baltimore 1988a,b).

The internalization of IL-1 may also be involved in signal transduction after binding of labeled IL-1 to its receptor label accumulates in the nucleus of T cells and fibroblasts (Mizel et al. 1987, Qwarnstrom et al. 1988). The identity of second messenger(s) for IL-1 is therefore not clear, but its elucidation is crucial to the understanding of how IL-1 works.

# XI. ACTIONS OF IL-1

The wide range of biological actions of IL-1 seem to be involved in the control of immune and inflammatory responses (di Giovine and Duff 1990) (Table 3).

**Table 3** Some Actions of IL-1 In Vivo

| |
|---|
| Metabolic Effects |
| Acute phase protein synthesis |
| Decreased albumin synthesis |
| Hypozincemia, hypoferremia, hypercupremia |
| Inhibition of lipoprotein lipase |
| Decreased cytochrome P450 |
| Increased sodium excretion |
| Endocrine Effects |
| Increased insulin, glucagon production |
| Increased corticosteroids and ACTH |
| Hemopoiesis |
| Neutrophilia |
| Lymphopenia |
| Stimulation of hemopoietic progenitor cells |
| Enhanced bone marrow recovery postradiation and post–cytotoxic drugs |
| Stimulation of GM-CSF production |
| Central Nervous System |
| Fever |
| Brain $PGE_2$ synthesis |
| Increased slow-wave sleep |
| Decreased appetite |
| Vascular System |
| Hypotension and shock |
| Capillary leak syndrome |
| Decreased vascular resistance |
| $PGE_2$ and $PGI_2$ production |

The multiple actions of IL-1 demonstrated in vitro (Table 4) should be interpreted with caution, since in many experiments very high concentrations of IL-1 have been used. Many of the apparent effects of IL-1 in vitro may of course be due to the induction of secondary cytokines, e.g., IL-1 stimulation of PDGF production by fibroblasts stimulating their mitogenesis (Raines et al. 1989).

## A. Actions of IL-1 in the Epidermis

Keratinocytes produce IL-1 and express high affinity receptors for it (Kupper 1988). The dead cells of the stratum corneum that contain high levels of IL-1 are therefore in close apposition to viable keratinocytes expressing IL-1 receptors. Release of IL-1 by trauma or ultraviolet irradiation (Kupper

**Table 4** Some Actions of IL-1 In Vitro

| |
|---|
| Immune System |
| B Cells: stimulation of proliferation, differentiation, chemotaxis, and antibody production |
| T Cells: acts as a comitogen inducing growth, differentiation, and production of IL-2 and IL-2R |
| TH1 cells: unresponsive to IL-1 or TH2 cells have absolute requirement |
| Monocytes: induction of $PGE_2$, cytotoxicity, and chemotaxis Nk cell activation |
| Hemopoiesis: induction of GM-CSF, G-CSF, M-CSF, IL-3 production by stromal cells |
| IL-1 acts synergistically with CSFs to stimulate proliferation of stem cells and progenitor cells |
| Effects on Vascular Tissue |
| Induction of adhesion molecules in endothelial cells |
| Proliferation of vascular smooth muscle cells |
| Induction of endothelial plasminogen activator synthesis |
| Induction of procoagulant activity in endothelial cells |
| Induction of Cytokine Gene Expression |
| IL-1, IL-2, IL-3, IL-4, IL-5, IL-6, IL-7, IL-8, TNF-$\alpha$, TNF-$\beta$1, GM-CSF, G-CSF, M-CSF, IL-2R (tac Ag) |
| Inflammatory Effects |
| Induction and procollagenase synthesis |
| Bone resorption |
| Induction of $PGE_2$ in fibroblasts, macrophages, and endothelial cells |
| Eosinophil degranulation |
| Basophil histamine release |
| Neutrophil and monocyte thromboxane release |
| Cytotoxic Effects |
| Some tumor cells, pancreatic $\beta$-islets |

et al. 1987) can therefore induce autocrine paracrine and possibly endocrine effects.

Keratinocytes grown in vitro under conditions inhibiting their differentiation release very low levels of IL-1 and express IL-1 receptors. If recombinant IL-1$\alpha$ is added to these cultures, it appears to be chemotactic and mitogenic for keratinocytes and also stimulates their production of GM-CSF, IL-6, and interferon-$\beta$2 (IFN-$\beta$2) (Kupper 1988, 1990b, Kupper et al. 1989). These actions of IL-1 released in response to trauma would therefore stimulate both reepithelialization and inflammation. Macrophages and monocytes in the papillary dermis are another significant source of IL-1 which may stimulate keratinocytes in response to inflammation in the dermis (Fig. 3).

In normal epidermis IL-1 is contained within cells, therefore its actions depend on stimuli that induce its release and the expression of its receptor. The production of GM-CSF and IL-6 by keratinocytes is related to the number of IL-1 receptors they are expressing. IFN-$\gamma$ is a potent stimulator of keratinocyte IL-1 receptor expression (Kupper 1990a,c) and is released by activated T cells in psoriasis (Nickoloff et al. 1990). Thus T cells via IFN-$\gamma$ can up-regulate IL-1R on keratinocytes and so permit their activation by IL-1 and release of proinflammatory cytokines.

IL-1$\alpha$ mRNA expression in a keratinocyte cell line can be induced by IL-1$\alpha$, IL-1$\beta$, TNF-$\alpha$ and GM-CSF (Ansel et al. 1988a,b, 1990b). All of these cytokines are produced by keratinocytes, and therefore it has been postulated that they can act in an autocrine manner to further increase IL-1 production.

Keratinocytes produce IL-6 (Kock et al. 1988, Kirnbauer et al. 1989, Kupper et al. 1989), and its production is stimulated by IL-1 (Ansel et al. 1990a). The actions of IL-1 and IL-6 overlap, and as IL-1 can induce IL-6 production, actions attributed to IL-1 may therefore be mediated by IL-6.

IL-1 released from keratinocytes also has effects on many dermal and epidermal cells (Fig. 3) and is thought to have a pivotol role in the initiation of the local and systemic inflammatory responses. The local release of IL-1 from keratinocytes following skin injury (trauma or UVB radiation), infection, or inflammation causes an autocrine and paracrine activation of keratinocytes, which then release further IL-1, GM-CSF, M-CSF, G-CSF, IL-6, IL-8, and monocyte-chemotactic and -activating factor (MCAF) (Kupper et al. 1988a,b, Larsen et al. 1989, Kupper 1990b, Camp et al. 1990a, Nozaki et al. 1991). These cytokines then initiate the production of an inflammatory infiltrate and activate fibroblasts to proliferate and produce collagen for wound healing.

## B. IL-1 Effects on Adhesion Molecule Expression

Endothelial cell leukocyte adhesion molecule-1 (ELAM-1), intercellular adhesion molecule-1 (ICAM-1), and vascular cell adhesion molecule-1 (VCAM-1) are cytokine-regulated cell surface molecules involved in leukocyte adhesion (Springer 1990, Nickoloff et al. 1990). The expression of adhesion molecules, especially the "selectin" ELAM-1, is markedly increased by IL-1 (Pober et al. 1986, Norris 1990, Carlos and Harlan 1990, Shimizu et al. 1990, Swerlick et al. 1991).

IL-1 also induces the production by keratinocytes and fibroblasts of the leukocyte chemotactic cytokines IL-8 and MCAF (Matsushima et al. 1988a,b, Matsushima and Oppenheim 1989, Westwick et al. 1989). Thus IL-1 can induce both the endothelial cell–binding sites and the chemotactic cytokine

(IL-8), which together mediate migration of T lymphocytes, monocytes, and neutrophils out of blood vessels and towards sites of injury and/or inflammation (Fig. 3).

## C. IL-1 Effects on the Extracellular Matrix

The extracellular matrix (ECM) is composed of an insoluble mixture of collagens, proteoglycans, hyaluronic acid, elastin, and adhesive glycoproteins including laminin, fibronectin, and thrombospondin (Hay 1981) and is produced by fibroblasts and other connective tissue cells (Wahl 1985, Freundlich et al. 1986). The ECM binds to cells via integrins (Hynes 1987) and is crucial to the regulation of cell proliferation and differentiation. Production of the ECM is regulated by cytokines including IL-1 and TNF-$\alpha$ (Larrick and Kunkel 1988, Mauviel et al. 1991).

Wound healing involves complex interactions between cells, cytokines, and the ECM. After injury there is inflammation followed by proliferation of fibroblasts and deposition of ECM. The collagen/glycosaminoglycan (GAG) matrix is then continually remodeled as healing progresses (Shosman 1981). IL-1 increases the production of hyaluronic acid (Bronson et al. 1987) and proteoglycans (Bartold 1988) by dermal and gingival fibroblasts.

IL-1 suppresses the expression of collagen types 2 and 4 by chondrocytes and increases their production of collagen types 1 and 3 (Mauviel et al. 1991). IL-1 also stimulates dermal fibroblasts to produce collagenase and stromelysin, which break down the ECM (Postlethwaite et al. 1983, Saus et al. 1988), and is presumably involved in the process of remodeling.

## D. IL-1 and the Regulation of Hair Growth

In the rat the dermal papilla is crucial to the control of growth and differentiation of the hair bulb epithelium (Oliver 1970). The extracellular matrix of the dermal papilla contains high levels of basement membrane proteins and chondroitin proteoglycans, and its volume and composition varies with the phase of the hair growth cycle (Couchman and Gibson 1985, Westgate et al. 1989). This is most marked for chondroitin-sulfate proteoglycan, and this basement membrane component may be crucial for dermo-epidermal interactions that lead to the growth of skin appendages (Couchman et al. 1990). Disturbed proteoglycan metabolism has been implicated in abnormal development of feather follicles (Goetinick and Carlone 1988) and alopecia areata (McDonagh et al. 1990). The control of ECM production and remodeling by IL-1 and TNF-$\alpha$ suggests that they may have a role in the regulation of hair growth.

In mice treated with cell cycle–specific cytotoxic drugs (cytosine arabinoside or daunorubicin) daily for 7 days, total alopecia develops. This can be prevented if they are given IL-1$\beta$ concurrently (Hussein et al. 1990, Jimenez et al. 1991). IL-1 may prevent entry of the hair bulb cells into cycle, protecting them from the drug; whether this is a direct effect or mediated via the extracellular matrix awaits elucidation. A similar effect of IL-1 is seen in its radioprotection of bone marrow cells (Neta et al. 1987).

## E. IL-1 in Psoriasis

Normal skin contains high levels of IL-1 (Fincham et al. 1988, Hammerberg et al. 1989), and in most studies this appears to be predominantly IL-1$\alpha$ (Kupper et al. 1986, Camp et al. 1990b), although others have reported an excess of IL-1$\beta$ (Didierjean et al. 1987). In psoriasis the levels of IL-1$\alpha$ are reduced up to 12-fold while IL-1$\beta$ is increased (Hammerberg et al. 1990, Gearing et al. 1990, Cooper et al. 1990). Although IL-1$\beta$ mRNA and immunoreactivity is increased in psoriatic lesional skin, it is not biologically active, although it is in its 17 kd active form (Cooper et al. 1990).

Although the levels of biologically active IL-1 are reduced in psoriatic lesional skin, they are sufficient to induce an inflammatory reaction when a comparable quantity is injected into normal skin (Dowd et al. 1988). The biological activity of IL-1 in psoriatic skin may be increased by the increased number of IL-1 receptors present (Sherman et al. 1990). IL-1 itself and IFN-$\gamma$ from infiltrating T cells both up-regulate their expression (Dower et al. 1990). It is possible that aberrant IL-1 receptor expression is an early event in the development of psoriatic lesions, but it could occur secondary to abnormal T-cell function.

As keratinocytes become more differentiated, the production of IL-1$\alpha$ falls (Ansel et al. 1988a) and the production of the intracellular IL-1 receptor antagonist increases (Bigler et al. 1992). In psoriasis where there is keratinocyte hyperproliferation and reduced differentiation, there is therefore less icIL-1ra. When combined with increased IL-1 receptor expression on keratinocytes (Sherman et al. 1990), this can lead to increased keratinocyte activation by the autocrine and paracrine effects of IL-1. Activated keratinocytes could then produce secondary cytokines such as GM-CSF, G-CSF, TGF-$\alpha$, IL-8 (Camp et al. 1990b), IL-6 (Schroder et al. 1987, Kupper et al. 1988, Schroder 1992), and further IL-1, all of which enhance keratinocyte proliferation and produce an inflammatory infiltrate of neutrophils, monocyte/macrophages, and T cells. These cells then release further cytokines, inducing the T-cell lymphokines such as IFN-$\gamma$ and IL-2 and perpetuating the inflammatory process.

The balance between the transcription of IL-1 mRNA, IL-1 mRNA half-life (Ansel et al. 1990a,b), expression of IL-1 receptors (Sherman et al. 1990, Kupper 1990c) and the production of IL-1 inhibitors such as icIL-1ra (Haskill et al. 1991, Bigler et al. 1992) and the soluble IL-1 receptor (Symons et al. 1990, 1991) is crucial to the production of a biological response. The initial triggering event in psoriasis is unknown, but T-cell production of IFN-$\gamma$ which up-regulates IL-1 receptor expression in the presence of low levels of icIL-1ra may be part of the answer. The results of sequential analysis of IL-1$\alpha$, IL-1$\beta$, IL-1R1, IL-1R2, icIL-1ra, sIL-1r, and secondary cytokines as psoriatic lesions develop may provide useful insights (Cork et al. 1992).

### F. Pathological Role of IL-1 in Other Diseases

Several diseases are characterized by apparent dysregulation of IL-1. This can be due to increased transcription (Dinarello et al. 1987), increased release of preformed protein, e.g., from damaged keratinocytes (Kupper 1990a), increased expression of IL-1 receptors, e.g., in psoriasis (Sherman et al. 1990), and decreased levels of IL-1 inhibitors.

In diseases such as rheumatoid arthritis there is a clear correlation between disease activity and the elevation of IL-1$\beta$ levels both locally in the synovial fluid and in the plasma (Eastgate et al. 1988, Symons et al. 1988, 1989, Duff, 1989, Rooney et al. 1990). Of relevance to rheumatoid arthritis, IL-1 augments release of prostanoids, proteinases, and oxygen metabolites and is a potent inducer of bone and cartilage resorption. IL-1 activation of T cells to produce IL-2 and IL-2 receptors may underlie the increased levels of soluble IL-2 receptors in rheumatoid arthritis and their good correlation with disease activity (Symons et al. 1988).

In scleroderma there is increased collagen production by fibroblasts producing fibrosis and a mononuclear cell infiltrate (Fleishmajer et al. 1977). A reported increased production of IL-1 by unstimulated mononuclear cells has been demonstrated in patients with scleroderma, suggesting a role for IL-1 in its pathogenesis (Alocer-Varela et al. 1985, Sandborg et al. 1985), while other groups have found reduced levels of IL-1 in scleroderma (Sandborg et al. 1985). Reduced levels of IL-1 are also associated with systemic lupus erythematosis (Boswell et al. 1988).

## XII. THERAPEUTIC IMPLICATIONS OF IL-1 ANTAGONISM

In diseases where high levels of IL-1 correlate with disease activity, IL-1 may have an important pathogenic role. The use of specific IL-1 antagonists is a new therapeutic approach. In an animal model of immune complex–induced colitis, the degree of inflammation and tissue damage correlated with systemic IL-1 levels. These changes could be markedly reduced if the animals were pretreated with the IL-1 receptor antagonist (Cominelli et al. 1990). The IL-1ra can also inhibit IL-1–induced synovial cell $PGE_2$ synthesis and collagenase synthesis from chondrocytes (Arend et al. 1990). The IL-1ra also blocks the production of IL-1, IL-6, and TNF-$\alpha$ from IL-1–induced PBMC (Granowitz et al. 1991).

Soluble IL-1 receptors bind to IL-1$\beta$ in solution and therefore prevent its binding to cell surface IL-1 receptors (Eastgate et al. 1990, Symons et al. 1990, 1991, Symons and Duff 1990, Maliszewski and Fanslow 1990). Recombinant soluble IL-1 receptors inhibit the rejection of heart allografts in mice (Fanslow et al. 1990) and IL-1–induced B-cell activation (Maliszewski et al. 1990). The demonstration that these inhibitors occur naturally has enormous therapeutic implications (Symons and Duff 1990).

The vitamin D metabolite 1,25-$(OH)_2D_3$ and its analog calcipotriol inhibit the proliferation of keratinocytes from normal and psoriatic patients in culture and enhance their differentiation (Kragballe et al. 1991). They also inhibit the actions of IL-1 in vitro (Muller et al. 1988) and IL-1–induced IL-8 production by keratinocytes (Larsen et al. 1991). Their actions are mediated via the vitamin D nuclear receptor, a transcriptional regulator. The therapeutic actions of calcipotriol in psoriasis (Kragballe et al. 1991) may be mediated in part by its actions on IL-1.

## XIII. IL-1 FUTURE PERSPECTIVES

The balance between IL-1 production, the expression of its receptors, and production of specific inhibitors determines the biological response. IL-1 also stimulates the production of several secondary cytokines that amplify inflammation, such as IL-6 and IL-8. Sequential dynamic systems involving multiple biopsies and assay of all of these parameters are needed to establish physiological control mechanisms (Cork et al. 1992).

The investigation of the genetic basis for variations in the production rates of IL-1$\alpha$, IL-1$\beta$, IL-1rt1, IL-1rt2, IL-1ra, and sIL-1R is a new area of research. Genetic polymorphism has been demonstrated at specific loci in the IL-1$\beta$ (di Giovine et al. 1991b, IL-1$\alpha$ (Bailly and Duff 1992), and IL-1ra (Tarlow et al. 1993) genes. Whether the genetic polymorphisms are related to cytokine producer phenotypes and are susceptibility or severity factors for chronic inflammatory diseases remains to be seen.

## ACKNOWLEDGMENT

We thank Andrew Brown of the medical illustration department, Royal Hallamshire Hospital, for producing excellent computer graphics.

## NOTE ADDED IN PROOF

Inflammatory dermatoses such as psoriasis, atopic eczema, dermatitis herpetiformis, SLE and scleroderma are probably polygenic. We would therefore expect to see small changes in the allelic frequencies of several genes.

The numerous abnormalities of cytokine production, receptor expression and inhibitor levels demonstrated in these diseases have not previously been related to their genetic component. Stable inter-individual production rates have been demonstrated for several cytokines IL-1alpha, IL-1beta, TNF-alpha and IL-1ra suggesting that there may be a genetic basis for different cytokine producer phenotypes, i.e., high producer or low producer (Molvig et al. 1988). We postulated that polymorphisms in the regulatory regions of cytokine and related genes may be associated with different cytokine producer phenotypes.

We have demonstrated in serial biopsies across the advancing edge of psoriatic plaques that the levels of mRNA for IL-1alpha decrease into the plaque while mRNA for IL-1beta and the IL-1 receptor type (IL-1R1) increase into the plaque. The IL-1ra mRNA levels are unchanged in the plaque but there is a marked decrease in the amount of IL-1ra protein (Cork et al. 1992, Mee et al. 1992). A similar decrease in IL-1ra protein within the psoriatic plaque has also been reported by two other groups (Hammerberg et al. 1992, Kristensen et al. 1992). These observations suggested that the IL-1ra gene could be a candidate gene in psoriasis.

We have characterised a 5 allele polymorphism due to a variable number of an 86bp tandem repeat in intron 2 of the IL-1 receptor antagonist (IL-1ra) gene. Mendelian segregation of the alleles has been demonstrated in four extensive pedigrees (Tarlow et al. 1993). We have determined allelic frequencies for the IL-1ra polymorphism in a control population and compared this with that in psoriasis, SLE, dermatitis herpetiformis, systemic sclerosis and alopecia areata. Allele 2 had a frequency of 24.1% in the control population. In type 1 psoriasis (early onset, positive family history and CW6+) (Hensler and Christophers 1985) allele 2 was increased to 35% while in type 2 psoriasis (late onset, no family history) allele 2 was decreased to <5% (Cork et al. 1993a,b).

In patients with SLE, allele 2 was increased to 35% overall, but subgroup analysis revealed much larger changes. Allele 2 was increased to 60% in patients with SLE and discoid rash and 40% in those with SLE and photosensitivity (Blakemore et al. 1993, Cork et al. 1993a). There was a direct relationship with disease severity from 25% (ARA criteria =4) to 48% (ARA =8). Allele 2 was also increased in alopecia areata (Cork et al. 1993b) and dermatitis herpetiformis. We are currently performing functional studies to test the hypothesis that allele 2 of this IL-1ra polymorphism is associated with low production of the IL-1 receptor antagonist.

## REFERENCES

L. A. Aarden, T. K. Brunner, J. C. Cerottini, et al., *J. Immunol. 123*, 2928 (1979).
R. T. Abraham et al., *J. Biol. Chem. 262*, 2719 (1987).
T. Akahoshi, J. J. Oppenheim, and K. Matsushima, *J. Exp. Med. 167*, 924 (1988).
J. Alocer-Varela et al., *Exp. Immunol. 59*, 666 (1985).
H. S. I. Anittila, S. Reitamo, P. Erkko, et al., *J. Invest. Dermatol. 95*, 31 (1990).

J. C. Ansel, T. A. Luger, D. R. Roop, et al., *J. Immunol. 140*, 2274 (1988a).
J. C. Ansel, P. Perry, M. Heinrich, et al., *Clin. Res. 36*, 630A (1988b).
J. C. Ansel, P. Perry, H. Heinrich, et al., *Clin. Res. 38*, 221A (1990a).
J. C. Ansel, P. Perry, J. Brown, et al., *J. Invest. Dermatol. 94*, 101S (1990b).
W. P. Arend, F. G. Joslin, R. C. Thompson, et al., *J. Immunol. 143*, 1851 (1989).
W. P. Arend, H. G. Welgus, R. C. Thompson, et al., *J. Clin. Invest. 85*, 1694 (1990).
W. P. Arend and B. P. Coll, *Cytokine 5*, 407 (1991).
E. Atkins, *Physiol. Rev. 40*, 580 (1960).
P. E. Auron and A. C. Webb, *Proc. Natl. Acad. Sci. USA 81*, 7907 (1984).
P. E. Auron et al., *J. Immunol. 138*, 1447 (1987).
P. A. Baeuerle and D. Baltimore, *Cell 53*, 211 (1988a).
P. A. Baeuerle and D. Baltimore, *Science 242*, 540 (1988b).
S. Bailly and G. W. Duff, *Eur. J. Immunol.* in press (1993).
O. Bakouche, D. C. Brown, and L. B. Lachman, *J. Immunol. 138*, 4249 (1987).
J. F. Balavoine, B. de Rochemonteix, and K. Williamson, *J. Clin. Invest. 78*, 1120 (1986).
V. Barack, A. J. Treves, P. Yani, et al., *Eur. J. Immunol. 16*, 1449 (1986).
M. Bartold, *Connective Tiss. Res. 17*, 287 (1988).
G. Beck and G. Habicht, *Proc. Natl. Acad. Sci. 83*, 7429 (1986).
I. L. Bennett and P. B. Beeson, *J. Exp. Med. 98*, 477 (1953).
G. Bensi et al., *Gene 52*, 95 (1987).
H. U. Beuscher et al., *J. Biol. Chem. 263*, 4023 (1988).
C. F. Bigler, D. A. Norris, W. L. Weston, et al., *J. Invest. Dermatol. 98*, 38 (1992).
T. A. Bird and J. Saklatvala, *Nature 324*, 263 (1986).
T. A. Bird et al., *FEBS Lett. 225*, 21 (1987).
A. I. F. Blakemore, J. K. Tarlow, M. J. Cork, et al. submitted. *Arthritis and Rheum. Res.* (1993).
R. A. Blanton et al., *Proc. Natl. Acad. Sci. USA 86*, 1273 (1989).
K. Bomsztyk, K. Sims, J. E. Stanton, et al., *Proc. Natl. Acad. Sci. USA 86*, 8034 (1989).
P. D. Bonin et al., *J. Biol. Chem. 263*, 11052 (1988).
W. Borth and T. A. Luger, *J. Biol. Chem. 264*, 5818 (1989).
D. Boraschi, L. Nencioni, L. Villa, et al., *J. Exp. Med. 168*, 675 (1988).
J. M. Boswell et al., *J. Immunol. 141*, 3050 (1988).
P. N. Bouchelouche et al., *Leukaemia 2*, 691 (1988).
R. E. Bronson, C. Bertolami, and E. P. Siebert, *Collagen Rel. Res. 7*, 323 (1987).
J. L. Browning and A. Ribolini, *J. Immunol. 138*, 2857 (1987).
S. L. Bursten et al., *J. Clin. Invest. 82*, 1479 (1988).
A. B. Cady, G. Riveau, L. Chedid, et al., *Int. J. Immunopharmacol. 11*, 887 (1989).
R. D. R. Camp et al., *J. Invest. Dermatol. 94*, 735 (1990a).
R. D. R. Camp, N. J. Fincham, J. S. Ross, et al., *J. Invest. Dermatol. 95*, 108S (1990b).
D. Caput et al., *Proc. Natl. Acad. Sci. USA 83*, 1670 (1986).
T. M. Carlos and J. M. Harlan, *Immunol. Rev. 14*, 6 (1990).
G. J. Carroll, *Br. J. Rheum. 25*, 359 (1986).
D. B. Carter, M. R. J. Deibel, C. J. Dunn, et al., *Nature 344*, 633 (1990).
M. C. Casagli et al., *Biochem. Biophys. Res. Commun. 162*, 357 (1989).
R. Chizzonite, T. Truitt, P. L. Kilian, et al., *Proc. Natl. Acad. Sci. USA 86*, 8029 (1989).
B. D. Clark et al., *Nucleic Acid Res. 14*, 7897 (1986).
B. D. Clark, M. J. Fenton, H. L. Rey, et al., in *Monokines and Other Non-lymphocytic Cytokines* (M. C. Powanda, J. J. Oppenheim, M. J. Kluger, and C. A. Dinarello, eds.), Alan R. Liss, New York, 1988, pp. 47–53.

B. D. Clark, T. Ikejima, J. Mancilla, et al., in *Molecular and Cellular Biology of Cytokines* (J. J. Oppenheim, M. C. Powanda, M. J. Kluger, and C. A. Dinarello, eds.), Wiley-Liss, New York, 1990, p. 131.
F. Cominelli, C. C. Nast, B. D. Clark, et al., *J. Clin. Invest. 86*, 972 (1990).
K. D. Cooper, C. Hammerberg, O. Baadsgaard, et al., *J. Invest. Dermatol. 95*, 24S (1990).
M. J. Cork, J. B. Mee, J. K. Tarlow, et al., *Brit. Jnl. Dermatol. 127*, 428 (1992).
M. J. Cork, J. B. Mee, J. K. Tarlow, et al., *Jnl. Invest. Dermatol. 100*, 448 (1993a).
M. J. Cork, J. K. Tarlow, A. I. F. Blakemore, et al., *Jnl. Invest. Dermatol. 100*, 522 (1993b).
J. R. Couchman and W. T. Gibson, *Dev. Biol. 108*, 290 (1985).
J. R. Couchman, J. L. King, and K. J. McCarthy, *J. Invest. Dermatol. 94*, 65 (1990).
B. Curtis, B. Gallis, R. Overell, et al., *Proc. Natl. Acad. Sci. USA 86*, 3045 (1989).
B. M. Curtis, M. B. Widmer, P. deRoos, et al., *J. Immunol. 144*, 1295 (1990).
M. M. D. Dayer, C. B. Wollheim, P. Seckinger, et al., *J. Autoimmun. 2*, 163 (1989).
M. O. Dayoff, W. C. Barker, and L. T. Hunt, *Methods Enzymol. 91*, 524 (1983).
L. B. Deeter, L. W. Martin, and J. M. Lipton, *Peptides 9*, 1285 (1988).
F. E. Dewhurst, P. P. Stshenko, J. E. Mole, and T. Tsuramachi, *J. Immunol. 135*, 2562 (1985).
M. Didier, C. Amsel, C. Pelassy, et al., *J. Immunol. 141*, 3078 (1988).
L. Didierjean, J. H. Saurat, C. Ucla, et al., *J. Invest. Dermatol. 89*, 322 (1987).
L. Didierjean, D. Solomon, Y. Merot, et al., *J. Invest. Dermatol. 92*, 809 (1989).
F. S. di Giovine and G. W. Duff, *Immunol. Today 11*, 13 (1990).
F. S. di Giovine et al., *J. Immunol. 138*, 3213 (1987).
F. S. di Giovine, J. A. Symons, and G. W. Duff, *Immunol. Lett. 29*, 211 (1991a).
F. S. di Giovine, G. Zhang, E. Takhish, et al., *Cytokine 3*, 5, 452 (1991b).
F. S. di Giovine, E. Takhsh, A. I. F. Blakemore, G. W. Duff, *Hu. Mol. Gen. 1*, 6,450 (1992).
G. M. Dillard and P. J. Bodel, *Clin. Immunol. 49*, 2418 (1989).
C. A. Dinarello et al., *Trans. Assoc. Am. Physicians 81*, 334 (1968).
C. A. Dinarello, L. J. Rossenwasser, and S. M. Wolff, *J. Immunol. 127*, 2517 (1981).
C. A. Dinarello, T. Ikejima, S. J. Warner, et al., *J. Immunol. 139*, 1902 (1987).
C. A. Dinarello et al., *Immunol. Today 10*, 49 (1989).
C. A. Dinarello, *Blood 77*(5), 1627 (1991).
P. M. Dowd, R. D. R. Camp, and M. W. Greaves, *Skin Pharmacol. 1*, 30 (1988).
S. K. Dower et al., *J. Exp. Med. 162*, 501 (1985).
S. K. Dower, E. E. Qwarnstrom, R. C. Page, et al., *J. Invest. Dermatol. 94*, 68S (1990).
D. Dripps, B. Brandhuber, R. C. Thompson, et al., *J. Biol. Chem. 266*, 10331 (1991).
G. W. Duff and E. Atkins, *J. Immunol. Methods 52*, 333 (1982).
G. W. Duff et al., *Br. J. Rheumatol. 24*, 94 (1985).
G. W. Duff, *Lancet 1*, 1432 (1989).
J. A. Eastgate, J. A. Symons, N. C. Wood, et al., *Lancet 2*, 706 (1988).
J. A. Eastgate, J. A. Symons, and G. W. Duff, *FEBS Lett. 260*, 213 (1990).
S. P. Eisenberg, R. J. Evans, W. P. Arend, et al., *Nature 343*, 341 (1990).
J. Elias, M. Reynolds, R. Kotloff, et al., *Proc. Natl. Acad. Sci. USA 86*, 6171 (1989).
E. Espel, C. Fromental, P. Reichenbach, et al., *EMBO 9*, 929 (1990).
W. C. Fanslow, J. E. Sims, H. Sassenfield, et al., *Science 248*, 739 (1990).
N. J. Fircham, R. D. R. Camp, A. J. H. Gearing, et al., *J. Immunol. 140*, 4294 (1988).
R. Fleischmajer, J. S. Perlish, and W. P. West, *Arch. Dermatol. 113*, 1661 (1977).
A. Flynn et al., *Science 218*, 475 (1982).
A. Fontana et al., *J. Immunol. 129*, 2413 (1982).

A. Fontana et al., *J. Immunol. 132*, 1837 (1984).
J. C. Foreman, *Skin Pharmacol. 1*, 77 (1988).
A. S. Freedman et al., *J. Immunol. 141*, 3398 (1988).
B. Freundlich, J. S. Bomalaski, J. S. Neilson, et al., *Immunol. Today 7*, 303 (1986).
Y. Furutani et al., *Nucleic Acid Res. 14*, 3167 (1986).
B. Gallis, K. Prickett, J. Jackson, et al., *J. Immunol. 143*, 3235 (1989).
A. J. H. Gearing, N. J. Fincham, C. R. Bird, et al., *Cytokine 2*, 68 (1990).
G. Gehr, T. Braun, and W. Lesslauer, *Clin. Invest. 70*, 164 (1992).
K. Georgilis et al., *J. Immunol. 138*, 3403 (1987).
I. Gery and B. H. Waksman, *J. Exp. Med. 136*, 143 (1972).
I. Gery and J. L. Lepe Zuniga, *Lymphokines 9*, 109 (1983).
P. Ghezzi and C. A. Dinarello, *J. Immunol. 140*, 4238 (1988).
D. Giulian et al., in *The Physiologic, Metabolic and Immunologic Actions of IL-1* (M. J. Kuger, J. J. Oppenheim, and M. C. Powanda, eds.), Alan R. Liss, New York, 1985, pp. 133–142.
P. F. Goetinick and D. L. Carlone, *Dev. Biol. 127*, 179 (1988).
D. Goldminz et al., *J. Invest. Dermatol. 88*, 97 (1987).
M. B. Goldring and S. M. Krane, *J. Biol. Chem. 262*, 16724 (1987).
K. Goto et al., *Br. J. Exp. Pathol. 65*, 94 (1984).
P. E. Gottschall, G. Katsuura, and A. Arimura, *Biochem. Biophys. Res. Commun. 163*, 764 (1989).
G. Grabner et al., *Invest. Opthalmol. Visual Sci. 23*, 757 (1982).
E. V. Granowitz, A. A. Santos, D. D. Poutsiaka, et al., *Lancet 338*, 1423 (1991).
E. V. Granowitz, B. D. Clark, E. Vannier, et al., *Blood 79*, 2356 (1992).
P. W. Gray et al., *J. Immunol. 137*, 3644 (1986).
F. Guesdon, N. Freshney, and J. Saklatvala, *Cytokine 3*, 484 (1991).
C. Hammerberg, W. P. Arend, G. J. Fisher, et al., *Jnl. Clin. Invest. 90*, 571 (1992).
C. Hammerberg, G. Fisher, O. Baadsgaard, et al., *J. Invest. Dermatol. 92*, 439 (1989).
C. Hammerberg, G. Fisher, J. J. Voorhees, et al., *J. Invest. Dermatol. 94*, 4 532 (1990).
C. H. Hannum, C. J. Wilcox, W. P. Arend, et al., *Nature 343*, 336 (1990).
S. Haskill, G. Martin, L. Van Le, et al., *Proc. Natl. Acad. Sci. USA 88*, 3681 (1991).
E. D. Hay, *J. Cell. Biol. 91*, 205s (1981).
D. J. Hazuda et al., *J. Biol. Chem. 263*, 8473 (1988).
T. Henseler and E. Christophers, *J. Am. Acad. Dermatol. 13*, 450 (1985).
T. R. Hesketh et al., *J. Biol. Chem. 258*, 4876 (1983).
M. E. Hiltz and J. M. Lipton, *FASEB J. 3*, 2282 (1989).
M. E. Hiltz and J. M. Lipton, *Peptides 11*, 979 (1990).
R. Horuk, J. J. Huang, M. Covington, et al., *J. Biol. Chem. 262*, 16275 (1987).
R. Horuk and J. A. McCubrey, *Biochem. J. 260*, 657 (1989).
M. Hurme, *J. Immunol. 139*, 1168 (1987).
M. Hurme, T. Palkama, and M. Sihvola, *Biochem. Biophys. Res. Commun. 157*, 861 (1988).
A. M. Hussein, J. J. Jimenez, et al., *Science 249*, 1564 (1990).
R. O. Hynes, *Cell 48*, 549 (1987).
M. Ikeda, U. Ikeda, and S. Kano, *Cytokine 3*, 2 131 (1991).
H. Iribe et al., *J. Exp. Med. 157*, 2190 (1983).
N. Isono and K. Kumagai, *Microbiol. Immunol. 33*, 43 (1989).
R. W. Janson, K. R. Hance, and W. P. Arend, *J. Immunol. 147*, 12 4218.
J. J. Jimenez, G. H. Wong, and A. A. Yunis, *FASEB 5*, 2456 (1991).
S. A. Jobling, P. E. Auron, G. Gurka, et al., *J. Biol. Chem. 31*, 16372 (1988).
R. Kirnbauer, A. Kock, T. Schwarz, et al., *J. Immunol. 142*, 1922 (1989).
P. J. Knudsden, C. A. Dinarello, and T. B. Strom, *J. Immunol. 137*, 3189 (1986).

P. J. Knudsden, C. A. Dinarello, and T. B. Storm, *J. Immunol. 139*, 4129 (1987).
Y. Kobayashi et al., *J. Immunol. 140*, 2279 (1988).
A. Kock, T. A. Luger, and J. C. Ansel, *Clin. Res. 36*, 3 (1988).
E. J. Kovacs, D. Radzioch, H. A. Young, et al., *J. Immunol. 141*, 3101 (1988).
K. Kragballe, B. T. Gjertsen, D. De Hoop, et al., *Lancet 337*, 193 (1991).
S. M. Krane, J. M. Dayer, L. S. Simon, and S. Byrne, *Collagen Relat. Res. 5*, 99 (1985).
M. Kristensen, B. Deleuran, D. J. Eedy, et al., *Brit. Jnl. Dermatol. 127*, 305 (1992).
R. Kroggel et al., *FEBS Lett. 229*, 59 (1988).
S. L. Kunkel, S. W. Chensue, and S. H. Phan, *J. Immunol. 136*, 186 (1986).
T. S. Kupper, *Adv. Dermatol. 3*, 293 (1988).
T. S. Kupper, *Arch. Dermatol. 125*, 1406 (1989).
T. S. Kupper, in *Immunophysiology* (J. J. Oppenheim and E. M. Shevach, eds.), Oxford University Press, Oxford, 1990a, pp. 285-305.
T. S. Kupper, *J. Invest. Dermatol. 94*, 146S (1990b).
T. S. Kupper, *J. Clin. Invest. 86*, 1783 (1990c).
T. S. Kupper et al., *J. Exp. Med. 164*, 2095 (1986).
T. S. Kupper et al., *J. Invest. Dermatol. 80*, 340 (1987).
T. S. Kupper, F. Lee, N. Birchall, et al., *J. Clin. Invest. 82*, 1787 (1988a).
T. S. Kupper, D. Coleman, J. Chodakewitz, et al., *J. Invest. Dermatol. 91*, 185 (1988b).
T. S. Kupper, K. Min, P. Sehgal, et al., *Ann. N.Y. Acad. Sci. 557*, 454 (1989).
E. A. Kurt-Jones, J. M. Kiely, and E. R. Unanue, *J. Immunol. 135*, 1548 (1985).
E. A. Kurt-Jones, W. Fiers, and J. S. Pober, *J. Immunol. 139*, 2317 (1987).
M. Lafarge et al., *Blood 73*, (1989).
J. W. Larrick and S. L. Kunkel, *Pharm. Res. 5*, 129 (1988).
C. G. Larsen, A. O. Anderson, J. J. Oppenheim, et al., *Immunology 68*, 31 (1989).
C. G. Larsen, M. Kristensen, K. Paludan, et al., *Biochem. Biophys. Res. Comm. 176*, 1020 (1991).
M. A. Lazare, *Endocrinol. Metab. Clin. North. Am. 20*, 4, 681 (1991).
J. M. Le, D. Weinstein, U. Gubler, et al., *J. Immunol. 138*, 2137 (1987a).
P. T Le, D. T. Tuck, C. A. Dinarello, et al., *J. Immunol. 138*, 2520 (1987b).
S. W. Lee, A. P. Tsou, H. Chan, et al., *Proc. Natl. Acad. Sci. USA 85*, 1204 (1988).
M. J. Lenardo and D. Baltimore, *Cell 58*, 227 (1989).
A. Lennard, P. Gorman, M. Carrier, et al., *Cytokine 4*, 2 83 (1992).
W. Lew, J. J. Oppenheim, and K. J. Matsushima, *J. Immunol. 140*, 1895 (1988).
C. Lewis, G. Mazzei, and A. Shaw, *Eur. J. Immunol. 20*, 207 (1990).
Z. Liao, R. S. Grimshaw, and D. L. Rosenstreich, *J. Exp. Med. 159*, 125 (1984).
P. Libby et al., *J. Clin. Invest. 78*, 1432 (1986).
R. M. Locksley et al., *J. Clin. Invest. 82*, 2097 (1988).
P. T. Lomedico, U. Gubler, C. P. Hellman, et al., *Nature 312*, 458 (1984).
H. Loppnow et al., *Eur. J. Immunol. 16*, 1263 (1986).
M. Lotz et al., *J. Immunol. 136*, 3643 (1986).
D. H. Lovett et al., *J. Immunol. 130*, 1796 (1983).
T. A. Luger, B. M. Stadler, S. I. Katz, and J. J. Oppenheim, *J. Immunol. 127*, 1493 (1981).
T. A. Luger et al., *J. Immunol. 128*, 2147 (1982).
H. R. MacDonald, *J. Immunol. 139*, 1546 (1987).
C. R. Maliszewski and W. C. Fanslow, *Tibtech. 8*, 324 (1990).
C. R. Maliszewski, C. R. Sato, T. V. Bos, et al., *J. Immunol. 144*, 3028 (1990).
J. Mancilla, I. Ikejima, B. D. Clark, et al., *Cytokine 1*, 95 (1989).
J. C. Manson, J. A. Symons, F. S. di Giovine, et al., *Eur. J. Immunol. 19*, 261 (1989).

C. L. March, B. Mosley, A. Larsen, et al., *Nature 315*, 641 (1985).
K. Matsushima, M. Bano, W. Kidwell, et al., *J. Immunol. 134*, 904 (1985a).
K. Matsushima et al., *J. Immunol. 135*, 1132 (1985b).
K. Matsushima, T. Akahoshi, M. Yamada, et al., *J. Immunol. 136*, 4496 (1986a).
K. Matsushima, J. Yodoi, Y. Tagaya, et al., *J. Immunol. 137*, 3183 (1986b).
K. Matsushima, K. Morishita, T. Yoshimura, et al., *J. Exp. Med. 167*, 1883 (1988a).
K. Matsushima, M. Shiroo, H. Kung, et al., *Biochemistry 27*, 3765 (1988b).
K. Matsushima and J. J. Oppenheim, *Cytokine 1*, 2 (1989).
A. Mauviel, J. Heino, K. Veli-Matti, et al., *J. Invest. Dermatol. 96*, 243 (1991).
G. J. Mazzei, P. L. Seckinger, J. M. Dayer, et al., *Eur. J. Immunol. 20*, 683 (1990).
A. J. G. McDonagh, L. Cawood, and A. G. Messenger, *Br. J. Dermatol. 123*, 717 (1990).
J. B. Mee, M. J. Cork, F. S. di Giovine, et al., in *Proceedings of the World Congress of Immunology*, Budapest, 1992.
C. R. Merriman, L. A. Pulliman, and R. F. Kampschmidt, *Proc. Soc. Exp. Biol. 154*, 224 (1977).
S. B. Mizel et al., *J. Immunol. 138*, 2906 (1987).
S. B. Mizel, *Immunol. Today 11*, 390 (1990).
H. Mizutani, R. Black, and T. Kupper, *Cytokine 1*, 78 (1989).
H. Mizutani, M. R. Black, and T. S. Kupper, *J. Clin. Invest. 87*, 3 1066 (1991).
J. Molvig, L. Baek, P. Christensen, et al., *Scand. J. Immunol. 27*, 705 (1988).
M. A. Moore and D. J. Warren, *Proc. Natl. Acad. Sci. USA 84*, 7134 (1987).
A. V. Muchmore and J. M. Decker, *J. Biol. Chem. 261*, 13404 (1986).
K. Muegge, T. Williams, J. Kant, et al., *Science 246*, 249 (1989).
N. Mukaida et al., *J. Immunol. 139*, 3321 (1987).
K. Muller, M. Stevenson, and K. Bendtzen, *Immunol. Lett. 17*, 361 (1988).
P. A. Murphy et al., *J. Immunol. 124*, 2498 (1980).
R. Neta et al., *J. Immunol. 139*, 1861 (1987).
B. J. Nickoloff, C. E. M. Griffiths, and J. N. W. N. Barker, *J. Invest. Dermatol. 94* (Suppl), 151 (1990).
D. A. Norris, *J. Invest. Dermatol. 95*, 115S (1990).
S. Nozaki, J. S. Abrahams, M. K. Pearce, et al., *J. Invest. Dermatol. 97*, 10 (1991).
R. F. Oliver, *J. Embryol. Exp. Morphol. 23*, 219 (1970).
F. Ollivierre et al., *Biochem. Biophys. Res. Commun. 141*, 904 (1986).
L. A. J. O'Neil, T. A. Bird, and J. Saklatvala, *Immunol. Today 11*, 392 (1990).
L. Osborn, S. Kunkel, and G. Nabel, *Proc. Natl. Acad. Sci. USA 86*, 2336 (1989).
M. Patarroyo, J. Prieto, J. Rincon, et al., *Immunol. Rev. 114*, 67 (1990).
M. E. Pierart, T. Najdovski, T. E. Appelboom, et al., *J. Immunol. 140*, 3808 (1988).
J. S. Pober, M. P. Bevilacqua, D. L. Mendrick, et al., *J. Immunol. 136*, 1680 (1986).
A. E. Postlethwaite, L. B. Lachman, C. L. Mainard, et al., *J. Exp. Med. 157*, 801 (1983).
J. P. Priestle, H. P. Schar, and M. G. Grutter, *Proc. Natl. Acad. Sci. USA 86*, 9667 (1989).
E. E. Qwarnstrom et al., *J. Biol. Chem. 263*, 8261 (1988).
E. W. Raines et al., *Science 243*, 393 (1989).
R. S. Rappaport and G. R. Dodge, *J. Exp. Med. 155*, 943 (1982).
K. Resch et al., *Immunobiology 172*, 336 (1986).
H. J. Ristow, *Proc. Natl. Acad. Sci. USA 84*, 194 (1987).
N. J. Roberts et al., *J. Exp. Med. 163*, 511 (1986).
B. C. Rodgers et al., *Trans. Assoc. Am. Phys. 98*, 334 (1985).
L. Romero, T. Ikejima, S. H. Pincus, et al., *J. Invest. Dermatol. 93*, 518 (1989).

M. Rooney, J. A. Symons, and G. W. Duff, *Rheumatol. Int. 10*, 217 (1990).
D. L. Rosenstreich, J. H. Tu, P. R. Kincade, et al., *J. Exp. Med. 168*, 1767 (1988).
P. M. Rosoff et al., *Cell 54*, 73 (1988).
A. Rubartelli, F. Cozzolino, M. Talio, et al., *Embo. J. 9*, 1503 (1990).
J. Saklatvala, S. J. Sarsfield, and Y. Townsend, *J. Exp. Med. 162*, 1208 (1985).
C. I. Sandborg et al., *Clin. Exp. Immunol. 60*, 294 (1985).
D. N. Sauder, *J. Invest. Dermatol. 85*, 1765 (1985).
D. N. Sauder, C. S. Carter, S. I. Katz, and J. J. Oppenheim, *J. Invest. Dermatol. 79*, 34 (1982).
D. N. Sauder et al., *J. Invest. Dermatol. 82*, 605 (1984a).
D. N. Sauder, N. L. Mounessa, S. I. Katz, et al., *J. Immunol. 132*, 828 (1984b).
J. Saus, S. Quinones, Y. Otani, et al., *J. Biol. Chem. 263*, (14) 6742 (1988).
G. Scala et al., *Nature 309*, 56 (1984).
G. Scapigliati, G. Ghiara, M. Bertalini, et al., *FEBS Lett. 243*, 394 (1989).
J. A. Schmidt et al., *J. Immunol. 128*, 2177 (1982).
A. Schmitt et al., *Lymphokine Res. 5*, 105 (1986).
J. A. Schmidt and M. J. Tocci, in *Peptide Growth Factors and their Receptors*, vol 1 (M. A. Sporn and A. B. Roberts, eds.), Springer-Verlag, Berlin, 1990, p. 473.
J. M. Schroder, *Exp. Dermatol. 1*, 12 (1992).
J. M. Schroder, U. Mrowietz, E. Morita, et al., *J. Immunol. 139*, 3474 (1987).
M. Schultzberg et al., *Neuroscience 30*, 805 (1989).
P. Seckinger and J. M. Dayer, *Ann. Inst. Pasteur/Immunol. 138*, 461 (1987).
S. Shaldon, K. M. Koch, M. Bingel, et al., *Kidney Int. 31*, 245 (1987).
G. Shaw and R. Kamen, *Cell 46*, 659 (1986).
L. Sherman, R. Ghiselli, and T. S. Kupper, *J. Invest. Dermatol. 94*, 578 (1990).
Y. G. A. Shimizu, K. van Seventer, K. Hogan, et al., *Immunol. Rev. 114*, 109 (1990).
F. Shirakawa and S. B. Mizel, *Mol. Cell. Biol. 9*, 2424 (1989).
F. Shirakawa, M. Chedid, J. Suttles, et al., *Mol. Cell. Biol. 9*, 959 (1989).
S. Shosman, *Int. Rev. Conn. Tiss. Res. 9*, 1 (1981).
P. L. Simon et al., *J. Immunol. 126*, 1534 (1981).
J. E. Sims, C. J. March, D. Cosman, et al., *Science 241*, 585 (1988).
J. E. Sims et al., *Proc. Natl. Acad. Sci. USA 86*, 8946 (1989).
R. Solari, *Cytokine 2*, 1, 21 (1990).
R. Solari, N. Smithers, K. Page, et al., *Cytokine 2*, 129 (1990).
T. A. Springer, *Nature 346*, 425 (1990).
M. J. Staruch and D. D. Wood, *J. Leukocyte Biol. 37*, 193 (1985).
A. Steinkasserer, K. Koelble, and R. B. Sim, *Nucleic Acid Res. 19*, 5095 (1991).
E. Stylianou, L. A. J. O'Neil, M. Edbrooke, et al., *Cytokine 3*, 478 (1991).
R. A. Swerlick, E. Garcia-Gonzalez, Y. Kubota, et al., *J. Invest. Dermatol. 97*, 190 (1991).
J. A. Symons, N. C. Wood, F. S. di Giovine, and G. W. Duff, *J. Immunol. 141*, 2612 (1988).
J. A. Symons, T. L. McDowell, F. S. di Giovine, et al., *Lymphokine Res. 8*, 365 (1989).
J. A. Symons and G. W. Duff, *FEBS Lett. 272*, 133 (1990).
J. A. Symons, J. A. Eastgate, and G. W. Duff, *Cytokine 2*, 190 (1990).
J. Symons, J. A. Eastgate, and G. W. Duff, *J. Exp. Med. 174*, 1251 (1991).
J. A. Symons, W. L. Warg, M. A. Palladino, and G. W. Duff, *Scand. J. Rheumatol. 21*, 92 (1992).
L. Takacs, H. Stockinger, O. Majdie, et al., *J. Immunol. Methods 141*, 3081 (1988).
J. K. Tarlow, A. I. F. Blakemore, A. Lennard, et al., *Human. Mol. Gen.* in press (1993).

B. Tartakovsky et al., *J. Immunol. 137*, 160 (1986).
J. L. Telford, G. Macchia, A. Massone, et al., *Nucleic Acid Res. 14*, 9955 (1987).
M. G. Tocci et al., *J. Immunol. 8*, 1109 (1987).
M. G. Tovey et al., *J. Immunol. 141*, 3106 (1988).
A. Uehara, A. Gottschall, P. E. Dahl, et al., *Biochem. Biophys. Res. Commun. 146*, 1286 (1987).
J. Uhl, R. C. Newton, J. G. Giri, et al., *J. Immunol. 142*, 1576 (1989).
C. R. Wagner et la., *Cell. Immunol. 93*, 91 (1985).
S. M. Wahl, *Ann. NY Acad. Sci. 460*, 224 (1985).
S. M. Wahl et al., *J. Immunol. 140*, 3026 (1988).
S. J. Warner, K. R. Auger, and P. J. Libby, *J. Exp. Med. 165*, 1316 (1987a).
S. J. Warner, K. R. Auger, and P. J. Libby, *J. Immunol. 139*, 1911 (1987b).
A. C. Webb et al., *Lymphokine Res. 5*, 77 (1986).
G. E. Westgate, L. P. Lewis, A. G. Messenger, et al., *J. Invest. Dermatol. 92*, 540A (1989).
J. Westwick, S. W. Li, and R. D. Camp, *Immunol. Today 10*, 146 (1989).
B. A. Wolf et al., *FEBS Lett. 248*, 35 (1989).
D. D. Wood et al., *Arthritis Rheum. 28*, 853 (1985).
P. R. Young, D. J. Hazuda, and P. L. Simon, *J. Cell. Biol. 107*, 447 (1988).
A. Zlotnik and K. W. Moore, *Cytokine 3*, 366 (1991).

# 2
# Interleukin 6

**Kazuyuki Yoshizaki and Tadamitsu Kishimoto**
*Osaka University Medical School*
*Osaka, Japan*

## I. INTRODUCTION

As the functional analysis of epidermal cells in the fields of biochemical and molecular biology has developed, the skin has been recognized as the largest defense system in the human body. The epidermis protects the body not only as a physicoanatomical organ but also as a first-level lymphoid organ. The skin consists of epidermal keratinocytes, which produce several kinds of cytokines, Langerhans cells, which process and present the antigens, recirculating T cells, most of which express $T\gamma\delta$ receptors, tissue macrophages, and other immunocompetent cells. In 1978, Streilein described the epidermis as skin-associated lymphoid tissues (SALT) [1].

Since Luger et al. [2] proposed and Kupper et al. [3] identified the epidermal cell–derived thymocyte-activating factor (ETAF) as interleukin 1 (IL-1), the epidermal keratinocyte, a main constituent of the skin, has been recognized as an immunoregulatory cell in immune response and inflammatory phenomena. Since then it has been found that more than 10 types of cytokines are produced by keratinocytes, e.g., IL-1, IL-3, IL-6, IL-8, granulocyte colony-stimulating factor (G-CSF), macrophage colony-stimulating factor (M-CSF), granulocyte/macrophage colony-stimulating factor (GM-CSF), tumor necrosis factor-alpha (TNF-$\alpha$), tumor growth factor-alpha (TGF-$\alpha$), TGF-$\beta$, and platelet-derived growth factor (PDGF). Growth of keratinocytes has been shown to be regulated by several cytokines, e.g., IL-1, epidermal cell growth factor (EGF), TGF-$\alpha$, TGF-$\beta$, and TNF-$\alpha$.

Although IL-6 was originally identified as a B-cell differentiation factor [4], subsequent researchers have shown that IL-6 is a pleiotropic cytokine which functions not only in the immune response [5] but also in inflammation [6], hematopoiesis [7], and neuroendocrine phenomena [8–10]. IL-6 has also been shown to react as an autocrine growth factor in several tumor cells including multiple myelomas/plasmacytomas [11] and renal cell carcinomas [12]. IL-6 has so far been found to be produced by immunoregulatory cells [13, 14], fibroblasts [13], endothelial cells [13], synovial cells [15], astrocytes [13], stromal cells [16], renal mesangial cells [17], as well as epidermal keratinocytes [18, 19].

Psoriasis is a chronic nonmalignant skin disease featuring epidermal hyperproliferation and accumulation of acute and chronic inflammatory cells. Although the etiology of this disease is unknown, some cytokines including IL-6 may be involved in the pathogenesis of psoriasis, especially in the process of the proliferation and differentiation of keratinocytes.

In this chapter we discuss the involvement of IL-6 in the physiological reactions of keratinocytes and its significance for the pathogenesis of epidermal proliferative skin diseases.

## II. IL-6 PRODUCTION BY KERATINOCYTES

Figure 1 shows the expression of interleukin 6 (IL-6) in cultured epidermal keratinocytes obtained from normal adult skin [20]. A thin section of the sheet of cultured keratinocytes is stained with a monoclonal anti–IL-6 antibody. The expression of IL-6 in the stratified keratinocytes is enhanced by stimulation with TNF-$\alpha$. This immunohistological analysis represents the function of normal human epidermal keratinocytes in the production of IL-6.

Kupper et al. [18] and Yamada et al. [21] in 1988 first reported IL-6 secretion from some keratinocyte cell lines (A431, KB). Although analysis using cell lines has the advantage of noncontamination with other cells, most of the cell lines do not represent the normal functions of the original normal cells. Kirnbauer et al. [19] in 1989 suggested the secretion and expression of IL-6 by normal human cultured keratinocytes following addition of IL-1 and phorbol myristate acetate (PMA). Strictly speaking, however, their observations posed some problems, because they could not deny the possibility that a small portion of epidermal fibroblasts and melanocytes was contaminated in the keratinocyte fraction that they used. Even so, their in vitro observations strongly suggest that unstimulated keratinocytes expressing a small amount of IL-6 can increase their production of IL-6 in the activated stages with the aid of various kinds of stimulators. Finally, immunohistochemical analysis utilizing anti–IL-6 antibody and in situ hybridization method

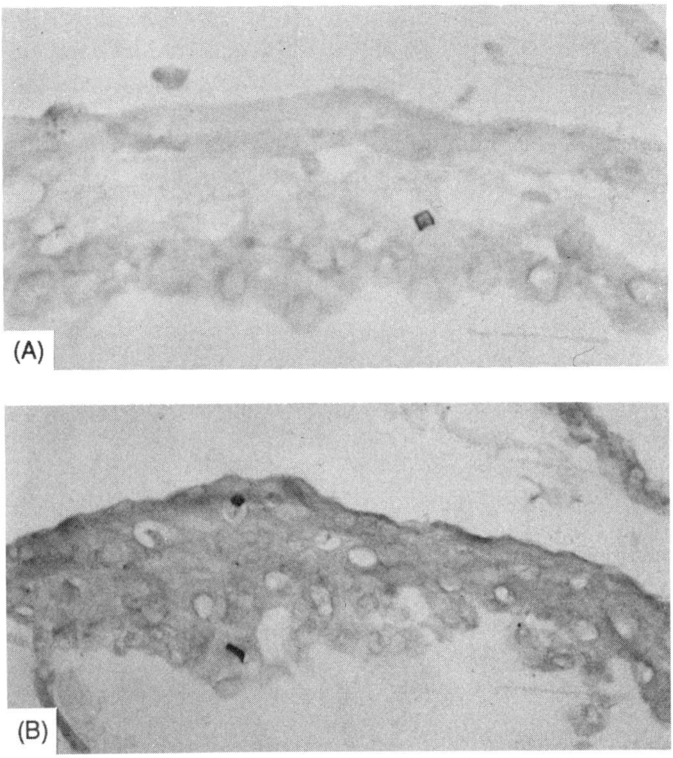


**Fig. 1** Enhancing effect of TNF-$\alpha$ on the expression of IL-6 in stratified cultured keratinocytes obtained from the normal human skin. The secretion of keratinocytes sheets were stained with a monoclonal anti–IL-6 antibody. (A) Low amount of IL-6 in nonstimulated keratinocytes. (B) Increase of IL-6 production in TNF-$\alpha$–stimulated keratinocytes.

using IL-6 cDNA has revealed IL-6 production by normal human keratinocytes both in vitro and in vivo [20, 22].

It is known that epidermal keratinocytes, the principal source of cytokines, are able to produce a number of cytokines. These cytokines derived from keratinocytes are IL-1$\alpha$, IL-1$\beta$, IL-3, IL-6, IL-8, G-CSF, M-CSF, GM-CSF, TGF-$\alpha$, TGF-$\beta$, TNF-$\alpha$, and PDGF, at least as far as we know at present [23, 24]. Therefore, when the keratinocytes are activated, it is possible that many types of cytokines, including IL-6, are produced. The synthesis and secretion of keratinocyte-derived IL-6 are enhanced by a variety of stimulators, which can be divided into four groups. The first group consists of bacterial products such as lipopolysaccharide (LPS) or *Staphylococcus* toxins [25–27]. These products of microorganisms may generate an early defense signal to the body through the induction of inflammatory cytokines either locally by the epidermis or systemically by macrophages and lymphocytes. This induction initiates the mobilization of a wide range of inflammatory and immunocompetent cells whose function is to destroy the invading bacteria. This IL-6–inducing activity of LPS in keratinocytes is considered the indirect effect of LPS through other cytokines such as IL-1 [19]. The second group of stimulators consists of physical stimulators such as ultraviolet (UV) radiation, heat injury, and mechanical injury. Kirnbauer et al. [28] directly observed the IL-6–inducing activity of UV irradiation in cultured normal human keratinocytes and the human epidermoid carcinoma cell line KB. UV light can be divided into three distinct wavelengths: UVA (320–400 nm), UVB (280–320 nm), and UVC (254–280 nm). Only UVB irradiation is able to induce IL-6 in keratinocytes. However, UVA induces the production of IL-6 in macrophages/monocytes, while UVC shows no IL-6–inducing activity in either keratinocytes or macrophages/monocytes. The third group consists of the virus itself. It is well known that macrophages can induce IL-6 production through human immunodeficiency virus (HIV) infection [29]. In the case of keratinocytes, Malejczyk et al. [30] demonstrated constitutive IL-6 secretion from a keratinocyte cell line (SK-V cells) harboring and expressing integrated human papillomavirus type 16 (HPV16) DNA sequences. This IL-6–inducing mechanism caused by infection with the virus is still unclear; however, it seems that viral infection may simultaneously induce the activation of IL-6 promoters and the viral replication itself. The final group of stimulators consists of inflammatory cytokines derived from keratinocytes [19, 20, 27, 31]. IL-1$\alpha$, IL-1$\beta$, TNF-$\alpha$, interferon beta (IFN-$\beta$), and IFN-$\gamma$, which are involved in embryogenesis, wound healing, infection, immune reaction, and inflammatory processes of the skin, significantly increase IL-6 production by both cell lines and normal keratinocytes. In contrast to other cell types, IL-4 induces IL-6 in keratinocytes only [32]. Induction of IL-6 by IL-1 or GM-CSF is greater than that by TGF-$\beta$ or TNF-$\alpha$ [27].

The inhibition of IL-6 production by keratinocytes, on the other hand, was reported only by Kirnbauer et al. [28]. IL-6 production by KB cells, a keratinocyte cell line either untreated or UVB irradiated, was inhibited by the addition of hydrocortisone. The inhibitory effect of dexamethasone on IL-6 production seemed to be more effective than that of hydrocortisone or prednisolone when the same concentration of $10^{-8}$ M was used in an in vitro experiment.

This inhibition by glucocorticoid is particularly interesting for the regulation of IL-6 gene expression because of the location of glucocorticoid-responsive elements (GREs) in the IL-6 promoter region. Since expression of the IL-6 gene may take part in the pathogenesis of epidermal hyperplasia, it is important to know the regulatory mechanism of the IL-6 gene expression. IL-6 is produced by various types of lymphoid and nonlymphoid cells, such as T cells, B cells, macrophages, and keratinocytes. As shown in Figure 2, the IL-6 promoter region at 5′ upstream of the IL-6 genes contains several potential transcriptional elements, such as an NF-IL6–responsive element (NF-IL6 RE), an NF-$\kappa$B RE, an AP-1–binding site, a cyclic AMP–responsive element, and GREs. Three nuclear factor–binding sites, namely, the NF-IL6 RE, the NF-$\kappa$B RE, and the 23 bp multiresponsive element (MRE), have been shown to be involved in the regulation of IL-6 gene expression [33–35]. Furthermore, the keratinocyte-inducing cytokines, e.g., IL-1, TNF-$\alpha$, and IL-6, are able to induce the transcription of IL-6 through the activation of these transcriptional nuclear factors (NF-IL6 and NF-$\kappa$B), resulting in association with the inflammatory state of psoriatic epidermis. However, the meaning of the presence of GREs in the promoter region is still unclear, although they may be involved in the suppression of IL-6 gene expression. Stimulators and inhibitors of IL-6 production in keratinocytes are summarized in Table 1.

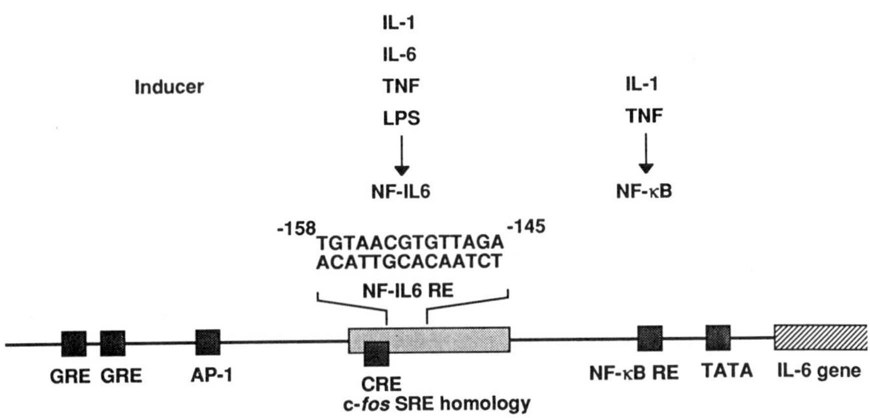


**Fig. 2** Promoter region of 5′ upstream of IL-6 gene. GRE, glucocorticoid-responsive element; NF-IL6 RE, NF-IL6–responsive element; NF-$\kappa$B RE: NF-$\kappa$B–responsive element.

**Table 1** Modulation of IL-6 Production in Keratinocytes

| | Effect | Ref. |
|---|---|---|
| Bacterial product | | |
| lipopolysaccharide | ↑↑ | 27 |
| Staphylococcus toxins | | |
| UV irradiation | | |
| UVA | ↑ | 19 |
| UVB | ↑↑ | 19 |
| UVC | (−) | |
| Virus | | |
| Papillomavirus | ↑ | 30 |
| Measles | ↑ | 31 |
| Poly(rI)poly(rC) | ↑ | 27, 31 |
| Protein kinase C activator | | |
| PMA | ↑ | 27 |
| Cytokine | | |
| IL-1$\alpha$ | ↑↑ | 19, 27 |
| IL-1$\beta$ | ↑ | 19, 31 |
| TNF-$\alpha$ | ↑ | 20, 27 |
| IFN-$\gamma$ | ↑ | 20 |
| TGF-$\beta$ | ↑ | 27 |
| GM-CSF | ↑↑ | 27 |
| Glucocorticoid | | |
| dexamethasone | ↓↓ | 19 |
| prednisolone | ↓ | 19 |
| hydrocortisone | ↓ | 19 |
| Vitamin D analog | | |
| MC903 | ↓ | 44 |

## III. PROLIFERATION OF KERATINOCYTES BY IL-6

It is known that IL-6 is an autocrine growth factor in myeloma cells [11], renal carcinoma cells [12], and mesangial cells [17]. Hancock et al. [36] demonstrated the stimulation of proliferation of cultured keratinocytes by several growth factors or cytokines. Following this, the stimulation by IL-6 of the proliferation of cultured keratinocytes was reported by Grossman et al. [37]. The effects of IL-1, (EGF), IFN-$\gamma$, and IL-6 on the proliferation of human keratinocytes were observed in a special culture medium, KBM, which contains EGF, insulin, hydrocortisone, and bovine pituitary extract [38]. The growth enhancement of normal human keratinocytes by IL-6 was confirmed with the cell number, in which the cells were allowed to grow for one week in the presence of recombinant human IL-6 (rIL-6) [20]. The cell growth of normal keratinocytes was increased 1.5- and 3.6-fold by 1 U/ml and 10 U/ml of rIL-6, respectively, as shown in Figure 3. These results show that IL-6 is a growth stimulator of human keratinocytes. However, it could not be said that the stimulation of proliferation was directly mediated by IL-6 until IL-6 receptors are found on the surface of keratinocytes. Expression of IL-6 receptors on keratinocytes was first suggested by the binding of $^{125}$I–IL-6 to keratinocyte monolayers by Krueger et al. [38]. Scatchard analysis of their data showed 6100 binding sites per cell with kd of 1.3 nM for IL-6. They proposed that fewer keratinocyte receptors per cells for IL-6 may be compatible with growth stimulation by IL-6 at lower molar concentrations than stimulation by EGF or TGF-$\alpha$ [37, 39]. Both EGF receptors and IL-6 receptors on keratinocytes show high affinity binding for their appropriate ligands. The expression of receptors for IL-6 on monolayered keratinocytes has been proved by two immunohistochemical analyses utilizing the monoclonal anti–IL-6R antibody MT-18 [20]. At first the presence of IL-6 receptors was observed in fixed single cells as shown in Figure 4. More directly, IL-6 receptors were detected on the cell surface of live keratinocytes with an Interactive Laser Cytometer (ACAS 470, Median Instruments, Inc., MI) as shown in Figure 5. Furthermore, IL-6 receptors are expressed on the cells in the lower layer in vertical sections of stratified keratinocytes (Fig. 6).

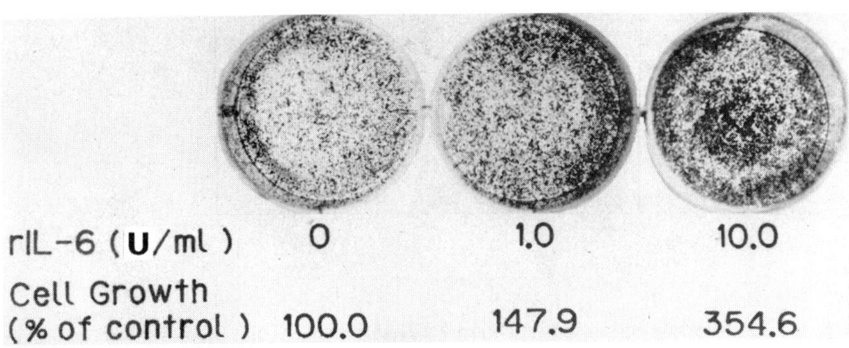


**Fig. 3** Growth-promoting activity of IL-6 on normal keratinocytes. Normal keratinocytes were cultured with 1 and 10 U/ml of rIL-6 for a week in the well. Cells were stained with crystal violet, and staining areas were measured with a computer-aided video camera. Cell growth in each group is presented as a percentage of that of non-stimulated control.

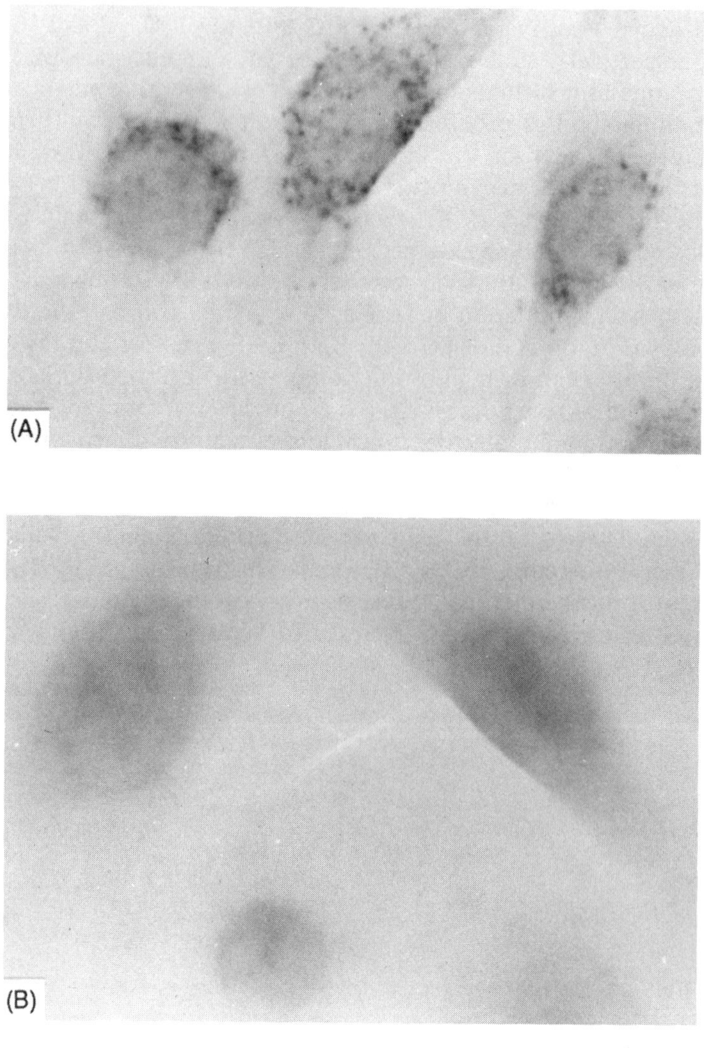


**Fig. 4** Immunocytochemical staining of IL-6 receptor on normal cultured keratinocytes. Cells were stained with (A) anti-IL-6 receptor antibody and (B) normal mouse IgG. Counterstaining was performed with methyl green.

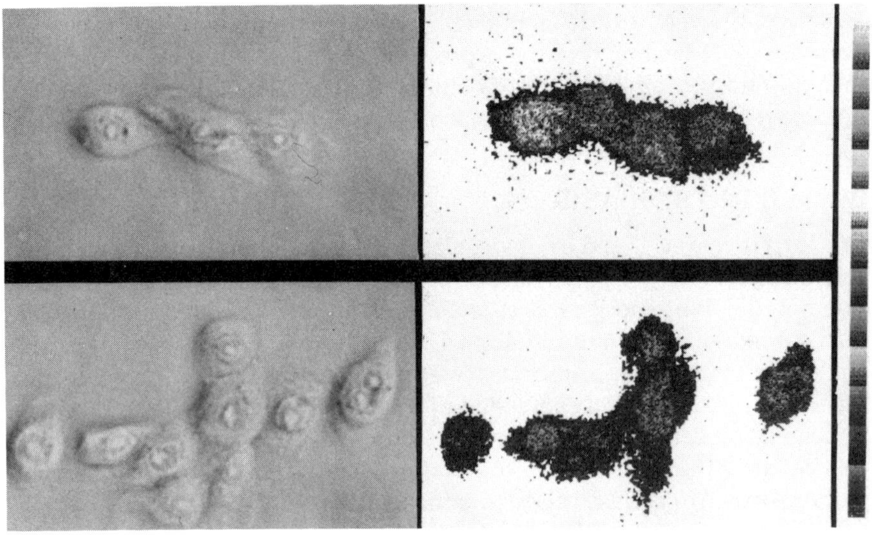

**Fig. 5** Detection of IL-6 receptors on live cultured keratinocytes by Interactive Laser Cytometer. Normal keratinocytes were lively stained with monoclonal anti-IL-6 receptor antibody (upper photographs) or not stained with normal mouse IgG (lower photographs). Left figures were obtained by optical microscopy, right figures by Interactive Laser Cytometer, ACAS 470.

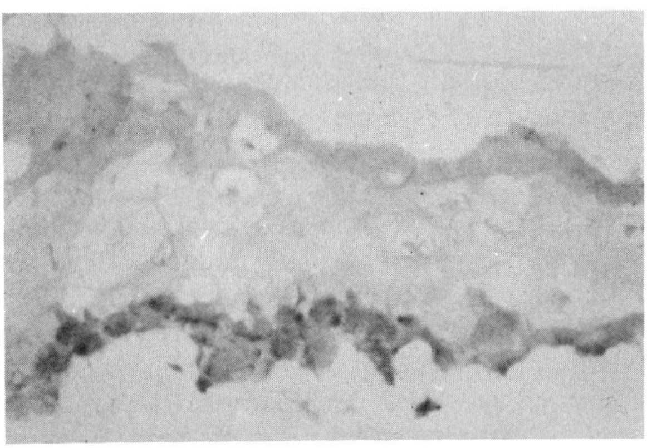

**Fig. 6** Immunohistochemical straining of IL-6 receptor in stratified cultured keratinocytes. The cells in the lower position expressed the receptors for IL-6.

However, the enlarged differentiated cells in the uppermost layers showed no staining, indicating that the expression of IL-6 receptors is restricted to the proliferative compartment of cultured epidermal keratinocytes and does not occur in the differentiated compartment [20].

## IV. IL-6 IN PSORIASIS

Psoriasis is characterized by dysregulation of keratinocyte growth with profound epidermal hyperplasia, altered epidermal maturation, capillary elongation and dilation, and local accumulation of neutrophils and mononuclear cells within the epidermis and dermis of the lesional skin. It is thought that epidermal hyperplasia in psoriasis may be partly related to increased production of cytokines and expression of their receptors. Therefore, it became important to detect specific growth factors or growth-promoting factors that regulate the proliferation of keratinocytes and may be involved in the pathogenesis of psoriasis through abnormal cytokine production.

Grossman et al. [37] and Sehgal [40] observed the expression of IL-6 in patients with active psoriasis. They showed increased levels of IL-6 in epidermal keratinocytes and in inflammatory dermal cells from active psoriatic plaques when compared to normal, nonlesional skin in the same patients. Prens et al. [41] also reported high levels of IL-6 in suction blister fluid from psoriatic plaque. IL-6 production by the keratinocytes in psoriatic lesions was detected by in situ hybridization with cDNA specific for IL-6 and by the detection of a higher percentage of IL-6–producing keratinocytes cultured from lesional skin than in those of cultured from uninvolved skin. In addition, Neuner et al. [42] reported that IL-6 was produced and secreted by monocytes that had infiltrated psoriatic epidermal lesions. Furthermore, not only locally infiltrating monocytes in psoriatic epidermis but also peripheral blood mononuclear cells (PBMNCs) in psoriatic patients secrete almost five times more IL-6 than healthy controls in vitro. The plasma levels of IL-6 in patients with psoriasis are higher than those of normal controls [42]. This elevation of plasma IL-6 may be caused by local production from lesional epidermis and by systemic secretion from mononuclear cells.

Psoralen plus UVA (PUVA) therapy is usually administered and seems to be effective in the treatment of psoriasis. It is believed that the beneficial effect of PUVA treatment may be due to the inhibition of DNA synthesis of keratinocytes, inactivation of lysosomal enzyme activity, modulation of polyamine synthesis, inactivation of psoriasis leukotactic factor, inhibition of lymphocyte proliferation, and so on.

The effect of PUVA therapy on the expression of IL-6 in psoriatic epidermis was first reported by Oxholm et al. [43], who employed immunohistochemistry utilizing anti-MK antiserum. Although the expression of IL-6 in the epidermis was neither enhanced nor suppressed at 48 h after the first dose of UVA, tissue-bound IL-6 decreased towards the levels found in unaffected skin with the clinical improvement of psoriasis. Neuner et al. [42] found the reduction of IL-6 production in in vitro PBMNCs with improvement at skin lesion at about 20 days after application of PUVA therapy. Finally, we have reported a patient with psoriasis who recently suffered from pneumonia with high fever as well as elevated levels of C-reactive protein (CRP) and IL-6 in the serum. A week after the start of antibiotic therapy, the number of platelets started to increase in association with the exacerbation of psoriasis in another week. This exacerbation of psoriatic skin after an infectious disease is frequently observed in patients with psoriasis. One of the causes of the exacerbation may be an inhancement of cytokine production by acute inflammation, which stimulates the induction of IL-6 derived from keratinocytes and the proliferation of the keratinocytes themselves. All evidence indicates that IL-6 may play an important role in the pathogenesis of psoriasis.

## V. CONCLUSION

The skin is the primary interface between the host and the environment and has been shown to be involved in the defense system as skin-associated lymphoid tissues. IL-6, an epidermal cytokine, is thought to be a multifunctional defense molecule in the body, because it displays a variety of biological effects on different cells, such as B-cell maturation, plasmacytoma-cell proliferation, T-cell activation, killer-cell induction, megakariocyte differentiation, activation of stem cells, and induction of the acute phase proteins. In this review we have focused on the possible role of IL-6 as an epidermal cytokine and a growth factor in cutaneous physiological and pathogenic processes. IL-6, originally isolated from immunocompetent cells, is produced by not only keratinocytes but also melanocytes and macrophages in the skin. The production of IL-6 by keratinocytes is enhanced by cytokines during the processes of immune reaction and inflammation. The enhancement of the proliferation of keratinocytes by IL-6 might be one of the defense activities of the IL-6 molecule. Ultimately, IL-6 is physically and pathologically involved with the growth of epidermal cells and the immunological phenomena in local epidermis. Furthermore, IL-6 produced in the skin may contribute to the immune and inflammatory phenomena in the whole body. Further studies are necessary to investigate the possible effect of IL-6 on the defense mechanisms in the skin.

## ACKNOWLEDGMENTS

We thank Dr. H. Yamada, Department of Dermatology, Kinki University Medical School, and Drs. K. Hashimoto, N. Okada, and K. Satoh, Department of Dermatology, Osaka University Medical School, for their helpful suggestions. We are grateful to Miss Ayumi Nobuhara for preparation of the manuscript.

## REFERENCES

1. J. W. Streilein, *J. Invest. Dermatol. 71*, 167 (1978).
2. T. A. Luger, B. M. Stadler, S. I. Katz, and J. J. Oppenheim, *J. Immunol. 127*, 1493 (1981).
3. T. S. Kupper, D. W. Ballard, A. O. Chua, J. S. McGuire, P. M. Flood, M. C. Horowitz, R. Langdon, L. Lightfoot, and U. Gubler, *J. Exp. Med. 164*, 2095 (1986).
4. T. Hirano, K. Yasukawa, H. Harada, T. Taga, Y. Watanabe, T. Matsuda, S. Kashiwamura, K. Nakajima, K. Koyama, A. Iwamatsu, S. Tsunasawa, F. Sakiyama, H. Matsui, Y. Takahara, T. Taniguchi, and T. Kishimoto, *Nature 324*, 73 (1986).
5. A. Muraguchi, T. Hirano, B. Tang, T. Matsuda, Y. Horii, K. Nakajima, and T. Kishimoto, *J. Exp. Med. 167*, 332 (1988).
6. J. Gauldie, C. Richards, D. Harnish, P. Landsdorp, and H. Baumann, *Proc. Natl. Sci. USA 84*, 7251 (1987).
7. K. Ikebuchi, G. G. Wong, S. C. Clark, J. N. Ihle, Y. Hirai, and M. Ogawa, *Proc. Natl. Acad. Sci. USA 84*, 9035 (1987).
8. T. Satoh, S. Nakamura, T. Taga, T. Matsuda, T. Hirano, T. Kishimoto, and Y. Kaziro, *Mol. Cell. Biol. 8*, 3546 (1987).
9. B. L. Spangelo, A. M. Judo, P. C. Isakson, and R. M. MacLeod, *Endoclinology 125*, 575 (1989).
10. H. Vankelecom, P. Carmeliet, J. Van Damme, J. Billiau, and C. Dennof, *Neuroendocrinology 49*, 102 (1989).
11. M. Kawano, T. Hirano, T. Matsuda, T. Taga, Y. Horii, K. Iwano, K. Asaoku, B. Tang, O. Tanabe, H. Tanaka, A. Kuramoto, and T. Kishimoto, *Nature 332*, 83 (1988).
12. S. Miki, M. Iwano, Y. Miki, M. Yamamoto, B. Tang, K. Yokokawa, T. Sonoda, T. Hirano, and T. Kishimoto, *FEBS Lett. 250*, 607 (1989).
13. T. Kishimoto and T. Hirano, *Ann. Rev. Immunol. 6*, 485 (1988).
14. Y. Horii, A. Muraguchi, S. Suematsu, T. Matsuda, K. Yoshizaki, T. Hirano, and T. Kishimoto, *J. Immunol. 141*, 1529 (1988).
15. T. Hirano, T. Matsuda, M. Turner, N. Miyasaka, G. Buchan, B. Tang, K. Sato, M. Shimizu, R. Maini, M. Feldman, and T. Kishimoto, *Eur. J. Immunol. 18*, 1797 (1988).
16. C-P. Chiu, C. Moulds, R. L. Cottman, D. Rennik, and F. Lee, *Proc. Natl. Acad. Sci. USA 85*, 7099 (1988).

17. Y. Horii, A. Muraguchi, M. Iwano, T. Matsuda, T. Hirayama, H. Yamada, Y. Fujii, K. Dohi, H. Ishikawa, Y. Ohmoto, K. Yoshizaki, T. Hirano, and T. Kishimoto, *J. Immunol. 143*, 3949 (1989).
18. T. Kupper, L. May, N. Birchall, and P. Segal, *J. Invest. Dermatol. 90*, 578 (1988).
19. R. Kirnbauer, A. Köck, T. Schwarz, A. Urbanski, J. Krutman, W. Borth, D. Damm, G. Shipley, J. C. Ansel, and T. A. Luger, *J. Immunol. 142*, 1922 (1989).
20. K. Yoshizaki, N. Nishimoto, K. Matsumoto, H. Tagoh, T. Taga, Y. Deguchi, T. Kuritani, T. Hirano, K. Hashimoto, N. Okada, and T. Kishimoto, *Cytokine 2*, 381 (1990).
21. H. Yamada, T. Matsuda, and M. Harada, *J. Invest. Dermatol. 90*, 619 (1988).
22. A. Oxholm, M. Diamant, P. Oxholm, and K. Bendtzen, *APMIS 99*, 58 (1991).
23. J. Ansel, P. Perry, J. Brown, D. Damm, T. Phan, C. Hart, T. Luger, and S. Hefeneider, *J. Invest. Dermatol. 94*, 101S (1990).
24. T. A. Luger and T. Schwarz, *J. Invest. Dermatol. 95*, 100S (1990).
25. T. S. Kupper, *Adv. Dermatol. 3*, 293 (1988).
26. T. A. Luger, J. A. Ansel, and T. Baba, in *Dermatology in Five Continents* (C. E. Orfanos, R. Stadler, H. Gallnick, eds.), Springer-Verlag, Berlin, 1988, p. 665.
27. M. Patridge, D. Chantry, M. Turner, and M. Feldmann, *J. Invest. Dermatol. 96*, 771 (1991).
28. R. Kirnbauer, A. Köck, P. Neuner, E. Förster, J. Krutmann, A. Urbanski, E. Schauer, J. C. Ansel, T. Schwarz, and T. Luger, *J. Invest. Dermatol. 96*, 484 (1991).
29. K. Nakajima, O. Martinez-Maza, T. Hirano, P. Nishanian, J. F. Salazar-Gonzalez, J. L. Fahey, and T. Kishimoto, *J. Immunol. 142*, 144 (1989).
30. J. Malejczyk, M. Malejczyk, A. Urbanski, A. Köck, S. Jablonska, G. Orth, and T. Luger, *Cell. Immunol. 136*, 155 (1991).
31. J. Van Damme and G. Opdenakker, *J. Invest. Dermatol. 95*, 90S (1990).
32. T. S. Kupper, K. Mink, P. B. Sehgal, H. Mizutani, N. Birchall, A. Ray, and L. May, *Ann. N.Y. Acad. Sci. 557*, 454 (1989).
33. K. Yasukawa, T. Hirano, Y. Watanabe, K. Muratani, T. Matsuda, S. Nakai, and T. Kishimoto, *EMBO J. 6*, 2939 (1987).
34. O. Tanabe, S. Akira, T. Kamiya, G. G. Wong, T. Hirano, and T. Kishimoto, *J. Immunol. 141*, 3875 (1988).
35. H. Isshiki, S. Akira, O. Tanabe, T. Nakajima, T. Shimamoto, T. Hirano, and T. Kishimoto, *Mol. Cell. Biol. 10*, 2757 (1990).
36. G. E. Hancock, G. Kaplan, and Z. A. Cohn, *J. Exp. Med. 168*, 1395 (1988).
37. R. M. Grossman, J. Krueger, D. Yourish, A. Granelli-Peperno, D. P. Murphy, L. T. May, T. S. Kupper, P. B. Sehgal, and A. B. Gottlieb, *Proc. Natl. Acad. Sci. USA 86*, 6367 (1989).
38. J. G. Krueger, J. F. Krane, M. Carter, and A. B. Gottlieb, *J. Invest. Dermatol. 94*, 135S (1990).
39. J. Krueger, J. Krane, A. B. Gottlieb, D. Yourish, P. Sehgal, L. May, S. Dicker, and T. Kupper, *J. Invest. Dermatol. 92*, 464 (1989).

40. P. B. Sehgel, *J. Invest. Dermatol. 94*, 2S (1990).
41. E. P. Prens, K. Benne, J. Van Damme, M. Bakkus, K. Brakel, R. Benner, and T. Van Joost, *J. Invest. Dermatol. 95*, 121S (1990).
42. P. Neuner, A. Urbanski, F. Trautinger, A. Möller, R. Kirnbauer, A. Kapp, E. Schöpt, T. Schwarz, and T. A. Luger, *J. Invest. Dermatol. 97*, 27 (1991).
43. A. Oxholm, P. Oxholm, B. Staberg, and K. Bendtzen, *Acta. Derm. Venereol. (Stockh.) 69*, 195 (1989).
44. A. Oxholm, P. Oxholm, B. Staberg, and K. Bendtzen, *Acta. Derm. Venereol. (Stockh.) 69*, 385 (1989).

# 3
# Tumor Necrosis Factor

**Günther R. Adolf**
*Bender & Co. GmbH*
*Vienna, Austria*

**Matthias Grell and Peter Scheurich**
*Institute for Cell Biology and Immunology*
*University of Stuttgart*
*Stuttgart, Germany*

## I. INTRODUCTION

Two independent lines of research have converged in the discovery of the protein now generally known as tumor necrosis factor (TNF). In studies on endotoxin-induced hemorrhagic necrosis of tumors in a mouse model, Carswell et al. identified a protein present in serum of bacille Calmette-Guérin (BCG)-primed, endotoxin-treated mice that mediated endotoxin activity and was toxic for tumor cells, but not normal cells, in vitro [1]. Concurrently, characterization of a serum factor mediating dramatic changes in the metabolism of animals suffering from parasitic infections resulted in the identification of a protein termed cachectin [2]. Sequence analysis of TNF and cachectin purified from cell cultures and molecular cloning of the respective cDNAs revealed the identity of these proteins [3]. Subsequently, the availability of DNA probes, essentially pure human and murine recombinant TNF proteins, highly specific antibodies, and sensitive immunoassays led within a few years to a wealth of information on the multifaceted biology of TNF, documented in thousands of publications. The therapeutic potential of TNF in cancer is currently being explored in clinical trials; moreover, following recognition of the involvement of TNF in the pathogenesis of various diseases, agents that inhibit TNF activity (e.g., monoclonal antibodies, soluble TNF receptor fragments) are under development.

A protein related to TNF, originally termed lymphotoxin, was also discovered independently by two groups in the course of studies on delayed-type hypersensitivity and a cytotoxic factor present in supernatants of activated lymphocytes, respectively [4, 5]. Following purification of this protein and subsequent cloning of its cDNA, the structural similarity of lymphotoxin and TNF was recognized [6, 7] and a modified nomenclature accounting for this relationship was suggested (TNF = TNF-$\alpha$; lymphotoxin = TNF-$\beta$).

Numerous reviews have in recent years attempted to provide a general overview on the biology of TNF [8, 9] or have emphasized specific aspects like the historical development [10], structure-function relationship [11], receptors and signal transduction [12, 13], the role of TNFs in physiological responses and pathological conditions [14–17], their mechanism of action [18, 19], and their potential as therapeutic agents [20–22]. Two books devoted entirely to TNFs were published recently [23, 24].

## II. GENES AND PROTEINS

### A. Genes: Structure, Location, Polymorphism

The human TNF-$\alpha$ and TNF-$\beta$ genes are closely linked and located on the short arm of chromosome 6 within the major histocompatibility complex. The TNF-$\beta$ gene is found about 200 kb centromeric to the HLA-B gene, separated by only about 1 kb from the TNF-$\alpha$ gene, which in turn is situated 350 kb telomeric to the class III gene cluster. Each gene comprises about 2–3 kb; in both cases, the coding regions are interrupted by three introns [25, 26]. In mice, the TNF genes show the same organization and are also localized in the major histocompatibility complex (MHC) region on chromosome 17 [27].

The close linkage of TNF and MHC genes led several groups to investigate whether MHC-linked autoimmune diseases are related to genetic variation in the TNF locus. In a mouse strain (NZW) predisposed to autoimmune nephritis, a restriction fragment length polymorphism (RFLP) in the TNF-$\alpha$ gene was found to correlate with low TNF-$\alpha$ production; replacement therapy with exogeneous TNF-$\alpha$ significantly delayed disease development [28]. Microsatellite tagging was used to identify a TNF allele unique for the NZW mouse that may be associated with a defect in TNF gene expression [29]. A mouse allele of the TNF-$\alpha$ locus, defined by an RFLP, is responsible for the failure to develop contact sensitivity following UVB exposure of the skin and development of hapten-specific tolerance (‘‘UVB susceptibility’’) [30]. In humans, only a low degree of polymorphism was observed at the RFLP level [31]. In systemic lupus erythematosus (SLE) patients, susceptibility to nephritis is associated with HLA-DR2 and DQw1 alleles and low TNF-$\alpha$ production; it is not known, however, in which way MHC class II genes might affect TNF production [32]. Recently, numerous human alleles were identified by microsatellite tagging, but the functional significance of this polymorphism is unclear [33, 34].

## B. Protein Structure

The 1.7 kb human TNF-$\alpha$ mRNA is translated into a protein consisting of 233 amino acids (26 kd). The 76 N-terminal amino acids constitute a putative signal sequence of unusual length (see below). Mature, secreted TNF-$\alpha$ is an acidic protein (156 amino acids, 17 kd, pl about 5) that contains a single intramolecular disulfide bond and is unglycosylated [7]. The primary translation product of the 1.4 kb human TNF-$\beta$ mRNA comprises 205 amino acids; the 34-amino-acid signal peptide is typical for secretory proteins. The mature protein (171 amino acids) does not contain cystein residues, but is N-glycosylated on asparagine 62 and probably also O-glycosylated (molecular mass 25 kd) [6, 35, 37]. Sequence comparison of TNF-$\alpha$ and TNF-$\beta$ shows that 28% of the residues are identical; TNF-$\beta$ has 18 additional N-terminal amino acids.

X-ray crystallography has recently provided a detailed three-dimensional structure of human TNF-$\alpha$ [36, 37]. In agreement with earlier reports on the solution structure of TNF, three TNF molecules were found to associate noncovalently to form a compact, wedge- or bell-shaped, stable trimer. The individual subunit represents a $\beta$-sandwich structure composed of two antiparallel $\beta$-pleated sheets. Analysis of conserved amino acids suggests a very similar structure for TNF-$\beta$. Interestingly, similar structural motifs ("jelly roll") have so far only been found in viral coat proteins. Putative receptor-binding sites are located near the base of the trimer at the interface between two subunits; the trimeric TNFs may thus be able to bind three receptor molecules simultaneously. Studies using soluble receptor fragments have recently provided direct evidence in support of this hypothesis [38].

The unusual length and structure of the putative TNF-$\alpha$ signal peptide suggest that TNF-$\alpha$ may not be secreted via the pathway established for typical secretory proteins; indeed, the peptide is not removed by the signal peptidase in a cotranslational process. In activated human and murine monocytes (but not in quiescent cells), the full-length TNF-$\alpha$ precursor is detectable as an integral membrane protein. The soluble 17 kd protein is liberated following cleavage of the precursor, probably by a serine protease [39, 40]. Importantly, membrane TNF is able to activate TNF receptors and kill target cells by direct cell-to-cell contact, and thus may play a role in local inflammatory responses [41]. A membrane-associated form of TNF-$\beta$ has recently been identified on a human T-cell hybridoma; however, as this molecule apparently did not contain a leader peptide, the anchoring mechanism must be different [42]. The occurrence of both membrane and soluble forms is not limited to TNF-$\alpha$. Other soluble polypeptide mediators, including CSF-1, the c-kit ligand, and the epidermal growth factor (EGF) family of growth factors, are also released from membrane-anchored pro-proteins by proteolytic cleavage [43].

## III. ASSAYS

Most laboratories employ cytotoxicity bioassays for quantitation of the biological activity of TNFs in culture supernatants and biological fluids (reviewed in Ref. 44). Murine L929 or L-M cells are most frequently used; the sensitivity of these cells is markedly increased in the presence of actinomycin D or other metabolic inhibitors [45]. The murine fibrosarcoma cell line WEHI 164 clone 13 is highly sensitive to the cytotoxic activity of TNF even in the absence of metabolic inhibitors [46]. Two human cell lines, BT-20 and KYM-1, were recently shown to be suitable for cytotoxicity bioassays [47, 48]. The potency of a TNF preparation is usually expressed in units/ml (U/ml); a preparation that results in lysis of 50% of the assay cells contains 1 U/ml. Other bioassay systems have been described, but their use has been rather limited [44].

The absolute sensitivity of the assay systems used in different laboratories varies enormously. To enable interlaboratory comparison of assay results, reference preparations for human TNF-$\alpha$ have been made available by the National Institute for Biological Standards and Control (UK), the National Cancer Institute (USA), and the National Institute of Health (Japan).

A general problem of TNF bioassays is their inherent lack of specificity. Most assay systems do not differentiate between TNF-$\alpha$ and TNF-$\beta$; in addition, other cytokines may have direct TNF-like activity (e.g., IL-1) or may potentiate the effects of TNF (e.g., IFN-$\gamma$). Further, soluble fragments of TNF receptors can be present in cell culture supernatants and human biological fluids; these proteins are still able to bind TNFs and thus inhibit their biological activities [49].

TNF immunoassays using antisera or monoclonal antibodies were developed by several groups. In addition to the general advantages of immunoassays, such assays are highly specific for either TNF-$\alpha$ or TNF-$\beta$. However, it should be kept in mind that soluble TNF receptors may again influence the assay results if the antibodies used recognize epitopes related to the receptor-binding site [49].

An important point to consider in the determination of plasma TNF-$\alpha$ levels is the possibility that endotoxin may be present in the tubes used for blood collection; this may induce TNF production by monocytes, resulting in artificially high plasma concentrations [50].

# IV. CELLULAR SOURCES AND REGULATION OF TNF PRODUCTION

## A. TNF Production In Vitro

In view of the multiple and potent biological activities of TNFs, it is hardly surprising that production of these proteins is tightly regulated. TNF-$\alpha$ synthesis is primarily controlled at the level of transcription, but regulation of mRNA stability and translational efficiency, mediated by UA-rich sequences in the 3′-untranslated region of the mRNA, may be even more important. Regulation of TNF-$\alpha$ production has been studied in detail in cells of the monocyte/macrophage lineage that represent a major source of this protein. Untreated cells contain undetectable or low levels of TNF-$\alpha$ mRNA, but no detectable protein. Treatment with lipopolysaccharide (LPS) results in a rapid but relatively small increase in transcriptional activity, a strong increase in steady-state mRNA levels, and secretion of large amounts of TNF protein [51, 52]. Peripheral blood monocytes, alveolar macrophages, Kupffer cells, tumor-infiltrating macrophages, and other types of tissue macrophages have all been shown to produce TNF-$\alpha$. Besides LPS, a variety of agents are able to induce TNF-$\alpha$ production in monocytes/macrophages in vitro, including phorbol myristate acetate (PMA) [53], bacterial components other than LPS [54], viruses [55–57], yeast [58], and parasites [59]. Further, immune complexes and antibody-coated phagocytizable particles strongly induce secretion of TNF-$\alpha$ [60], and a variety of tumor cell lines stimulate TNF-$\alpha$ release [61].

Many other cell types are also able to secrete TNF-$\alpha$, including B and T lymphocytes stimulated by mitogens, PMA, or calcium ionophores [62–65]; large granular lymphocytes/natural killer (NK) cells release TNF-$\alpha$ after contact with sensitive target cells [66]. Cultured neutrophil granulocytes spontaneously release low levels of TNF-$\alpha$; following LPS stimulation, significantly larger quantities are secreted [67]. Vascular smooth muscle cells treated with LPS and astrocytes treated with LPS or infected with viruses are further sources of TNF-$\alpha$ [68, 69]. An apparently unique situation is found in dermal and peritoneal mast cells that store TNF-$\alpha$ within granules and release the protein upon IgE-induced degranulation [70, 71]. Cultured human keratinocytes as well as epidermoid carcinoma cell lines stimulated with LPS or irradiated with UVB light secrete TNF-$\alpha$ [72].

In contrast to the wide spectrum of cell types able to produce TNF-$\alpha$, TNF-$\beta$ production seems to be limited to B and T lymphocytes activated by mitogens and, possibly, NK cells [62, 63, 73]. The only other cells reported to secrete TNF-$\beta$ are virus-infected astrocytes [69].

Although spontaneous production of TNFs does not usually occur in primary cells, a surprising number of permanent cell lines of various origins constitutively secrete TNFs. EBV-transformed B-lymphoblastoid cell lines, myeloma cell lines, and T-cell lines transformed by HTLV I or HTLV II produce TNF-$\beta$ [74–76]; T-lymphoid, B-lymphoid, and myeloid cell lines as well as various nonhematopoietic tumor cell lines selected for resistance to TNF can produce TNF-$\alpha$ [64, 65, 77, 78].

## B. Modulation of TNF Production

A number of mediators have positive or negative regulatory effects on TNF production. Cytokines including IFN-$\gamma$, IL-1, IL-3, M-CSF, GM-CSF, and, unexpectedly, TNF-$\alpha$ itself, although unable to directly induce TNF-$\alpha$, markedly stimulate TNF-$\alpha$ production induced by LPS [79–81]. In monocytes, $PGE_2$ inhibits LPS-induced TNF synthesis; as LPS also induces $PGE_2$ production in these cells, $PGE_2$ may function as a negative feedback regulator [82]. Glucocorticoids also exert negative effects on TNF synthesis; again, as TNF rapidly increases cortisol and corticosterone blood levels in vivo, these hormones may represent negative feedback regulators for TNF production (reviewed in Ref. 8). Similarly, TNF-$\alpha$ stimulates production of IL-6 by fibroblasts and other cell types; IL-6, in contrast, reduces LPS-induced TNF-$\alpha$ production by monocytes [83]. TGF-$\beta$ blocks production of TNF-$\alpha$ by mononuclear leukocytes induced by LPS [84], and also inhibits production of TNF-$\alpha$ and TNF-$\beta$ during IL-2–induced generation of LAK cells [85]. As TNF-$\alpha$ and TGF-$\beta$ have opposing immunoregulatory effects (e.g., on cytotoxic T-lymphocyte (CTL) development and thymocyte and B-cell proliferation), these two cytokines may represent further components of a homeostatic mechanism controlling the immune response.

## C. TNF Production In Vivo

Many studies have sought to quantitate TNF concentrations in biological fluids in humans or experimental animals. In view of the diversity of biological and immunological assay systems used by different groups, the lack—until recently—of international reference preparations, variable degrees of interference by soluble TNF receptors, and possible artifacts due to induction of TNF production by endotoxin-contaminated collection tubes, it is hardly surprising that the results of these experiments are not always consistent. Nevertheless, it seems clear now that serum or plasma of healthy human individuals contains very little, if any, TNF-$\alpha$ ($<50$ pg/ml). In an experimental setting, intravenous administration of endotoxin to humans results in a rapid rise in TNF-$\alpha$ levels that peak after about 2 h and return to background concentrations within 4 h [86]; similar studies—with similar results—were performed in several animal species, including mice, rabbits, and monkeys [8]. Total body UV irradiation of human volunteers results in the appearance of TNF-α in the serum; in this case, the concentrations increase for at least 24 h [72]. In normal human skin, immunofluorescence studies detected expression of TNF-α on keratinocytes, but not on Langerhans cells; TNF-α expression was increased after UVB irradiation, but not in allergic or irritant patch test reactions [87, 88].

TNF-α has been detected in sera from patients with a variety of infectious diseases, including gram-negative septicemia and septic shock [89–91], bacterial meningitis [92, 93], and leprosy [94], as well as in parasitic infections (Leishmaniasis, malaria) [94–96], AIDS-related complex, and AIDS [97]. In patients with septic shock, meningitis, and malaria, high serum concentrations are positively correlated with disease severity or unfavorable prognosis.

The evidence for elevated TNF-α serum levels in malignant diseases is controversial. Balkwill et al. [98] using a monoclonal antibody-based ELISA, found a "TNF-like factor" in 50% of patients with carcinomas, myelomas, and lymphomas, but not in normal subjects. However, the apparent concentrations determined (mean, 5.4 ng/ml, individual samples with up to 40 ng/ml !) were very high compared with levels determined by others in septic shock (most samples < 1 ng/ml); moreover, the "factor" was not biologically active and remarkably unstable. It is thus not clear whether the "TNF-like factor" is indeed identical with TNF. Using different assay systems, other authors failed to detect TNF in serum from cancer patients (see Ref. 99). Saarinen et al. [100] observed elevated TNF-α levels in 94% of children with malignancies; however, the concentrations measured (median 140 pg/ml) were much lower than those determined by Balkwill et al. Further studies are thus clearly required to determine the relevance of TNF production in malignancies.

Enhanced production of TNF is also associated with a variety of other diseases. Elevated serum concentrations were detected in patients with rheumatoid arthritis [101], progressive (but not stable) multiple sclerosis [102], Kawasaki disease [103], severe chronic heart failure [104], allograft rejection [105], and graft-versus-host disease [106].

In addition to disease states characterized by elevated levels of circulating TNF, local production of this cytokine may be associated with other diseases where spillover to the circulation is limited and thus serum TNF is not detectable. For example, whereas 15 out of 18 children suffering from bacterial meningitis had elevated TNF-α levels in their cerebrospinal fluid, only one of 11 tested had a concomitant increase in serum TNF [93]. In patients with adult respiratory distress syndrome, TNF-α was detected in broncoalveolar lavage fluid, but not in plasma samples [102].

In animal models, infection with influenza virus [55], gram-positive or gram-negative bacteria (including *E. coli, Listeria,* and *Legionella*) [107–

109], or parasites (e.g., *Plasmodium*) [110] results in the appearance of TNF in the circulation or in bronchoalveolar washings, depending on the route of infection.

## V. RECEPTORS AND SIGNAL TRANSDUCTION

### A. Receptor Structure

Purification of soluble TNF-binding proteins [111–113] and cellular TNF receptors (TNF-Rs) [114] recently facilitated cloning of cDNAs coding for two distinct types of human TNF-Rs, a 55–60 kd receptor with 455 amino acids (TR60) and a 75–80 kd TNF-R (TR80) with 461 amino acids [113, 115–117] (reviewed in Ref. 12). Both receptors bind TNF-$\alpha$ as well as TNF-$\beta$. mRNA analyses suggest near ubiquitous expression of both receptors with a single 2.3 kb transcript for TR60 in many tissues, but alternatively sized transcripts in certain cell types [113, 115, 118]. TR80 mRNA shows some size heterogeneity with transcripts of 4.5–5 kb, depending on the tissue [117, 118].

Single-copy genes code for both types of TNF-R. Recent data show that each of the four repeats that constitute the extracellular domain of TR60 (see below) is interrupted by an intron. The complete coding region and 3′-untranslated region of TR60 is distributed over 10 exons [119]. In contrast to genes coding for the ligands, the receptor genes are not linked and do not map to the MHC; the TR60 gene is located at chromosome 12p13 [119, 120], whereas the TR80 gene is located at 1p36 [121].

Both TNF-R chains can be subdivided into four structural elements: a hydrophobic signal peptide, an extracellular region, a single transmembrane segment, and an intracellular domain. The most intriguing feature of the extracellular regions is their high cysteine content of 24 and 22 residues in TR60 and TR80, respectively. These regions, containing the ligand-binding sites, form four structurally related pseudo-repeats of about 40 amino acids, each including 6 cysteines at conserved positions. Interestingly, the extracellular regions of human and rat nerve growth factor receptor (NGF-R) possess a similar structure; a new family of cytokine receptors can thus be defined [12, 122–124]. Further members of this family include the putative human cytokine receptor CD40, a murine B-lymphocyte activation antigen (4-1BB), and the human CD27 antigen [125]; the ligands for these receptors have not yet been defined. Further, OX40, a surface antigen present on activated rat CD4+ T lymphocytes, and the human Fas antigen contain three of these repeat sequences in their extracellular domains [124, 126, 127]. In addition, a protein of Shope fibroma virus, a tumorigenic poxvirus of rabbits, also contains four related repeats and is capable of binding TNF [124, 128]. Surprisingly, the structural similarity between the two types of TNF receptors (27% identity over 152 residues) is no more pronounced than between other members of the family (e.g., 30% identity between human TR60 and NGF) and is restricted in each case to the extracellular domains. Despite this similarity, no high-affinity binding of TNF or NGF to the heterologous receptors has been demonstrated.

In contrast to the extracellular parts, the cytoplasmic domains of the TNF-Rs show very little similarity to each other or any other receptor. However, TR60, the Fas antigen, and CD40 show homologies within a short stretch of about 40 amino acids located at different positions of the cytoplasmic domain of the respective molecule [127]. In the case of CD40, this region is essential for signal transduction [129]. No resemblance to the catalytic domains of tyrosine- or serine/threonine-specific protein kinases was found in the TNF-Rs. With the exception of the Fas antigen, receptor-associated components lacking intrinsic TNF-binding capacity have so far not been described. As Fas antigen comodulates with TNF-Rs and is able to induce apoptosis when stimulated by specific antibodies, it has been suggested that TNF-induced cytotoxicity may be mediated via TNF-R coupling to Fas [126].

Soluble TNF-binding proteins isolated from human urine have been identified as extracellular fragments of both TNF-Rs [111, 112, 130]. The soluble fragment of TR60 (and presumably also of TR80) is generated by proteolytic cleavage of the transmembrane receptor protein. TNF-binding proteins are present in serum and urine of healthy individuals; elevated levels have been observed in patients with renal failure, SLE, burns, and rheumatoid arthritis [112, 131–134]. A physiological function of these proteins, e.g., in protection against unphysiologically high levels of the ligands or in prolonging the half-life of TNFs, has yet to be demonstrated.

## B. Regulation of Receptor Expression

While many tissues and cell lines constitutively express TR60 as well as TR80, expression on certain cell types is subject to regulation. In human T and B lymphocytes, TNF-R expression is activation dependent and reversible [135, 136]; the majority of binding sites is provided by TR80 [147, M. Grell, unpublished). Both receptor types are up-regulated upon activation of $CD56^+$ NK cells and are involved in the generation of lymphokine-activated killer (LAK) cells [137].

Modulation of TNF-R expression by cytokines has been demonstrated in vitro in a variety of cell types. IFN-$\alpha$, -$\beta$, and -$\gamma$ enhance TNF-R numbers in several cell lines [138, 139]. TR60 mRNA levels in LAK cells are increased by IL-1$\beta$, IL-4, and IL-6 [140]. In vivo, TNF-R expression in hairy cells is strongly increased upon treatment of patients with IFN-$\alpha$ [141]. Increases in TNF-binding capacity are of interest as a quantitative relationship between receptor-ligand interactions and cellular responses is generally observed [142].

Other compounds regulating TNF-R expression include activators of protein kinase A (PKA), e.g., db cAMP and the phosphodiesterase inhibitor IBMX, that induce a selective increase in TR80 expression [13]. On the other hand, activators of protein kinase C (PKC), e.g., phorbol esters, diacylglycerols, rapidly decrease the number of TNF-binding sites in different cell types and concomitantly induce TNF resistance (reviewed in Refs. 13, 18, 19). The mechanisms by which receptor down-regulation occurs are not fully understood but most likely include proteolytic cleavage of both types of receptor [143, 144]. IL-1 also down-regulates TNF-Rs; whether protein kinase C is involved is still unclear [145].

## C. Signal Transduction

The multitude of different, but not necessarily independent, TNF signal transduction pathways identified so far includes typical second messenger systems. As the sequences of both receptors do not provide evidence for instrinsic kinase activity or any other enzymatic activity, receptor-associated components are thought to represent or activate intracellular enzymes like phospholipases (PLs). Results from several laboratories demonstrate TNF-mediated stimulation of $PLA_2$ in different cell types, resulting in production of arachidonic acid [13, 18, 19]. Arachidonate metabolites may then affect expression of TNF-sensitive genes as demonstrated for c-*fos* [146]. In addition, arachidonate metabolites, such as lysolipids, may function as effector molecules in TNF toxicity. In human neutrophils, TNF acts as a costimulator for $PLA_2$ activation, increasing the sensitivity of the cells for secondary stimuli (e.g., fMLP) of leukotriene production [147]; similarly, TNF treatment primes PLD, resulting in enhanced phosphatidic acid formation upon secondary stimulation [148].

A second major signaling pathway involves specific C-type phospholipase(s) which cleave phosphatidylcholine (rather than phosphatidylinositol-4,5-bisphosphate), resulting in production of the PKC activator diacylglycerol [149, 150]. In several cell lines, PKC activation and rapid translocation from cytosol to the cell membrane was observed [151]. No raise in intracellular calcium was seen, obviously due to lack of inositol triphosphate release. Most likely additional protein kinases, distinct from PKC, PKA, or casein kinase, are activated in response to TNF [152]. The role of PKC in TNF signal transduction is still unclear, as several typical TNF effects are not blocked when PKC is eliminated by persistent stimulation with phorbol ester. It is thus possible that at least in some cases redundant signal pathways can compensate for a lack of PKC [153, 154]. In some cell lines, TNF induces a rapid increase in cAMP formation, resulting in activation of PKA [13].

A well-characterized substrate for TNF-activated PK activity is the EGF receptor. TNF, like IL-1 and phorbol esters, causes an increase in EGF-R serine and threonine phosphorylation. Again, depletion of PKC does not block this effect, indicating TNF signal transduction independent of PKC [155, 156]. In addition, several cytosolic proteins are phosphorylated exclusively at serine residues within minutes of TNF treatment; these include low molecular weight heat shock proteins, mRNA cap-binding proteins, and a 26 kd cytosolic protein [13, 19]. The role of these proteins is so far unknown.

Involvement of sphingolipid turnover in TNF signal transduction has recently been described. In HL60 cells, TNF triggers activation of sphingomyelinase, which subsequently cleaves its substrate to phosphocholine and ceramide. A functional role of ceramide is strongly suggested by results demonstrating that this molecule, similar to TNF treatment, induces HL60 differentiation and c-*myc* proto-oncogene down-regulation [157]. The ceramide cleavage product, sphingosine, also shows strong synergy with TNF in $PLA_2$ activation [158].

Only limited data are so far available that distinguish the roles of the two types of TNF receptors in signal transduction and cell activation. Functional studies with receptor transfectants are often difficult to interpret because of expression of endogeneous receptors. Approaches to circumvent this problem have utilized the species specificity of human TNF-$\alpha$, which binds to mouse TR60 but not to mouse TR80, and antibodies specific for either TR60 or TR80 that may either act as agonists or as antagonists. Taken together, these results indicate that both types of receptor are functional and may mediate distinct cellular responses: TR60 is involved in cytotoxicity and induction of the transcription factor NF-$\kappa$B and of manganese superoxide dismutase, whereas TR80 mediates the growth-promoting activity for thymocytes and cytotoxic T cells [159–164].

Various transcription factors are activated by TNF. Among these, NF-$\kappa$B has been shown to influence expression of several TNF-responsive genes. The nuclear factor AP-1 is newly synthesized upon TNF treatment; one of its genes, c-*fos*, is activated by TNF via the arachidonate cascade, whereas expression of c-*jun* is controlled by as yet undefined mechanisms. Additional proteins involved in TNF signaling are the interferon response factors [13, 18, 19].

TNF-activated intracellular signaling finally results in the activation of multiple genes that include proto-oncogenes (see above) and genes coding for cytokines and enzymes (see, e.g., Ref. 165). Of particular interest is the induction of manganese superoxide dismutase, an enzyme that protects cells against the cytotoxic effects of TNF [166].

# VI. BIOLOGICAL ACTIVITIES, PHYSIOLOGY, AND PATHOPHYSIOLOGY

## A. Immunity and Inflammation—General Aspects

T lymphocytes express TNF receptors only after activation [135]. On activated T cells, TNF-$\alpha$ exerts multiple stimulatory activities, including enhancement of HLA-DR antigen and IL-2 receptor expression, enhancement of the proliferative response to IL-2 and of IL-2–induced IFN-$\gamma$ production [135, 167]. Further, TNF-$\alpha$ is a growth factor for thymocytes and promotes development of cytotoxic T cells [168, 169]. Similarly, TNF-$\alpha$ enhances the proliferative response of mitogen-activated B lymphocytes and stimulates the generation of immunoglobulin-secreting cells in response to mitogen and IL-2 by direct effects on the B cells [170]. The mixed lymphocyte reaction is also enhanced by exogeneous TNF-$\alpha$; neutralization of endogeneously produced TNF by antibodies suppresses the response [171, 172]. Further, TNF-$\alpha$ synergizes with IL-2 in the generation of LAK cells [173].

In vivo low doses of TNF-$\alpha$ enhance the antibody response of mice to a T-cell–dependent antigen (sheep erythrocytes) but have no effect on T-cell–independent antigen (polysaccharide) [174]. TNF has adjuvant activity on both the induction of specific T-cell toxicity to a tumor cell vaccine and the induction of specific antibodies [172]; mice that reject tumors after TNF treatment develop specific immunity for this tumor cell type [175].

The function of monocytes/macrophages, the major source of TNF-$\alpha$, is altered by TNF. Treatment with TNF enhances human monocyte and macrophage cytotoxicity, induces production of IL-1, $PGE_2$, and platelet-activating factor (PAF) and synergistically enhances LPS-stimulated IL-1 production [176–178]. In murine peritoneal macrophages stimulated with PMA, treatment with TNF-$\alpha$ results in production of increased amounts of hydrogen peroxide and enhanced Fc receptor expression [179]. TNF-treated macrophages show an increased capacity for killing of tumor cells [176], mycobacteria [179], and *Leishmania* [180, 181].

TNF-$\alpha$ as well as TNF-$\beta$ profoundly affect the activity of granulocytes, rapidly stimulating phagocytic activity, respiratory burst and degranulation, aggregation, and adherence to endothelial cells [182–187]; a possible chemotactic activity for granulocytes is controversial [188, 189]. Consequently, the toxicity of neutrophils and eosinophils, e.g., towards yeasts [190], protozoa [191, 192], amebae [193], and helminths [194], is enhanced. Treatment of human platelets with TNF-$\alpha$ or TNF-$\beta$ transforms them into efficient killer cells for *Schistosoma mansoni* larvae [195].

On endothelial cells, TNF-$\alpha$ stimulates expression of adhesion molecules, including ICAM-1 and ELAM-1. Consequently, granulocytes, monocytes, and lymphocytes can bind to the vessel walls, a prerequisite for subsequent migration into tissues. A further effect of TNF on endothelial cells is their conversion from an anticoagulant into a procoagulant state, mediated by increased expression of plasminogen activator inhibitor and suppression of thrombomodulin and plasminogen activator expression. Additional effects on endothelial cells include induction of IL-1, platelet-derived growth factor (PDGF), GM-CSF, prostacyclin, and PAF production and enhanced expression of MHC antigens (for reviews, see Refs. 16, 196). Further, TNF treatment induces growth inhibition, morphological changes, and, on endothelial cells derived from capillaries, cytotoxicity [197]. Toxic effects were also observed when TNF-$\alpha$ was added to endothelial cells together with neutrophils [198].

In addition to its direct effects on leukocytes, endothelial cells, and other cell types, TNF-$\alpha$ indirectly affects the immune response by inducing the production of several cytokines and low molecular weight mediators in a variety of cell types, including IL-1 (monocytes, endothelial cells, smooth muscle cells), IL-6 (fibroblasts), IL-8 (many cell types), IFN-$\beta$ (fibroblasts), and GM-CSF (fibroblasts, endothelial cells), prostaglandins (monocytes, endothelial cells), and PAF (monocytes, neutrophils, endothelial cells) (reviewed in Ref. 8). TNF thus participates in the network of signals that regulate immunoinflammatory reactions.

## B. Viral Infections

In vitro, infection with DNA and RNA viruses induces production of both TNF-$\alpha$ and TNF-$\beta$ in a variety of cell types [199, 200]. Both proteins inhibit replication of lytic RNA viruses and DNA viruses, and this activity is synergistically enhanced in combination with IFNs. In some experimental systems, the antiviral activity of TNFs may be mediated at least in part by induction of IFN-$\beta$ [200–202]. A combination of TNF-$\alpha$ and IFN-$\gamma$ markedly inhibits HIV replication [203]; however, TNF-$\alpha$ in the absence of IFNs may also stimulate HIV replication in cell lines as well as in blood cells of AIDS patients tested in vitro [204, 205]. Virus-infected cells show increased sensitivity to the cytotoxic activity of TNFs, and the selective toxicity of NK cells for virus-infected cells is mediated by secreted TNF [75, 200, 203, 206]. Additional evidence for the importance of TNF-$\alpha$ in viral infections comes from a study on herpesvirus infection in mice, in which low doses of TNF protected the animals against a lethal HSV-1 challenge, an effect not due to increased interferon production [207].

## C. Bacterial and Parasitic Infections

As outlined above, TNF can activate phagocytes to kill bacteria, yeast, protozoa, and helminths in in vitro experiments. Evidence that TNF indeed plays a physiological role in the resistance to infection is contributed by three experimental approaches: TNF-$\alpha$ is induced by inoculation of experimental animals with the infectious agent, administration of neutralizing antibodies exacerbates infection, and exogeneous TNF-$\alpha$ increases host resistance. This is illustrated nicely in a murine model of listeriosis: a sublethal infection with *Listeria monocytogenes*, a gram-positive, facultative intracellular bacterium, results in local production of TNF in the spleen early in the course of infection; TNF can be detected in the serum when a larger, lethal inoculum is used. Antibodies to TNF delay the elimination of bacteria from spleen and liver, and high doses convert a sublethal infection to a lethal one; finally, recombinant murine TNF administered early after infection protects the animal against a lethal dose of bacteria [208, 209].

Beneficial effects of TNF-$\alpha$ have also been demonstrated or implied in various other infection models. Endotoxin-resistant mice unable to produce TNF in response to endotoxin (C3H/HeJ) are more likely to be infected with virulent *E. coli* compared with normal mice (C3H/HeN) [210]. In the liver of mice infected with BCG, injection of antibody to TNF inhibits the formation of granulomas and subsequent elimination of the bacteria [211]. Intratracheal infection of mice with *Legionella pneumophila* results in production of TNF in the lung; administration of exogeneous TNF enhances clearance of the bacteria and protects from mortality [111]. Low doses of TNF improve survival of mice following experimental infection with *Klebsiella pneumoniae* [212], and a combination of TNF and antibiotics improves the condition of rats infected with *Staphylococcus aureus* [213]. Treatment of mice with antibodies to TNF abolishes both early and late immunity induced by an attenuated strain of *Salmonella typhimurium* [214]. Administration of TNF-$\alpha$ to *Plasmodium yoelii*-infected mice results in slower increase in parasitemia and prolonged survival [215].

## D. Tumors

A variety of tumor cell lines are able to stimulate release of TNF-$\alpha$ from macrophages [216], and TNF-$\alpha$ is one of the effector molecules responsible for tumor cell killing by activated macrophages [217], as suggested by studies showing a correlation between the susceptibility of tumor cells to the toxic effects of macrophages and TNF as well as experiments using neutralizing antibodies. Using recombinant TNF-$\alpha$ and TNF-$\beta$, numerous studies have shown that these proteins are able to inhibit the proliferation of a wide range of tumor cell lines in vitro. However, relatively high concentrations are often required to achieve significant cytostasis; further, many cell lines do not respond, and in some cases, proliferation may even be enhanced [218,

219]. Synergistic enhancement of the cytostatic effect was observed in some cell lines by simultaneous treatment with TNFs and IL-1 or IFNs, particularly IFN-$\gamma$; by combining TNF and IFN-$\gamma$, it is possible to overcome resistance to the cytostatic effect of TNF [218–220]. By continuous culture of TNF-sensitive tumor cell lines in low concentrations of TNF, resistant sublines can be developed; interestingly, these cells often produce TNF themselves [80, 221].

In a variety of animal models, TNF-$\alpha$ has been shown to suppress tumor growth (see, e.g., Refs. 222–224). However, the direct antiproliferative effect of TNF is of questionable relevance; for example, antitumor efficacy in vivo can be seen with cell lines that are insensitive to TNF in vitro. The importance of indirect, host-mediated effects has been demonstrated in several studies [175, 225]. The hemorrhagic necrosis of some tumors induced by TNF-$\alpha$, an effect that led to the discovery of this cytokine, is probably mediated by destruction of the tumor cell vasculature due to direct toxicity for endothelial cells or activation of PMNs [226]. The complexity of the in vivo situation is illustrated by a study on the effects of TNF-$\alpha$ on sarcomas growing intradermally in mice: administration of TNF-$\alpha$ resulted in hemorrhagic necrosis in the center of the tumor in all animals, whereas the surviving peripheral tumor cells regressed only in some of them. In T-cell–deficient mice, the hemorrhagic reaction was strongly reduced, and regression of the residual tumor was not observed. In general, near-lethal doses of TNF had to be applied to generate antitumor effects [226].

In other mouse models, the effects of local TNF production on tumor formation were studied using TNF-resistant tumor cells transfected with a TNF-$\alpha$ gene [227, 228]. In comparison with the untransfected parental cell lines, tumor development by TNF-secreting cells was strongly suppressed; neutralizing antibodies to TNF-$\alpha$ abolished the suppression. Massive infiltration of the tumor tissue by macrophages was observed in one of these studies; the suppressive effect was clearly weaker in T-cell–deficient nude mice. In both studies, TNF production by the tumor cells was low, and antitumor activity was observed in the absence of detectable side effects.

The results available from a number of clinical phase I/II trials of TNF-$\alpha$ in cancer patients (systemic administration) confirm the unimpressive efficacy observed in animal studies. The antitumor effects were generally poor, and considerable toxicity precluded further dose escalation (reviewed in Refs. 20–22, 229). However, in patients suffering from melanomas and sarcomas of the extremities, isolated perfusion with high doses of TNF-$\alpha$ in combination with melphalan and pretreatment with IFN-$\gamma$ resulted in dramatic antitumor effects (89% complete remissions) [230]. These results demonstrate that TNF-$\alpha$, in combination with other therapeutic regimens, may be useful in cancer therapy, provided that the systemic toxicity can be controlled.

## E. Metabolic Effects

TNF-$\alpha$ has originally been identified as the mediator responsible for cachexia and concomitant triglyceridemia associated with chronic trypanosome infection [2]. In vitro studies using adipocytes have identified suppressive effects of TNF-$\alpha$ on several enzymes of the lipogenic pathway, including lipoprotein lipase, and stimulating effects on catabolic, lipolytic pathways (reviewed in Ref. 9). Prolonged administration of sublethal doses of TNF-$\alpha$ to rats causes anorexia, weight loss, and depletion of lipid and protein stores, in addition to anemia and inflammatory changes in several organs, reminiscent of changes seen in cachexia related to infections and malignant diseases [231]. In other, similar studies, however, sustained cachexia was not observed; this discrepancy may be due to the development of tolerance to the anorexia-inducing effects of TNF [231, 232]. Oliff et al. [233] developed an animal model that was expected to mimic more closely the long-term effects of low doses of TNF in tumor-bearing hosts. A recombinant hamster cell line secreting TNF-$\alpha$ was inoculated into nude mice; the majority of animals developed severe cachexia. Tachyphylaxis was not observed; factors other than TNF associated with the presence of tumor cells may—together with TNF-$\alpha$—be responsible for this difference with respect to models that use TNF in the absence of tumors.

Evidence that TNF-$\alpha$ mediates some, but not all, of the derangements observed in cancer cachexia was derived from mouse models in which antibodies were used to block the activity of endogeneously produced TNF. The results show that endogeneous TNF contributed to anorexia and changes in lipid and protein metabolism, whereas hematological and acute phase protein responses were not affected [234].

Although the experimental evidence clearly shows that TNF can induce cachexia in tumor models and enhanced production of TNF is observed in human infectious diseases associated with weight loss, such as AIDS, it is still unclear whether TNF contributes to cachexia in human cancer (reviewed in Ref. 235). Clinical trials with TNF antagonists may be able to provide a definitive answer.

In conclusion, the catabolic state induced by TNF that may provide improved nutrient supply during acute infections may result in deleterious effects during prolonged exposure to infectious agents and, possibly, tumors.

## F. Tissue Remodeling

Through effects on osteoblasts, osteoclasts, chondrocytes, and fibroblasts, TNF-$\alpha$ and TNF-$\beta$ participate in the regulation of bone and cartilage remodeling and are involved in the destruction of tissues in chronic inflammation. In bone cultures, both cytokines cause an increase in the number of osteoclasts, a decrease in mineralized bone matrix, and inhibition of collagen synthesis [236]. In cartilage explants, TNF-$\alpha$ stimulates chondrocytes to degrade proteoglycan and inhibits proteoglycan biosynthesis by these cells [237]. Synovial cells and dermal fibroblasts in culture respond to TNF treatment with enhanced production of $PGE_2$ and metalloproteinases (collagenase, gelatinase, stromelysin) [238]. In addition to direct effects, TNF may also indirectly affect bone and cartilage by stimulating the production of IL-1 in monocytes and fibroblasts; IL-1, itself a potent stimulator of bone resorption, synergizes with TNF at suboptimal concentrations [239]. The relevance of these experimental findings for the in vivo situation is underlined by the detection of IL-1 and TNF-$\alpha$ in synovial fluid from arthritis patients; the cytokines seem to be derived from synovial macrophages [240].

TNF-$\alpha$ is a weak mitogen for fibroblasts and cooperates with EGF by up-regulating EGF receptors [241]. Further effects of TNF on fibroblasts in vitro include inhibition of collagen and fibronectin synthesis [242]. Although TNF-$\alpha$ inhibits the proliferation of endothelial cells in vitro and may even by cytotoxic for cells derived from capillaries, it is angiogenic in vivo in both a rabbit cornea model and in chick chorioallantoic membranes [243–245]. In a mouse model, subcutaneous administration of low amounts of TNF-$\alpha$ delivered by a minipump over several days induced neoformation of tissue, composed mainly of fibroblasts, collagen fibrils, and capillaries; the covering epidermis showed a hyperplastic reaction. Perfusion with higher doses led to massive coagulation necrosis [246].

Taken together, TNFs may participate in the regulation of physiological repair mechanisms, whereas prolonged production of these proteins may contribute to tissue destruction, e.g., in chronic joint inflammation (TNF-$\alpha$) or bone destruction in myeloma patients (TNF-$\beta$) (see below).

## G. Toxicity

Infusion of humans or animals with endotoxin or live gram-negative bacteria induces TNF-$\alpha$ production; administration of TNF-$\alpha$ results in a similar pattern of toxicity as observed in septicemia and septic shock, and neutralizing antibodies protect animals from endotoxin toxicity. It is thus generally accepted now that TNF-$\alpha$ plays a central role in the pathogenesis of septic shock (reviewed in Refs. 15, 17). Whereas direct effects of TNF-$\alpha$ and cells activated by TNF-$\alpha$ (e.g., neutrophils) [247] are important, it is increasingly becoming clear that additional mediators that are induced by TNF, including IL-1, IL-6, and PAF, contribute to toxicity. In animal models of endotoxin shock, an antagonist of IL-1 reduces lethality, but does not affect TNF serum levels [248]; antibodies to IL-6 increase serum TNF activity induced by *E. coli*, but nevertheless protect against shock [249]; antibodies to TNF-$\alpha$ block endotoxin-induced increases in IL-1 and IL-6 production [15]; synthetic PAF antagonists also are able to prevent endotoxin- and TNF-induced shock [250].

Pathological changes induced by administration of high doses of TNF-$\alpha$ to animals are seen in multiple organ systems and include vascular leaking, intravascular coagulation, hypotension, pulmonary inflammation and hemorrhage, and necrosis of the liver, kidney, and intestinal tract. Metabolic effects include acidosis, hyperglycemia, and hyperkalemia (reviewed in Refs. 8, 15, 16). In clinical trials in cancer patients, common side effects of TNF-$\alpha$ therapy were fever, chills, fatigue, headache, nausea, and anorexia; dose-limiting toxicity included hypotension, thrombocytopenia and leukopenia, hepatotoxicity, and fluid retention [229].

In a number of animal disease models, experiments using neutralizing antibodies have confirmed the role of TNF-$\alpha$ as a mediator of toxicity. Antibodies to TNF-$\alpha$ are able to inhibit cerebral malaria in mice [251], prolong graft survival following heart or liver transplantation in rats [252], prevent the development of lesions and decrease mortality in graft-versus-host disease in mice [253], and reduce pulmonary lesions and fibrosis induced by bleomycin [254]. Further, antibodies to TNF-$\alpha$ inhibit autoimmune demyelination induced by passive transfer of myelin-specific T cells [255].

## VII. BIOLOGY OF TNF-$\beta$

As discussed above, the genes for TNF-$\alpha$ and TNF-$\beta$ are closely linked; the proteins are distantly related in structure and compete with each other for binding to the same receptors. Production of TNF-$\beta$ is limited to lymphoid cells; the regulation of TNF-$\beta$ production in these cells differs from that of TNF-$\alpha$ [64]. Human (but not murine) TNF-$\alpha$ and TNF-$\beta$ can be distinguished easily as they are antigenically unrelated; however, in studies performed before the availability of antibodies, it is often unclear whether the biological activity observed was due to TNF-$\alpha$ or TNF-$\beta$.

Compared with the enormous amount of information available on the biology of TNF-$\alpha$, much less is known about the biological effects and the physiological and possible pathophysiological roles of TNF-$\beta$ (reviewed in Ref. 256). One of the reasons may be that recombinant human and mouse TNF-$\beta$, appropriate antibodies, and immunoassays are less readily available than the respective TNF-$\alpha$ reagents. Most studies that have compared the biological effects of TNF-$\alpha$ and TNF-$\beta$ have come to the conclusion that both molecules have qualitatively the same and quantitatively very similar activities. However, a few notable exceptions have been reported. TNF-$\alpha$, but not TNF-$\beta$, induces M-CSF production in purified blood monocytes; pretreatment of the cells with TNF-$\beta$ blocks TNF-$\alpha$–induced M-CSF secretion [257]. Similarly, TNF-α stimulates secretion of G-CSF and GM-CSF production in human fibroblasts, whereas TNF-β is at least 1000-fold less potent [258]. Human endothelial cells treated with low concentrations of TNF-α acquire the ability to bind neutrophils, whereas at least 100-fold higher levels of TNF-β are required to obtain the same effect; in addition, TNF-α induces hematopoietic growth factor production, whereas TNF-β is inactive [259]. Large quantitative differences in the potencies of TNF-α and TNF-β were also observed in the induction of MHC class I antigens on a human T-lymphocyte hybridoma [260] and the cytostatic effects on various human carcinoma cell lines [261]. It is not clear whether all these differences can be explained by different affinities of the two TNFs for the two types of membrane receptors and the differential expression of these receptors on different cell types; other factors, e.g., receptor-associated accessory molecules, may be involved [260].

Very little is known about a potential pathophysiological role of TNF-β. In myeloma patients, TNF-β produced by the tumor cells probably is the mediator of osteoclastic bone destruction and hypercalcemia [77]. A possible role in diseases characterized by overproduction of TNF-α has so far not been established.

In conclusion, although TNF-β is most probably involved in the regulation of immunoinflammatory reactions in a manner quite similar to TNF-α, its precise role in physiology remains to be determined. Inactivation of the TNF-β gene in mice by homologous recombination may provide a useful model for addressing this question.

## VIII. CONCLUSIONS

TNF-α/cachectin is produced upon appropriate stimulation (immune complexes, viruses, bacteria, parasites, tumor cells, UV light) mainly by monocytes/macrophages, but also by a variety of other hematopoietic and nonhematopoietic cell types. Its production is enhanced by several cytokines, including IFN-γ, and inhibited by $PGE_2$, glucocorticoid hormones, IL-6, and TGF-β. The protein interacts with target cells through two distinct cell membrane receptors, inducing changes in cell proliferation and/or functional activity in multiple cell types, including lymphocytes, macrophages, granulocytes, and endothelial cells. Effects of TNF-α on cytokine and lipid mediator production (e.g., IL-1, IL-6, PG, PAF) and additive or synergistic interactions with other cytokines (IL-1, IFN-γ) establish its role in the cytokine regulatory network; effects on glucocorticoid hormone production link immune and endocrine systems. Further activities include effects on lipid and protein metabolism and a shift in the coagulation balance towards a procoagulant state. TNF-α thus plays an important role in specific and unspecific immunity and inflammation; beneficial effects were observed in animal models of viral, bacterial, and parasitic infections. A crucial pathophysiological role for TNF-$\alpha$ has been demonstrated in sepsis and septic shock, cerebral malaria, and cachexia in parasitic infections (and possibly cancer) as well as in the joint destruction in arthritis. Graft rejection and lesions in graft-versus-host disease are also mediated by TNF-$\alpha$. TNF-$\beta$/lymphotoxin, distantly related to TNF-$\alpha$ in structure, is produced by lymphocytes only; it binds to and activates the same cell membrane receptors as TNF-$\alpha$. The biological activities of TNF-$\beta$ in many experimental systems are very similar to those of TNF-$\alpha$, however, much less is known about its possible pathophysiological role.

## REFERENCES


1. E. A. Carswell, L. J. Old, et al., *Proc. Natl. Acad. Sci. USA 72*, 3666 (1975).
2. B. Beutler, J. Mahoney, et al., *J. Exp. Med. 161*, 984 (1985).
3. B. Beutler, D. Greenwald, et al., *Nature 316*, 552 (1985).
4. N. H. Ruddle and B. H. Waksman, *Science 157* (1967).
5. G. A. Granger and T. W. Williams, *Nature 218*, 1253 (1968).
6. P. W. Gray, B. B. Aggarwal, et al., *Nature 312*, 721 (1984).
7. D. Pennica, G. E. Nedwin, et al., *Nature 312*, 724 (1984).
8. B. Beutler and A. Cerami, *Ann. Rev. Immunol. 7*, 625 (1989).
9. M. Jäättelä, *Lab. Invest. 64*, 724 (1991).
10. L. J. Old, *Science 230*, 630 (1985).
11. C. R. Goh and A. G. Porter, *Protein Eng. 4*, 385 (1991).
12. S. R. Sprang, *Trends Biochem. Sci. 15*, 366 (1990).
13. M. Krönke, S. Schütze, et al., *Cell. Signal. 2*, 1 (1990).
14. J. W. Larrick and S. L. Kunkel, *Pharmaceut. Rev. 5*, 129 (1988).
15. Y. Fong and S. F. Lowry, *Clin. Immunol. Immunopathol. 55*, 157 (1990).
16. C. S. Rock and S. F. Lowry, *J. Surg. Res. 51*, 434 (1991).
17. K. J. Tracey, *Circ. Shock 35*, 123 (1991).
18. J. Vilcek and T. H. Lee, *J. Biol. Chem. 266*, 7313 (1991).
19. G. Camussi, E. Albano, et al., *Eur. J. Biochem. 202*, 3 (1991).
20. K. Haranaka, *J. Biol. Resp. Mod. 7*, 525 (1988).
21. E. Frei and D. Spriggs, *J. Clin. Oncol. 7*, 291 (1989).
22. A. G. Porter, *Trends Biotech. 9*, 158 (1991).
23. B. B. Aggarwal and J. Vilček, eds., *Tumor Necrosis Factor: Structure, Function, and Mechanism of Action*, Marcel Dekker, New York, 1991.
24. B. Beutler, ed., *Tumor Necrosis Factor. The Molecules and Their Emerging Role in Medicine*, Raven Press, New York, 1991.
25. G. E. Nedwin, S. L. Naylor, et al., *Nucl. Acids Res. 13*, 6361 (1985).
26. M. C. Carroll, P. Katzman, et a.., *Proc. Natl. Acad. Sci. USA 84*, 8535 (1987).
27. S. M. Gardner, B. A. Mock, et al., *J. Immunol. 139*, 476 (1987).
28. C. O. Jacob and H. O. McDevitt, *Nature 331*, 356 (1988).
29. C. V. Jongeneel, H. Acha-Orbea, et al., *J. Exp. Med. 171*, 2141 (1990).

30. T. Yoshikawa and J. W. Streilein, *Immunogenetics 32*, 398 (1990).
31. G. C. Webb and D. D. Chaplin, *J. Immunol. 145*, 1278 (1990).
32. C. O. Jacob, Z. Fronek, et al., *Proc. Natl. Acad. Sci. USA 87*, 1233 (1990).
33. S. A. Nedospasov, I. A. Udalova, et al., *J. Immunol. 147*, 1053 (1991).
34. C. V. Jongeneel, L. Briant, et al., *Proc. Natl. Acad. Sci. USA 88*, 9717 (1991).
35. B. B. Aggarwal, W. J. Henzel, et al., *J. Biol. Chem. 260*, 2334 (1985).
36. M. J. Eck and S. R. Sprang, *J. Biol. Chem. 264f*, 17595 (1989).
37. E. Y. Jones, D. I. Stuart, and N. P. C. Walker, *Nature 338*, 225 (1989).
38. H. Loetscher, R. Gentz, et al., *J. Biol. Chem. 266*, 18324 (1991).
39. M. Krieger, C. Perez, K. DeFay, I. Albert, and S. D. Lu, *Cell 53*, 45 (1988).
40. P. Scuderi, *J. Immunol. 143*, 168 (1989).
41. C. Perez, I. Albert, et al., *Cell 63*, 251 (1990).
42. J. L. Browning, M. J. Androlewicz, et al., *J. Immunol. 147*, 1230 (1991).
43. J. Massague, *J. Biol. Chem. 265*, 21393 (1990).
44. A. Meager, H. Leung, and J. Wooley, *J. Immunol. Methods 116*, 1 (1989).
45. S. M. Kramer and M. E. Carver, *J. Immunol. Methods 93*, 201 (1986).
46. T. Espevik and J. Nissen-Meyer, *J. Immunol. Methods 95*, 99 (1986).
47. J. Yen and S. M. Kramer, *J. Immunotherapy 10*, 174 (1991).
48. A. Meager, *J. Immunol. Methods 144*, 141 (1991).
49. I. Engelberts, S. Stephens, et al., *Lancet 338*, 515 (1991).
50. G. Leroux-Roels, F. Offner, et al., *Clin. Chem. 34*, 2373 (1988).
51. B. Beutler, N. Krochin, et al., *Science 232*, 977 (1986).
52. J. Han, T. Brown, and B. Beutler, *J. Exp. Med. 171*, 465 (1990).
53. E. Sariban, K. Imamura, et al., *J. Clin. Invest. 81*, 1506 (1988).
54. P. F. Barnes, S. J. Fong, et al., *J. Immunol. 145*, 149 (1990).
55. F. Vacheron, A. Rudent, et al., *J. Gen. Virol. 71*, 477 (1990).
56. A. E. Goldfeld and T. Maniatis, *Proc. Natl. Acad. Sci. USA 86*, 1490 (1989).
57. D. Aderka, H. Holtmann, et al., *J. Immunol. 136*, 2938 (1986).
58. J. Y. Djeu, D. K. Blanchard, et al., *J. Immunol. 141*, 4047 (1988).
59. S. Picot, F. Peyron, et al., *Infect. Immun. 58*, 214 (1990).
60. J. M. H. Debets, C. J. Van der Linden, et al., *J. Immunol. 141*, 1197 (1988).
61. R. Feinman, D. Hendriksen-Destefano, et al., *J. Immunol. 138*, 635 (1987).
62. M. C. Cuturi, M. Murphy, et al., *J. Exp. Med. 165*, 1581 (1987).
63. U. Andersson, G. Adolf, et al., *J. Immunol. Methods 123*, 233 (1989).
64. S. S. J. Sung, J. M. Bjorndahl, et al., *J. Exp. Med. 167*, 937 (1988).
65. S. S. J. Sung, L. K. L. Kung, et al., *J. Exp. Med. 168*, 1539 (1988).
66. P. M. Peters, J. R. Ortaldo, et al., *J. Immunol. 137*, 2592 (1986).
67. D. B. Dubravec et al., *Proc. Natl. Acad. Sci. USA 87*, 6758 (1990).
68. S. J. C. Warner and P. Libby, *J. Immunol. 142*, 100 (1989).
69. A. P. Lieberman, P. M. Pitha, et al., *Proc. Natl. Acad. Sci. USA 86*, 6348 (1989).
70. L. J. Walsh, G. Trinchieri, et al., *Proc. Natl. Acad. Sci. USA 88*, 4220 (1991).
71. J. R. Gordon and S. J. Galli, *Nature 346*, 274 (1990).
72. A. Köck, T. Schwarz, et al., *J. Exp. Med. 172*, 1609 (1990).
73. C. V. Paya, N. Kenmotsu, et al., *J. Immunol. 141*, 1989 (1988).
74. B. D. Williamson et al., *Proc. Natl. Acad. Sci. USA 80*, 5397 (1983).
75. I. R. Garrett, B. G. M. Durie, et al., *N. Engl. J. Med. 317*, 526 (1987).
76. E. Tschachler, M. Robert-Guroff, et al., *Blood 73*, 194 (1989).

77. B. B. Aggarwall, W. J. Kohr, et al., *J. Biol. Chem. 260*, 2345 (1985).
78. B. Y. Rubin, S. L. Anderson, et al., *J. Exp. Med. 164*, 1350 (1986).
79. M. K. Warren and P. Ralph, *J. Immunol. 137*, 2281 (1986).
80. G. E. Gifford and M. L. Lohmann-Matthes, *J. Natl. Cancer Inst. 78*, 121 (1987).
81. S. A. Cannistra, E. Vellenga, et al., *Blood 71*, 672 (1988).
82. S. L. Kunkel et al., *Biochem. Biophys. Res. Comm. 137*, 404 (1986).
83. D. Aderka, J. Le, and J. Vilcek, *J. Immunol. 143*, 3517 (1989).
84. D. Chantry, M. Turner, et al., *J. Immunol. 142*, 4295 (1989).
85. T. Espevik, I. S. Figari, et al., *J. Immunol. 140*, 2312 (1988).
86. H. R. Michie, K. R. Manogue, et al., *N. Engl. J. Med. 318*, 1481 (1988).
87. A. Oxholm, M. Diamant, P. Oxholm, and K. Bendtzen, *APMIS 99*, 58 (1991).
88. A. Oxholm, P. Oxholm, et al., *Acta Derm. Venereol. 71*, 93 (1991).
89. F. Offner, J. Philippé, et al., *J. Lab. Clin. Med. 116*, 110 (1990).
90. E. Girardin, G. E. Grau, et al., *N. Engl. J. Med. 319*, 397 (1988).
91. T. Calandra, J. D. Baumgartner, et al., *J. Infect. Dis. 161*, 982 (1990).
92. A. Waage, A. Halstense, and T. Espevik, *Lancet i*, 355 (1987).
93. D. Nadal, D. Leppert, et al., *Arch. Dis. Child. 64*, 1274 (1989).
94. P. Pisa, M. Gennene, et al., *J. Infect. Dis. 161*, 988 (1990).
95. P. Scuderi, K. E. Sterling, et al., *Lancet ii*, 1364 (1986).
96. G. E. Grau, T. E. Taylor, et al., *N. Engl. J. Med. 320*, 1586 (1989).
97. J. Lähdevirta, C. P. J. Maury, et al., *Am. J. Med. 85*, 289 (1988).
98. F. Balkwill, R. Osborne, et al., *Lancet ii*, 1229 (1987).
99. P. J. Selby, S. Hobbs, et al., *Lancet i*, 483 (1988).
100. U. M. Saarinen, E. K. Koskelo, et al., *Cancer Res. 50*, 592 (1990).
101. C. P. J. Maury and A. M. Teppo, *Arthritis Rheum. 32*, 146 (1989).
102. D. J. Roberts, J. M. Davies, et al., *Lancet ii*, 1043 (1989).
103. C. P. J. Maury, E. Salo, and P. Pelkonen, *J. Lab. Clin. Med. 113*, 651 (1989).
104. B. Levine, J. Kalman, et al., *N. Engl. J. Med. 323*, 236 (1990).
105. C. P. Maury and A. M. Teppo, *J. Exp. Med. 166*, 1132 (1987).
106. F. W. Symington, M. S. Pepe, et al., *Transplantation 50*, 518 (1990).
107. D. G. Hesse, K. J. Tracey, et al., *Surg. Gynecol. Obstet. 166*, 147 (1988).
108. E. A. Havell, *J. Immunol. 139*, 4225 (1987).
109. D. K. Blanchard, J. Y. Djeu, et al., *Infect. Immun. 55*, 433 (1987).
110. G. E. Grau, L. F. Fajardo, et al., *Science 237*, 1210 (1987).
111. H. Engelmann, D. Novick, and D. Wallach, *J. Biol. Chem. 265*, 1531 (1990).
112. I. Olsson, M. Lantz, et al., *Eur. J. Haematol. 42*, 270 (1989).
113. A. Himmler, I. Maurer-Fogy, et al., *DNA Cell Biol. 9*, 705 (1990).
114. H. Loetscher, E. Schlaeger, et al., *J. Biol. Chem. 265*, 20131 (1990).
115. T. J. Schall, M. Lewis, et al., *Cell 61*, 361 (1990).
116. H. Loetscher, Y. C. E. Pan, et al., *Cell 61*, 351 (1990).
117. C. A. Smith, T. Davis, et al., *Science 248*, 1019 (1990).
118. R. G. Goodwin, D. Anderson, et al., *Mol. Cell. Biol. 11*, 3020 (1991).
119. P. Fuchs, S. Strehl, et al., *Genomics 13*, 219 (1992).
120. J. Derré, O. Kemper, et al., *Hum. Genet. 87*, 231 (1991).
121. O. Kemper, J. Derré, et al., *Hum. Genet. 87*, 623 (1991).
122. K. I. Arai, F. Lee, et al., *Ann. Rev. Biochem. 59*, 783 (1990).

123. S. Gillis, *Curr. Opin. Immunol. 3*, 315 (1991).
124. S. Mallett and A. N. Barclay, *Immunol. Today 12*, 220 (1991).
125. R. Q. Hintzen, R. de Jong, et al., *J. Immunol. 147*, 29 (1991).
126. S. Yonehara, A. Ishii, and M. Yonehara, *J. Exp. Med. 169*, 1747 (1989).
127. N. Itoh, S. Yonehara, et al., *Cell 66*, 233 (1991).
128. C. A. Smith, T. Davis, et al., *Biochem. Biophys. Res. Comm. 176*, 335 (1991).
129. S. Inui, T. Kaisho, et al., *Eur. J. Immunol. 20*, 1747 (1990).
130. P. Seckinger, J. H. Zang, et al., *Proc. Natl. Acad. Sci. USA 87*, 5188 (1990).
131. D. Aderka, H. Engelmann, et al., *Cytokine 3*, 473 (1991).
132. G. Adolf and I. Apfler, *J. Immunol. Methods 143*, 127 (1991).
133. M. Lantz, H. Thysell, et al., *J. Clin. Invest. 88*, 2026 (1991).
134. P. Roux-Lombard and J. M. Dayer, *Cytokine 3*, 494 (1991).
135. P. Scheurich, B. Thoma, et al., *J. Immunol. 13*, 1786 (1987).
136. B. K. Erikstein, E. B. Smeland, et al., *Eur. J. Immunol. 21*, 1033 (1991).
137. B. Naume, R. Shalaby, et al., *J. Immunol. 146*, 3045 (1991).
138. B. B. Aggarwal, T. Eessalu, and P. E. Hass, *Nature 318*, 665 (1985).
139. M. Tsujimoto, Y. K. Yip, and J. Vilcek, *J. Immunol. 136*, 2441 (1986).
140. C. A. Dett, M. Gatanaga, et al., *J. Immunol. 146*, 1522 (1991).
141. C. Billard, F. Sigaux, and J. Wietzerbin, *J. Immunol. 145*, 1713 (1990).
142. K. Pfizenmaier, M. Krönke, P. Scheurich, and G. A. Nagel, *Blut 55*, 1 (1987).
143. M. Lantz, U. Gullberg, et al., *J. Clin. Invest. 86*, 1396 (1990).
144. T. Kohno, M. T. Brewer, et al., *Proc. Natl. Acad. Sci. USA 87*, 8331 (1990).
145. H. Holtmann and D. Wallach, *J. Immunol. 139*, 1161 (1987).
146. E. M. Haliday, C. S. Ramesha, and G. Ringold, *EMBO J. 10*, 109 (1991).
147. S. A. Bauldry, C. E. McCall, et al., *J. Immunol. 146*, 1277 (1991).
148. S. A. Bauldry, D. A. Bass, et al., *J. Biol. Chem. 266*, 4173 (1991).
149. P. W. Majerus, T. S. Ross, et al., *Cell 63*, 459 (1990).
150. S. Schütze, D. Berkovic, et al., *J. Exp. Med. 174*, 975 (1991).
151. S. Schütze, S. Nottrott, et al., *J. Immunol. 144*, 2604 (1990).
152. S. Shiroo and K. Matsushima, *Cytokine 2*, 13 (1990).
153. A. Meichle, S. Schütze, et al., *J. Biol. Chem. 265*, 8339 (1990).
154. A. J. Ritchie, D. R. Johnson, et al., *J. Immunol. 146*, 3056 (1991).
155. T. A. Bird and J. Saklatvala, *J. Biol. Chem. 265*, 235 (1990).
156. T. A. Bird and J. Saklatvala, *J. Immunol. 142*, 126 (1989).
157. M. Y. Kim, C. Linardic, et al., *J. Biol. Chem. 266*, 484 (1991).
158. M. Candela, S. C. Barker, and R. L. Ballou, *J. Exp. Med. 174*, 1363 (1991).
159. M. Krönke, K. Wiegemann, and S. Schütze, *Cytokine 3*, 475 (1991).
160. B. Thoma, M. Grell, et al., *J. Exp. Med. 172*, 1019 (1990).
161. H. Engelmann, H. Holtmann, et al., *J. Biol. Chem. 265*, 14497 (1990).
162. H. P. Hohmann, R. Remy, et al., *J. Biol. Chem. 264*, 14927 (1989).
163. M. R. Shalaby, A. Sundan, et al., *J. Exp. Med. 172*, 1517 (1990).
164. L. A. Tartaglia, R. F. Weber, et al., *Proc. Natl. Acad. Sci. USA 88*, 9292 (1991).
165. T. H. Lee, G. W. Lee, E. B. Ziff, and J. Vilcek, *Mol. Cell. Biol. 10*, 1982 (1990).
166. G. H. W. Wong and D. V. Goeddel, *Science 242*, 941 (1988).

167. S. Yokota, T. D. Geppert, and P. E. Lipsky, *J. Immunol. 140*, 531 (1988).
168. G. E. Ranges, A. Zlotnik, et al., *J. Exp. Med. 167*, 1472 (1988).
169. G. E. Ranges, I. Figari, et al., *J. Exp. Med. 166*, 991 (1987).
170. D. F. Jelinek and P. E. Lipsky, *J. Immunol. 139*, 2970 (1987).
171. R. M. Shalaby, T. Espevik, et al., *J. Immunol. 141*, 499 (1988).
172. J. E. Talmadge, H. Phillips, et al., *Cancer Res. 48*, 544 (1988).
173. S. Chouaib, J. Bertoglio, et al., *Proc. Natl. Acad. Sci. USA 85*, 6875 (1988).
174. P. Ghiara, D. Boraschi, et al., *J. Immunol. 139*, 3676 (1987).
175. M. A. Palladino, M. R. Shalaby, et al., *J. Immunol. 138*, 4023 (1987).
176. R. Philip and L. B. Epstein, *Nature, 323*, 86 (1986).
177. P. R. Bachwich et al., *Biochem. Biophys. Res. Comm. 136*, 94 (1986).
178. G. Camussi, F. Bussolini, et al., *J. Exp. Med. 166*, 1390 (1987).
179. M. Hoffmann and J. B. Weinberg, *J. Leuk. Biol. 42*, 704 (1987).
180. L. E. M. Bermudez and L. S. Young, *J. Immunol. 140*, 3006 (1988).
181. L. M. Kumaratilake, A. Ferrante, et al., *J. Immunol. 146*, 762 (1991).
182. J. W. Larrick, D. Graham, et al., *Blood 69*, 640 (1987).
183. Y. Ozaki, T. Ohashi, Y. Niwa, and S. Kume, *Inflammation 12*, 297 (1988).
184. I. S. Figari, N. A. Mori, and M. A. Palladino, *Blood 70*, 979 (1987).
185. B. Perussia, M. Kobayashi, et al., *J. Immunol. 138*, 765 (1987).
186. W. K. Seow, Y. H. Tong, and A. Ferrante, *Immunology 62*, 357 (1987).
187. M. R. Shalaby, B. B. Aggarwal, et al., *J. Immunol. 135*, 2069 (1985).
188. W. J. Ming, L. Bersan, and A. Mantovani, *J. Immunol. 138*, 1469 (1987).
189. E. Kownatzki, A. Kapp, and S. Uhrich, *Clin. Exp. Immunol. 74*, 143 (1988).
190. J. Y. Djeu, D. K. Blanchard, et al., *J. Immunol. 137*, 2980 (1986).
191. E. H. DeTitto, J. R. Catterall, et al., *J. Immunol. 137*, 1342 (1986).
192. L. M. Kumaratilake, A. Ferrante, et al., *J. Immunol. 146*, 762 (1991).
193. A. Ferrante, *Infect. Immun. 57*, 3110 (1989).
194. D. S. Silberstein and J. R. David, *Proc. Natl. Acad. Sci. USA 83*, 1055 (1986).
195. M. Damonneville, J. Wietzerbin, et al., *J. Immunol. 140*, 3962 (1988).
196. S. L. Kunkel, D. G. Remick, et al., *CRC Crit. Rev. Immunol. 9*, 93 (1989).
197. N. Sato, T. Goto, et al., *J. Natl. Cancer Inst. 76*, 1113 (1986).
198. E. J. U. von Asmuth et al., *Scand. J. Immunol. 34*, 197 (1991).
199. D. Aderka, H. Holtmann, et al., *J. Immunol. 136*, 2938 (1986).
200. G. H. W. Wong and D. V. Goeddel, *Nature 323*, 819 (1986).
201. T. K. Hughes, T. A. Kaspar, and D. H. Coppenhaver, *Antiviral Res. 10*, 1 (1988).
202. J. Mestan, W. Digel, et al., *Nature 323*, 816 (1986).
203. G. H. W. Wong, J. F. Krowka, et al., *J. Immunol. 140*, 120 (1988).
204. G. Poli, A. Kinter, et al., *Proc. Natl. Acad. Sci. USA 87*, 782 (1990).
205. S. Michihiko, N. Yamamoto, et al., *Lancet i*, 1206 (1989).
206. P. Durksen-Huges, W. S. M. Wold, et al., *J. Immunol. 143*, 4193 (1989).
207. R. Rossol-Voth, S. Rossol, et al., *J. Gen. Virol. 72*, 143 (1991).
208. E. A. Havell, *J. Immunol. 143*, 2894 (1989).
209. A. Nakane, T. Minagawa, and K. Kato, *Infect. Immun. 56*, 2563 (1988).
210. S. Cross, J. C. Sadoff, et al., *J. Exp. Med. 169*, 2021 (1989).
211. V. Kindler, A. P. Sappino, et al., *Cell 56*, 731 (1989).

212. M. J. Hershman, J. D. Pietsch, et al., *Br. J. Surgery 76*, 1282 (1989).
213. D. H. Livingston, M. A. Malangoni, et al., *J. Trauma 29*, 967 (1989).
214. J. P. Tite, G. Dougan, and S. N. Chatfield, *J. Immunol. 147*, 3161 (1991).
215. J. Taverne, J. Tavernier, et al., *Clin. Exp. Immunol. 67*, 1 (1987).
216. J. D. Hasday, E. M. Shah, and A. P. Lieberman, *J. Immunol. 145*, 371 (1990).
217. J. L. Urban, H. M. Shepard, et al., *Proc. Natl. Acad. Sci. USA 83*, 5233 (1986).
218. B. J. Sugerman, B. B. Aggarwal, et al., *Science 230*, 943 (1985).
219. B. D. Williamson et al., *Proc. Natl. Acad. Sci. USA 80*, 5397 (1983).
220. V. Ruggiero and C. Baglioni, *J. Immunol. 138*, 661 (1987).
221. D. Spriggs, K. Imamura, et al., *Proc. Natl. Acad. Sci. USA 84*, 6563 (1987).
222. A. A. Creasey, M. T. Reynolds, and W. Laird, *Cancer Res. 46*, 5687 (1986).
223. F. R. Balkwill, A. Lee, et al., *Cancer Res. 46*, 3990 (1986).
224. I. Gresser, F. Belardelli, et al., *Int. J. Cancer 38*, 771 (1986).
225. T. Manda, K. Shimomura, et al., *Cancer Res. 47*, 3707 (1987).
226. E. A. Havell, W. Fiers, and R. J. North, *J. Exp. Med. 167*, 1067 (1988).
227. M. N. Teng, B. H. Park, et al., *Proc. Natl. Acad. Sci. USA 88*, 3535 (1991).
228. T. Blankenstein, Z. Qin, et al., *J. Exp. Med. 173*, 1047 (1991).
229. M. Schleuning and R. Munker, *Klin. Wochenschr. 68*, 841 (1990).
230. D. Lienard, F. Lejeune, and P. Ewalenko, *Cytokine 3*, 491 (1991).
231. K. J. Tracey, H. Wei, et al., *J. Exp. Med. 167*, 1211 (1988).
232. S. H. Socher, A. Friedman, and D. Martinez, *J. Exp. Med. 167*, 1957 (1988).
233. A. Oliff, D. Defeo-Jones, et al., *Cell 50*, 555 (1987).
234. B. A. Sherry, J. Gelin, et al., *FASEB J. 3*, 1956 (1989).
235. M. J. Tisdale, *Br. J. Cancer 63*, 337 (1991).
236. D. R. Bertolini, G. E. Nedwin, et al., *Nature 319*, 516 (1986).
237. J. Saklatvala, *Nature 322*, 547 (1986).
238. J. M. Dayer, B. Beutler, and A. Cerami, *J. Exp. Med. 162*, 2163 (1985).
239. P. Stashenko, F. E. Dewhirst, et al., *J. Immunol. 138*, 1464 (1987).
240. K. L. Macnaul, N. I. Hutchinson, et al., *J. Immunol. 145*, 4154 (1990).
241. V. J. Palombella, J. Mendelsohn, et al., *J. Cell. Physiol. 135*, 23 (1988).
242. A. Mauviel, M. Daireaux, et al., *FEBS Lett. 236*, 47 (1988).
243. N. Sato, T. Goto, et al., *J. Natl. Cancer Inst. 76*, 1113 (1986).
244. M. Frater-Schröder et al., *Proc. Natl. Acad. Sci. USA 84*, 5277 (1987).
245. S. J. Leibovich, P. J. Polverini, et al., *Nature 329*, 630 (1987).
246. P. F. Piguet, G. E. Grau, and P. Vassalli, *Am. J. Pathol. 136*, 103 (1990).
247. A. A. Mallick, A. Ishizaka, et al., *Chest 95*, 1114 (1989).
248. H. R. Alexander, G. M. Doherty, et al., *J. Exp. Med. 173*, 1029 (1991).
249. H. F. Starnes, M. K. Pearce, et al., *J. Immunol. 12*, 4185 (1990).
250. R. Rabinovici, T. L. Yue, et al., *J. Pharmacol. Exp. Ther. 255*, 256 (1990).
251. G. E. Grau, L. F. Fajardo, et al., *Science 237*, 1210 (1987).
252. D. K. Imagawa, J. M. Millis, et al., *Transplantation 51*, 57 (1991).
253. P. F. Piguet, G. E. Grau, et al., *J. Exp. Med. 166*, 1280 (1987).
254. P. F. Piguet, M. A. Collart, et al., *J. Exp. Med. 170*, 655 (1989).
255. K. Selmaj, C. S. Raine, and A. H. Cross, *Ann. Neurol. 30*, 694 (1991).
256. N. L. Paul and N. H. Ruddle, *Ann. Rev. Immunol. 6*, 407 (1988).

257. W. Oster, A. Lindemann, et al., *Blood 70*, 1700 (1987).
258. H. P. Koeffler, J. Gasson, et al., *Blood 70*, 55 (1987).
259. V. C. Broudy, J. M. Harlan, and J. W. Adamson, *J. Immunol. 138*, 4298 (1987).
260. J. S. Andrews, A. E. Berger, and C. F. Ware, *J. Immunol. 144*, 2582 (1990).
261. J. Browning and A. Ribolini, *J. Immunol. 143*, 1859 (1989).

# 4

# Interleukin 8 and Structurally Related Cytokines

**Jens-Michael Schröder, Michael Sticherling, Pavel Smid, and Enno Christophers**

*University of Kiel*
*Kiel, Germany*

## I. INTRODUCTION

A number of inflammatory skin diseases are characterized by neutrophil and/or lymphocyte infiltration of the epidermis. This observation led to the suggestion that epidermal cells may actively respond to different injuries by secretion of leukocyte chemotactic factors. Among epidermal cells, keratinocytes represent the major cell population. Therefore a number of studies have been performed to evaluate whether these cells are able to produce leukocyte attractants of either lipid or peptide nature.

12-Hydroxyeicosatetraenoic acid (12-HETE) was detected as one of the major lipid mediators in psoriatic lesions [1, 2] and subsequently shown to be the most important leukocyte attractant secreted by keratinocytes. Another lipid chemoattractant, $LTB_4$, was thought to be of keratinocyte origin [3–5], but several studies have now shown that keratinocytes produce only very little if any $LTB_4$ [6, 7].

Apart from lipidlike leukocyte chemotactic factors, keratinocytes also produce different proteinaceous attractants. Partially purified preparations of keratinocyte-derived interleukin 1 (epidermal cell–derived thymocyte-activating factor, or ETAF) were reported to be chemotactically active for neutrophils and monocytes [8, 9]. With the availability of recombinant IL-1, however, it was shown that this cytokine exerts neither of these activities [10]. Consequently, ETAF preparations apparently contained at that time not yet clearly defined leukocyte attractants. Since then, several different chemoattractants have been detected which belong to a family of closely related peptides, the so-called IL-8 supergene family, and will be described in the following paragraphs.

## II. KERATINOCYTE-DERIVED LEUKOCYTE-ATTRACTING PROTEINS

### A. Interleukin 8

Supernatants of growing human keratinocytes are known to induce neutrophil chemotaxis when tested by the Boyden chamber system [8]. When these culture supernatants were directly applied to a G-75 gel column, the majority of neutrophil chemotactic activity eluted in the 5–20 kd area (Fig. 1). A second peak of activity could sometimes be observed in the 50–80 kd area, apart from minor activity in the lower $M_r$ area (0–1 kd).

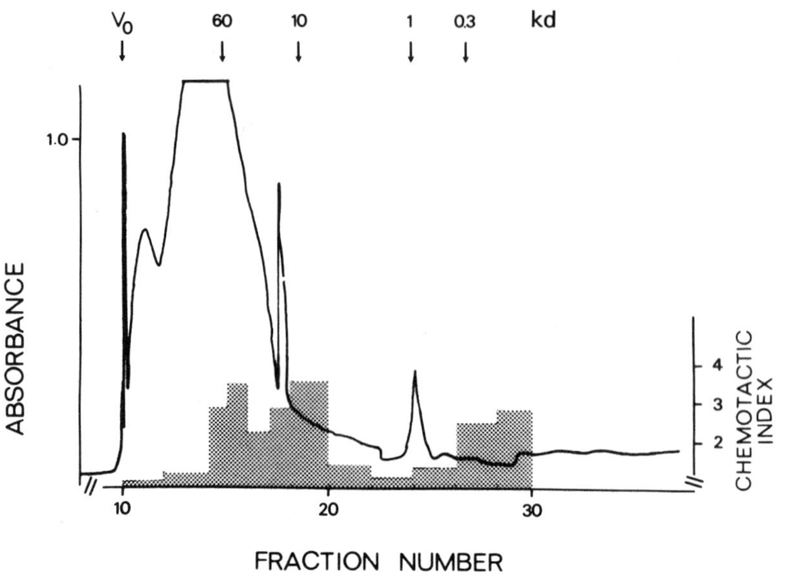


**Fig. 1** Molecular sieve chromatography analysis of neutrophil chemotactic peptides in conditioned keratinocyte growth media. Tenfold concentrated media obtained from growing foreskin-derived keratinocytes (second passage) were applied to a Pharmacia Hi Load 16/60 Superdex column. Proteins were eluted with 0.05 M ammonium formate buffer (pH 5.0) and monitored at 280 nm. The shaded area represents neutrophil myeloperoxidase-releasing activity in column fractions.

When column fractions were tested for IL-1 activity using an in vitro mouse thymocyte stimulation assay system, some of them overlap; no co-elution, however, of neutrophil chemotactic and IL-1 activity was observed (data not shown). When the 5–20 kd peak of polymorphonuclear leukocyte (PMN) chemotactic activity was further purified by size-exclusion high performance liquid chromatography (HPLC), peak PMN chemotactic activity eluted in fractions corresponding to 10 kd. On the other hand, major IL-1 activity elutes in fractions corresponding to a $M_r$ of 15 kd. This dissociation of both activities clearly indicates that PMN chemotaxis cannot be attributed to IL-1/ETAF as originally suggested [8, 9].

Further sequential purification of the putative PMN chemotactic proteins by ion exchange and reversed-phase HPLC revealed the presence of at least three biochemically distinct peaks of activity (Fig. 2). Upon high resolu-

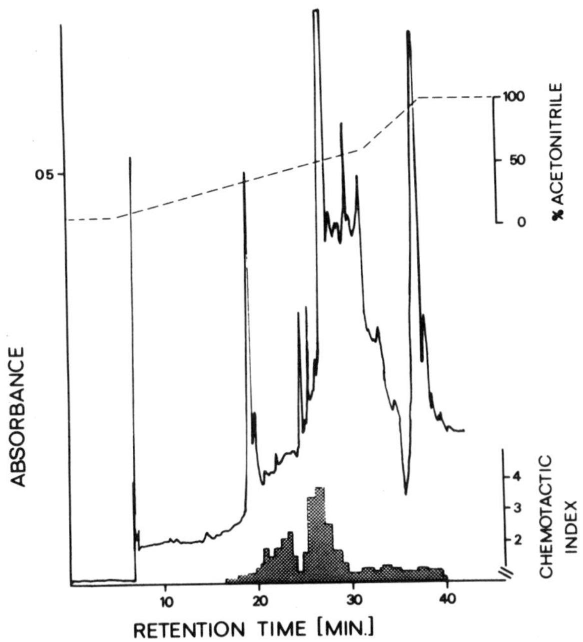


**Fig. 2** Preparative reversed-phase (RP-8) HPLC of partially purified keratinocyte-derived neutrophil attractants. Pooled 5–20 kd chemotactic material off molecular sieve chromatography separated, partially purified, keratinocyte-derived neutrophil attractants were further separated by preparative RP-8 HPLC (300–7C8 Nucleosil, 250 × 12.6 mm, Macherey and Nagel, Düren, Germany) using a gradient of acetonitrile for elution of proteins. PMN chemotactic activity in HPLC fractions is indicated by the shaded area.

tion SDS-PAGE analysis, these PMN chemotactic proteins show $M_r$s near 8 kd [11]. When Western blot analyses using monoclonal anti–IL-8 antibodies are performed, two bands are visible [11] indicating antigenic similarities of these two polypeptides to IL-8.

When compared to known variants of IL-8, the band corresponding to a molecular weight of 8.3 kd migrates with higher mobility than authentic 77-residue IL-8 (endothelial cell–derived IL-8) [25], whereas the second band comigrates with authentic 69-residue IL-8 (Fig. 3). Therefore there is ample evidence that without any stimulation by exogenous agents, growing keratinocytes secrete two variants of the neutrophil chemotactic IL-8, namely, the 72- and the 69-residue forms.

Biological activities of the 72- and 69-residue forms of IL-8 are similar with respect to potency ($ED_{50}$) as well as efficacy (number of migrating cells)

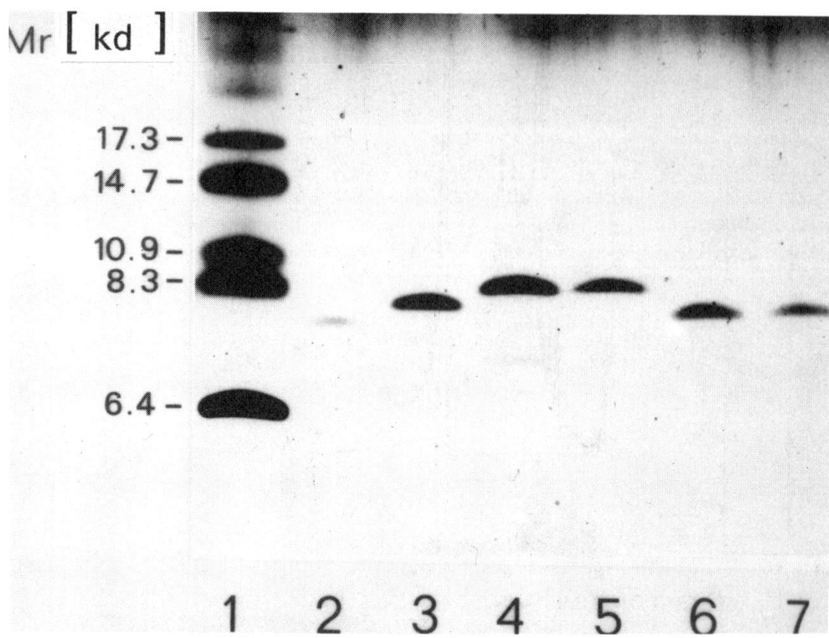


**Fig. 3** SDS-PAGE analysis of the two major KENAPs. SDS-PAGE analyses were performed in the presence of 8 M urea [19]. Whereas lane 1 contains cyanogen bromide cleavage products of myoglobine for calibration, in lane 3 $\alpha_1$-KENAP and in lane 6 $\alpha_2$-KENAP were applied. Lanes 2 and 7 contained authentic [Glu-IL-8]$_{69}$. In lanes 4 and 5 authentic fibroblast-derived [Ala-IL-8]$_{77}$ were loaded. $\alpha_1$-KENAP showed identity in mobility with [Ser-IL-8]$_{72}$ (not shown).

(Fig. 4). In addition to eliciting chemotactic responses selectively in neutrophils—not, however, in eosinophils and monocytes—both IL-8 variants also activate other functions of human neutrophils. These include degranulation and release of myeloperoxidase, elastase, or $\beta$-glucuronidase from primary granules (only after pretreatment of the PMN with cytochalasin B) [12, 13] as well as vitamin $B_{12}$-binding protein and lactoferrin from secondary granules [13, 14]. Apart from a rise of intracellular calcium after receptor binding, activation of neutrophil 5-lipoxygenase is effected by IL-8 [17]. $LTB_4$, however, is only produced in the presence of exogenous arachidonic acid. Therefore, IL-8 apparently does not activate the release of cellular arachidonate [17]. All these effects are mediated by specific receptors on neutrophils, which originally were postulated [12, 13] and have recently been cloned [15, 16].

As outlined above, keratinocytes secrete as major neutrophil attractants the 69- and 72-residue forms of IL-8 [11, 18]. Other cell types, however, produce a different set of amino-terminally modified variants of IL-8: dermal fibroblasts nearly exclusively secrete the 77-residue form [19], which is

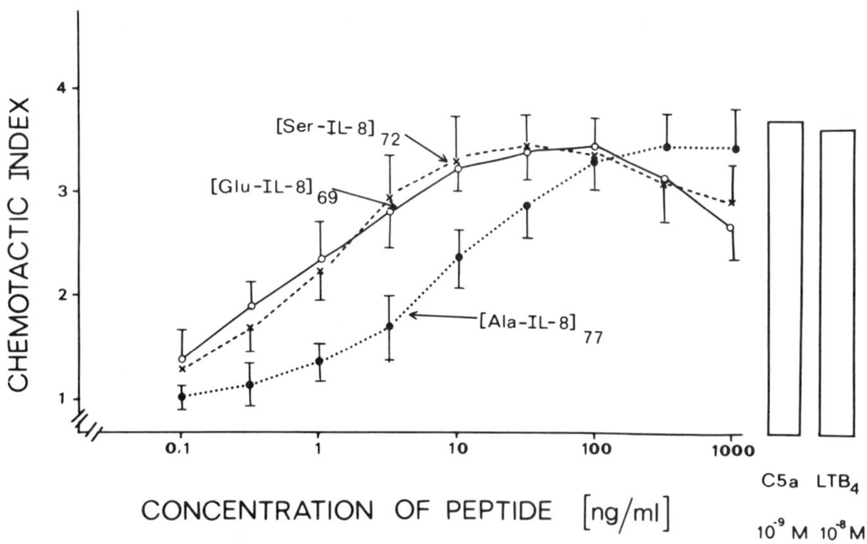


**Fig. 4** PMN chemotactic activity of the two major KENAPs. PMN chemotactic activity of purified KENAPs identified as the 72-residue form of IL-8 (×) or 69-residue form of IL-8 (○) as well as the 77-residue form of IL-8 (●) is shown. Bars indicate PMN chemotactic activity of other potent attractants at optimal concentration.

known to be of 8- to 10-fold lower potency than the 72-residue form of IL-8 [19, 20]. Blood monocytes, on the other hand, release the 72-residue form [21–23], whereas lymphocyte preparations produce a mixture of both the 72- and 77-residue forms [23]. In our experience, endothelial cells mainly secrete the 69-residue form [19, 24], whereas Gimbrone et al. detected the 77-residue form as the major variant [25].

Enzymatic amino-terminal truncation by cell-bound enzymes could be an important mechanism of potentiation of IL-8 activity. A degradation of the 77-residue to the 72-residue form is effected, e.g., by thrombin [19, 20], and results in an 8- to 10-fold increase of biological activity [19, 20].

When freshly isolated keratinocyte preparations are used for investigation into which specific forms of IL-8 are produced, contamination by dermal fibroblasts is of critical importance: as mentioned above, fibroblasts produce upon stimulation with IL-1$\alpha$, IL-1$\beta$, or TNF-$\alpha$ large amounts of IL-8 [19, 26, 27] and its 77-residue form. When cultured keratinocytes were incubated in vitro with the purified 77-residue form of IL-8, after more than 24 h could we detect partial degradation to the 72-residue form, not, however, to the 69-residue form. Therefore, the different IL-8 forms released by keratinocyte preparations could provide insight as to whether contaminating fibroblasts contribute to IL-8 production of these preparations or not. Any 77-residue IL-8 present in this set of experiments appears to derive from contaminating fibroblasts. Moreover, keratinocytes do not significantly contribute to transcellular potentiation of this specific IL-8 activity, but do produce 72- and 69-residue forms.

Several studies have shown that the production of IL-8 in keratinocytes can be induced by different cytokines. A dose of 1000 U IL-1$\alpha$ elicited a slight but significant induction of IL-8 mRNA [26]. In another study, IL-8 mRNA was undetectable in unstimulated keratinocytes, whereas TNF-$\alpha$ induced little IL-8 gene transcription, an effect strongly amplified by pretreatment of keratinocytes with IFN-$\gamma$ [28]. Responses to TNF-$\alpha$ were found to be rapid and transient with maximal expression 2–8 h after stimulation [28]. This was in contrast to IFN-$\gamma$–pretreated keratinocytes in which IL-8 mRNA was still detectable at 18 h [28]. Apart from IL-8 gene expression, the release of biologically active IL-8 can also be induced: when supernatants of TNF-$\alpha$–stimulated cultured keratinocytes were analyzed by preparative reversed-phase HPLC and gradient elution, the majority of PMN chemotactic activity eluted at 50% acetonitrile. Peak IL-8 immunoreactivity, analyzed by an IL-8 ELISA, could be detected at the same time point (Fig. 2).

When compared to other cells such as monocytes, umbilical vein endothelial cells, or dermal fibroblasts [29], IL-8 gene expression as well as release of biologically active IL-8 by cultivated keratinocytes was low even after stimulation with cytokines such as TNF-$\alpha$ or IL-1$\alpha$. In order to evaluate conditions for strong induction of IL-8 release in cultured normal keratinocytes, we have studied the effects of various stimuli under different culture conditions on the release of IL-8–like immunoreactivity.

As shown in Table 1, the most efficient inducers of IL-8 release so far appear to be phorbolesters like phorbol myristate acetate (PMA), which is in agreement with recent observations [30]. Pretreatment of keratinocytes with IFN-$\gamma$ prior to TNF-$\alpha$ does not significantly enhance IL-8 release in contrast to the IL-8 message, which is elevated sixfold when compared to treatment with TNF-$\alpha$ alone [28]. In agreement with recent observations [26], both IL-1$\alpha$ and IL-1$\beta$ were found to be only weak inducers of IL-8. Bacterial lipopolysaccharides apparently do not induce the release of IL-8 in keratinocytes [26]. Accordingly, keratinocytes show similar activation of IL-8 release as seen for dermal fibroblasts [19], which do not, however, respond to PMA (our unpublished results). So far it is not known whether other bacterial products directly activate IL-8 release in keratinocytes. Interestingly, the toxic principle of poison ivy (*Rhus radicans* L.), urushiol, which is known to induce rhus dermatitis, represents an efficient inducer of IL-8 release in keratinocytes, possibly via induction of TNF-$\alpha$ and subsequent autoinduction of IL-8 [31]. In respect to the lymphocyte-attracting properties of IL-8 in vitro [32], it has been speculated that lymphocytes seen in the affected tissue of rhus dermatitis may be attracted by keratinocyte-derived IL-8 [31].

## B. Melanoma Growth Stimulatory Activity

Another low molecular weight neutrophil attractant that could be important in skin inflammation is a peptide with melanoma growth stimulatory activity called MGSA/gro [33, 34]. It is structurally related to IL-8 (Fig. 5), and

**Table 1** Induction of IL-8 in Keratinocytes[a]

| | None | TNF-$\alpha$ (100 ng/ml) | TNF-$\alpha$ + IFN-$\gamma$ (100 ng/ml/ 100 U/ml) | IL-1$\alpha$ (100 U/ml) | IL-1$\beta$ (10 ng/ml) | LPS (100 ng/ml) | PMA (10 ng/ml) |
|---|---|---|---|---|---|---|---|
| IL-8 (ng/ml) | 8 ± 3 | 36 ± 7 | 43 ± 8 | 12 ± 4 | 11 ± 5 | 11 ± 2 | 104 ± 23 |

[a] $2 \times 10^5$ normal keratinocytes were incubated with the stimuli for 18 h. In supernatants IL-8 was measured by the use of a Sandwich-ELISA.

```
                1          10         20         30         40         50         60         70
IL-8        AVLPRSAKELRCQCIKTYSKPFHP-KFIKELRVIES-GPHCANTEIIVKL-SDGRELCLDPKENWVQR-VVEKFLKRAENS
NAP-2               AELRCMCIKTTSG-IHP-KNIQSLEVIGK-GTHCNQVEVIATL-KDGRKICLDPDAPRIKK-IVQKKLAGDESAD
MGSA/groα       ASVATELRCQCLQTLQG-IHP-KNIQSVMVKSP-GPHCAQTEVIATL-KNGRKACLNPASPIVKK-IIEKMLNSDKSN
ENA 78     AGPAAAVLRELRCVCLQTTQG-VHP-KMISNLQVFAI-GPQCSKVEVVASL-KNGKEICLDPEAPFLKK-VIQKILDGGNKEN
IP-10           VPLSRTVRCTCISISNQPVNP-RSLEKLEIIPA-SQFCPRVEIIATMKKKGEKRCLNPESKAIKN-LL-KAVSKEMSKRSP

HuMIP-1α          ADTPTAC-CFSYTSRQI-PQNFIAD-Y-FETSSQ-CSKPGVIF-LTKRSRQVCADPSEEWVQKYV--SDLELSA
HuMIP-1β      APMGSDPPTSC-CFSYTARKL-PHNFVVD-Y-YETSSL-CSQPAVVF-QTKRGKQVCADPSESWVQEYV--YDLELN
MCP-1/MCAF    QPDAINAPVTC-CYNFTNRKI-SVQRLAS-YRRITSSK-CPKEAVIF-KTIVAKEICADPKQKWVQDSM--DHLDKQTQTPKT
I-309       VDSKSMQVPFSRC-CFSFAEQEI-PLRAILC-Y-RNTSSI-CSNEGLIF-KLKRGKEACALDTVGWVQRHR--KMLRHCPSKRK
RANTES          SPYSSDTTPC-CFAYIARPL-PRAHIKE-Y-FYTSGK-CSNPAVVF-VTRKNRQVCANPEKKWVREYI--NSLEMS
```

**Fig. 5** Alignment of the amino acid sequences of some members of the C-X-C and the C-C branches of IL-8–like cytokines. The single-letter code for amino acids has been used. Note the presence of four cysteines at identical relative positions (shaded area).

both belong to the same so-called "C-X-C" subfamily of host defense cytokines (for review see Ref. 35). Apart from sequence homologies of about 45%, they share as a common structural characteristic four half-cysteines, the first two of which are separated by another amino acid (C-X-C).

MGSA was originally detected as an autocrine growth factor in melanoma cells [39] and was structurally characterized in 1988 [33]. The peptide represents the gene product of the oncogene *gro*, which was found to be overexpressed in some human fibroblast cell lines [34]. It is secreted as yet another neutrophil-activating cytokine by IL-1–stimulated fibroblasts [19] as well as LPS-stimulated monocytes [40]. The same applies to LPS-stimulated umbilical cord endothelial cells, which produce in addition to the 69-residue form of IL-8 a second neutrophil attractant ($\alpha$-ENAP) with biochemical and biological properties similar to MGSA/gro [24].

In respect to keratinocytes, MGSA/gro immunoreactivity could be detected in the basal layer of normal epidermis [41] using a monoclonal antibody raised against the peptide. We could in fact isolate MGSA/gro as another major constituent of psoriatic scale–derived anionic neutrophil-activating peptide, or ANAP [36] by sequential purification via HPLC and subsequent amino acid sequencing [37, 38]. The presence of large amounts of MGSA/gro in scales of psoriatics as well as MGSA/gro immunoreactivity in basal epidermal cells raises the question of whether it can indeed be secreted by keratinocytes.

When culture supernatants of growing keratinocytes were investigated for neutrophil chemotactic activity, apart from IL-8 a second peak eluting prior to the bulk of IL-8–like activity is detectable (Fig. 2). Upon further purification it became clear that this activity is of similar molecular weight as IL-8 by size exclusion HPLC as well as SDS-PAGE analyses [11]. It was tentatively called $\beta$-keratinocyte-derived neutrophil-activating peptide, or $\beta$-KENAP. Coinjection with authentic MGSA obtained from psoriatic scales led to coelution of part of the chemotactic activity. In assays of PMN chemotaxis, $\beta$-KENAP showed a dose response profile identical to that found for MGSA obtained from different sources and presented the typical bell-shaped curve [11]. The maximal number of migrating PMN in vitro is, however, lower when compared to IL-8 [19, 40], implicating that the efficacy of MGSA in the in vitro chemotaxis system is lower than that of IL-8. In summary, normal proliferating keratinocytes can most likely produce MGSA/gro, in lower amounts, however, than IL-8. So far, it is not known which cytokines (such as IL-1 or TNF-$\alpha$) induce the release of MGSA/gro in keratinocytes. Furthermore, it is not known which type of gro is secreted. By now, three related gro genes termed gro $\alpha$, gro $\beta$, and gro $\gamma$ have been identified, which are induced on at least two distinct pathways: a growth-related serum response pathway and an IL-1– or TNF-$\alpha$–induced pathway [42].

## C. Other Members of the C-X-C Cytokine Family

Apart from IL-8 and MGSA/gro, two other structurally related neutrophil chemotactic proteins have been identified. One of these is the neutrophil-activating protein 2 (NAP-2), which is, however, not directly released by cells [43]. It is processed by enzymatic cleavage from its original precursor, the platelet basic protein (PBP) via its truncation products connective tissue-activating peptide III (CTAP III) and $\beta$-thromboglobulin [44].

If, however, enzymatic truncation of NAP-2 precursors occurs in cells other than leukocytes as demonstrated is presently unknown. So far, no evidence for secretion of NAP-2 or its precursors by keratinocytes has been presented. Consequently, the importance of NAP-2–related cytokines in inflammatory skin diseases has to be further elucidated.

Recently an additional member of the IL-8 C-X-C subfamily exhibiting neutrophil chemotactic properties has been identified which is produced by a human type II epithelial cell line, A 549, when stimulated with cytokines. This novel peptide was called epithelial neutrophil-activating peptide (ENA-78) [45] (Fig. 5) and is secreted concomitantly with IL-8, gro $\alpha$, and gro $\gamma$ [45]. Like the aforementioned peptides, ENA-78 induces neutrophil chemotaxis and exocytosis as well as a rise in intracellular free calcium [45]. Moreover, cross-desensitization experiments with these cytokines reveal that all of them bind to the same IL-8 receptors, which in fact have recently been detected and characterized [15, 16]. It is not known so far whether, apart from lung epithelial cells, ENA-78 is produced by other epithelial cells such as keratinocytes. There is evidence that supernatants of cytokine-stimulated keratinocytes produce more than two IL-8–related neutrophil chemotactic peptides in that upon reversed-phase HPLC analysis, minor peptide neutrophil attractants can be seen. Further purification and sequence analysis is, however, necessary to demonstrate identity with ENA-78.

$\gamma$-Interferon–induced protein (IP-10) represents yet another member of the C-X-C subfamily of IL-8–like host defense proteins [46]. The gene encoding IP-10 was originally detected in mononuclear cells and fibroblasts when stimulated with IFN-$\gamma$ [46]. Its homology to IL-8 and related peptides (Fig. 5) suggests biological functions in inflammatory response, which so far have, however, not been characterized. In immunoprecipitation analysis of biosynthetically labeled material, stimulated endothelial cells and keratinocytes were found to be the most potent producers of IP-10 [46, 48] when compared to fibroblasts and monocytes.

After intradermal injection of IFN-$\gamma$, distinct epidermal IP-10–like immunoreactivity could be found, none, however, in dermal cells [47]. Furthermore, IP-10 protein was immunohistochemically detected in delayed type hypersensitivity reaction of the skin. These results suggest an association between IP-10 and the development of a cellular immune response and thus an important role in a number of different skin inflammatory reactions.

## D. Monocyte Chemotactic Protein 1/Monocyte Chemotactic Activation Factor

Apart from neutrophil-activating properties, which have by now been attributed to IL-8, Luger and coworkers demonstrated monocyte chemotactic activity in partially purified human epidermal cell–derived thymocyte-activating factor (ETAF) preparations [8]. Again, IL-1 was originally suggested to be the biologically active protein. Recombinant IL-1, however, did not show any monocyte chemotactic activity [49], indicating that this activity in ETAF preparations originated from another, at that time unidentified monocyte chemotactic protein.

Purification and characterization of the monocyte chemotactic factor was finally achieved when glioma cell lines were available that secrete this protein constitutively [52] apart from a human myelomonocytic cell line that secretes the peptide upon stimulation with LPS [53]. The resulting peptide was eventually termed monocyte chemotactic protein 1 (MCP-1) [50] or monocyte chemotactic activation factor (MCAF) [51].

MCP-1/MCAF is a relatively basic protein [54], which upon cation exchange HPLC falls into two separate peaks and migrates in SDS-PAGE as 15 and 13 kd proteins, respectively (MCP-1$\alpha$ and 1$\beta$) [55]. Based on amino acid sequence and cloning data [54], the molecular mass of MCP-1/MCAF is 8.7 kd. These differences of apparent molecular weight are supposedly based on as yet unidentified posttranslational modifications.

MCP-1/MCAF represents an additional member of the IL-8 supergene family (Fig. 5) (for review see Ref. 54). In contrast to the previously mentioned peptides—IL-8 itself as well as MGSA/gro, NAP-2, ENA-78, and IP-10—this cytokine shows as structural characteristics two adjacent cysteine residues (C-C) and thus represents a second subfamily of IL-8–related cytokines (Fig. 5). MCP-1/MCAF selectively attracts monocytes, not, however, neutrophils or eosinophils [54]—in contrast to IL-8, which acts solely on neutrophils, but not on monocytes or eosinophils [12, 21].

The finding that monocytes accumulate in the epidermis and along the dermo-epidermal junction in a number of different inflammatory skin disorders led to the suggestion that epidermal cells may also be capable of producing MCP-1/MCAF. As shown recently, cultivated normal keratinocytes are indeed potent producers of the cytokine. Interestingly, however, production and release occurred only upon stimulation with IFN-$\gamma$, not, however, with TNF-$\alpha$, IL-1$\beta$, TGF-$\beta$, or phorbolesters [56].

In contrast, MCP-1/MCAF mRNA was found to be constitutively expressed in cultivated keratinocytes and up-regulated only in the presence of IFN-$\gamma$ [56]. MCP-1/MCAF therefore shows an expression and release pattern that is completely different to that seen for IL-8 where constitutive gene expression is absent [28] and expression can be induced by TNF-$\alpha$ and phorbolesters, not, however, by IFN-$\gamma$ [28, 31]. It is likely that keratinocyte-derived MCP-1/MCAF is important in the regulation of cutaneous monocyte trafficking, which appears to be in part linked to T-lymphocyte invasion and release of IFN-$\gamma$.

### E. Other Members of the C-C Cytokine Family

Apart from MCP-1/MCAF, the C-C-cytokine subfamily comprises several other distinct molecules like macrophage inflammatory proteins MIP-1$\alpha$ and -1$\beta$, which were originally detected in mice [57, 58], RANTES (regulated on activation, normal T expressed and secreted) [59], first found in T-lymphocyte clones [60], as well as HC 14 [59] and I-309 [59] (Fig. 5).

So far there is no published information on gene expression or peptide release of any of these cytokines by human keratinocytes or other epidermal cells. In the murine system, however, freshly isolated in contrast to cultivated epidermal Langerhans cells express the MIP-1$\alpha$ gene [61]. Interestingly, in addition to inhibiting bone marrow stem cells, murine MIP-1$\alpha$ was found to inhibit keratinocyte colony formation [61].

Each of the above-mentioned cytokines of the C-C family seems to represent a selective attractant for specific leukocyte subsets: RANTES exerts its effects on CD4+/CD45R0+ phenotype T lymphocytes (memory T cells) and monocytes, not, however, on neutrophils [62], whereas MIP-1$\beta$ acts primarily on naive helper T cells [59] and MIP-1$\alpha$ on killer T cells and B lymphocytes [59]. These activities point towards a possibly potential role of these cytokines in chronic skin inflammation and a variety of autoimmune diseases. Future studies will show if mRNA expression as well as release of these novel C-C-branch cytokines can be induced in keratinocytes under certain conditions and if they exert signals for specific subsets of mononuclear blood cell resulting in inflammatory tissue infiltration.

## III. KERATINOCYTE-DERIVED CHEMOTACTIC CYTOKINES IN DERMATOLOGICAL DISEASES

### A. Neutrophil Chemotactic Cytokines in Psoriasis Vulgaris

Neutrophil accumulation in the upper part of the epidermis is a striking feature of the developing psoriatic lesion [63]. The location of the cellular infiltrate as well as the predominance of neutrophils led to the working hypothesis that in psoriasis epidermal cells are a source of specific or preferential neutrophil attractants. Initial work on this hypothesis led to the detection of complement-derived chemotaxins like C5a [64], which are, however, of blood origin. Later, lipidlike attractants such as 12-HETE [1], $LTB_4$ [65], or platelet-activating factor (PAF) [66] were found in lesional scale material of psoriatics and appeared to be important inducers of neutrophil accumulation in the psoriatic epidermis. None of these factors, however, shows a preference or selectivity for neutrophils. All of them are in fact chemotactic for eosinophils and monocytes as well. Therefore the presence of other, more specific neutrophil attractants in the psoriatic lesion has been considered. In a most extensive analysis of neutrophil attractants in psoriatic scales, we detected peptides of around 10–12 kd [36]. As this activity was distinct from the more cationic chemotactic complement fragment $C5a_{des\ arg}$, we tentatively termed the newly discovered activity anionic neutrophil-activating peptide (ANAP) because of its relatively more anionic behavior [36]. ANAP is identical to the "IL-1-like neutrophil chemotactic activity" described at the same time by another group [67, 68]. In contrast to the chemotactic factors detected earlier in psoriatic scale material, ANAP appeared to fulfill the criterion of neutrophil selectivity or specificity because it lacked any chemotactic activity for other leukocytes such as monocytes, lymphocytes, or eosinophils [69]. Further HPLC purification of ANAP obtained from psoriatic scales revealed the presence of at least nine distinctly different neutrophil-activating peptides [70]. The three major ANAP components, termed $\beta_1$-ANAP, $\beta_2$-ANAP, and $\alpha_2$-ANAP, were purified to homogeneity. Amino-terminal amino acid sequence analysis of these components revealed identity of the major ANAP, $\beta_1$-ANAP, with the 69-residue form of IL-8, whereas a minor ANAP, $\beta_2$-ANAP, represents the 72-residue form of IL-8 (monocyte-derived IL-8) [38, 71]. The other major ANAP, $\alpha_2$-ANAP, is identical with the so-called 16 kDa moiety of melanoma growth stimulatory activity (MGSA).

Apart from these cytokines, we were able to separate another six polypeptides. In the PMN enzyme-release assay system, they show cross-desensitization with IL-8, which indicates binding to the same IL-8 receptors on neutrophils (Table 2). So far, two of these ANAPs, $\beta_3$-ANAP and $\beta_4$-ANAP, have been found to represent carboxy-terminally truncated forms of IL-8 [72]. These are of 50- to 100-fold lower potency in inducing PMN chemotaxis when compared to IL-8 [73]. The other ANAP components have so far not been structurally characterized. Since these components elute at low ion strength from cation exchange HPLC columns, it is likely that they exhibit lower isoelectric points. This may result from partial hydrolysis of glutamine and asparagine residues in both IL-8 and MGSA, as has been shown for IL-1 [74].

**Table 2** Biological and Biochemical Characteristics of Some ANAPs

| ANAP | $M_r$[a] (kd) | $ED_{50}$ (Chemotaxis)[b] (ng/ml) | Deactivation[c] (% of control) | Relative abundance[d] |
|---|---|---|---|---|
| $\alpha_{1a}$-ANAP | 7.8 | 1.8 | 6 | 2 |
| $\alpha_{1b}$-ANAP | 8.0 | 5.8 | 0 | 3 |
| $\alpha_2$-ANAP | 7.5 | 1.0 | 0 | 80 |
| $\alpha_{3a}$-ANAP | 8.0 | 1.0 | 11 | 10 |
| $\alpha_{3b}$-ANAP | 8.0 | 1.5 | 8 | 10 |
| $\beta_1$-ANAP | 7.8 | 0.8 | 13 | 100 |
| $\beta_2$-ANAP | 8.0 | 0.7 | 15 | 30 |
| $\beta_3$-ANAP | 6.0 | 55 | 0 | 50 |
| $\beta_4$-ANAP | 5.6 | 63 | 0 | 10 |

[a]Estimated using high resolution SDS-PAGe analyses as described in Ref. 19.
[b]Chemotaxis was determined with the endogeneous component chemotaxis assay [12].
[c]$\beta$-Glucuronidase release of IL-8 (50 ng/ml)–treated neutrophils as percentage of the $\beta$-glucuronidase release in buffer treated PMN is shown. PMN treated with C5a as control stimulus showed >80% of control enzyme release. For experimental details, see Ref. 12.
[d]Relative abundance is estimated from cation exchange HPLC–purified material via determination of the titer in eliciting PMN chemotactic responses.

IL-8 has been detected in psoriatic scales in large quantities when measured by either ELISA [75] or HPLC/bioassay [38]. Approximately 3 ng/ml scale [38] were found, which is nearly 150-fold more than detected in normal heel callus control. These findings point toward a correlation of IL-8 content with this inflammatory disease.

Northern blot analysis demonstrated IL-8 mRNA in epidermis, not, however, in dermis of plaque-type psoriasis [76]. Whereas Barker et al. [28] using Northern blot analysis were able to locate IL-8 mRNA in basal keratinocytes, Gillitzer et al. [77] used in situ hybridization techniques and detected IL-8 transcripts mainly clustered in a spotty pattern between the tips of elongated papillae. In their study, the lower epidermal region and the dermal compartment were devoid of IL-8 mRNA [77].

Immunohistochemical staining for IL-8 using polyclonal antibodies raised against recombinant IL-8 showed two different epidermal patterns. The first included mainly basal cells above or adjacent to the dermal papillae in the area called the "squirting papillae," and the second pattern included intense epidermal staining of the uppermost portion of the epidermis in the vicinity of spongiform pustules [76].

Using monoclonal antibodies raised against natural IL-8 [78], a completely different IL-8 immunostaining pattern was observed: in contrast to the results mentioned above, with the monoclonal anti–IL-8 antibody 52E8 suprabasal keratinocytes of both normal and nonaffected psoriatic skin was stained [79, 80] (Fig. 6). On the other hand, in diseased skin there is an inverse relation of epidermal immunostaining to inflammatory state, in that immunoreactivity is decreased or absent above dense inflammatory infiltrates or beneath parakeratosis [79] (Fig. 6). Interestingly, upon clinical resolution of lesions, normal IL-8 immunostaining is regained (unpublished results).

Reasons for this inverse immunostaining pattern as well as the presence of large amounts of IL-8 immunoreactivity in normal skin are so far unknown and a matter of discussion [81, 82]. It could be shown, however, that IL-8 immunoreactivity can be extracted from normal skin. Upon partial purification and Western blot analysis, it was found to be represented by 50–60 kd protein(s) [83], which are not biologically active. Neither genuine IL-8, which is a 8.5 kd protein, nor its precursor with a calculated molecular weight of 11 kd are likely to cause this IL-8 immunoreactivity pattern. It may, however, represent a biologically inactive and protein-bound form of IL-8 [83]. Consequently, during epidermal inflammation such as in psoriasis, apart from direct cellular synthesis, biologically active IL-8 may be released from an intracellular pool of protein-bound IL-8 by a yet unknown enzymatic process.

## B. Neutrophil Chemotactic Cytokines in Other Inflammatory Skin Diseases

The presence of large amounts of IL-8 and MGSA/gro in psoriatic lesions raises the question of whether this finding is specific for psoriasis vulgaris. We therefore investigated scale material obtained from other inflammatory skin diseases for content of these cytokines.

Surprisingly, in scaling material obtained from patients with ichthyosis congenita, similar amounts of both IL-8–related and MGSA/gro-related cytokines were found, as detected in psoriatic scales. Since a neutrophilic tissue infiltrate is absent in this skin disorder, it is interesting to speculate about the role of these two cytokines in ichthyosis. Obviously, the in vivo presence of IL-8–related cytokines in the tissue appears to be necessary, but *not* sufficient for a tissue infiltration by neutrophilic granulocytes.

As has been shown recently by in vitro experiments [84], neither IL-8 nor MGSA/gro are able to activate endothelial cells for enhanced adherence and diapedesis of leukocytes. The absence of distinct endothelium stimulation by these cytokines may explain why injection of IL-8 into human skin leads mainly to a perivascular but not dermal or epidermal infiltrate by neutrophils exclusively [89, 90]. On the other hand, absence of any lymphocyte

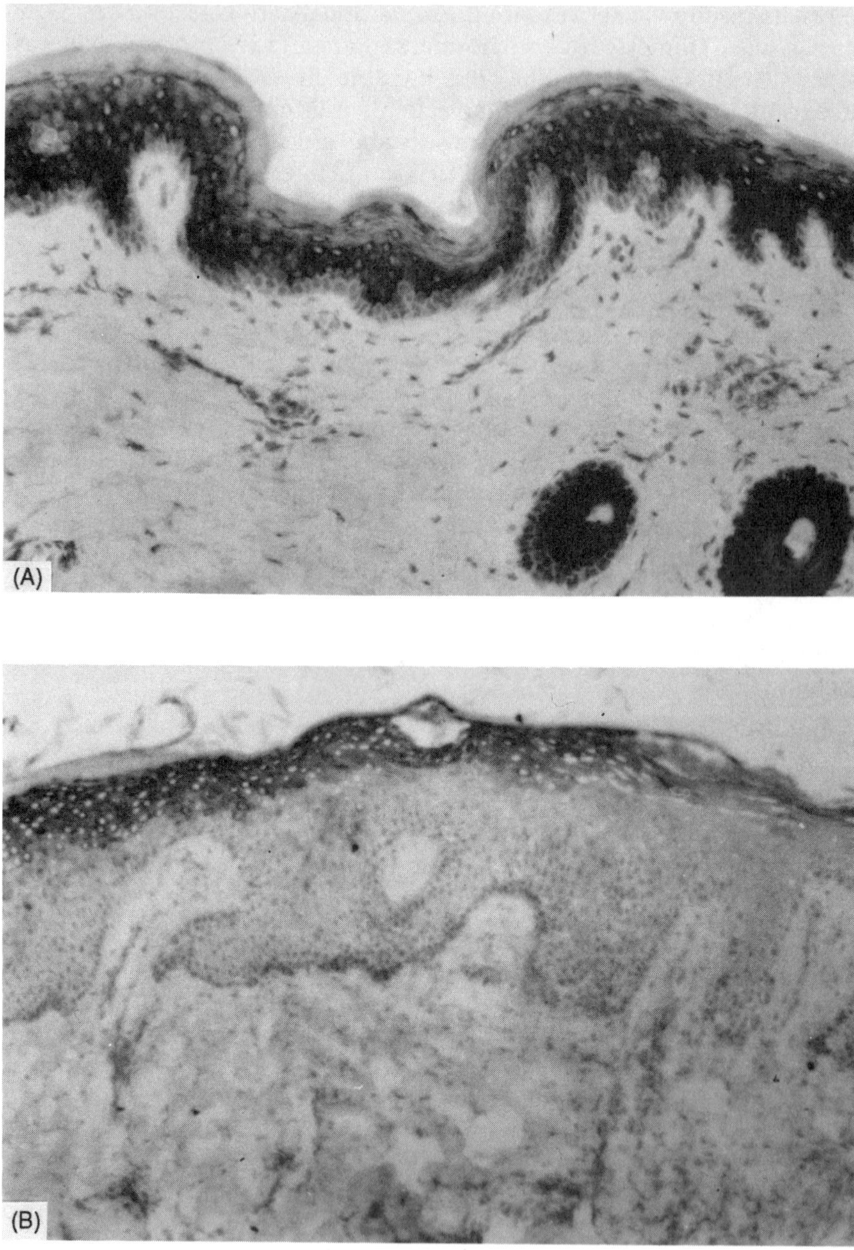


**Fig. 6** Immunoperoxidase staining of normal skin (A) and psoriatic skin (B) with monoclonal anti-IL-8 antibody 52E8 [78, 79].

infiltrate upon injection of IL-8 into human skin makes it unlikely that IL-8, known to be a T-lymphocyte chemotactic factor in vitro [32], is responsible for the T-lymphocyte infiltrate seen in ichthyosis congenita.

In contrast to absent effects on endothelial cells, IL-8 effectively activates expression of $CD_{11b}/CD_{18}$ integrins on neutrophils, which has been demonstrated for other chemotactic factors as well [85]. Accordingly, IL-8, e.g., in its endothelial cell–derived form, may play a critical role in the regulation of adherence of neutrophils to the endothelium and subsequent diapedesis of leukocytes [86, 87].

For tissue infiltration by neutrophils, at least two steps seem to be necessary: first, expression of adherence-promoting proteins as well as stimulation of IL-8 production in endothelial cells, which may be effected by other inflammatory cytokines such as TNF-$\alpha$ or IL-1 [88], and second, activation of neutrophils by secreted IL-8 to adhere to and pass through the endothelium.

This sequence of events may, in contrast to other inflammatory skin diseases, be different in ichthyosis congenita. It is, however, tempting to speculate upon the presence of both cytokines in affected epidermis and the formation of scales in hyperproliferative skin diseases: mitogenic properties of IL-8 for keratinocytes but not for fibroblasts have been reported in the past [92, 93]. In addition, MGSA/gro was originally detected as an autocrine growth factor for some melanoma cell lines [39].

Apart from above-mentioned skin diseases, IL-8 as well as MGSA/gro have been found in large amounts in scale material obtained from patients with eczema and atopic dermatitis [71]. Neither of them could, however, be detected in blister roofs or scaling material obtained from patients with UV burn, drug reactions, or Lyell's syndrome [71].

## C. Monocyte Chemotactic Proteins in Inflammatory Skin Disorders

In contrast to IL-8 and MGSA/gro, there is so far very little information available on the role of monocyte chemotactic cytokines; such as MCP-1/MCAF or RANTES in different skin diseases. The presence of dermal macrophages/dendrocytes in the papillary dermis of psoriasis vulgaris and along the basement membrane of the cubbing rete ridges led to the assumption that MCP-1/MCAF could be important in this phenomenon. Recently, by in situ hybridization using MCP-1 antisense probes, the majority of transcripts could be located to the basal epidermal cell layer at the tips of rete ridges [97].

In cellular immune reactions, local production of monocyte attractants is thought to effect accumulation of monocytes. This hypothesis was supported by the finding that after addition of antigen, sensitized lymphocytes produce a monocyte attractant [93], which was shown to be identical to MCP-1/MCAF [94]. In a number of different tumor types, infiltration and destruction of tumor cells by macrophages can be seen. The accumulation of these cells may well be mediated by attractants generated directly by tumor cells. It has in fact been shown that MCP-1/MCAF is spontaneously produced and secreted by a number of different tumor cells (for review see Ref. 54). Furthermore, both MCP-1 mRNA transcripts and protein have been found in Kaposi's sarcoma by radioactive in situ hybridization using $^{35}S$-labeled probes [95, 96]. mRNA expression was, however, not confined to the tumor, but was also present in the overlying basal epidermal cell layer [96]. It is therefore tempting to speculate about MCP-1 being produced by basal keratinocytes as an important cytokine that induces macrophage infiltration not only in psoriasis but possibly in other inflammatory skin diseases as well.

In respect to the involvement of other chemotactic cytokines, such as RANTES or macrophage inflammatory proteins (MIPs), only circumstantial evidence has been provided so far. RANTES [62], for example, could be relevant in skin diseases such as cutaneous late-phase reactions or atopic dermatitis, which show infiltrates with prominently memory T lymphocytes. Availability of mRNA probes and both monoclonal and polyclonal antibodies to the increasing number of peptides belonging to the IL-8/RANTES supergene family will in the future give insight into the precise role of each of these peptides in different skin diseases.

## IV. CONCLUSIONS

The presence of different subsets of leukocytes in tissue of inflammatory skin diseases led to the working hypothesis that apart from pan-leukocyte chemotactic factors such as C5a, $LTB_4$, F-Met-Leu-Phe, or PAF, more cell-specific attractants do exist, which are locally produced and selectively influence the pattern of leukocyte tissue infiltrate. Recently, several members of a novel supergene family of 6–10 kd cytokines have been detected, which fulfill the criterion of selective or cell-specific chemotactic factors. Cytokines of this supergene family show close sequence and structural similarities, but in fact can be allocated to two subfamilies with two half-cysteines in the immediate vicinity (C-C subfamily) or separated by another amino acid (C-X-C subfamily), respectively.

The most prominent examples of the C-X-C subfamily are the neutrophil-activating protein 1, now generally termed IL-8, and melanoma growth stimulatory activity, both of which are selective attractants for neutrophils. In vitro lymphocyte chemotactic activity as shown for IL-8 has so far not been demonstrated for MGSA/gro.

Members of the C-C subfamily such as MCP-1/MCAF or RANTES as well as MIP-1$\alpha$ and MIP-1$\beta$ are apparently not chemotactic for neutrophils, but stimulate chemotaxis for other leukocytes such as monocytes (MCP-1/MCAF), memory T lymphocytes (RANTES), cytotoxic T lymphocytes (MIP-1$\alpha$), or naive T lymphocytes (MIP-1$\beta$) [59]. Keratinocytes as well as other epidermal cells such as melanocytes [98] or Langerhans cells [99] are under certain conditions able to produce and secrete IL-8, MCP-1/MCAF, and possibly MGSA/gro as well. Consequently, these cytokines may well be responsible for neutrophil and monocyte infiltration, respectively, into the epidermis under inflammatory conditions.

An interesting aspect in this context is the effect of well-established antipsoriatic drugs on IL-8, MGSA/gro, and MCP-1/MCAF production by epidermal cells. Very recent reports do indeed indicate that corticosteroids, cyclosporin A, 1,25-$(OH)_2D_3$, and anthralin distinctly inhibit IL-8 and/or MCP-1/MCAF gene expression and peptide release in blood leukocytes as well as other tissue cell types [100–103].

The development of new drugs, which either specifically inhibit the production of these cytokines or block cellular responses elicited by them, is an attractive perspective for future work on antiinflammatory therapy. The selective inhibition of tissue infiltration by subsets of leukocytes, which are known or suggested to play an important role in the pathogenesis of different inflammatory skin disorders, may help in a more effective treatment of these often tenacious diseases.

## NOTE ADDED IN PROOF

Members of the IL-8 supergene family (chemokine family [104]) have been shown to be selective chemotaxins for several leukocyte types and subsets, except eosinophils. Recently we could identify the C-C cytokine RANTES as potent and efficient chemotaxin for human eosinophils [105]. Due to its selective chemotactic properties for memory T-lymphocytes and eosinophils but not neutrophils it could be an important cytokine in late phase allergic reactions and atopic dermatitis.

## ACKNOWLEDGMENTS

The experimental work was supported in part by Deutsche Forschungsgemeinschaft grants Schr 308/1-2 and Sti 95/2-1. We are indebted to Christine Gerbrecht-Gliessmann, Jutta Quitzau, Anke Rose, and Claudia Mehrens for their excellent technical assistance and to Mrs. Ilse Brandt for expert secretarial help.

## REFERENCES


1. S. Hammarström, M. Hamberg, B. Samuelsson, E. A. Duell, M. Stawiski, and J. J. Voorhees, *Proc. Natl. Acad. Sci. USA 72*, 5130 (1975).
2. E. J. Goetzl and W. C. Pickett, *J. Immunol. 125*, 1789 (1980).
3. V. A. Ziboh, T. L. Casebolt, C. L. Marcelo, and J. J. Voorhees, *J. Invest. Dermatol. 83*, 425 (1984).
4. S. D. Brain, R. D. R. Camp, I. M. Leigh, and A. W. Ford-Hutchinson, *J. Invest. Dermatol. 78*, 328 (abstract).
5. T. Rosenbach and B. Czarnetzki, in *Eicosanoids and the Skin* (T. Ruzicka, ed.), CRC Press, Boca Raton, FL, 1990, p. 127.
6. M. J. Holtzman, J. Turk, and A. Pentland, *J. Clin. Invest. 84*, 1446 (1989).
7. H. H. Henneicke-von Zepelin, J.-M. Schröder, P. Smid, M. K. Reusch, and E. Christophers, *J. Invest. Dermatol. 97*, 291 (1991).
8. T. A. Luger, J. A. Charon, M. Colot, M. Micksche, and J. J. Oppenheim, *J. Immunol. 131*, 816 (1983).
9. D. N. Sauder, N. L. Mounessa, S. I. Katz, C. A. Dinarello, and J. I. Gallin, *J. Immunol. 132*, 828 (1984).
10. D. W. Hunninghake, A. J. Glazier, M. M. Monick, and C. A. Dinarello, *Am. Rev. Respir. Dis. 135*, 66 (1987).
11. J.-M. Schröder, P. Smid, M. Sticherling, H. H. Henneicke-von Zepelin, M. Herlyn, and E. Christophers, manuscript in preparation.
12. J.-M. Schröder, U. Mrowietz, E. Morita, and E. Christophers, *J. Immunol. 139*, 3474 (1987).
13. P. Peveri, A. Walz, B. Dewald, and M. Baggiolini, *J. Exp. Med. 167*, 1547 (1988).
14. J. Willems, M. Joniau, S. Cinque, and J. van Damme, *Immunology 67*, 540 (1989).
15. W. E. Holmes, J. Lee, W. J. Kuang, G. C. Rice, and W. I. Wood, *Science 253*, 1278 (1991).
16. P. M. Murphy and H. L. Tiffany, *Science 253*, 1280 (1991).
17. J.-M. Schröder, *J. Exp. Med. 170*, 464 (1989).
18. J.-M. Schröder, M. Sticherling, H. H. Henneicke-von Zepelin, P. Smid, M. Herlyn, and E. Christophers, *Arch. Dermatol. Res. 283*, 57 (abstract) (1991).
19. J.-M. Schröder, M. Sticherling, H. H. Henneicke-von Zepelin, W. C. Pressner, and E. Christophers, *J. Immunol. 144*, 2223 (1990).
20. C. A. Hèbert, F. W. Luscinskas, J.-M. Kiely, E. A. Luis, W. C. Darbonne, G. L. Bennett, C. C. Lin, M. S. Obin, M. A. Gimbrone Jr., and J. B. Baker, *J. Immunol. 145*, 3033 (1990).
21. T. Yoshimura, K. Matsushima, S. Tanaka, E. A. Robinson, E. Appella, J. J. Oppenheim, and E. J. Leonard, *Proc. Natl. Acad. Sci. USA 84*, 9233 (1987).
22. A. Walz, P. Peveri, H. Aschauer, and M. Baggiolini, *Biochem. Biophys. Res. Commun. 149*, 755 (1987).
23. H. Gregory, J. Young, J.-M. Schröder, U. Mrowietz, and E. Christophers, *Biochem. Biophys. Res. Commun. 151*, 883 (1988).
24. J.-M. Schröder and E. Christophers, *J. Immunol. 142*, 244 (1989).

25. M. A. Gimbrone, M. S. Obins, A. F. Brock, E. A. Luis, P. E. Hass, C. A. Hèbert, Y. K. Yip, D. W. Leung, D. G. Lowe, W. J. Kohr, W. C. Dabronne, K. B. Bechtal, and J. B. Baker, *Science 246*, 1601 (1989).
26. C. Gronhoj-Larsen, A. O. Anderson, J. J. Oppenheim, and K. Matsushima, *Immunology 68*, 31 (1989).
27. R. Strieter, S. H. Phan, H. J. Showell, D. G. Remick, J. P. Lynchz, M. Genord, C. Raiford, M. Escandari, R. M. Marks, and S. L. Kunkel, *J. Biol. Chem. 264*, 10621 (1989).
28. J. N. W. N. Barker, V. Sama, R. S. Mitra, V. M. Dixit, and B. J. Nickoloff, *J. Clin. Invest. 85*, 605 (1990).
29. M. S. Kristensen, K. Paludan, C. G. Larsen, C. O. C. Zachariae, B. W. Beleuran, P. K. A. Jensen, P. Jorgensen, and K. Thestrup-Pedersen, *J. Invest. Dermatol. 97*, 506 (1991).
30. J. N. W. N. Barker, R. S. Mitra, C. E. M. Griffiths, V. M. Dixit, and B. J. Nickoloff, *Lancet 337*, 211 (1991).
31. C. E. M. Griffiths, J. N. W. N. Barker, S. Kunkel, and B. J. Nickoloff, *Br. J. Dermatol. 124*, 519 (1991).
32. C. Gronhoj-Larsen, A. O. Anderson, E. Appella, J. J. Oppenheim, and K. Matsushima, *Science 243*, 1464 (1989).
33. A. Richmond, E. Balentien, H. G. Thomas, G. Flaggs, D. E. Barton, J. Spiess, R. Bardoni, U. Francke, and R. Drynck, *EMBO J. 7*, 2025 (1988).
34. A. Anisowicz, L. Bardwell, and R. Sager, *Proc. Natl. Acad. Sci. USA 84*, 7188 (1987).
35. M. Baggiolini, A. Walz, and S. L. Kunkel, *J. Clin. Invest. 84*, 1045 (1989).
36. J.-M. Schröder and E. Christophers, *J. Invest. Dermatol. 87*, 53 (1986).
37. J.-M. Schröder, J. Young, H. Gregory, and E. Christophers, *J. Invest. Dermatol. 92*, 515 (abstract) (1988).
38. J.-M. Schröder, H. Gregory, J. Young, and E. Christophers, *J. Invest. Dermatol. 98*, 241 (1992).
39. A. Richmond and H. G. Thomas, *J. Cell. Physiol. 129*, 375 (1986).
40. J.-M. Schröder, N. Persoon, and E. Christophers, *J. Exp. Med. 171*, 1091 (1990).
41. A. Richmond and H. G. Thomas, *J. Cell. Biochem. 36*, 185 (1988).
42. S. Haskill, A. Peace, J. Morris, S. A. Sporn, A. Anisowicz, S. W. Lee, T. Smith, G. Martin, P. Ralph, and R. Sager, *Proc. Natl. Acad. Sci. USA 87*, 7732 (1990).
43. A. Walz and M. Baggiolini, *Biochem. Biophys. Res. Commun. 159*, 969 (1989).
44. A. Walz, B. Dewald, V. von Tscharner, and M. Baggiolini, *J. Exp. Med. 170*, 1745 (1989).
45. A. Walz, R. Burgener, B. Car, M. Baggiolini, S. L. Kunkel, and R. M. Strieter, *J. Exp. Med. 174*, 1355 (1991).
46. A. D. Luster and J. V. Ravetch, *J. Exp. Med. 166*, 1084 (1987).
47. G. Kaplan, A. D. Luster, G. Hancock, and Z. A. Cohn, *J. Exp. Med. 166*, 1098 (1987).
48. J. G. Krueger, J. F. Krane, D. M. Carter, and A. B. Gottlieb, *J. Invest. Dermatol. 94* (Suppl), 135S (1990).
49. J. I. Kuratsu, E. J. Leonard, and T. Yoshimura, *J. Natl. Cancer Inst. 81*, 347 (1989).

50. E. A. Robinson, T. Yoshimura, E. J. Leonard, S. Tanaka, P. R. Griffin, J. Shabanowitz, D. R. Hunt, and E. Appella, *Proc. Natl. Acad. Sci. USA 86*, 1850 (1989).
51. K. Matsushima and J. J. Oppenheim, *Cytokine 1*, 2 (1989).
52. T. Yoshimura, E. A. Robinson, S. Tanaka, E. Appella, J.-I. Kuratsu, and E. J. Leonard, *J. Exp. Med. 169*, 1449 (1989).
53. K. Matsushima, C. G. Larsen, G. C. DuBois, and J. J. Oppenheim, *J. Exp. Med. 169*, 1485 (1989).
54. E. J. Leonard and T. Yoshimura, *Immunol. Today 11*, 97 (1990).
55. T. Yoshimura, E. A. Robinson, S. Tanaka, E. Appella, and E. J. Leonard, *J. Immunol. 142*, 1956 (1989).
56. J. N. W. N. Barker, M. L. Jones, C. L. Swenson, V. Sarma, R. S. Mitra, P. A. Ward, K. J. Johnson, J. C. Fantone, V. M. Dixit, and B. J. Nickoloff, *J. Immunol. 146*, 1192 (1991).
57. S. D. Wolpe, G. Davatelis, B. Sherry, B. Beutler, D. G. Hesse, H. T. Naguyen, L. L. Moldawer, C. G. Nathan, S. F. Lowry, and A. Cerami, *J. Exp. Med. 167*, 570 (1988).
58. B. Sherry, P. Tekamp-Olson, C. Gallegos, D. Bauer, G. Davatelis, S. D. Wolpe, A. Masiarz, D. Coit, and A. Cerami, *J. Exp. Med. 168*, 2251 (1988).
59. T. J. Schall, *Cytokine 3*, 165 (1991).
60. T. J. Schall, J. Jongstra, B. J. Dyer, J. Jorgensen, C. Clayberger, M. M. Davis, and A. M. Krensky, *J. Immunol. 141*, 1018 (1988).
61. C. Heufler, F. Koch, E. K. Parkinson, G. J. Graham, B. Trockenbacher, E. Kämpgen, N. Romani, I. B. Pragnell, and G. Schuler, *Arch. Dermatol. Res.* in press.
62. T. J. Schall, K. Bacon, K. J. Toy, and D. V. Goeddel, *Nature 347*, 669 (1990).
63. O. Braun-Falco and E. Christophers, *Arch. Dermatol. Forsch. 251*, 95 (1974).
64. H. Tagami and S. Ofuji, *Br. J. Dermatol. 97*, 509 (1977).
65. S. D. Brain, R. D. R. Camp, P. M. Dowd, M. W. Greaves, A. K. Black, A. I. Mallet, and P. M. Woollard, *Br. J. Pharmacol. 83*, 313 (1983).
66. A. I. Mallet, F. M. Cunningham, and R. Daniel, *J. Chromatogr. 309*, 160 (1984).
67. R. D. R. Camp, N. J. Fincham, F. M. Cunningham, M. W. Greaves, J. Morris, and A. Chu, *J. Immunol. 137*, 3469 (1986).
68. N. J. Fincham, R. D. R. Camp, A. J. H. Gearing, C. R. Bird, and F. M. Cunningham, *J. Immunol. 140*, 4294 (1988).
69. U. Mrowietz, J.-M. Schröder, E. Morita, T. Ternowitz, and E. Christophers, *J. Invest. Dermatol. 89*, 330 (abstract) (1987).
70. J.-M. Schröder and E. Christophers, *J. Invest. Dermatol. 91*, 395 (abstract) (1988).
71. J.-M. Schröder, in *Interleukin-8 (NAP-1) and Related Chemotactic Cytokines* (M. Baggiolini and C. Sorg, eds.), Karger, Basel, 1992, p. 54.
72. J.-M. Schröder and E. Christophers, *Arch. Dermatol. Res. 284*, 12 (abstract) (1990).
73. I. J. D. Lindley, H. Aschauer, C. Lam, J. Besemer, and A. Rot, in *Molecular and Cellular Biology of Cytokines* (J. J. Oppenheim, M. C. Powanda, M. J. Kluger, C. A. Dinarello, eds.), Wiley-Liss, New York, 1990, p. 345.

74. T. P. Hopp, S. K. Dower, and C. J. March, *Immunol. Res. 5*, 271 (1986).
75. A. J. H. Gearing, N. J. Fincham, C. R. Bird, M. Wadhawa, A. Meager, J. E. Cartwright, and R. D. R. Camp, *Cytokine 2*, 68 (1990).
76. B. J. Nickoloff, G. D. Karabin, J. N. W. N. Barker, C. E. M. Griffiths, V. Sarma, R. S. Mitra, J. T. Elder, S. L. Kunkel, and V. M. Dixit, *Am. J. Pathol. 138*, 129 (1991).
77. R. Gillitzer, R. Berger, V. Mielke, K. Wolff, and G. Stingl, *J. Invest. Dermatol. 97*, 73 (1991).
78. M. Sticherling, J.-M. Schröder, and E. Christophers, *J. Immunol. 143*, 1628 (1989).
79. M. Sticherling, E. Bornscheuer, J.-M. Schröder, and E. Christophers, *J. Invest. Dermatol. 96*, 26 (1991).
80. M. Sticherling, J.-M. Schröder, and E. Christophers, *J. Invest. Dermatol. 96*, 1025 (1991).
81. J. N. W. N. Barker, C. E. M. Griffiths, and B. J. Nickoloff, *J. Invest. Dermatol. 97*, 606 (1991).
82. M. Sticherling, J.-M. Schröder, and E. Christophers, *J. Invest. Dermatol. 97*, 607 (1991).
83. M. Sticherling, J.-M. Schröder, and E. Christophers, *J. Invest. Dermatol. 95*, 491 (1990).
84. M. S. Obin, J. M. Kiely, C. Hébert, J. Baker, and M. A. Gimbrone, *FASEB J. 4*, A625 (1990).
85. P. A. Detmers, S. L. Lo, E. Elsen-Egbert, A. Walz, M. Baggiolini, and Z. A. Cohn, *J. Exp. Med. 171*, 1155 (1990).
86. A. R. Huber, S. L. Kunkel, R. F. Todd, and S. J. Weiss, *Science 254*, 99 (1991).
87. D. H. Hechtman, M. I. Cybulsky, H. J. Fuchs, J. B. Baker, and M. A. Gimbrone, Jr., *J. Immunol. 147*, 883 (1991).
88. M. I. Cybulsky, D. J. McComb, and H. Z. Movat, *J. Immunol. 140*, 3144 (1988).
89. O. Swensson, C. Schubert, E. Christophers, and J.-M. Schröder, *J. Invest. Dermatol. 95*, 682 (1991).
90. E. J. Leonard, T. Yoshimura, S. Tanaka, and M. Raffeld, *J. Invest. Dermatol. 95*, 690 (1991).
91. G. Krueger, C. Jörgensen, C. Miller, J.-M. Schröder, M. Sticherling, and E. Christophers, *J. Invest. Dermatol. 94*, 545 (abstract) (1990).
92. M. K. Reusch, M. Studtmann, J.-M. Schröder, M. Sticherling, and E. Christophers, *J. Invest. Dermatol. 95*, 485 (abstract) (1990).
93. L. C. Altman, in *Chemotactic Lymphokines* (C. J. I. Gallin and P. G. Quie, eds.), Raven Press, New York, 1978, p. 267.
94. T. Yoshimura and E. J. Leonard, in *Interleukin-8 (NAP-1) and Related Chemotactic Cytokines* (M. Baggiolini and E. Sorg, eds.), Karger, Basel, 1992, p. 131.
95. R. Gillitzer, G. Burg, K. Wolff, G. Stingl, and R. Berger, *J. Invest. Dermatol. 96*, 1011 (abstract) (1991).
96. R. Gillitzer, D. Tong, G. Burg, A. A. Hartmann, K. Wolff, G. Stingl, and R. Berger, *Arch. Dermatol. Res. 284*, 18 (abstract) (1990).
97. R. Gillitzer, K. Wolff, G. Stingl, A. A. Hartmann, and R. Berger, *Arch. Dermatol. Res. 284,* 24 (abstract) (1990).

98. C. O. C. Zachariae, K. Thestrup-Pedersen, and K. Matsushima, *J. Invest. Dermatol. 97*, 593 (1991).
99. T. Bieber, M. Sticherling, R. Rupec, and J.-M. Schröder, *J. Invest. Dermatol. 96*, 1013 (abstract) (1991).
100. N. Mukaida, C. C. O. Zachariae, G. L. Gusella, and K. Matsushima, *J. Invest. Dermatol. 146*, 1212 (1991).
101. M. Kristensen, K. Paludan, C. Gronhoj-Larsen, B. Deleuran, C. Zachariae, P. K. A. Jensen, and K. Thestrup-Pedersen, *J. Invest. Dermatol. 96*, 1023 (abstract) (1991).
102. C. Gronhoj-Larsen, M. Kristensen, K. Paludan, B. Deleuran, M. K. Thomsen, C. O. C. Zachariae, K. Kragballe, K. Matsushima, and K. Threstrup-Pedersen, *J. Invest. Dermatol. 96*, 1008 (abstract) (1991).
103. U. Mrowietz, H. Jessat, A. Urbanski, T. Schwarz, J.-M. Schröder, T. Luger, and E. Christophers, *Arch. Dermatol. Res. 284*, 12 (abstract) (1990).
104. I. J. D. Lindley, J. Westwick, and S. L. Kunkel, *Immunology Today 14*, 24 (1993).
105. Y. Kameyoshi, A. Dörschner, A. I. Mallet, E. Christophers, and J.-M. Schröder, *J. Exp. Med. 176*, 587 (1992).

# 5
# Interleukin 10

**Alexander H. Enk***
*National Cancer Institute*
*National Institutes of Health*
*Bethesda, Maryland*

## I. INTRODUCTION

A major advance in cellular immunology occurred in 1986, when Mosmann et al. defined two subsets of murine CD4+ Th cells (Th1 and Th2 cells) that could be differentiated from each other functionally and by their distinctive cytokine profiles [1, 2]. With regard to cytokines, Th1 clones mainly produce IFN-$\gamma$, IL-2, and lymphotoxin, whereas Th2 cells are sources of IL-4, IL-5, IL-6, and express mRNA for P600, a gene of as yet unknown function [3]. Both Th1 and Th2 clones secrete IL-3, GM-CSF, and TNF-$\alpha$ (Table 1). Functionally, Th1 cells have been shown to mediate delayed-type hypersensitivity reactions and to provide help for B-cell production of $IgG_{2a}$, in contrast to Th2 cells that provide B-cell help for antibody secretion for all classes (especially IgE and $IgG_1$ [1, 2]). Gajewski and Fitch [4] and Fernandez-Botran et al. [5] subsequently demonstrated that the Th1 cell product IFN-$\gamma$ inhibited the proliferation of Th2 cells but not Th1 cells, and suggested that possible cross-regulatory mechanisms between the two Th cell types existed. The observation that a product of the D10.G4.1 Th2 clone suppressed the proliferation of Th1 cells by Janeway et al. [6] led to the search for a Th2 cell product that inhibited Th1 function. Preliminary characterization of this factor, from then on called cytokine synthesis inhibitory factor (CSIF), was achieved in 1989 by Fiorentino et al. [7]. These investigators demonstrated that the Th2 product CSIF inhibited production of IFN-$\gamma$ by Th1 cells and that this inhibition occurred at the transcriptional level. This activity was dependent on the presence of antigen-presenting cells (APC) and was distinct

**Current affiliation*: University of Mainz, Mainz, Germany.

**Table 1** Cytokines Produced by Th Precursor Cells (Thp), Indeterminate Th Cells (Th0), Th1 and Th2 Cells, as Well as Cytotoxic T Cells (CTL)

| | Thp | Th0 | Th1 | Th2 | CTL |
|---|---|---|---|---|---|
| IL-2 | + + | + + | + + | − | +/− |
| IFN-$\gamma$ | − | + + | + + | − | + + |
| LT | | | + + | − | + |
| IL-3 | − | + + | + + | + | + |
| IL-4 | − | + + | − | + + | − |
| IL-5 | − | + + | − | + + | − |
| IL-6 | | | − | + + | − |
| IL-10 | − | + + | − | + + | − |
| P600 | | | − | + + | − |
| GM-CSF | − | + + | + + | + | + |
| TNF-$\alpha$ | | | + + | + | + |
| TY5 | | | + + | + | + + |
| P500 | | | + + | + | + + |
| H400 | | | + + | + | |
| Met-enk. | | | + | + + | + |

from all the other known cytokines [7]. In 1990 Moore et al. [8] cloned the cDNA encoding murine CSIF from concanavalin A (ConA)–stimulated D10 cells and named the gene product interleukin 10 (IL-10). This chapter presents a synopsis of IL-10 biochemistry and biology, with emphasis on the role that IL-10 may play in the regulation of immune responses in skin.

## II. MOLECULAR ASPECTS OF IL-10

### A. The IL-10 Gene

The nucleotide sequence encoding murine IL-10 was determined by expression cloning [8]. mRNA derived from the Th2 clone D10 was reverse-transcribed and cDNAs were transfected into COS cells with the expression vector pcDSR$\alpha$. Stable transfectants secreting IL-10 were identified based on their ability to secrete an activity that inhibited IFN-$\gamma$ production by the Th1 clone HDK, and the relevant cDNA was isolated and sequenced [8]. Analysis of the sequence revealed extensive homology of murine IL-10 on the nucleic acid and amino acid level with an uncharacterized open reading frame, BCRF1, in the Epstein-Barr virus (EBV) genome. Further characterization of a 7.2 kb segment of genomic DNA containing the mouse IL-10 gene (Fig. 1) revealed five exons that spanned ~5.1 kb of genomic DNA.

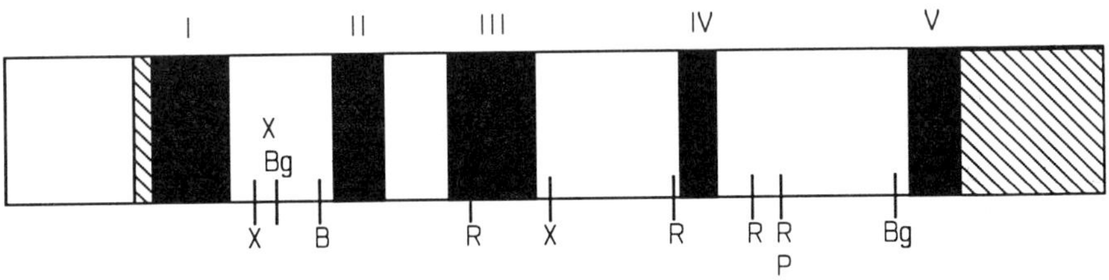


**Fig. 1** Schematic and partial restriction map of the IL-10 gene. Exons are labeled I–V, containing coding (black) and untranslated sequences (hatched). B, BamHI; Bg, BglII; R, EcoRI; P, PstI; X, Xbal. (Adapted from Ref. 9.)

Both murine and (with some certainty) human IL-10 genes have been mapped to the long arm of chromosome 1. In addition, Southern blot analysis and sequence data suggest that IL-10 is a single-copy gene, whose first exon encodes the 5′-untranslated sequence, the signal sequence, and approximately 34 amino acids comprising the N-terminus of the mature protein. Exon V encodes the C-terminal 30 amino acids of mIL-10 and the entire 3′-untranslated region of the ~1.4 kb mIL-10 mRNA. Because exon-intron junctions do not disrupt amino acid codons, alternative splicing events are possible without disruption of the open-reading frame (ORF). The strong homology of mIL-10 to the EBV BCRF1 ORF (also called viral IL-10 [vIL-10]) is not restricted to any particular exon, suggesting that BCRF1 was originally derived from a cellular IL-10 gene. Candidate regulatory sequence motifs including a TATA box centered at −30 bp from the 5′-end of the mIL-10 cDNA sequence, putative glucocorticoid responsive elements, a cAMP-responsive element, and consensus AP-1 and NF-$\kappa$B–binding sites have been identified in the 5′-untranslated region of the mIL-10 cDNA.

The human IL-10 cDNA sequence has been published more recently [10]. The overall DNA sequence homology between hIL-10 and mIL-10 is 81% and occurs throughout the entire sequence, except for a region between nucleotide position 1162 and 1477, where a repetitive element of the human *Alu* family is inserted. The amino acid homology between the two is 73%. In contrast, the predicted amino acid sequence homology between hIL-10 and BCRF1 is greater (84%) than their nucleic acid homology (71%). No significant homology of hIL-10 or mIL-10 to proteins other than BCRF1 has been detected.

## B. The IL-10 Protein

The murine IL-10 gene contains an ORF encoding a 178-amino-acid polypeptide with an $NH_2$-terminal hydrophobic leader sequence of 18 residues.

The calculated molecular weight of mature IL-10 is 18.7 kd and the calculated pI 8 [8]. Although the mIL-10 sequence contains two consensus N-linked glycosylation sites, experiments with tunicamycin and glycosidase suggest that only one of these sites is glycosylated on some IL-10 molecules, so that natural as well as recombinant mIL-10 each consist of polypeptides of 16 and 20 kd. Molecular sieving suggests that mIL-10 exists as homodimer of 35–40 kd in solution. The mature protein is acid-labile [12].

Unlike mIL-10, hIL-10 (18 kd) and vIL-10 (17 kd) have little or no N-linked carbohydrate and can be distinguished from each other by apparent molecular mass in SDS-PAGE despite extensive sequence homology [10]. Whereas hIL-10 is similarly active on murine cells, mIL-10 has virtually no effect on human cells. Although vIL-10 and hIL-10 share some functional activities, there are some important differences. Whereas hIL-10 is a potent mast cell growth cofactor, vIL-10 neither expresses such an activity nor does it support the viability of mast cells, or thymocyte proliferation, or the MHC class II induction on B cells [11]. vIL-10 is, on the other hand, fully capable of blocking IFN-γ production by T cells. Perhaps IL-10 possesses several distinct functional domains, some of which are lost in BCRF1.

At least seven monoclonal antibodies of mIL-10 and one for hIL-10 have been developed [12] and used to develop sensitive and unambiguous assay systems (ELISA, immunoprecipitation, Western blot). These antibodies as well as the availability of rIL-10 will facilitate future experiments (including the detection of an IL-10 receptor).

## III. CELLULAR SOURCES OF IL-10

IL-10 was originally described as a product of Th2 cell clones. Since then other bone marrow–derived cells have been demonstrated to produce IL-10. Today the list of IL-10 sources includes B cells (especially Ly-1 B cells [13]), monocytes [14], mast cell lines [15], and Th0 cells [16]. Our laboratory [17] has recently shown that IL-10 is also produced by activated murine keratinocytes, indicating that bone marrow–derived cells are not the only sources of this pleiotropic cytokine.

## IV. EFFECTS OF IL-10

### A. Effects of IL-10 on T Lymphocytes

The effect that IL-10 has on T cells depends on the nature of the T cell and the species from which it is derived. In the murine system, MacNeil et al. [18] have shown that IL-10, together with IL-2 and IL-4, is a growth cofactor for both adult and 15-day fetal thymocytes. This effect was, to some extent, also seen in combination with IL-7. IL-10 alone was without effect.

Fetal thymocyte proliferation in this system was mostly attributable to IL-2 and IL-10 and seemed to be a direct effect of IL-10 on the T cells. When adult thymocytes were sorted based on their expression of CD4 and CD8 molecules, double negative and single positive cells proliferated in response to IL-10 in the presence of IL-2/IL-4, whereas double positive thymocytes did not proliferate to this cytokine combination. In addition, IL-10 alone did not significantly alter the viability of adult thymocytes in culture, whereas the combination of IL-10 with IL-2/IL-4 resulted in a significantly higher viability of thymocytes than IL-2/IL-4 alone. In phenotypic analyses of double and triple negative adult and 15-day fetal thymocytes, IL-10 in combination with IL-2 and IL-4 significantly up-regulated CD3 but not CD4 expression and only minimally enhanced CD8 expression [18]. The proliferative response of adult peripheral T cells was also enhanced by IL-10 in combination with IL-2/IL-4, to some extent. In aggregate, these data support findings by Bendelac and Schwartz [19] that IL-10 is being produced during certain phases of thymic development and that IL-10 plays an important role in the proliferation and maturation of certain thymic T-cell subsets.

Another direct effect of IL-10 on T cells reflects its activity as a cytotoxic T-cell differentiation factor. Chen and Zlotnik [20] showed that IL-10 augmented the proliferation of ConA-stimulated CD8 + T cells in combination with IL-2. Again, IL-10 alone had no effect. IL-10 also enhanced the IL-2–induced lectin-dependent, antigen-nonspecific cytotoxicity of effector cytotoxic T lymphocytes (CTL) in a dose-dependent fashion. Time-course studies showed that IL-10 was most effective when added at the initiation of the cultures, but also significantly enhanced cytotoxicity when added at later times, suggesting an effect of IL-10 on both early and late stages of CTL differentiation. In addition, IL-10 in combination with IL-2 significantly increased the CTL-precursor frequency of sorted CD8 + T lymphocytes in a filler cell-free system using solid-phase anti-CD3 monoclonal antibodies (mAb) as activator [20]. On the other hand, IL-10 did not enhance the ability of IL-2 or IL-4 to induce lymphokine-activated killer (LAK) cells [20]. Taken together these data indicate a significant role for IL-10 in CTL induction and development.

Apart from these reports of direct effects on T lymphocytes, most IL-10 effects on T cells seem to be mediated via APC. In the mouse, Fiorentino et al. [21] reported that IL-10–blocked macrophage supported IFN-γ production by a peptide-specific Th1 cell clone only if metabolically active APC were present. IL-10 also did not exert any effect on IFN-γ production if fixed APC were used in the assay. IL-10 had no effect on the cytokine production by Th2 cell clones or Th1 cell clones when B cells were used as APC. These findings suggest an effect of IL-10 on T-cell function that may be dependent on the presence or absence of APC-derived costimulatory signals.

In the human system, Taga and Tosato [22] have shown that hIL-10 inhibited production of IFN-$\gamma$ by peripheral T cells, and also blocked mitogen- and anti-CD3–induced T-cell proliferation in the presence of APC by ~90%. Inhibition of proliferation was more pronounced when suboptimal amounts of mitogen or cross-linking mAb were used and was similar for CD4+, CD8+, CD45RA high, and CD45RA low T cells. Dose-response experiments demonstrated that IL-10 inhibited production of IFN-$\gamma$ more readily than T-cell proliferation. In addition, exogenously added IL-2 or IL-4 completely reversed the IL-10–induced inhibition of T-cell proliferation, but not IFN-$\gamma$ production. These data suggest that the effect of IL-10 on T-cell proliferation is at least partially mediated via suppression of endogenous IL-2 production, whereas the impact of IL-10 on IFN-$\gamma$ secretion seems to be IL-2–independent. The exact mechanism of action of IL-10 remains unknown, however.

## B. Effects of IL-10 on B Cells

IL-10 has been known to be produced by B cells and B-cell lymphomas for some time [23]. O'Garra et al. reported that CD5+ (Ly-1) B cells are primarily responsible for IL-10 production [13]. In contrast to normal splenic B cells, Ly-1 B cells are a self-replenishing population that is relatively abundant in the peritoneal cavity and is minimally represented in spleen and lymph nodes of normal adult mice. In older mice, clonal expansions of Ly-1 B cells have been observed giving rise to speculation about a possible bias of immune reactivity in older mice towards a Th2 response. In a recent report, Ishida et al. [24] demonstrated that IL-10 acts as an autocrine growth factor for Ly-1 B cells. Mice treated continuously from birth to 8 weeks of age with a neutralizing anti–IL-10 mAb lacked peritoneal-resident Ly-1 B lymphocytes, exhibited greatly reduced serum IgM levels, and were unable to generate significant in vivo antibody responses to bacterial determinants $\alpha$1,3-dextran or phosphorylcholine, antigens known to activate the Ly-1 B-cell subset. In contrast, conventional splenic B cells of anti-IL-10–treated mice were normal with respect to total numbers, phenotype, and function. The mechanism of Ly-1 B-cell depletion appeared to be related to elevation of endogenous IFN-$\gamma$ levels in anti-IL-10–treated mice, since coadministration of neutralizing anti–IFN-$\gamma$ antibodies substantially restored the number of peritoneal Ly-1 B cells in these mice. These results implicate IL-10 as a regulator of Ly-1 B-lymphocyte development and an important modulator of humoral immune responses.

IL-10 not only is a growth factor for Ly-1 B cells, but also exerts various effects on conventional B cells. Highly purified, small, dense splenic B cells from unstimulated mice show increased expression of class II MHC antigens and enhanced viability when cultured with affinity-purified recombinant

IL-10, compared with B cells cultured in medium alone [11]. Unlike IL-4, IL-10 did not up-regulate the expression of Fcε receptors (CD23) or induce proliferation of small resting B cells, indicating differential mechanisms of action of the two cytokines [11]. Interestingly, IL-10 did not up-regulate class II MHC antigens on B cells from X chromosome–linked immunodeficiency (XID) mice, while the same cells showed normal up-regulation of class II antigens in response to IL-4. The related molecule BCRF1 enhanced viability, but not MHC class II expression on B cells, suggesting at least two functional domains of IL-10.

In the human system, hIL-10 and vIL-10 are potent growth and differentiation factors for activated B cells [10]. IL-10 and vIL-10 enhanced the proliferation of *Staphylococcus aureus* strain Cowan (SAC)–activated B cells, but had no activity on unstimulated cells. Even at optimal concentrations, the IL-10 effect in this system was less pronounced than when B cells were costimulated with IL-2 or IL-4. When B lymphocytes were stimulated with anti-CD40 mAb, IL-4 and IL-10 were equally active, whereas IL-2 was inactive.

With regard to B-lymphocyte differentiation, IL-10 induced SAC-preactivated B cells to produce high levels of IgM, IgG, and IgA more effectively than IL-2 or IL-4 [10]. When B cells were activated via the CD40 molecule, addition of IL-10 augmented production of IgM, IgG, and IgA. Again, IL-10 was much more efficient than IL-2 or IL-4. Unlike IL-4, neither vIL-10 nor hIL-10 induced anti-CD40–activated B lymphocytes to secrete IgE. All four isotypes were detected when IL-4 and IL-10 were added simultaneously, however. Whereas the combination of IL-4 and IL-10 had additive effects on B-cell proliferation, the levels of secreted IgM, IgG, and IgA in response to both cytokines were less than those observed with IL-10 alone [10].

In another report, Defrance et al. [25] assessed the effects of hIL-10 and TGF-β on naive, surface $IgD^+$ ($sIgD^+$) B cells as compared with more differentiated, $sIgD^-$ B lymphocytes. Both vIL-10 and hIL-10 dramatically increased the Ig secretion by both types of B cells preactivated by SAC or anti-CD40 mAb. Whereas $sIgD^+$ B cells mainly produced IgM, IgG constituted the predominant Ig isotype produced by $sIgD^-$ B cells in response to IL-10. Furthermore, naive B cells produced IgA when cultured with TGF-β and IL-10 in the presence of anti-CD40 mAb and CDw32-transfected L cells. In contrast TGF-β suppressed the IL-10–mediated IgG, IgM, and IgA secretions by $sIgD^-$ B cells. Naive B cells could not be induced to secrete IgA by TGF-β and IL-10 after cross-linking of sIg, suggesting that ligation of CD40 was an obligatory signal required for commitment of $sIgD^+$ B lymphocytes to IgA secretion. IL-10 and TGF-β therefore seem to functionally cooperate as switch factors for naive human B lymphocytes to secrete IgA. In aggregate, the data suggest an important role for IL-10 in regulating B-cell proliferation and differentiation. The nature of this effect seems to be dependent upon the way that B cells are activated (e.g., CD40 vs. sIg), on the presence or absence of other cytokines, and on the state of differentiation of the B cell.

In a different system, Pecanha et al. [26] demonstrated that IL-10 inhibited Ig secretion by dextran-conjugated, anti-$\delta$-antibody–activated B cells as well as the Ag-specific responses of B cells to TNP-Ficoll (a T-independent type 2 Ag) in the presence of IL-5. IL-10 did not inhibit on IL-2–stimulated responses, indicating that its inhibitory effect was selective for a specific mode of B-cell activation. IL-10 also did not inhibit anti-$\delta$-dextran–stimulated B-cell proliferation, and the IL-10–induced inhibition of Ig secretion did not result from suppression of IFN-$\gamma$ production. These data suggest that IL-10 exerts different effects on B cells depending on their maturation stage. IL-10 seems to promote early phases in B-cell differentiation and suppress the late steps in the pathways of Ag-stimulated B-cell activation.

## C. Effects of IL-10 on Mast Cells

IL-10 also enhanced the IL-3– and IL-4–dependent growth of mast cell lines [15], most dramatically if all three cytokines were added simultaneously. IL-10 alone had no significant effect on proliferation, but seemed to enhance mast cell viability. IL-10 also enhanced colony formation by mast cell progenitors, but only in combination with IL-3 and/or IL-4. In addition, Ghildyal et al. [27] recently showed that IL-10 enhanced expression of the mucosal MC protease MMCP-2 gene in IL-3–pretreated bone marrow–derived mast cells. Withdrawal of IL-10 from the culture medium resulted in the complete suppression of MMCP-2 induction, indicating that IL-10 is also an important regulator of transcription of genes encoding secretory granule neutral proteases.

## D. Effects of IL-10 on Macrophages and Monocytes

In their initial studies, Mosmann et al. reported that IL-10 exerted its effect on the production of IFN-$\gamma$ by Th1 cells only when macrophages were utilized as APC [21]. These studies have since been confirmed in different (but related) systems by other groups. De Waal Malefyt et al. [28] reported that hIL-10 and vIL-10 strongly reduced monocyte-dependent antigen-specific proliferation of human T-cell clones via down-regulation of class II MHC on monocytes. Inhibition was most efficient when monocytes were preincubated with IL-10, but significant reductions were also observed without pretreatment [28]. While the reduction of class II MHC on monocytes was reversed by IL-4 and to some extent by IFN-$\gamma$, neither IL-4 nor IL-2 reversed the effects of IL-10 on T-cell proliferation. This indicates that the proliferation-inhibiting activity of IL-10 in this system was not solely mediated by MHC class II down-regulation on APC. In addition to inhibiting T-cell proliferation, IL-10 also attenuated Ag-induced $Ca^{2+}$ flux in T-cell clones as compared to controls [28], suggesting an influence of IL-10 on rather early events in T-cell activation. All of these inhibitory effects of IL-10 were dependent on the presence of metabolically active monocytes as APC; IL-10 was without effect when B cells were used as APC or if requirements for APC were bypassed.

Work by Taga and Tosato [22] also showed that IL-10 inhibited the IL-2 production and proliferation of naive human T lymphocytes in the presence of monocytes. This effect of IL-10 on T-cell function was not limited to selected subtypes of T cells, but affected CD4+, CD8+, CD45RA high, and CD45RA low T cells to a similar degree. In contrast to observations by de Waal Malefyt et al. [14], Taga and Tosato reported complete reversal of IL-10 effects on T-cell proliferation by exogenously added IL-2 or IL-4. This treatment did not reverse the suppression of IFN-$\gamma$ production, however. Taken together, the data indicate that IL-10 exerts suppressive effects on T-cell proliferation and IFN-$\gamma$ production via monocytes/macrophages as APC. These effects may be only partially mediated by down-regulation of MHC class II antigens and might also be mediated via regulation of costimulatory factors as well.

In addition to serving as an inhibitor of monocyte function, IL-10 has been shown to be produced by activated monocytes and to autoregulate endogenous cytokine synthesis. De Waal Malefyt et al. [14] demonstrated that LPS-activated human monocytes produced high levels of IL-10 and that IL-10 inhibited the production of IL-1$\alpha$, TNF-$\alpha$, GM-CSF, G-CSF by 80–100% in monocytes. Effects on IL-1$\beta$ and IL-6 production were less dramatic, and IL-10 had no influence on monocyte IL-8 production. IL-10 inhibited monocyte cytokine production by inhibiting gene transcription. Because neutralizing mAbs for IL-10 enhanced MHC class II antigen expression, IL-10 may act as an autoregulator of monocyte function. Effects of IL-10 on the production of TNF-$\alpha$ or IL-1 by monocytes or macrophages have been confirmed by several other groups [29, 30], emphasizing the importance of IL-10 as a modulator of inflammatory immune responses.

In addition to effects of IL-10 on cytokine production and monocyte/macrophage APC function, IL-10 has been shown to inhibit parasite killing and nitrogen oxide production by activated macrophages [31], presumably by inhibiting IFN-$\gamma$–induced synthesis of nitric oxide synthetase in activated macrophages [32]. In addition, IL-10 synergizes with IL-4 and TGF-$\beta$ to inhibit macrophage cytotoxic activity [33].

### E. Effects of IL-10 on Langerhans Cells and Dendritic Cells

Effects of IL-10 on Langerhans cells (LC) and dendritic cells (DC) have not been extensively studied to date. Because we [17, 34, 35] and subsequently others [36] have established that activated keratinocytes are a source of IL-10, it is important to assess the effect of this cytokine on the APC function of epidermal Langerhans cells. Recent data from our laboratory demonstrate that IL-10 inhibits the production of IFN-$\gamma$ in a LC-supported anti-CD3 proliferation assay by 50–60% when naive peripheral lymph node CD4+ T lymphocytes are used as responder cells. Effects on IFN-$\gamma$ production by T cells were completely reversed by a neutralizing anti–IL-10 mAb. As reported in other systems [7], IL-10 was most efficient when LC were precultured with the cytokine for at least 24 h, although addition of the cytokine directly into cultures containing LC and T cells also resulted in significant inhibition of IFN-$\gamma$ production. IL-10 had similar inhibitory effects on the production of IL-2 by peripheral CD4+ T cells in a LC-supported anti-CD3 assay. Other cytokines (including GM-CSF and TNF-$\alpha$) did not exert similar effects on LC-induced IFN-$\gamma$ production. In contrast to effects of IL-10 on MHC class II expression by B cells or monocytes (enhancement or inhibition, respectively), IL-10 did not significantly alter class II expression on LC after a 48-h culture period. IL-10 also did not seem to enhance or decrease LC survival in vitro. Furthermore, IL-10 did not enhance or inhibit proliferation of peripheral lymph node CD4+ T lymphocytes induced by allogeneic LC, or anti-CD3 mAb in the presence of syngeneic LC.

One report has dealt with the effects of IL-10 on blood dendritic cells. Ding and Shevach [37] showed that IL-10 had no suppressive effect on the lectin-driven response of mesenteric lymph node T cells in a dendritic cell (or B cell)–supported proliferation assay [37]. In contrast, macrophage-induced proliferation of CD4+ and CD8+ T lymphocytes was inhibited significantly and to a similar extent. Taken together these data indicate that LC and DC are probably unlike monocytes and B cells in their response towards IL-10 in that they show no MHC class II changes, no cellular proliferation, and no change in viability. Still it was shown at least for the LC that IL-10 exerts a significant influence on the IFN-$\gamma$ production of T cells stimulated with IL-10–treated LC. More studies will be necessary to determine how IL-10 acts on cells of the dendritic lineage.

## V. IN VIVO EFFECTS OF IL-10

It is well established that antibody production and delayed type hypersensitivity (DTH) responses are mutually exclusive during many immune responses [38]. As mentioned earlier, there is good evidence that Th1 and Th2 cells appear to be differentially responsible for antibody and DTH responses and that these functional differences are reflected by the cytokines that they secrete. Several actions of Th1 and Th2 cell–derived cytokines are consistent with these mutually inhibitory and/or self-stimulatory effects. Gajewski and Fitch have shown that IFN-$\gamma$ is an essential growth factor for Th1 cells [4] and Fernandez-Botran et al. [5] demonstrated that IFN-$\gamma$ inhibited proliferation responses of Th2 cells induced by IL-2 and IL-4. These investigators [5] and others [39] have also provided evidence that IL-4 preferentially stimulates growth of Th2 cells in vitro. Existing data regarding IL-10 suggest that IL-10 inhibits Th1 function and indirectly augments Th2 growth in mixed T-cell populations, perhaps as a result of decreased IFN-$\gamma$ production. These effects of IL-10 are, on the other hand, partially counteracted by IL-4, a cytokine known to stimulate Th1 cell growth and cytokine production [4, 5]. This situation is analogous to the effects of the Th1 cell products IL-2 and IFN-$\gamma$ that have opposite effects on Th2 clones [4, 5]. It seems likely that it is the balanced production of various cytokines at different times in the course of an immunological reaction that prevents the immune system from becoming locked in either the Th1 or Th2 mode. Such a lock would certainly be ultimately harmful to the individual in that it would deprive the body of the overall important flexibility needed to react to different stimuli. The role that individual cytokines play in immune responses in vivo can be best studied in knock-out transgenic mice where complete (cytokine) genes are rendered nonfunctional by gene-targeting. Indeed W. Müller has developed IL-10 knock-out transgenic mice recently [40]. Although detailed analyses of these animals are not yet available, it seems that IL-10–deficient mice tend to be smaller than their normal littermates and may die prematurely. In contrast to results of Ishida et al. [24], where continuous postnatal administration of anti–IL-10 mAb resulted in elimination of their CD5+ (Ly-1) B cells and caused IgM deficiency, IL-10–deficient mice had normal IgM levels. These results emphasize the importance of these knock-out experiments, which are thus far the only existing tools for studying the physiological effects of cytokines.

Studies on the involvement of cytokines in pathological events are more straightforward. For IL-10, the type of immune response that reflects vigorous Th2 cell stimulation is of greatest interest. One of the earliest of these studies was performed by Heinzel et al. [41], who studied production of IL-10 and other CD4+ T cell–derived cytokines during resolving and progressing murine leishmaniasis in vivo. These investigators observed distinct patterns of Th1- and Th2-derived cytokines in leishmaniasis-resistant and -susceptible mice, respectively. Whereas C57BL/6 (resistant) mice developed a Th1-like response (as determined by extracting RNA from draining lymph node cells and assessing IFN-$\gamma$ and IL-2 mRNAs), BALB/c (susceptible) mice showed a Th2-type response by expressing IL-4 and IL-10 mRNAs. Since IFN-$\gamma$ is believed to be critical for the activation of monocytes in parasitic infection, it is probably the down-regulation of this cytokine by IL-10 that is responsible for the inefficient host response of susceptible animals to leishmania. This mechanism is supported by studies performed by Silva et al. [42] in mice infected with *Trypanosoma cruzi* that revealed that susceptible mouse strains mounted a much stronger IL-10 response than resistant strains. These investigators also demonstrated that preincubation of murine peritoneal macrophages with IL-10 significantly reduced the inhibitory effects of IFN-$\gamma$ on the intracellular replication of *T. cruzi*. Administration of anti–IFN-$\gamma$ mAb in vivo made resistant mice susceptible to fatal *T. cruzi* infection, confirming the importance of IFN-$\gamma$ in maintaining host resistance in this setting. Similar findings have been reported by Mosmann et al. in *Nippostrongylus brasiliensis* infection [43] and by Vella and Pearce in mice infected with *Schistosoma mansoni* [44].

This concept has been extended to humans infected with *Mycobacterium leprae* by Yamamura et la. [45]. Whereas IFN-$\gamma$ and IL-2 mRNAs were most abundant in lesions of patients with the benign (tuberculoid) form of leprosy, IL-4, IL-5, and IL-10 were dominant in lesions of lepromatous leprosy. These data correlate well with the aforementioned concept of a poor host response against chronic infectious diseases in the setting of a predominate Th2 response.

Surprisingly, similar findings were reported by Gazzinelli et al. [46] in the murine AIDS model. These investigators reported that spleen cells from virally infected mice released cytokines characteristic of a Th0 (IFN-$\gamma$, IL-2, IL-4, IL-5, IL-10) pattern in the early stages of infection and converted to a Th2 pattern after 2–4 weeks. This is accompanied by high serum IgE levels in these mice. These findings may help explain some of the clinical manifestations of the disease in that these lymphokines can induce chronic B-cell activation, a central feature of the disorder. In addition, the ability of IL-10 to inhibit cytokine production by CD4+ Th1 cells, as well as CD8+ T cells, may be responsible for the progressive loss of CTL responses to self plus X and alloantigens in vitro, and also loss of the ability of AIDS mice to reject allogeneic skin grafts.

## VI. IL-10 AND SKIN

Because IL-10 is a recent entrant in the field of epidermal cytokines, comparatively little is known about the effects of this cytokine in the skin. We initially identified IL-10 as an epidermal-derived cytokine involved in the induction of contact sensitivity in mice [17, 34, 35]. While investigating the early changes in the cytokine pattern of the epidermis in the induction phase of contact sensitivity, we observed that IFN-γ and interferon-induced protein 10 were selectively and reproducibly decreased 6 or 8 h after hapten application, respectively, although the inflammatory process persisted [34]. We reasoned that epidermis-derived IL-10 might be responsible for the rapid reduction in the mRNA signals of these two cytokines. Making use of a sensitive, quantitative RT-PCR technique, we detected IL-10 mRNA in epidermal cells. Whereas the baseline level of production was found to be rather low, stimulation of the cells by contact sensitizers like trinitrochlorobenzene (TNCB) led to induction of high levels of specific IL-10 mRNA. A time-course analysis of the IL-10 mRNA changes is shown in Figure 2. Induction of IL-10 mRNA occurred within 4 h of hapten application, reached maximum levels after 12 h, and was down-regulated by 24 h after application of allergen. Cell de-

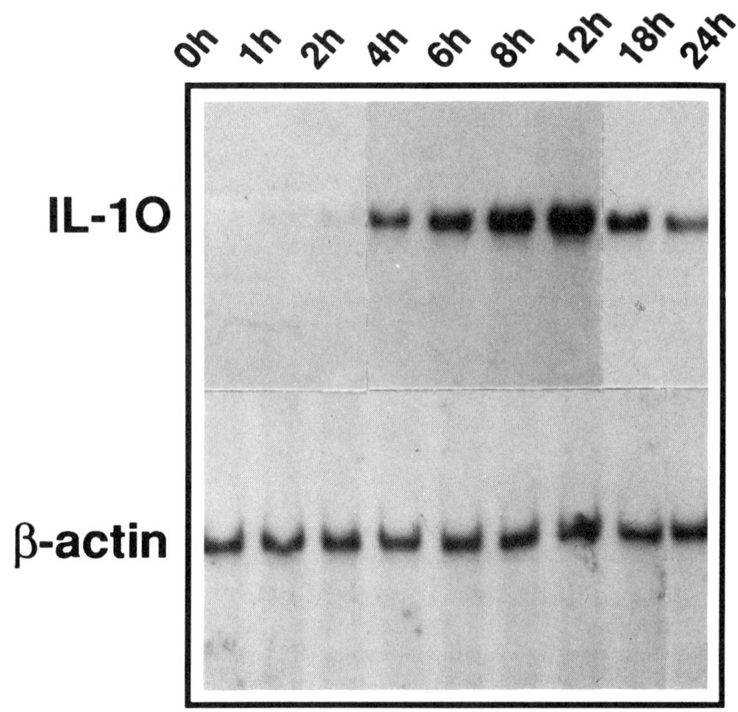


**Fig. 2** Time course of IL-10 up-regulation following application of 3% TNCB to murine skin. Mouse ears were treated with 3% trinitrochlorobenzene and RNA extracted at various times [3]. RNA was subjected to reverse-transcriptase PCR using primers specific for IL-10 or β-actin control, followed by a liquid hybridization with specific, internal oligonucleotides. Time points are as shown.

pletion assays using cocktails of mAb and complement to selectively deplete LC, Thy1$^+$ dendritic epidermal cells (DEC), or infiltrating CD4+/CD8+ T lymphocytes revealed that epidermal keratinocytes were the major cellular source of IL-10 mRNA (Fig. 3). This finding was supported by studies demonstrating that PAM 212 cells (a spontaneously transformed murine keratinocyte cell line) also contained IL-10 mRNA after stimulation with phorbol ester (Fig. 3). The enhancement of IL-10 mRNA levels in epidermis was specific for allergens and did not occur when tolerogens, irritants, or vehicle control were applied to skin. To determine if epidermal cells could also produce IL-10 protein, a solid phase immunoadsorption technique was used to precipitate IL-10 protein from $^{35}$S-labeled epidermal cell supernatants with a specific mAb for IL-10. As shown in Figure 4, significant amounts of IL-10 protein were specifically immunoprecipitated from the supernatants of

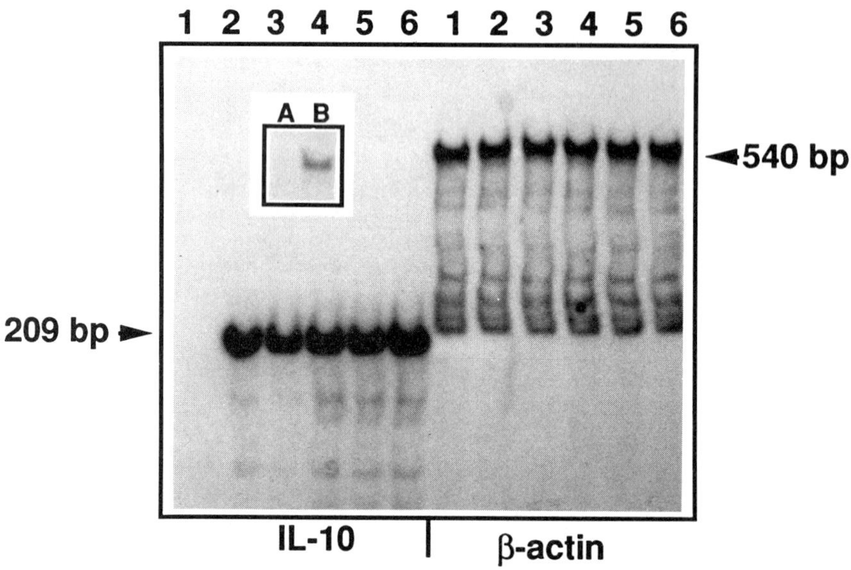


**Fig. 3** Cell depletion assay for IL-10. Epidermal RNA was extracted from epidermal cell suspensions following: no treatment (lane 1), 4 h after application of 3% TNCB only (lane 2), 4 h after application of 3% TNCB plus control mAb and complement treatment (lane 3), 4 h after 3% TNCB plus depletion of LC (lane 4), 4 h after 3% TNCB plus depletion of Thy1$^+$ dendritic epidermal cells (lane 5), and 4 h after 3% TNCB plus depletion of CD4+/CD8+ T cells (lane 6). RNA was then subjected to RT-PCR and liquid hybridization [4]. β-Actin controls are shown on the right side. The insert shows signals derived from untreated (lane A) or phorbolester-treated PAM212 cells (a spontaneously transformed keratinocyte cell line).

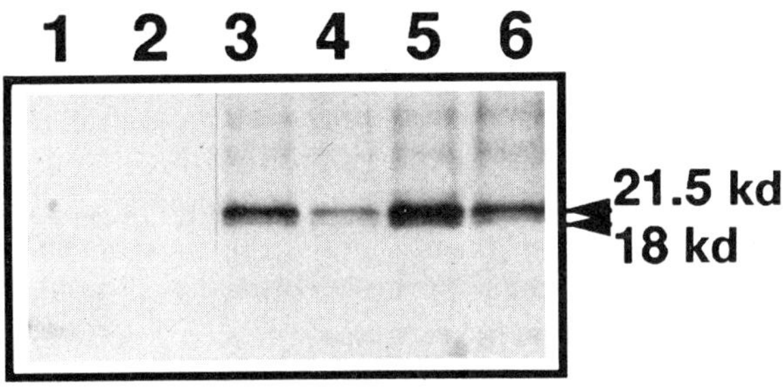


**Fig. 4** Immunoprecipitation of IL-10 protein from epidermal cell suspensions. Epidermal cell suspensions were stimulated with allergens, and IL-10 was specifically immunoprecipitated after 12 h [3]. Lane 1, untreated epidermal cell supernatants; lane 2, $TNBSO_3$-treated epidermal cell supernatants preincubated with mIL-10; lane 3, $TNBSO_3$-treated epidermal cell supernatants; lane 4, $DNBSO_3$-treated epidermal cell supernatants; lane 5, epidermal cell supernatants preincubated with mock supernatants; lane 6, epidermal cell supernatants preincubated with mIL-1$\alpha$.

allergen-stimulated epidermal cells; only minimal amounts were produced by nonstimulated epidermal cells. Rivas and Ullrich later confirmed our results when they showed that PAM 212 cells irradiated with UV light contained mRNA and protein for IL-10 [36].

In aggregate, these data indicate that activated keratinocytes produce both IL-10 mRNA and protein. These findings are important to immunodermatologists for several reasons. First, IL-10 is known to be an antiinflammatory cytokine [14, 29]. Our data suggest that IL-10 may exert analogous antiinflammatory effects in the epidermis in the initiation phase of contact sensitivity. IL-10 is up-regulated later than all other cytokines tested, may inhibit IFN-$\gamma$ and IP-10 production, and may potentially have similar effects on IL-1$\alpha$, IL-1$\beta$, or TNF-$\alpha$ (as has been shown for monocytes and macrophages [14]). One role of IL-10 may be to prevent severe damage to the skin by damping the risk of necrosis by an ongoing inflammatory process. Other relevant mechanisms may include direct effects of IL-10 on the APC activity of epidermal LC, as summarized earlier. In the microenvironment of the epidermis IL-10 may promote induction of a Th2 response by inhibiting IFN-$\gamma$ production by Th1 cells, thereby facilitating the outgrowth of Th2 cells. Another possible mechanism of action of IL-10 on LC may involve the down-regulation of a costimulatory molecule needed for the activation of Th1 cells. IL-10 production by epidermal KC may explain earlier findings in our laboratory that LC selectively promoted outgrowth of Th2 cell clones [47]. Further studies will be needed to address these questions.

## VII. CONCLUSIONS

Although comparatively little is known about the details of the mechanisms of action of IL-10, this novel cytokine certainly is already of great interest to immunologists and (after having been described as a product of activated keratinocytes) immunodermatologists. IL-10's activity as an inhibitor of cytokine production and as potential regulator of inflammatory skin reactions is particularly intriguing. The possible mechanisms of action of IL-10 have been discussed and include effects on the cytokine release of keratinocytes, as well as direct effects on the APC function of epidermal LC. Contact of LC with IL-10 or with cytokines induced by IL-10 may bias these important APC towards induction of a specialized subset of T cells in the regional lymph nodes. The goal of future experiments will be to define the mechanisms of action of IL-10 more precisely and to elucidate its role in the regulation of physiological (and pathological) immune and inflammatory reactions in the skin and elsewhere.

## ACKNOWLEDGMENTS

The author gratefully thanks Dr. Mark Udey for reviewing the manuscript and Dr. Stephen Katz for his continued support and mentorship. This work was supported by the Deutsche Forschungsgemeinschaft.

## REFERENCES

1. T. R. Mosmann, H. Cherwinski, M. W. Bond, M. A. Giedlin, and R. L. Coffmann, *J. Immunol. 136*, 2348 (1986).
2. D. J. Cher and T. R. Mosmann, *J. Immunol. 138*, 3688 (1987).
3. K. D. Brown, S. M. Zurawski, T. R. Mosmann, and G. Zurawski, *J. Immunol. 142*, 679 (1989).
4. T. F. Gajewski and F. W. Fitch, *J. Immunol. 140*, 4245 (1988).
5. R. Fernandez-Botran, V. M. Sanders, T. R. Mosmann, and E. Vitetta, *J. Exp. Med. 168*, 543 (1988).
6. J. B. Horowitz, J. Kaye, P. J. Conrad, M. Katz, and C. A. Janeway, *Proc. Natl. Acad. Sci. USA 83*, 1886 (1986).
7. D. F. Fiorentino, M. W. Bond, and T. R. Mosmann, *J. Exp. Med. 170*, 2081 (1989).
8. K. W. Moore, P. Vieira, D. F. Fiorentino, M. L. Trounstine, T. A. Khan, and T. R. Mosmann, *Science 248*, 1230 (1990).
9. J. M. Kim, C. I. Brannan, N. G. Copeland, N. A. Jenkins, T. A. Khan, and K. W. Moore, *J. Immunol. 148*, 3618 (1992).
10. F. Rousset, E. Garcia, T. Defrance, C. Peronne, N. Vezzio, D. H. Hsu, R. Kastelein, K. W. Moore, and J. Banchereau, *Proc. Natl. Acad. Sci. USA 89*, 1890 (1992).

11. N. F. Go, B. E. Castle, R. Barrett, R. Kastelein, W. Dang, T. R. Mosmann, K. W. Moore, and M. Howard, *J. Exp. Med. 172*, 1625 (1990).
12. T. R. Mosmann, J. H. Schumacher, D. F. Fiorentino, J. Leverah, K. W. Moore, and M. W. Bond, *J. Immunol. 145*, 2938 (1990).
13. A. O'Garra, R. Chang, N. Go, R. Hastings, G. Haughton, and M. Howard, *Eur. J. Immunol. 22*, 711 (1992).
14. R. de Waal Malefyt, J. Abrams, B. Bennett, C. G. Figdor, and J. de Vries, *J. Exp. Med. 174*, 1209 (1991).
15. L. Thompson-Snipes, V. Dhar, M. W. Bond, T. R. Mosmann, K. W. Moore, and D. M. Rennick, *J. Exp. Med. 173*, 507 (1991).
16. T. R. Mosmann and K. W. Moore, *Immunol. Today 12*, (1991).
17. A. H. Enk and S. I. Katz, *J. Invest. Dermatol. 98*, 578 (1992).
18. I. A. MacNeil, T. Suda, K. W. Moore, T. R. Mosmann, and A. Zlotnik, *J. Immunol. 145*, 4167 (1990).
19. A. Bendelac and R. H. Schwartz, *Nature 353*, 68 (1991).
20. W. F. Chen and A. Zlotnik, *J. Immunol. 147*, 528 (1991).
21. D. F. Fiorentino, A. Zlotnik, P. Vieira, T. R. Mosmann, M. Howard, K. W. Moore, and A. O'Garra, *J. Immunol. 146*, 3444 (1991).
22. K. Taga and G. Tosato, *J. Immunol. 148*, 1143 (1992).
23. A. O'Garra, G. Stapleton, V. Dhar, M. Pearce, J. Schumacher, H. Rugo, D. Barbis, A. Stall, J. Cupp, K. Moore, et al., *Int. Immunol. 2*, 821 (1990).
24. H. Ishida, R. Hastings, J. Kearney, and M. Howard, *J. Exp. Med. 175*, 1213 (1992).
25. T. Defrance, B. Vanbervliet, F. Briere, I. Durand, F. Rousset, and J. Banchereau, *J. Exp. Med. 175*, 671 (1992).
26. L. M. T. Pecanha, C. M. Snapper, A. Lees, and J. Mond, *J. Immunol. 148*, 3427 (1992).
27. N. Ghildyal, H. P. McNeil, M. F. Gurish, K. F. Austen, and R. L. Stevens, *J. Biol. Chem. 267*, 8473 (1992).
28. R. de Waal Malefyt, J. Haanen, H. Spits, M. G. Roncarolo, A. te Velde, C. Figdor, K. Johnson, R. Kastelein, H. Yssel, and J. de Vries, *J. Exp. Med. 174*, 915 (1991).
29. C. Bogdan, Y. Yodovotz, and C. Nathan, *J. Exp. Med. 174*, 1549 (1991).
30. P. Ralph, I. Nakoinz, A. Sampson-Johannes, S. Fong, D. Lowe, H. Y. Min, and L. Lin, *J. Immunol. 148*, 808 (1992).
31. R. T. Gazzinelli, I. P. Oswald, S. L. James, and A. Sher, *J. Immunol. 148*, 1792 (1992).
32. F. Q. Cunha, S. Moncada, and F. Y. Liew, *Biochem. Biophys. Res. Commun. 182*, 1155 (1992).
33. I. P. Oswald, R. T. Gazzinelli, A. Sher, and S. L. James, *J. Immunol. 148*, 3578 (1992).
34. A. H. Enk, J. Knop, and S. I. Katz, *Arch. Derm. Res.* (1991).
35. A. H. Enk and S. I. Katz, *J. Immunol. 149*, 92 (1992).
36. J. M. Rivas and S. E. Ullrich, *J. Invest. Dermatol. 98*, 578 (1992).
37. L. Ding and E. M. Shevach, *J. Immunol. 148*, 3133 (1992).
38. C. R. Parish, *Transplant. Rev. 13*, 35 (1972).

39. S. Swain, A. D. Weinberg, and M. English, *J. Immunol. 144*, 1788 (1989).
40. W. E. Paul, *Nature 357*, 16 (1992).
41. F. P. Heinzel, M. D. Sadick, S. S. Mutha, and R. M. Locksley, *Proc. Natl. Acad. Sci. USA 88*, 7011 (1991).
42. J. S. Silva, P. J. Morrissey, K. H. Grabstein, K. M. Mohler, D. Anderson, and S. G. Reed, *J. Exp. Med. 175*, 169 (1992).
43. A. Sher, D. Fiorentino, P. Caspar, E. Pearce, and T. Mosmann, *J. Immunol. 147*, 2713 (1991).
44. A. T. Vella and E. J. Pearce, *J. Immunol. 148*, 2283 (1992).
45. M. Yamamura, K. Uyemura, R. J. Deans, K. Weinberg, T. H. Rea, B. R. Bloom, and R. L. Modlin, *Science 254*, 277 (1991).
46. R. T. Gazzinelli, M. Makino, S. K. Chattopadhyay, C. M. Snapper, A. Sher, A. W. Hugin, and H. Morse, *J. Immunol. 148*, 182 (1992).
47. C. Hauser and S. I. Katz, *Proc. Natl. Acad. Sci. USA 85*, 5625 (1988).

# 6

# T-Cell–Derived Lymphokines

**Martin Röcken***
*National Institute of Allergy and Infectious Diseases, National Institutes of Health*
*Bethesda, Maryland*

**Kai M. Müller and Conrad Hauser**
*Hôpital Cantonal Universitaire*
*Geneva, Switzerland*

## I. INTRODUCTION

Antigen-specific immune responses are mediated by three types of cells: antigen-presenting cells (APC), T lymphocytes, and B lymphocytes. CD4+ T-helper/inducer lymphocytes are considered to be the principal regulatory cells in this network.

Antigen-specific immune responses are initiated when antigen is processed by APC and presented to antigen-specific T lymphocytes. T lymphocytes activated by APC, i.e., primed T lymphocytes, are capable of antigen-specific interaction either with B lymphocytes or with other antigen-loaded target cells. Thus, primed T lymphocytes may exert effector functions. The target cell–T-cell interaction can consist of direct cell-cell contact and/or be mediated by cytokines secreted by T cells in response to activation. In contrast, nonactivated, i.e., resting T lymphocytes, are thought not to be capable of acting as effector cells.

Cytokines are soluble polypeptides. They are potent hormonelike pleiotropic factors that control a wide range of biological functions in their target cells, such as cell growth, differentiation, and immunoglobulin production. One group of cytokines that originally was thought to act selectively between lymphocytes was named interleukins.

Because of their distinct effects and their high biological activity, T cell–derived lymphokines (LK) are considered to be among the most potent regu-

**Current affiliation*: Ludwig-Maximilians-University Munich, Munich, Germany.

lators of immune responses. Here we review some of the properties of LK with special reference to their function in effector target cell–T-cell interaction. Since CD4+ T cells are the main source of T-cell LK, we will focus on the LK produced by these cells. A brief account will be given of CD4+ T-cell subsets that have been defined according to their distinct lymphokine pattern. Furthermore, a short overview is given on the mechanisms involved in the differentiation of T-helper cell subsets.

## II. LYMPHOKINES AND T-CELL FUNCTION

### A. General Remarks

Nonprimed, resting CD4+ T lymphocytes produce IL-2 but no other LK when stimulated in vitro with T cell activators such as lectins, antigen-bearing APC, or ionomycine and phorbol esters. In contrast, previously activated CD4+ T lymphocytes may produce a large panel of LK, such as IL-2, IL-3, IL-4, IL-5, IL-6, IL-10 and IFN-$\gamma$ when restimulated with the same T cell activators [1–3]. It has also become clear that, after primary activation, CD4+ T cells have no effector functions other than the production of their autocrine growth factor IL-2. This stands in contrast to previously activated CD4+ T cells that become capable of subserving various effector functions upon reactivation. From these observations it was inferred that the production of LK other than IL-2 may be associated with effector functions exerted on other cell types.

### B. Lymphokines and the Definition of T-Helper Cell Subsets

In 1986 Mosmann and coworkers reported that many long-term cultured CD4+ T-cell clones did not produce a random pattern of LK [4]. They found that long-term cultured murine CD4+ T-cell clones could be divided into two distinct subsets, according to the LK profile they secreted upon activation. One group of CD4+ T-cell clones preferentially produced IL-2 and IFN-$\gamma$ as distinct LK and was named Th1. The other group of CD4+ T cell clones produced IL-4 and IL-5 but neither IL-2 nor IFN-$\gamma$. This second group was named Th2 [4]. Extension of the analysis to further LK confirmed that the two subsets produced soluble polypeptides unique for each subset but shared the release of others (Table 1) [5,6]. Studies in many experimental systems have subsequently demonstrated that the pattern of LK secreted by CD4+ T lymphocytes upon stimulation is biologically relevant since it was closely related to distinct functions both in vitro and in vivo. Later it was reported that clones exist that produce LK typical for both Th1 and Th2; they had an unrestricted LK pattern and were named Th0 [7]. The unrestricted

**Table 1** Lymphokines Secreted by Th1 and Th2 Cells

| Lymphokine | Th1 | Th2 |
|---|---|---|
| IL-2 | + + | — |
| IFN-$\gamma$ | + + | — |
| TNF-$\beta$ (LT) | + + | — |
| GM-CSF | + + | + |
| TNF-$\alpha$ | + + | + |
| IL-3 | + + | + + |
| IL-4 | — | + + |
| IL-5 | — | + + |
| IL-6 | — | + + |
| IL-10 (CSIF) | — | + + |

LT, lymphotoxin; CSIF, cytokine synthesis inhibiting factor.
*Source*: Ref. 6.

LK pattern of Th0 clones resembled polyclonal CD4+ T-cell populations that are restimulated after primary activation. A Th0-like LK pattern has also recently been reported for single CD4+ thymocytes after in vitro activation [8].

### C. Lymphokine Pattern and Function In Vitro

The in vitro effector functions of CD4+ T-cell clones and lines of the Th1 and Th2 type have been extensively studied. Since the interaction of most CD4+ T cells is restricted to MHC class II+ APC, these latter cells were chosen as targets.

MHC class II+ macrophages can serve as APC for CD4+ T cells. In turn, this interaction can modify effector functions or subsequent antigen presentation. Th1 but not Th2 clones were capable of inducing macrophage activation (tumor cytotoxicity) [9]. This activity was inhibited by antibodies to IFN-$\gamma$, indicating that this LK was the responsible T-cell–derived macrophage-activating factor [9]. As a consequence of interaction with Th2, the capacity of APC such as macrophages to present antigen to Th1 has been shown to be downregulated. IL-10, a recently cloned Th2 LK, was subsequently identified as the factor causing the decrease in antigen-presenting activity [6,10]. This implied that Th2 cells could indirectly influence the response of Th1 cells. When the two types of clones were tested for cytotoxic T-cell activity, Th2 clones were noncytolytic or weakly cytolytic. In contrast, Th1 clones showed both TNF-dependent and TNF-independent cytotoxicity [11].

The interaction of T-helper cell subsets and B cells attracted a wide interest. The production of immunoglobulin isotypes by B cells was most frequently measured as a B-cell response. While most Th1 clones were unable to induce immunoglobulin production [12], some Th1 clones with low-level IFN-$\gamma$ production stimulated IgG2A secretion by B cells [13,14]. The inability of most Th1 clones to stimulate immunoglobulin production was attributed to the high amounts of IFN-$\gamma$ produced by these cells, since IFN-$\gamma$ at high doses was previously shown to inhibit immunoglobulin production [15]. In contrast to Th1 clones, most Th2 clones were capable of inducing immunoglobulin synthesis in B cells [12–14]. However, the isotype pattern differed. High concentrations of IgG1 and IgE were observed. The addition of antibodies to IL-4 completely abrogated IgE but not IgG1 production, suggesting that IL-4 was an absolute requirement for IgE production [13]. IL-4 was later shown to switch B cells from IgG1 to IgE production by inducing a rearrangement of the immunoglobulin-constant region genes. IL-4 has remained until now the only known IgE-inducing factor. IL-5 and IL-6, two other Th2-characteristic LK, were shown to enhance immunoglobulin production including IgE but not to be essential for IgE synthesis [16].

Although both Th1 and Th2 are very efficiently stimulated by antigen-bearing epidermal Langerhans cells to proliferate and to produce LK [17], it is at present unknown what functions they modify within this cell, which is closely related to other types of dendritic cells. It is also unknown what functions T-helper cell subsets induce in nonprofessional APC that have been induced to express MHC class II molecules. One report, however, documented that Th1 clones can be rendered nonresponsive to restimulation after interaction with MHC class II+ keratinocytes [18].

In conclusion, many in vitro studies demonstrated the close relation between the LK pattern of T-helper cell subsets and the distinct functions they induce in target cells.

## D. Function of Murine T-Helper Cell Subsets and their Lymphokines In Vivo

As expected from the in vitro experiments, the occurrence of Th1- and Th2-like cells has been found to be associated with various appropriate and inappropriate immune responses in vivo.

Th1-like cells are thought to be responsible for inflammatory reactions such as contact sensitivity and delayed-type hypersensitivity [19–21]. The latter was shown to be partially dependent on IFN-$\gamma$ [22]. Acute GvH was also shown to be mediated by CD4+ T-cell clones with a Th1 phenotype

[23, 24]. It is conceivable that the high titers of virus-neutralizing isotype IgG2A observed in acute viral infections are induced by the activation of Th1-like cells [15]. Moreover, it has been demonstrated that the induction of Th1-like cells by infections and infestations is frequently associated with protective immunity [25]. For example, in murine disease models with *Leishmania major, Trichinella spiralis,* and *Schistosoma mansoni*, the induction of Th1 cells was followed by successful elimination of the parasites. Th1 cells have even been implicated in immunity against cancer since tumor-infiltrating CD4+ T lymphocytes were reported to show a predominant Th1 LK pattern [26].

Conversely, chronic GvH as well as some autoimmune diseases have been thought to be mediated by Th2-like cells [27, 28]. In the above-mentioned parasitic diseases the induction of an immune response characterized by predominant Th2-like cells has often been correlated with disease progression or persistence [25].

High IgE levels, commonly observed in parasitic diseases such as infestation with Nippostrongylus brasiliensis, were shown to be decreased by the administration of antibodies to IL-4 as well as by the injection of IFN-$\gamma$, the natural antagonist of IL-4 with regard to IgE synthesis. IL-5, another Th2 LK, also plays an important biological role in parasitic diseases because in N. brasiliensis infestation blood eosinophilia was prevented by the administration of antibodies to IL-5 [29].

## E. Evidence for Th-Cell Subsets in the Human

Initial analysis of human CD4+ T-cell clones has cast doubt upon the existence of Th1 and Th2 subsets in humans since most of them produced a Th0-like LK pattern. Recent reports, however, have shown that Th1- and Th2-like cells can be cloned from peripheral blood as well as from tissue lesions with lymphocytic infiltrations [30].

Antigen-specific clones producing a predominant Th1 profile were isolated from patients with allergic contact dermatitis [30] but also from patients with bacterial diseases such as Lyme borreliosis [31] or leprosy [32, 33]. Purified protein derivative (PPD)-specific Th-cell clones from BCG-vaccinated volunteers also had a Th1 phenotype [34].

Th2 cells were obtained from patients with parasitic infestations such as toxocariasis [34]. Th2-like cells also seem to play a role in atopic diseases since allergen-specific clones secreting IL-4 were prepared from atopic donors. Such clones were obtained from vernal conjunctivitis [35] and atopic dermatitis lesions [30]. Although Th2 clones were also isolated from the blood, their frequency was higher in skin lesions, indicating that allergen-specific Th2 cells accumulate preferentially at the lesional site [30]. Most of these clones were capable of stimulating IgE synthesis that was critically dependent on IL-4 production. IL-5 and IL-6, two other Th2-typic LK, were shown to amplify IL-4–induced IgE release [36]. Further support for the involvement of IL-4 in increased IgE synthesis in atopics was provided by the observation that spontaneous in vitro IgE synthesis by lymphocytes from patients with atopic dermatitis was partially inhibited by anti-IL-4 antibodies and IFN-$\gamma$ [37].

In vitro analysis of human lymphocytes, however, bears the disadvantage of possible artifacts. To resolve this problem, in situ hybridization for LK messenger RNA was performed in skin biopsies from cutaneous late-phase reactions of patients with allergic asthma [38]. Positive hybridization signals for IL-4 and IL-5 but not IL-2 and IFN-$\gamma$ were identified, suggesting a Th2-like response in vivo.

## III. LYMPHOKINE INDUCTION AND LYMPHOKINE MODULATION IN VITRO

### A. Factors Influencing the Production of Lymphokines by T-Helper Cells

Since Th1- and Th2-like cells appear to be responsible for distinct biological effects, the origin and development of these T-cell populations have become major fields of immunological research. Investigations were focused on two questions:

1. What are the signals required for the induction of Th1- or Th2-like cells?
2. Are Th1 and Th2 subsets derived from two mutually exclusive, postthymic CD4+ T-cell precursors that have a predetermined LK response pattern, or are they derived from a common precursor population that has the capacity to differentiate into either Th1 or Th2?

Experiments with long-term cultured T-cell clones did not allow the identification of the signals required for the preferential induction of Th1 or Th2. Therefore, several short-term culture systems have been established in order to determine the factors that regulate the LK pattern in CD4+ T cells. In vitro stimulation with mitogenic agents ("priming") was reported to be required for the induction of T cells capable of producing cytokines other than IL-2 [1–3]. Reactivation of primed T cells resulted in the secretion of a wide range of other cytokines, such as IFN-$\gamma$ and IL-3 to IL-6 by more than one order of magnitude. Subsequently, it was demonstrated that IL-2 and IL-4 were required for the induction of IL-4 secretion [39–41]. Furthermore, in vivo experiments have shown the induction of IL-4–producing cells after exposure to anti-CD3 monoclonal antibody (mAb) [42].

While the above studies suggested that several factors may influence the production of LK other than IL-2, the selective signals required for the development of either Th1-like or Th2-like cells were not identified by these systems. Some reports documented that the development of IL-4–producing cells by antigen plus APC was inhibited by IFN-$\gamma$ and that the majority of outgrowing cells had a Th1 phenotype [41, 43]. However, other investigators found that IL-4–producing cells could be induced, even in the presence of high amounts of IFN-$\gamma$ [40, 44].

In vivo experiments suggested that the natural ligands of the T cells, i.e., antigen and MHC-encoded proteins, could determine whether an animal reacts with a Th1 or a Th2 response [45–47]. This is in line with the report that the antigen used for priming in vivo determined the in vitro development of antigen-specific T-helper cell subsets [48].

We observed that nonprimed CD4+ T cells activated in a 3-day culture developed into Th1-like cells when subsequently cultured in medium supplemented with IL-2. In contrast, resting CD4+ T cells differentiated into Th2-like cells when activated and then cultured for 2 weeks in the permanent presence of a T-cell activator in addition to IL-2 [49]. Based on these findings, we have been investigating the signals that regulate the differentiation of CD4+ T cells toward a Th1 or Th2 phenotype and identified a postthymic precursor cell for Th1 and Th2.

## B. Induction of Th2-Like Cells Requires Prolonged Exposure to T-Cell Mitogens

In vitro activated, polyclonal CD4+ T cells produced large amounts of IL-2 but little or no IL-4 when restimulated after a culture period of 2 weeks in medium supplemented only with IL-2 as a T-cell growth factor (Fig. 1, Table 2). These cells therefore resembled Th1 cells. This observation was largely independent of the way the T cells were primed in vitro [49]. However, repetitive in vitro stimulation of these IL-2–producing, Th1-like CD4+ cells with antigen or polyclonal T-cell activators regularly induced CD4+ T cells that produced IL-4 but no IL-2 [13]. The data suggested that signals delivered during the stimulation of polyclonal CD4+ T cells favor the development of Th2-like cells. Thus the outgrowth of IL-4–producing T cells was most likely due to mitogenic signals or to cytokines released during the repetitive stimulation of T cells.

Since expansion of activated T cells in the presence of IL-2 alone induces a Th1-like phenotype within 2 weeks of culture (Table 2), this system allowed the investigation of signals capable of modulating the LK phenotype of CD4+ T cells. To this end, activated CD4+ T cells were expanded with IL-2 or with

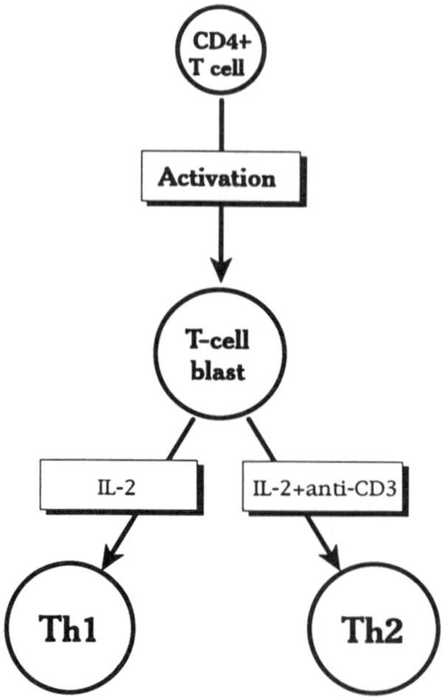


**Figure 1** Schematic representation of an in vitro culture system for the development of Th1 and Th2 cells. CD4+ T cells were prepared from nonimmunized mice and primarily activated with APC in the presence of a T-cell mitogen. Subsequent culture for 10–12 days with IL-2 yielded cells presenting with a Th1 phenotype upon reactivation, whereas Th2-like cells were obtained from cultures with IL-2 plus a T-cell mitogen present during the whole culture period.

**Table 2** Influence of Culture Conditions on LK Pattern of Th Cells

| Cell type | Culture condition | LK production | | | | |
|---|---|---|---|---|---|---|
| | | IFN-$\gamma$ | IL-2 | IL-3 | IL-4 | IL-5 |
| CD4+ TCR $\alpha\beta$ | IL-2 | + + + | + + + | + + + | — | — |
| CD4+ TCR $\alpha\beta$ | IL-2 + lectin | — | — | + + + | + + + | + + + |
| CD4+ TCR $\alpha\beta$ | IL-2 + anti-CD3 | — | — | + + + | + + + | + + + |
| CD4+ TCR $\alpha\beta$ | IL-2 + anti-TCR $\alpha\beta$ | nd | — | nd | + + + | nd |
| CD4+ TCR V$\beta$8+ | IL-2 + anti-TCR V$\beta$8 | nd | — | nd | + + + | nd |
| CD4+ TCR V$\beta$8− | IL-2 + anti-TCR V$\beta$8 | nd | + + + | nd | — | nd |

nd, not done.

IL-2 plus single defined agents that could be responsible for the modulation of the LK pattern toward a Th2 phenotype (Fig. 1). Potential agents that regulate the induction of the Th2 phenotype are cytokines. However, CD4+ T-cell blasts that were expanded for 2 weeks with IL-2 plus single defined cytokines (IL-1, IL-3, IL-4, IL-5, IL-6, IFN-$\gamma$, M-CSF, GM-CSF) as well as T cells that were expanded with supernatants of activated T cells produced the same LK pattern as T cells cultured with IL-2 alone [49].

These results suggested that mitogenic signals may be required for the induction of IL-4 and the downregulation of IL-2. To study the influence of mitogenic signals on the induction of IL-4, freshly isolated and activated CD4+ T cells were expanded in the presence of polyclonal T activators such as the plant lectins concanavalin A (ConA) or phytohaemagglutinin, which stimulate T-cell blasts even in the absence of APC or phorbol esters. In contrast to cytokines, ConA strongly influenced the LK response pattern of CD4+ T-cell blasts when added during the culture period with IL-2: CD4+ T cells that were expanded for 2 weeks in the presence of IL-2 and ConA produced up to 100 times more IL-4 and up to 100 times less IL-2 than cells of the same origin that were expanded with IL-2 alone (Table 2). The induction of IL-4 and the downregulation of IL-2 production required prolonged binding of the lectin to the T-cell surface, since $\alpha$-methyl-mannoside, which competes for the binding sites of Con A, completely abrogated its effect on the IL-2/IL-4 pattern [49].

Since ConA binds to the T-cell receptor (TCR) and since T-cell activation by ConA requires crosslinking of the TCR, these data suggested that the LK pattern of CD4+ T cells can be modulated via the TCR. However, lectins bind to a large number of other surface glycoproteins, which raised the possibility that surface molecules other than the TCR could be responsible for the modulation of the LK pattern.

## C. T-Cell Receptor–Mediated Differentiation Toward a Th1 or Th2 Phenotype

CD4+ T cells that had been activated with the superantigen staphylococcal enterotoxin B plus APC released large amounts of IL-2 when restimulated after culture with IL-2. These cells also produced IL-3 and IFN-$\gamma$ but neither IL-4 nor IL-5 and thus expressed a cytokine pattern that defines Th1 cells (Table 2) [44]. In contrast, when cultured with rIL-2 plus a mitogenic mAb to the TCR-associated CD3-complex, the cells released IL-3, IL-4, and IL-5, but neither IL-2 nor IFN-$\gamma$ (Table 2) [44]. This cytokine profile is characteristic for Th2 cells. Similarly, a mitogenic mAb to a common epitope of the $\alpha\beta$ TCR also modified the LK pattern toward a Th2 phenotype [44].

The ability to induce Th2-like cells appeared to be restricted to mitogenic mAb, since nonmitogenic antibodies to T cells were not capable of modulating the LK pattern. These data demonstrate that TCR-derived signals are critically involved in the generation of a specific LK response pattern.

## D. The Role of T-Cell Receptor Occupancy and IL-4 in the Induction of Th2

We observed that activated CD4+ T cells produced IFN-$\gamma$, IL-3, IL-4, and IL-5 during culture with IL-2 and antibodies to the TCR or to the CD3-complex. Thus, cytokines produced in autocrine fashion could alone be responsible for the induction of Th2. To address this point, TCR V$\beta$8+ and V$\beta$8− T-cell blasts were co-cultured in the presence of a mAb to V$\beta$8 (Fig. 2). After restimulation, V$\beta$8+ cells had a Th2-like phenotype and V$\beta$8− cells had a Th1-like LK profile similar to cells cultured with IL-2 alone (Table 2) [44]. This demonstrates that TCR ligation is required for the induction of Th2-like cells. TCR-mediated induction of Th2, however, was also dependent

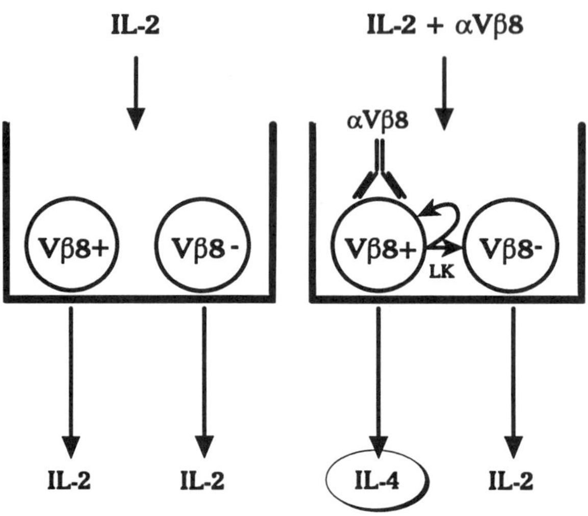


**Figure 2** Evidence for the requirement of prolonged TCR occupancy for T-cell differentiation toward a Th2 phenotype. Activated polyclonal CD4+ T cells, comprising both V$\beta$8+ and V$\beta$8− cells, were cultured either in the presence of IL-2 alone or with IL-2 plus a mAb specific for V$\beta$8. After 2 weeks, V$\beta$8+ and V$\beta$8− cells were separated by cell sorting and restimulated. Only V$\beta$8+ cells from cultures with anti-V$\beta$8 released IL-4. This demonstrates that TCR occupancy itself is necessary for the induction of a Th2 phenotype and that LK released by stimulated V$\beta$8+ cells are not sufficient to induce this phenotype in V$\beta$8− cells.

on IL-4 since the addition of an antibody to IL-4 prevented the development of Th2 cells. The resulting phenotype was Th1-like. Thus, we propose a model for the induction of Th2 cells that comprises at least two signals: one is provided by IL-4, either exogenously added or produced in an autocrine fashion, and the other consists of TCR ligation (Fig. 3).

## E. Th1- and Th2-Like Cells Can Be Derived from a Common CD4+ Precursor Cell

To analyze the precursor cell for Th1 or Th2 cells, pairs of subclones were derived from single CD4+ T cells by the split-clone technique. With this approach, it could be demonstrated that subclones expanded with IL-2 alone regularly give rise to a predominantly IL-2–producing phenotype. In contrast, sister clones derived from the same precursor but expanded with IL-2 and a mitogenic mAb to CD3 consistently gave rise to predominantly IL-4–producing subclones [50]. Analysis of 66 pairs of clones revealed that none of them was predetermined for a distinct LK response pattern. Sixty-eight percent of the clones gave rise to both one Th1-like and one Th2-like subclone. The latter released up to 50 times more IL-4 but 90 times less IL-2 than the corresponding Th1-like subclones. Less than 2% of the split clones gave a mixed LK pattern (Th0 phenotype) under both culture conditions.

These data demonstrate that one single, freshly isolated, postthymic CD4+ T cell can give rise to both Th1 and Th2. Since none of the investigated clones were predetermined for the production of either IL-2 or IL-4, the Th1 or Th2 phenotype of CD4+ T cells represents a functional differentiation state that is acquired during culture. Several of the described short-term IL-2–producing T-cell clones could be switched to IL-4 producers by prolonged stimulation with anti-CD3 plus IL-2 [50]. This demonstrates that Th1-like cells can function as precursors for Th2.

These results also show that recently isolated CD4+ T cells have a LK pattern that can be modulated. This stands in sharp contrast to long-term cultured T-cell clones, in which the LK pattern is fixed.

## F. Functional Properties of Th1- and Th2-Like Populations Obtained from Short-Term Culture

Short-term cultured Th1- or Th2-like polyclonal T-cell blasts share not only the LK pattern of established long-term clones, but also other biological properties of Th1 or Th2. Like Th2 clones, the IL-4–producing T-cell blasts were capable of providing B-cell help for IgG1, IgG2A and IgE synthesis under cognate conditions (44). In contrast, the IL-2 producing cells were not capable of providing B cell help. They however interacted with B cells since they produced LK in cognate interaction.

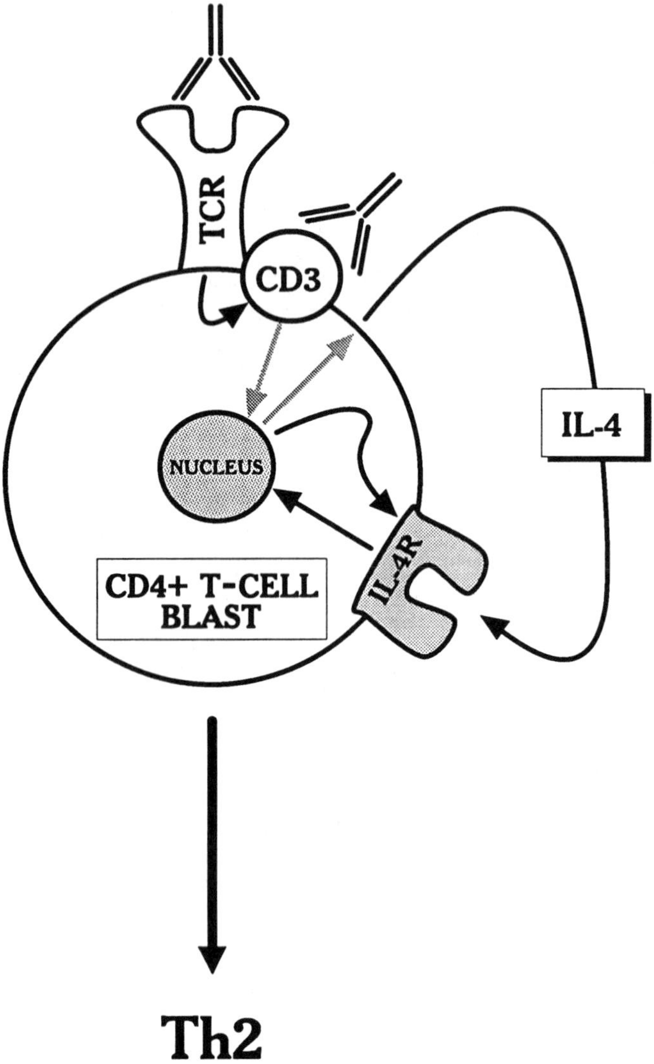


**Figure 3** A model for Th-cell differentiation toward a Th2 phenotype. The data shown so far suggest that prolonged TCR occupancy exerts a dual mode of action on activated Th cells: it induces the auto- or paracrine secretion of IL-4 in these cells, and it enables the cells to develop a Th2-like phenotype, at least partially in response to shed IL-4.

## IV. CONCLUSIONS

Long-term murine CD4+ T-cell clones can be classified into two distinct subsets that produce either IL-2 and IFN-$\gamma$ (Th1) or IL-4 and IL-5 (Th2). This functional separation of CD4+ T cell has subsequently been shown to be of great biological relevance, since these T-helper cells subsets can be associated with protective or pathogenic immune responses. While a large number of in vitro and in vivo experiments underlined the biological relevance of Th1 and Th2 phenotypes, the ontogeny of Th1 or Th2 cells remained unknown until recently. Experiments published during the last 3 years have shown that cytokines such as IL-2, IL-4, and IFN-$\gamma$ can influence the LK response pattern of CD4+ T cells. However, further investigations demonstrated that these cytokines alone had no effect on the modulation of the LK response pattern.

Prolonged TCR binding by mitogenic mAb delivered a signal required for the induction of the Th2 phenotype. Whereas this signal cannot be replaced by soluble factors, ligation of the TCR together with LK leads to the development of Th2. The fact that TCR-mediated induction of Th2 in vitro takes the same time as the antigen-mediated commitment of Th1- or Th2-like cells in vivo underlines the role of TCR mediated signals in T-helper cell subset differentiation. Since the two subsets can be derived from a common postthymic CD4+ precursor, the Th1 or Th2 phenotype is acquired during T-cell differentiation and is not secondary to the expansion of distinct subpopulations which are predetermined for the production of a specific LK pattern.

The structure of the natural ligands of the TCR, i.e., antigens and MHC class II–encoded molecules, have been shown to influence the development of T-helper cells with distinct LK profiles in vivo. This suggests that the TCR-ligand interaction is decisive for the commitment of a peripheral CD4+ T cell toward a Th1- or a Th2-like response pattern.

## ACKNOWLEDGMENTS

This work was supported in part by grants from the Deutsche Forschungsgemeinschaft to MR (RO 764/1-1) and from the Swiss National Foundation for Scientific Research to CH (3.115-0.88 and 32-27/59.89).

## REFERENCES

1. R. C. Budd, J.-C. Cerottini, and H. R. MacDonald, *J. Immunol.*, *138*, 3583 (1987).
2. S. L. Swain, D. T. McKenzie, A. D. Weinberg, and W. Hancock, *J. Immunol.*, *141*, 3445 (1988).

3. G. D. Powers, A. K. Abbas, and R. A. Miller, *J. Immunol.*, *140*, 3352 (1988).
4. T. R. Mosmann, H. Cherwinski, M. W. Bond, M. A. Giedlin, and R. L. Coffman, *J. Immunol.*, *136*, 2348 (1986).
5. T. R. Mosmann and R. L. Coffman, *Annu. Rev. Immunol.*, *7*, 145 (1989).
6. T. R. Mosmann and K. W. Moore, *Immunol. Today*, *12*, A49 (1991).
7. G. S. Firestein, W. D. Roeder, J. A. Laxer, K. S. Townsend, C. T. Weaver, J. T. Hom, J. Linton, B. E. Torbett, and A. L. Glasebrook, *J. Immunol.*, *143*, 518 (1989).
8. A. Bendelac and R. H. Schwartz, *Nature*, *353*, 68 (1991).
9. R. D. Stout and K. Bottomly, *J. Immunol.*, *142*, 760 (1989).
10. D. F. Fiorentino, A. Zlotnik, P. Vieira, T. R. Mosmann, M. Howard, K. W. Moore, and A. O'Garra, *J. Immunol.*, *146*, 3444 (1991).
11. S. T. Ju, N. H. Ruddle, P. Strack, M. E. Dorf, and R. H. DeKruyff, *J. Immunol.*, *144*, 23 (1990).
12. L. Killar, G. MacDonald, J. West, A. Woods, and K. Bottomly, *J. Immunol.*, *138*, 1674 (1987).
13. C. Hauser, C. M. Snapper, J. Ohara, W. E. Paul, and S. I. Katz, *Eur. J. Immunol.*, *19*, 245 (1989).
14. T. L. Stevens, A, Bossie, V. M. Sanders, R. Fernandez-Botran, R. L. Coffman, T. R. Mosmann, and E. S. Vitetta, *Nature*, *334*, 255 (1988).
15. C. M. Snapper, and W. E. Paul, *Science*, *236*, 944 (1987).
16. E. S. Vitetta, R. Fernandez-Botran, C. D. Myers, and V. M. Sanders, *Adv. Immunol.*, *45*, 1 (1989).
17. C. Hauser and S. I. Katz, *Immunol. Rev.*, *117*, 67 (1990).
18. A. A. Gaspari, M. K. Jenkins, and S. I. Katz, *J. Immunol.*, *141*, 2216 (1988).
19. D. J. Cher and T. R. Mosmann, *J. Immunol.*, *138*, 3688 (1987).
20. R. L. Wong, N. H. Ruddle, S. J. Padula, E. G. Lingenheld, C. M. Bergman, R. V. Rugen, D. I. Epstein, and R. B. Clark, *J. Immunol.*, *141*, 3329 (1988).
21. C. Hauser, *J. Invest. Dermatol.*, *95*, 436 (1990).
22. T. A. T. Fong and T. R. Mosmann, *J. Immunol.*, *143*, 2887 (1989).
23. P. V. Lehmann., G. Schumm, D. Moon, U. Hurtenbach, F. Falcioni, S. Muller, and Z. A. Nagy, *J. Exp. Med.*, *171*, 1485 (1990).
24. M. Tary-Lehmann, A. G. Rolink, P. V. Lehmann, Z. A. Nagy, and U. Hurtenbach, *J. Immunol.*, *145*, 2092 (1990).
25. P. Scott and S. H. E. Kaufmann, *Immunol. Today*, *12*, 346 (1991).
26. M. Nagarkatti, S. R. Clary, and P. S. Nagarkatti, *J. Immunol.*, *144*, 4898 (1990).
27. M. Goldman, P. Druet, and E. Gleichmann, *Immunol. Today*, *12*, 223 (1991).
28. J. M. Doutrelepont, M. Moser, O. Leo, D. Abramowicz, M. L. Vanderhaegen, J. Urbain, and M. Goldman, *Clin. Exp. Immunol.*, *83*, 133 (1991).
29. R. L. Coffman, B. W. P. Seymour, S. Hudak, J. Jackson, and D. Rennick, *Science*, *245*, 308 (1989).
30. M. L. Kapsenberg, E. A. Wierenga, J. D. Bos, and H. M. Jansen, *Immunol. Today*, *12*, 392 (1991).
31. H. Yssel, M. C. Shanafelt, C. Soderberg, P. V. Schneider, J. Anzola, and G. Peltz, *J. Exp. Med.*, *174*, 593 (1991).

32. J. B. A. G. Haanen, R. De Waal Malefijt, P. C. M. Res, E. M. Kraakman, T. H. M. Ottenhoff, R. R. P. De Vries, and H. Spits, *J. Exp. Med.*, *174*, 583 (1991).
33. P. Salgame, J. S. Abrams, C. Clayberger, H. Goldstein, J. Convit, R. L. Modlin, and B. R. Bloom, *Science*, *254*, 279 (1991).
34. G. F. Del Prete, M. De Carli, C. Mastromauro, R. Biagiotti, D. Macchia, P. Falagiani, M. Ricci, and S. Romagnani, *J. Clin. Invest.*, *88*, 346 (1991).
35. E. Maggi, P. Biswas, G. Del Prete, P. Parronchi, D. Macchia, C. Simonelli, L. Emmi, M. De Carli, A. Tiri, M. Ricci, and S. Romagnani, *J. Immunol.*, *146*, 1169 (1991).
36. D. Vercelli, H. H. Jabara, K. I. Arai, and R. S. Geha, *J. Exp. Med.*, *169*, 1295 (1989).
37. S. Vollenweider, J.-H. Saurat, M. Röcken, and C. Hauser, *J. Allergy Clin. Immunol.*, *87*, 1088 (1991).
38. A. B. Kay, S. Ying, V. Varney, M. Gaga, S. R. Durham, R. Moqbel, A. J. Wardlaw, and Q. Hamid, *J. Exp. Med.*, *173*, 775 (1991).
39. S. Z. Ben-Sasson, G. Le Gros, D. H. Conrad, F. D. Finkelman, and W. E. Paul, *J. Immunol.*, *145*, 1127 (1990).
40. G. Le Gros, S. Z. Ben-Sasson, R. Seder, F. D. Finkelman, and W. E. Paul, *J. Exp. Med.*, *172*, 921 (1990).
41. M. Betz and B. S. Fox, *J. Immunol.*, *145*, 1046 (1990).
42. V. Flamand, D. Abramowicz, M. Goldman, C. Biernaux, G. Huez, J. Urbain, M. Moser, and O. Leo, *J. Immunol.*, *144*, 2875 (1990).
43. T. F. Gajewski, J. Joyce, and F. W. Fitch, *J. Immunol.*, *143*, 15 (1989).
44. M. Röcken, K. M. Müller, J.-H. Saurat, I. Müller, J. A. Louis, J.-C. Cerottini, and C. Hauser, *J. Immunol.*, *148*, 47 (1992).
45. J. S. Murray, J. Madri, J. Tite, S. R. Carding, and K. Bottomly, *J. Exp. Med.*, *170*, 2135 (1989).
46. F. Y. Liew, S. M. Millott, and J. A. Schmidt, *J. Exp. Med.*, *172*, 1359 (1990).
47. A. Jardim, J. Alexander, H. S. Teh, D. Ou, and R. W. Olafson, *J. Exp. Med.*, *172*, 645 (1990).
48. N. E. Street, J. H. Schumacher, T. A. T. Fong, H. Bass, D. F. Fiorentino, J. A. Leverah, and T. R. Mosmann, *J. Immunol.*, *144*, 1629 (199).
49. M. Röcken, K. M. Müller, J.-H. Saurat, and C. Hauser, *J. Immunol.*, *146*, 577 (1991).
50. M. Röcken, J.-H. Saurat, and C. Hauser, *J. Immunol.*, *148*, 1031 (1992).

# 7
# Colony-Stimulating Factors and the Skin

**John W. Schrader**
*The Biomedical Research Centre*
*University of British Columbia*
*Vancouver, British Columbia, Canada*

## I. INTRODUCTION

The skin and the blood are two of the key organs in defense against microorganisms. Thus, it is not unexpected that the responses of these organs to infection or trauma are tightly coordinated and interlinked by a series of regulatory processes. Many of these involve cytokines, a loose group of polypeptides that act as paracrine, or less commonly endocrine, regulators of inflammatory responses. Dozens of such molecules have now been described. Cytokines fall into a number of broad structural families—in some cases the relationships within a family being more evident from the structure of their receptors than the cytokines—and their nomenclature is unsystematic and confusing. The colony stimulating factors (CSFs) are a functional subgroup that includes members of two of the main structural families of cytokines, and CSFs are defined by their common property of stimulating the generation and function of various types of cells of hemopoietic origin.

## II. CLASSIFICATION OF CSFs

Colony-stimulating factor is an operational term based on the original colony assay, which identified soluble factors that stimulated single hemopoietic progenitor cells to generate colonies of their progeny. In this procedure, pioneered in the 1960s by Pluznick and Sachs (1965) and Bradley and Metcalf (1966), a suspension of nucleated bone marrow cells was cultured in tissue-culture medium that had been gelled, for example, by the inclusion of agar. It was observed that over a period of 7–14 days, individual progenitor cells gave rise to colonies of hundreds or thousands of differentiated blood cells of various lineages. The multiplication and differentiation of these progenitor cells was absolutely dependent on the presence of soluble factors released by a variety of tissues or cell lines. These soluble factors were termed colony-stimulating activities (CSAs) or factors (CSFs). Different types of colonies were recognized in the initial experiments. Some contained neutrophils, others macrophages, and others mixtures of the two. It was recognized that different CSF's could be defined in terms of the types of colony stimulated. In many, but importantly, as discussed below, not all instances, CSFs that stimulated different colonies were eventually shown to be distinct molecular entities. Thus, the term granulocyte-CSF, G-CSF, became associated with a molecule that stimulated the growth of colonies of neutrophils, granulocyte-macrophage CSF (GM-CSF) with a molecule that stimulated colonies containing both neutrophils and macrophages, and macrophage CSF, M-CSF (more commonly termed CSF-1), with a molecule that stimulated the growth of colonies of macrophages. As shown in Table 1, it is now evident that these molecules actually affect a wider range of cell types than implied by their names.

**Table 1** Targets of CSFs

| | |
|---|---|
| G-CSF | Neutrophilic granulocytes<br>Progenitors of neutrophils<br>Pluripotential hemopoietic stem cells (synergy with other factors) |
| CSF-1 | Macrophages/Monocytes<br>Osteoclasts<br>Trophoblast |
| GM-CSF | Neutrophilic, eosinophilic, and basophilic granulocytes<br>Progenitors of neutrophils, eosinophils, basophils<br>Progenitors of megakaryocytes<br>Dendritic cells<br>Macrophages/Monocytes |
| IL-3 | Pluripotential hemopoietic stem cells<br>Progenitors of neutrophils, eosinophils and basophils<br>Progenitors of megakaryocytes, erythrocytes<br>Progenitors of mast cells<br>Mast cells, megakaryocytes, basophils, eosinophils, macrophages |

Colonies containing other cell types were also observed, and the existence of eosinophil-CSFs or megakaryocyte-CSFs were postulated. Likewise, colonies containing mixtures of many cell types, e.g., neutrophils, macrophages, megakaryocytes, and erythroid cells, were recognized, suggesting the existence of factors stimulating the growth of more primitive, less committed progenitor cells. All of these activities were shown to be properties of a single hemopoietin that targeted multiple hemopoietic lineages. This molecule is now termed interleukin 3 (IL-3) (Schrader et al., 1988). Reflecting its broad range of activities, major contributions to its characterization came from outside the field of experimental hematology, from immunologists working on the one hand on an enzyme at that time erroneously thought to be associated with T-lymphocyte differentiation (Ihle et al., 1981) and on mast cells (Schrader and Nossal, 1980; Clark-Lewis et al., 1984). As discussed below, combinations of CSFs and cytokines can also act synergistically to stimulate primitive progenitor cells and to generate various cell lineages.

It is important to recognize that, like most cytokines, CSFs have multiple cellular targets and bioactivities (Table 1). Likewise, hemopoietic progenitor cells are regulated by multiple CSFs and by other cytokines. GM-CSF, G-CSF, CSF-1, and IL-3 are the three hemopoietins that have been most intensely studied, were the first to be molecularly cloned, and are now in clinical trials. A number of other cytokines, however, also stimulate the proliferation and differentiation of hemopoietic progenitor cells. In some cases these can stimulate the growth of small colonies in standard cultures, whereas in others, they act synergistically with other cytokines.

One of the most important of these factors is a recently identified molecule variously called steel factor (SLF), stem-cell factor, mast-cell growth factor, or kit-ligand (Anderson et al., 1990; Copeland et al., 1990; Huang et al., 1990; Williams et al., 1990a). As the last name implies, SLF is the ligand for the c-kit molecule, a receptor that has a similar structure to the CSF-1 receptor and, like that molecule, also has tyrosine kinase activity.

SLF and c-kit are the products of genes at two loci: steel (SI) and white spotting (W) (Bernstein et al., 1990). Mutations at either of these loci result in the homozygous state in defects in pigmentation of the skin and hair, germ-cell migration, and hemopoiesis. Depending on the severity of the resulting deficit in functional SLF or c-kit, mice with mutations at these loci show varying degrees of anemia and deficiencies of mast cells in the skin, peritoneal cavity, mucosal membranes, and other tissues. Levels of neutrophils, macrophages, and lymphocytes seem unaffected. SLF and c-kit are also expressed at high levels in the brain, although their function in the brain is obscure, as mutant mice with deficits in SLF or c-kit function show no obvious neurological problems. SLF has relatively weak activity as a CSF when added alone to cultures of bone marrow cells (Metcalf, 1991). However, it exhibits strong synergistic colony-stimulating activity on more primitive hemopoietic stem and progenitor cells in the presence of other cytokines such as IL-3, GM-CSF, G-CSF, CSF-1, IL-6, or erythropoietin (see Moore, 1991).

Erythropoietin—the physiological regulator of erythrocyte levels—stimulates late erythroid progenitors to form small colonies of erythrocytes (Krantz, 1991). Erythropoietin can also synergize with other factors such as SLF in stimulating more primitive progenitor cells to develop erythroid colonies. There is also evidence that erythropoietin can increase the size of colonies of megakaryocytes (McLeod et al., 1976).

Interleukin-5 stimulates the limited division and differentiation of eosinophil progenitors and alone can stimulate the growth of small colonies of eosinophils (Clutterbuck and Sanderson, 1988). Interleukin 6 (IL-6) has very limited colony-stimulating activity. Interleukin 4 (IL-4), interleukin 1 (IL-1), interleukin 11, LIF, and tumor necrosis factor $\alpha$ can synergize with CSFs (see Moore, 1991).

## III. MOLECULAR STRUCTURE OF CSFs

The nomenclature of the CSFs reflects the history of their characterization, and not a systematic categorization according to function or structure. Recent progress in the elucidation of the structure of hemopoietins, and in particular of their receptors (Bazan, 1990), has established the existence of two major structural families. These families, shown in Table 2, highlight the evolutionary relationships of the CSFs with other cytokines involved in defense and repair responses and in some cases in the steady-state generation of lymphohemopoietic cells.

### A. Monomeric CSFs

GM-CSF, G-CSF, and IL-3 are members of a structural family of monomeric cytokines. Although there is little evidence of homology at the level of their amino acid sequences, all are globular glycoproteins, with polypeptide chains of about 120–180 amino acids. This family includes IL-7 and erythropoietin, which are important in the steady-state generation of B lymphocytes and erythrocytes, respectively, and leukemia inhibitory factor (LIF), which probably is important in embryogenesis but may also be involved in inflammation. Also in this family are a group of cytokines released only during inflammatory responses and includes interleukins 2, 4, 5, and 6.

The receptors for cytokines of this family are likely to be dimers (Bazan, 1990). The receptors for IL-3, GM-CSF, IL-5, IL-6, and LIF are heter-

**Table 2** Two Structural Families of Colony-Stimulating Factors

| Family | CSFs | Other members | Receptors |
|---|---|---|---|
| Monomeric CSFs | GM-CSF | Erythropoietin | Dimers or heterodimers |
| | | IL-4 | Hemopoietin receptor supergene family |
| | G-CSF | IL-5 | |
| | | IL-6 | No intrinsic enzymatic activity |
| | IL-3 | IL-7 | |
| | | LIF | |
| | | Growth hormone | |
| | | Prolactin | |
| Dimeric CSFs | CSF-1 | Platelet-derived growth factors | Dimers<br>Extracellular, Ig-like domains |
| | SLF | Fibroblasts-derived growth factors | Intrinsic tyrosine kinase activity |

odimers, in which both subunits share the structural features and are of members of the hemopoietin receptor family. The receptor for IL-2 is a heterotrimer, although the smaller $\alpha$-chain is not a member of the hemopoietin receptor family. The receptor for G-CSF appears to be a homodimer, resembling in this regard the receptor for growth hormone, also a member of this family. While receptors of this family lack intrinsic enzymatic activity, ligand binding results in activation of tyrosine kinases, the molecular nature of which remains largely uncharacterized. In the case of the IL-2 receptor, there is evidence that the lck kinase associates with and is activated by the receptor, although it appears that other kinases can be substituted for lck (Hatakeyama et al., 1991). It seems likely that other perhaps yet undescribed members of the src family of kinases may associate with other members of this receptor family.

## B. Dimeric CSFs

The second family of CSFs includes CSF-1 and the recently discovered SLF. CSF-1 and SLF are both homodimers. The subunits of each consist of a polypeptide of about 150 amino acids that is heavily glycosylated. Their interrelationship and their grouping with the platelet-derived growth factors (PDGF) and the fibroblast growth factors (FGF) became evident from the molecular similarities in the respective receptors. All consist of extracellular domains made up of a series of immunoglobulinlike domains—five in the case of the receptors for CSF-1 and SLF—a transmembrane segment, and structurally related intracellular segments that include tyrosine kinase domains.

Interestingly, both SLF and CSF-1 exist not only as soluble factors, but also as cell-bound, transmembrane proteins. In both cases there is good evidence that the cell-bound forms of the molecules are biologically active (Rettenmeir, 1989; Anderson et al., 1990). In fact, in the case of SLF there is good evidence that the membrane-bound form of the factor is more effective in stimulating its cellular targets than is the soluble form (Flanagan et al., 1991).

## IV. ACTIONS OF CSFs

CSFs of both the major structural families share three basic actions and stimulate survival, growth, and differentiation and function. CSFs enhance the survival of both progenitor cells and mature cells. In the absence of CSFs, progenitor cells (Williams et al., 1990a; Koury and Bondurant, 1990) as well as mature, effector cells like mast cells (Crapper et al., 1984), neutrophils (Savill et al., 1989), and macrophages (Mangan and Wahl, 1991) die by initiation of the process of apoptosis or programmed cell death.

This action of CSFs in preventing apoptosis and thus maintaining the viability of cells of hemopoietic origin probably serves an important physiological purpose. It would ensure that the rapid increase of progenitor cells and effector cells that results from the stimulation of hemopoiesis by the multiplicity of CSFs and other cytokines released by inflammatory stimuli such as microorganisms is rapidly reversed when the inflammatory stimuli has been removed and levels of stimulating cytokines have dropped.

As implied by their name, all CSFs stimulate the multiplication of progenitor cells and their differentiation into end cells in colony assays. The question of whether these effects are direct and due to the CSF alone or result from more complex interactions is not completely resolved. Because colony assays have usually been carried out in the presence of serum, which contains multiple hormones, as well as cytokines and other products released by blood clotting, it is not self-evident that the growth and differentiation of mature hemopoietic cells in these cultures is due to the actions of the added CSF. Serum-free culture-media offer an approach to excluding a cooperative effect of serum components, although usually these media still contain large amounts of proteins such as albumin, which could still be complexed with small amounts of hormones or growth factors. An additional source of uncertainty arises from the fact that CSFs could be acting in concert with other factors released by other cells in the culture, perhaps as a result of stimulation by the CSF under test. To some extent this question can be addressed by determining whether cloning efficiency or colony size drops as the density of cells in the culture is lowered or as progenitor cells are purified away from contaminating cells.

Another question is raised by the likelihood, discussed below, that hemopoietic cells themselves may be induced to produce CSFs and other cytokines. This makes it more complicated to demonstrate that a given effect, e.g., differentiation of a progenitor along a certain hemopoietic lineage, is the result of activation of the receptor for a particular CSF. Thus there are multiple instances where exposure of a cell to one cytokine induces release of a second, which in turn induces a particular effect.

## V. SOURCES OF CSFs AND STIMULI FOR PRODUCTION

Table 3 summarizes data on the known cellular sources of the four major CSFs. In the case of CSF-1 and SLF, there is good evidence for the constitutive production of these factors in normal adult animals not undergoing inflammatory responses. Not a great deal is known about the regulation of SLF by inflammatory stimuli. In contrast, the production of G-CSF, CSF-1, GM-CSF, and IL-3 are clearly increased by inflammatory stimuli. Increased synthesis of G-CSF, GM-CSF, and CSF-1 occurs in all of the cell

**Table 3** Sources of Colony-Stimulating Factors

| | |
|---|---|
| G-CSF | Activated macrophages |
| | Activated fibroblasts |
| | Activated epithelial cells |
| | Activated endothelial cells |
| GM-CSF | Activated T (B) lymphocytes |
| | Activated mast cells |
| | Activated eosinophils |
| | Activated macrophages |
| | Activated endothelial cells |
| | Activated fibroblasts |
| | Activated epithelial cells |
| | Activated vascular smooth muscle cells |
| IL-3 | Activated T lymphocytes |
| | Activated mast cells |
| CSF-1 | Activated macrophages |
| | Activated fibroblasts |
| | Activated endothelial cells |
| | Activated vascular smooth muscle cells |
| | Uterine columnar epithelial cells in pregnancy |

types listed in response to products of microorganisms—bacterial endotoxin being a strong stimulus—and in response to other cytokines or other products released in response to trauma, e.g., during blood clotting. The rapid induction of cytokine production by cytokines, e.g., of G-CSF, GM-CSF, and CSF-1 production in macrophages by IL-1, generates the cascade of cytokine release characteristic of inflammatory responses.

It is evident that many hemopoietic cells can be induced to release CSFs. For example, stimulation of mast cells by cross-linking of Fcε receptors (Plaut et al., 1989; Wodnar-Filipowicz et al., 1989) or of eosinophils by stimulation with cytokines results in the production by these cells of IL-3 and GM-CSF (Moqbel et al., 1991; Kita et al., 1991). Stimulation of macrophages by stimuli like cytokines or endotoxin results in the production of CSF-1, GM-CSF, and G-CSF (Kluck and Falkenburg, 1980). There is evidence suggesting that hemopoietic progenitors may produce IL-6 (Dy et al., 1991). Certainly we have observed that factor-dependent lines with many characteristics of hemopoietic progenitor cells can produce cytokines like IL-3 or IL-6.

There are reports of cell lines that produce cytokines and CSFs without apparent stimulation by agents like endotoxin. For example, we observed that cultured vascular smooth muscle cells produced high titers of CSF-1 and some GM-CSF apparently spontaneously (Schrader et al., 1991). Although there was no evidence that stimuli like endotoxin or serum components like PDGF were necessary, tissue culture systems involve other potential stimuli that are hard to exclude such as adhesion of the cells to artificial surfaces.

The interpretation of observations of the in vitro production of CSFs by transformed or immortalized cell lines rather than primary cultures is even more problematic. As noted above, multiple stimuli including CSFs and crosslinking of Fc receptors trigger hempoietic cells to release CSFs and cytokines. Some of the same signal transduction pathways activated by these stimuli, e.g., activation of $p21^{ras}$ (Duronio et al., 1992) are also often activated in transformed cells. It is not surprising that the same genetic changes that result in oncogenic growth may also result in cytokine production. In other instances, the constitutive production of a CSF by a transformed hemopoietic cell reflects a pathological oncogenic activation of a CSF gene by a mutation of the gene or its regulatory sequences, resulting in autostimulation and continuous growth (Leslie et al., 1991). For all of these reasons, great caution must be exercised in extrapolating from observations of constitutive production of CSFs by cells in cell line in vitro to the in vivo situation.

## VI. PHYSIOLOGICAL ROLE OF CSFs

It is important to recognize that like other cytokines, CSFs in general act locally as paracrine hormones in the immediate vicinity of their source. CSF-1 and SLF occur in the serum in normal animals, but GM-CSF and IL-3 only reach significant levels in the serum of severe infections or events activating the immune system, such as graft-versus-host disease.

GM-CSF, G-CSF, CSF-1, and IL-3 are clearly important components of the inflammatory response to microorganisms. As noted above, GM-CSF, G-CSF, and CSF-1 (like IL-1, TNF, IL-6) are also released as a result of direct stimulation of many cell byproducts of microorganisms or inflammatory mediators. IL-3 and GM-CSF, like IL-4, IL-5, and TNF, are also released as a result of immunological stimuli—either via direct activation of antigen-specific T lymphocytes or by activation of cells such as mast cells by complexing of antigen with preformed antibodies and crosslinking of Fc receptors (Plaut et al., 1989; Wodner-Filipowicz et al., 1989). These CSFs, together with other cytokines released during inflammation, serve to rapidly increase the production and function of the granulocytes and macrophages that are the key effector cells in defense and repair.

## A. CSFs and Steady-State Hemopoiesis

While CSFs are obviously key components of the response to infection, their role in the continuous steady-state generation of blood cells is much less clear. G-CSF may occur in small amounts in the plasma of apparently normal humans, while CSF-1 is present in plasma and urine (Stanley, 1990). In contrast, there is no evidence for the production of GM-CSF or IL-3 in normal animals. However, it is technically impossible to exclude the production of small but crucial amounts of CSFs, e.g., by rare stromal cells in the bone-marrow or by stem cells themselves by direct techniques. Thus the only convincing data on the importance of a particular CSF in normal hemopoiesis come from the analysis of mice where mutations in a particular CSF gene prevents any synthesis whatsoever of that molecule.

Two mouse strains with naturally occurring mutations have been identified. Analysis of these mice indicates that both CSF-1 and SLF are involved in steady-state regulation of hemopoietic cells.

Mice homozygous for the *op* mutation, which introduces a stop codon into the CSF-1 gene, exhibit osteopetrosis and defective tooth development (Wiktor-Jedrzejczak et al., 1990). These defects appear to reflect a role for CSF-1 in the normal development of osteoclasts. There are lower numbers of macrophages at some but not all sites in the body, suggesting that CSF-1 has an important although not absolutely essential role in the steady-state generation of macrophages.

Mice lacking SLF (or having a mutation at the W locus that encodes c-kit, thus resulting in a defective receptor for SLF) exhibit anemia, a deficiency of mast cells and evidence of a defective response of pluripotential hemopoietic stem cells to microenvironmental stimuli (Bernstein et al., 1968).

SLF thus clearly has a role in regulating the function of pluripotential hemopoietic stem cells and the progenitors of erythrocytes in normal steady-state conditions.

The use of homologous recombination in embryo stem cells to generate strains of transgenic mice with mutations in CSF genes (Capecchi, 1989) should clarify the role of other CSFs in normal hemopoiesis and in disease. A recent development will allow the generation of transgenic mice where CSF genes are deleted in particular cell lineages (Orban et al., 1992), allowing detailed analysis of the importance of particular cellular sources of CSFs.

## B. Mast Cells

The regulation of mast cell numbers in the skin appears to be complex. It is of both particular and general interest, however, as the mechanisms involved may mirror those regulating the survival and behavior of pluripotential hemopoietic stem cells in the bone marrow. Like mast cells, pluripotential hemopoietic stem cells respond to both IL-3 and SLF. However, these rare cells, in contrast to mast cells, are hard to identify and study in vivo.

Mice with mutations in c-kit or SLF genes also exhibit a deficiency mast cells and mast cell progenitors in the skin (Kitamura, 1989) and gut mucosa (Crapper et al., 1984), suggesting a role for SLF in the homing or survival of mast cell progenitors in the skin and at mucosal surfaces. These data suggest that SLF is expressed in these tissues, at least at the specific sites where mast cell progenitors and mast cells survive. There is evidence that SLF is expressed in the mesoderm but not the epidermal layers of developing skin (Matsui et al., 1990). Nishikawa et al. (1991) observed that anti-kit antibodies administered to fetal mice at day 15.5, after melanoblasts had entered the epidermal layer, had no effect on the development of coat color, in contrast to antibodies administered earlier. They interpreted this as indicating that the melanoblasts were quiescent and not being stimulated by SLF in the epidermis.

Several lines of evidence suggest that normal skin can only support the generation and survival of a limited number of mast cells, the precise density of mast cells varying in skin from different sites of the body. Mast cells that were generated by culturing mouse bone marrow in the presence of IL-3 then transplanted into the skin of $W^f/W^f$ mice disappeared over 3 weeks unless the animal was provided with a source of IL-3 (Crapper et al., 1984).

The injection of SLF into animals leads to large increases in connective tissue–type mast cells in the skin. However, when the administration of exogenous SLF is stopped, numbers of mast cells rapidly decline to those characteristic of the skin at a particular anatomical site (Tsai et al., 1991).

All of these observations suggest that the skin has a limited capacity to support the survival of mast cells. This might imply that the expression of SLF in the skin was normally limited to specific microenvironments that provided a fixed number of niches. Alternatively, based on the in vitro studies with the soluble form of SLF that indicate that SLF characteristically synergizes strongly with other growth factors (Moore, 1991), it is possible that, while there is a low generalized level of SLF expression in the dermis, additional synergistic signals, e.g., transmitted by adhesion molecules or other growth factors, have a more restricted, patchy distribution.

### C. Melanocytes

Another component of the skin affected by SLF are the melanocytes. In vitro SLF can induce proliferation of melanocytes (Halaban, 1991). Interestingly, the human piebald trait, characterized by a white hair forelock and areas of ventral cutaneous hypopigmentation, has been associated with a deletion of c-kit (Fleischman et al., 1991). Local injection of antibodies specific for the c-kit protein into the skin of black adult mice resulted in the development of patches of unpigmented hair, not at the injection site, but at sites where the hair had been shaved (Nishikawa et al., 1991). This result was interpreted as indicating that the anti-kit antibody blocked activation of the melanocytes in the initiation of the hair cycle. This observation suggests a role for SLF in the regulation of pigment cells in vivo. However, the effect of the anti-kit antibodies could also be trivial, in the sense that it reflected nonspecific interference with the function or migration of melanocytes by cell-bound antibodies, rather than a specific interference with a critical function of c-kit. Unfortunately, the study was not controlled by use of an irrelevant antibody that would also bind melanoblasts or melanocytes. A more conclusive experiment would investigate whether the local injection of antibodies specific for SLF would have a similar effect.

## VII. PRODUCTION OF CSFs IN THE SKIN DURING INFLAMMATION

### A. Keratinocytes

Many cellular components of the skin are potential sources of colony-stimulating factors. Keratinocytes in vitro can produce GM-CSF, G-CSF, and CSF-1 in response to stimuli such as endotoxin. Fibroblasts and endothelial cells have similar capabilities.

There have been a number of reports that keratinocytes produce IL-3 or IL-3–like molecules. The most compelling data are based on analysis of a transformed keratocyte cell line of murine origin, PAM 212 (Kupper et al., 1987). However, as discussed above, it can be misleading to extrapolate from data on cytokine production by transformed cell lines to the normal cells. Moreover, S1 nuclease production analysis suggested that the mRNA from murine keratinocytes did not contain an mRNA species that was totally homologous with T-cell–derived IL-3 mRNA (Kupper et al., 1987).

An activity from human epidermal cells termed human epidermal cell IL-3–like activity has been described (Danner and Luger, 1987). This activity was detected on murine factor–dependent hemopoietic lines. However, this biological activity clearly distinguishes it from human IL-3, which does not cross-react with the murine IL-3 receptor and thus fails to stimulate murine factor–dependent hemopoietic cell lines. Thus, while there is no unequivocal evidence that keratinocytes produce IL-3, there may be novel CSFs produced by these cells.

## B. Skin Cells of Hemopoietic Origin

Skin cells of hemopoietic origin such as Langerhans cells, the dendritic Thy-1$^+$ epidermal cells and mast cells and their progenitors, are also potential sources of CSFs. The importance of hemopoietin production by the Thy-1$^+$ epidermal cells has not been explored in detail. The $\gamma\delta$ T lymphocytes do produce IL-3 and GM-CSF when stimulated (Cron et al., 1989) and accumulate in the skin in disease (Modlin et al., 1989).

There is good evidence for the production of CSFs by T lymphocytes in inflamed skin. GM-CSF and IL-3 mRNA-producing cells can be detected in situ hybridization in particular in allergen-induced late-phase cutaneous reactions in atopic individuals (Kay et al., 1991), but also in delayed-type hypersensitive reactions in skin (Tsicopoulos et al., 1992). In both instances T cells are probably the major site of cytokine production. Increased numbers of mast cells that are present in a wide range of lesions, including those associated with viral infections, e.g., herpes varicella and potential autoimmune phenomena, e.g., lichen planus (G. Varigos and J. W. Schrader, unpublished data), probably reflect the local release of IL-3 from activated T cells.

As discussed above, mast cells (Plaut et al., 1989) and their progenitors (Dy et al., 1991) can be stimulated to release hemopoietins such as IL-3, IL-4, IL-5, and GM-CSF, as well as other cytokines following cross-linking of specific antibodies bound to Fc receptors.

There is also evidence suggesting a nonimmunologically cell-specific mechanism for upregulating cytokine production by mast cells. Thus mast cells accumulated IL-3 mRNA when cultured in contact with fibroblasts (Razin et al., 1991). It has not been determined whether this phenomenon requires activation of the fibroblasts; as serum was present in these cultures it is possible that factors that activate fibroblasts and are released in response to stress such as PDGF are involved.

## VIII. ACTIONS OF CSFs IN INFLAMED SKIN

A diversity of stimuli, products of microorganisms, trauma, UV light, and specific antigens initiate the local release of CSFs and other cytokines by the keratinocytes, fibroblasts, endothelial cells, mast cells, and T lymphocytes in the skin. These CSFs and cytokines contributed to adherence of leukocytes to local endothelial cells and their exit from the blood into the affected tissues. CSFs in inflamed skin then play an important role in prolonging the extravascular survival of the various granulocytes and phagocytes and enhancing their function by priming for respiratory bursts and enhancing phagocytosis.

CSFs can also stimulate the local generation of hemopoietic cells in the skin. The mast cells that accumulate in skin lesions in a wide variety of conditions are probably generated in situ. There is good evidence from the work of Kitamura and colleagues (1989) that undifferentiated mast cell progenitors are present in normal skin and can be activated to generate mast cells. Moreover, the blood normally contains circulating hemopoietic progenitor cells, the levels of which are increased by IL-3, G-CSF, or G-CSF and inflammatory stimuli (Siena et al., 1989; Du et al., 1988). It is possible that these progenitor cells lodge preferentially at sites of inflammation and there under the influence of high, local concentrations of CSFs generate their progeny in situ. This process may be important in chronic inflammation and contribute to the formation of granulomata.

The actions of CSF's on the specific components of the skin are discussed in detail elsewhere in this volume. GM-CSF enhances the viability and function of dendritic cells (Witmer-Pack et al., 1987). The recent demonstration that GM-CSF stimulates the growth and differentiation of colonies of dendritic cells from progenitors circulating in the blood is interesting (Inaba et al., 1992). It will be important to determine whether these bloodborne progenitors seed into and proliferate in inflammatory lesions as discussed above.

The administration of IL-3 to primates resulted not only in the accumulation of mast cells in the skin but ancanthosis and an increase in expression of a cell cycle–associated antigen in the basal layer (Volc-Platzer et al., 1991). This effect could involve direct stimulation of keratinocytes or an indirect effort dependent on factors released by other cell types responding to IL-3 (e.g., mast cells). In vitro experiments (Hancock et al., 1988) also indicated that IL-3 and GM-CSF stimulated the growth of human keratinocytes. There is some evidence that IL-3, GM-CSF, and G-CSF may bind to certain carcinomas (Berdel et al., 1989), but as yet receptors for CSFs have not been demonstrated on normal epithelial cells. At present it seems more likely that the effect of IL-3 and GM-CSF on keratinocytes is indirect, but further investigation of the question is required.

## IX. CONCLUSIONS

Colony-stimulating factors play important roles in the development of normal skin and in mediating the response of the skin to inflammatory stimuli. SLF regulates the development and function of melanocytes and mast cells in the skin. Other CSFs—notably GM-CSF, G-CSF, CSF-1, and IL-3—are synthesized in response to invasion of the skin by foreign materials. GM-CSF, G-CSF, and CSF-1 are produced by many cell types including keratinocytes and skin cells of hemopoietic origin. IL-3 is produced by activated T lymphocytes and mast cells. During inflammation, CSFs stimulate migration of leukocytes into the skin and enhance their survival, phagocytic, and bacteriocidal activity. Local production of CSFs may also result in production of hemopoietic cells such as mast cells in the skin. The development of antagonists of the various CSFs may provide selective means of modulating inflammatory or allergic reactions in the skin.

## REFERENCES

D. M. Anderson, S. D. Lyman, A. Baird, J. M. Wignal, J. Eisenmann, C. Rauch, C. J. March, et al., *Cell 63*, 235 (1990).

J. F. Bazan, *Immunol. Today 11*, 350 (1990).

W. E. Berdel, S. Danhauser-Riedl, G. Steinhauser, et al., *Blood 73*, 80 (1989).

S. E. Bernstein, E. S. Russell, and G. Keighley, *Ann. NY Acad. Sci. 149*, 475 (1990).

T. R. Bradley and D. Metcalf, *Aust. J. Exp. Med. Biol. Sci. 44*, 287 (1966).

M. R. Capecchi, *Science 244*, 1288 (1989).

E. J. Clutterbuck and C. J. Sanderson, *Blood 71*, 646 (1988).

N. G. Copeland, D. N. Gilbert, B. C. Cho, P. J. Donovan, N. A. Jenkins, et al., *Cell 63*, 175 (1990).

R. M. Crapper, W. R. Thomas, and J. W. Schrader, *J. Immunol. 133*, 2174 (1984).

R. Q. Cron, T. F. Gajewski, S. O. Sharrow, et al., *J. Immunol. 142*, 3754 (1989).

M. Danner and T. A. Luger, *J. Invest. Dermatol. 88*, 353 (1987).

P. Desreumaux, A. Janin, F. Colombel, et al., *J. Exp. Med. 175*, 293 (1992).

U. Du, J. O. Villeval, J. Boyd, et al., *Blood 72*, 2074 (1988).

V. Duronio, M. Welham, S. Abraham, P. Dryden, and J. W. Schrader, *Proc. Soc. Natl. Acad. Sci. USA 89*, 1587 (1992).

M. Dy, D. Jankovic, R. Ploemacher, J. Theze, and E. Schneider, *Exp. Hematol. 19*, 934 (1991).

J. G. Flanagan, D. C. Chan, and P. Leder, *Cell 64*, 1025 (1991).

R. A. Fleischman, D. L. Saltman, V. Stastny, and S. Zneimer, *Proc. Natl. Acad. Sci. USA 88*, 10885 (1991).

R. Halaban, *Cancer Metastasis Rev. 10*, 129 (1991).

G. E. Hancock, G. Kaplan, and Z. Cohn, *J. Exp. Med. 168*, 1395 (1988).

M. Hatakeyama, T. Kono, N. Kobayashi, et al., *Science 252*, 1523 (1991).

E. Huang, K. Nocka, D. Beyer, T. Y. Chu, H. W. Lam, D. Wellner, J. Buck, and P. Besmer, *Cell 63*, 225 (1990).
J. N. Ihle, L. Pepersack, and L. Rebar, *J. Immunol. 126*, 2184 (1981).
K. Inaba, R. M. Steinman, M. W. Pack, et al., *J. Exp. Med. 175*, 1157 (1992).
A. B. Kay, S. Ying, V. Varney, et al., *J. Exp. Med. 173*, 775 (1991).
H. Kita, T. Ohnishi, Y. Okubo, et al., *J. Exp. Med. 174*, 745 (1991).
Y. Kitamura, *Annu. Rev. Immunol. 7*, 59 (1989).
P. Kluck and J. H. F. Falkenburg, *Blood 68*, 1316 (1980).
M. J. Koury and M. C. Bondurant, *Science 248*, 378 (1990).
S. B. Krantz, *Blood 77*, 419 (1991).
T. S. Kupper, M. Horowitz, F. Lee, D. Coleman, and P. Flood, *Clin. Res. 35*, 697A (1987).
K. B. Leslie, F. Lee, and J. W. Schrader, *Mol. Cell. Biol. 11*, 5562 (1991).
D. F. Mangan and S. M. Wahl, *J. Immunol. 147*, 3408 (1991).
Y. Matsui, K. M. Zsebo, and B. L. M. Hogan, *Nature 347*, 667 (1990).
D. L. McLeod, M. M. Shreve, and A. A. Axelrad, *Nature 261*, 492 (1976).
D. Metcalf, *Proc. Natl. Acad. Sci. USA 88*, 11310 (1991).
R. L. Modlin, C. Pirmez, F. M. Hofman, et al., *Nature 339*, 544 (1989).
M. A. S. Moore, *Blood 78*, 1 (1991).
R. Moqbel, Q. Hamid, S. Ying, et al., *J. Exp. Med. 174*, 749 (1991).
S. Nishikawa, M. Kusakubo, K. Yoshinaga, et al., *EMBO J. 10*, 2111 (1991).
M. Plaut, J. H. Pierce, C. J. Watson, J. Hanley-Hyde, R. P. Nordan, and W. E. Paul, *Nature 339*, 64 (1989).
D. H. Pluznik and S. L. Sachs, *J. Cell. Comp. Physiol. 66*, 319 (1965).
E. Razin, K. Leslie, and J. W. Schrader, *J. Immunol. 146*, 981 (1991).
C. W. Rettenmier, *Curr. Topic Microbiol. Immunol. 149*, 129 (1989).
J. Savill, A. H. Wyllie, J. E. Henson, M. J. Walport, et al., *Clin. Invest. 83*, 865 (1989).
J. W. Schrader, I. Clark-Lewis, R. M. Crapper, et al., in *Lymphokines 15*; *Interleukin 3*: *The Panspecific Hemopoietin* (J. W. Schrader, ed.), Academic Press, San Diego, CA, 1988, pp. 281–311.
J. W. Schrader and G. J. V. Nossal, *Immunol. Rev. 53*, 61 (1980).
J. W. Schrader, H. J. Ziltener, and K. B. Leslie, *Proc. Natl. Acad. Sci. USA 83*, 2458 (1986a).
J. W. Schrader, I. Clark-Lewis, H. J. Ziltener, et al., in *Immune Regulation by Characterized Polypeptides* (G. Goldstein, J. F. Bach, and H. Wigzell, eds.), Liss, New York, 1986b, pp. 475–483.
J. W. Schrader, C. Moyer, H. J. Ziltener, and C. L. Reinisch, *J. Immunol. 146*, 3799 (1991).
S. Siena, M. Bregni, B. Brando, et al., *Blood 74*, 1905 (1989).
E. R. Stanley, in *Genetics of Pattern Formation and Growth Control* (A. P. Mahowald, ed.), Wiley-Liss, New York, 1990, pp. 165–180.
M. Tsai, L.-S. Shih, G. F. J. Newlands, et al., *J. Exp. Med. 174*, 125 (1991).
A. Tsicopoulos, Q. Hamid, V. Varney, et al., *J. Immunol. 148*, 2058 (1992).
B. Volc-Platzer, P. Valent, T. Radaszkiewicz, et al., *Lab. Invest. 64*, 557 (1991).

W. Wiktor-Jedrzeiczak, A. Barocci, W. Ferrante, A. Ahmed-Ansari, K. W. Sell, J. W. Pollard, and E. R. Stanley, *Proc. Natl. Acad. Sci. USA 87*, 4828 (1990).

D. E. Williams, J. Eisenman, A. Baird, C. Rauch, K. Van Ness, C. J. March, L. S. Park, U. Martin, D. Y. Mochizuki, H. S. Boswell, G. S. Burgess, D. Cosmann, and S. D. Lyman, *Cell 63*, 167 (1990a).

G. T. Williams, C. A. Smith, E. Spooncer, T. M. Dexter, and D. R. Taylor, *Nature 343*, 76 (1990b).

M. D. Witmer-Pack, W. Olivier, J. Valinsky, G. Schuler, and R. M. Steinman, *J. Exp. Med. 166*, 1484 (1987).

A. Wodnar-Filipowicz, C. H. Heusser, and C. Moroni, *Nature 339*, 150 (1989).

# 8
# The Interferons

**Sidney Pestka**
*Robert Wood Johnson Medical School*
*University of Medicine & Dentistry of New Jersey*
*Piscataway, New Jersey*

## I. INTRODUCTION

The interferons represent proteins with antiviral activity that are secreted from cells in response to a variety of stimuli (see Refs. 1–4 for detailed reviews). There are at least four classes of interferons (IFN): alpha ($\alpha$), beta ($\beta$), gamma ($\gamma$), and omega ($\omega$). In general, exposure of cells to viruses and double-stranded RNAs induce the production of IFN-$\alpha$ and IFN-$\beta$ species. Nevertheless, the ratio of these interferons produced by cells varies with the tissue of origin and the species of the organism. T lymphocytes produce IFN-$\gamma$ when stimulated with antigens to which they are immune or when stimulated with mitogens such as staphylococcal enterotoxin A or the combination of phytohemagglutinin and phorbol esters. Table 1 summarizes the production of the human interferons from natural sources. Most of the interferons in therapeutic use are produced through genetic engineering [1–5].

Many procedures have been described for the partial purification of human and animal interferons [1–6]. Although partial purification of the interferons as bands on SDS-polyacrylamide gels was reported by a number of groups, it was not until 1978 and thereafter that any interferon was purified to homogeneity in solution in sufficient amounts for its chemical and physical characterization [7–11]. The introduction of reverse phase and normal phase high performance liquid chromatography (HPLC) to the purification of proteins [8, 10, 11] led to the first successful purification of these proteins so that sufficient amounts were available in solution without detergent for their chemical, biological, and immunological studies. Various affinity purification techniques, particularly antibody affinity chromatography,

**Table 1** Production of Human Interferons from Natural Sources

| Source | Inducer | Interferon |
|---|---|---|
| Leukocytes | Virus | IFN-α (major) |
| | | IFN-β (minor) |
| | | IFN-ω (minor) |
| | Mitogen | IFN-γ |
| | Antigen | IFN-γ |
| Fibroblasts | dsRNA | IFN-β |
| | Virus | IFN-α and IFN-β |

were utilized to purify human leukocyte (α) and fibroblast (β) interferons [1, 12–21]. This review will concentrate on the purification of the human leukocyte and fibroblast interferons from natural sources as well as the leukocyte interferon produced by recombinant DNA technology. A short review of the purification of human immune (γ) interferon is also included. In the last section, the sequences of many of the interferons are summarized.

## II. PURIFICATION OF HUMAN LEUKOCYTE INTERFERON (Hu-IFN-α)

Since their discovery, many attempts were made to purify the interferons, with little success until recent years. In fact, interferon used in experiments as well as in initial human clinical trials was essentially a crude protein fraction less than 1% of which by weight consisted of interferon. Because of the use of such crude interferon-containing material, it was not clear what activities of these preparations were indeed due inherently to the interferon present and what activities were due to the numerous other contaminating proteins. By definition, the antiviral activity was due to the interferon. However, these crude preparations exhibited antiprotozoal and antibacterial activities, inhibited cellular growth (antiproliferative activity), blocked antibody synthesis, and were ascribed to have an enormous number of other activities. However, without essentially pure interferon, it was not possible to demonstrate definitively whether or not a particular activity was due to the interferon protein molecule itself. Accordingly, it was essentialy to obtain pure interferon to determine what activities were an inherent part of the interferon molecule. Since very little was known about the size and structure of the interferons, the isolation of pure interferons would establish their chemical composition and structure as well as their biological activities. Some of the activities ascribed to interferon turned out to be exhibited by the pure forms, but other properties were not demonstrable with pure preparations and were, therefore, due in whole or in part to one of the contaminants in the crude preparations. To obtain purified interferons, many groups began work on their purification shortly after their discovery.

## A. Production

We began purification of interferon from human leukocytes in 1977. This interferon was produced by incubating human white blood cells with Newcastle disease virus or Sendai virus for 6–24 hours [22–25]. The procedure was a combination of previously reported techniques [26, 27]. The antiviral activity was found in the cell culture medium after overnight incubation of the leukocytes as illustrated in Figure 1. We substituted milk casein for human or bovine serum in the culture medium as had been described [26]. The use of casein, a single protein, instead of serum, which contains many different and uncharacterized proteins, simplified the initial concentration and purification steps. We used leukocytes from normal donors as well as from patients with chronic myelogenous leukemia. These leukemic cells make large amounts of human leukocyte interferon when induced with Newcastle disease virus or Sendai virus [23, 28–30].

The cytopathic effect inhibition assay for interferon as originally described took 3 days. Other assays for interferon were even longer. It was necessary to develop a more rapid assay so that we could evaluate whether a puficiation step was useful. A cytopathic effect inhibition assay that could be done in 12–16 hours was developed [31, 32] and accelerated the purification immensely.

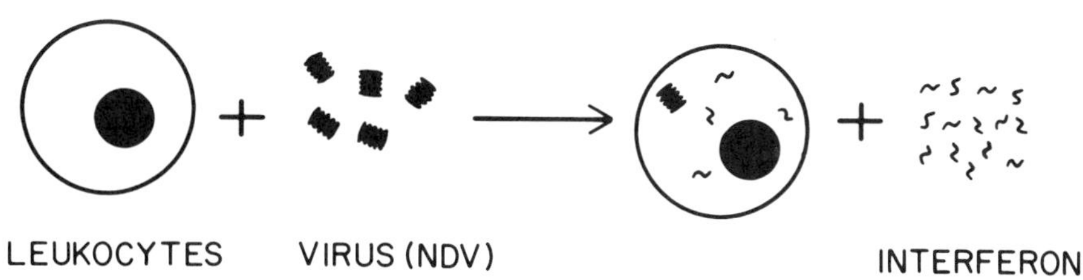


**Fig. 1** Production of interferon with Newcastle disease virus and leukocytes. Leukocytes, the white blood cells of peripheral blood, are obtained from normal donors or patients with chronic myelogenous leukemia. The cells are washed, placed in culture medium with Newcastle disease virus (or with Sendai virus), and incubated overnight at 37°C. Interferon is found in the culture medium after incubation. The cells and virus can be removed by centrifugation, leaving the culture medium containing interferon.

## B. HPLC for Protein Purification

Because we knew that classical techniques for protein purification, as applied by others, were not remarkably successful in purification of the human interferons, we applied HPLC to the purification of proteins. Udenfriend and co-workers [33–35] had developed sensitive fluorescent techniques for detection of amino acids and peptides and had achieved the separation of peptides by reverse-phase HPLC. However, separation of proteins had not yet been accomplished. In the early experiments, there was uniform failure to achieve any purification of proteins with reverse-phase HPLC because the interferon activity was continually lost. At the time, increasing ethanol concentration was used to elute proteins, and this was tried for interferon and other proteins without success. It was necessary to use a less polar solvent to elute interferon. Although there was initial hesitancy to use *n*-propanol above 20% (v/v) and other organic solvents because of the limited solubility

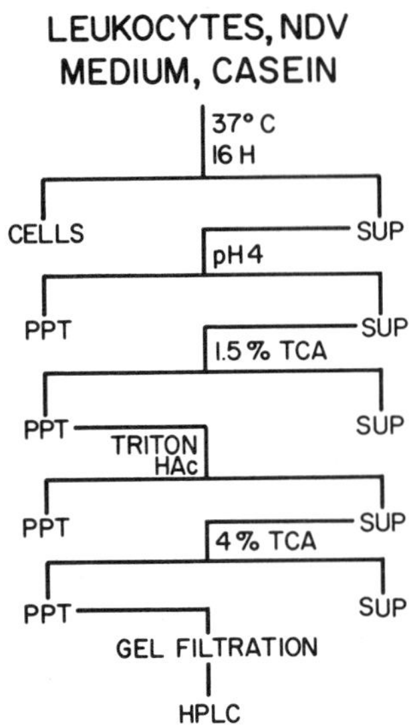


**Fig. 2** Flow chart of initial steps in purification of leukocyte interferon. Cells and debris were removed by low-speed centrifugation from the medium containing interferon. Casein was used as a serum substitute. By acidification of the medium to pH 4 with hydrochloric acid, the bulk of the casein, which precipitated, was removed from the interferon, which remained in solution. The interferon was concentrated by two steps, involving precipitation with trichloroacetic acid. The concentrated solution containing relatively crude interferon was separated into components of different sizes by gel filtration on Sephadex G-100 in the presence of 4 M urea. Details of these procedures have been described [8, 9, 25, 39].

of proteins in such solvents, it was found that *n*-propanol gradients effectively eluted interferon and other proteins without noticeable precipitation at the concentrations employed [7–9, 36]. Furthermore, by changing the pH of the elution buffer, a completely different separation could be achieved during elution of the same reverse-phase column with *n*-propanol. As subsequently demonstrated with fibroblast interferon [11], a large number of different columns and solvent systems could be used to effect resolution of proteins. By applying normal-phase chromatography with a diol silica col-

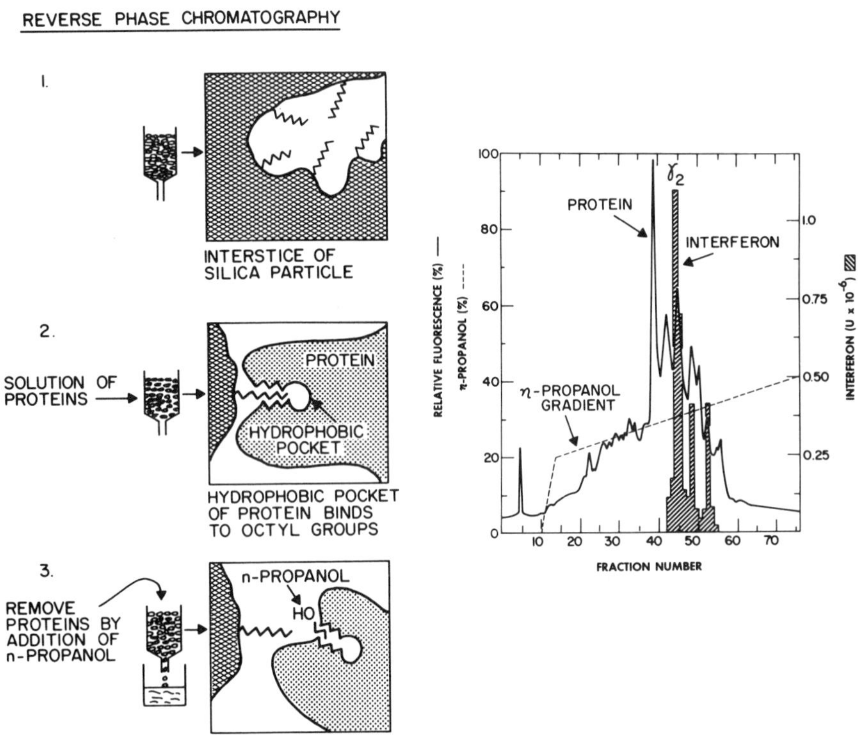


**Fig. 3** HPLC of leukocyte interferon on reverse-phase columns. Columns of porous silica to which octyl groups were bound were used to separate leukocyte interferons from other proteins and to resolve the individual leukocyte interferons. The proteins enter the interstices within the silica particles where the hydrophobic areas of the protein bind tightly to the octyl groups. The nonpolar portion of *n*-propanol can interact with interferon, releasing interferon and other proteins from the column. By eluting the proteins with an increasing gradient of *n*-propanol, the proteins are released in order of their increasing hydrophobicity. Those proteins binding most tightly are released only after high concentrations of *n*-propanol are used [5].

umn between the two reverse-phase columns, it was possible to use just three sequential HPLC steps to purify human leukocyte interferon to homogeneity. Sufficient amounts were purified in high yield for initial chemical characterization of the protein and for determination of amino acid composition. The amino acid composition of the human leukocyte interferon species $\gamma 2$ was the first reported for any purified interferon [8].

The initial steps included selective precipitations and gel filtration (Fig. 2) followed by HPLC. The HPLC steps were reverse-phase chromatography (Fig. 3) at pH 7.5 on LiChrosorb RP-8, normal partition chromatography on LiChrosorb Diol (Fig. 4), and reverse-phase chromatography at pH 4.0 on LiChrosorb RP-8. Gradients of *n*-propanol were used for elution of interferon from these columns (Figs. 3, 4, 5). The overall purification was about

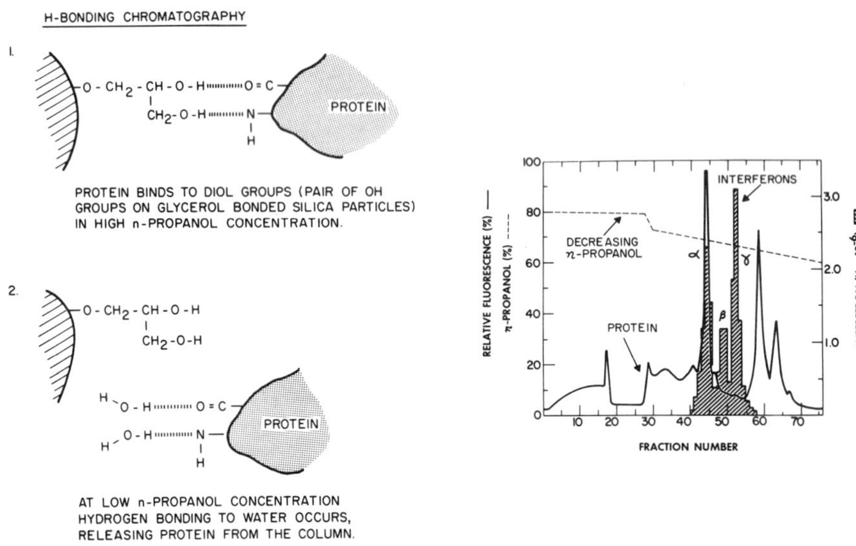


**Fig. 4** Hydrogen-bonding HPLC on diol-silica. Hydrogen bonding of proteins to columns containing glycerol covalently attached to silica was used to separate interferon species. Since hydrogen bonds are relatively weak bonds and are readily made to the water in which the protein is dissolved, in order to force proteins to bind to the diol-silica, it was necessary to use very high concentration of *n*-propanol. Upon reduction of the *n*-propanol concentration, proteins are released from the column in order of their increasing ability to form H-bonds with the diol groups of the column. Those proteins released first form the weakest H-bonds with the column. Multiple molecular species of human leukocyte interferon ($\alpha$, $\beta$, and $\gamma$) are shown in the figure. These designations should not be confused with the subsequent nomenclature of IFN-$\alpha$, IFN-$\beta$, and IFN-$\gamma$ assigned to leukocyte, fibroblast, and immune interferons, respectively.

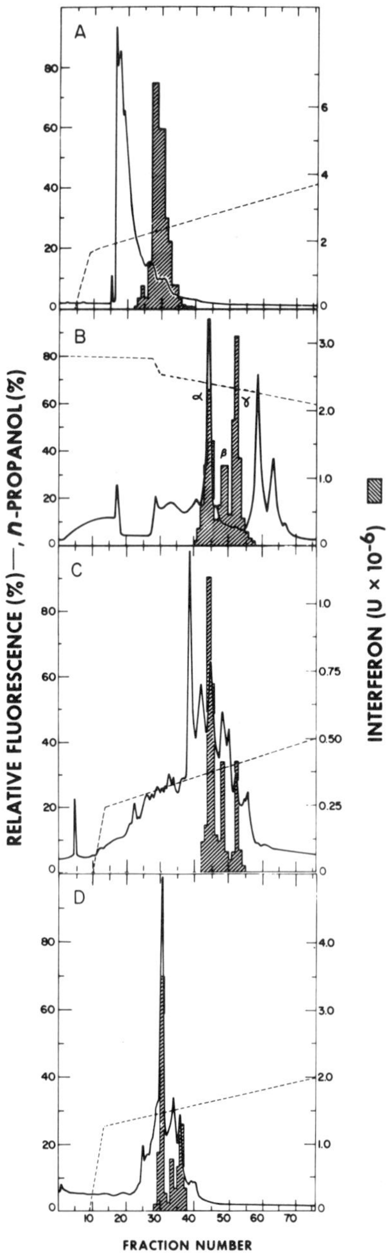


**Fig. 5** HPLC of interferon. (A) Chromatography on LiChrosorb RP-8 at pH 7.5. (B) Chromatography on LiChrosorb diol at pH 7.5. (C) Chromatography on LiChrosorb RP-8 at pH 4.0 of the $\gamma$ peak of part B. (D) Rechromatography on LiChrosorb RP-8 of the major activity peak of part C. The conditions were similar to those of step C. Several preparations carried through step C were pooled ($13 \times 10^6$ units) and applied to the last column. The gradations on the abcissa correspond to the end of the fractions. The solid lines on the graph represent protein as measured by the fluorescamine method [5, 8].

80,000-fold, and the specific activity of pure interferon was 2–4 × $10^8$ units/mg [8]. Interferon prepared by this procedure yielded a single band of MW 17,500 on polyacrylamide gel electrophoresis. The antiviral activity was associated with the single protein band [7]. The specific activity of this peak was 4 × $10^8$ units/mg, and those of some other leukocyte interferons are shown in Table 2.

Several reports had previously described HPLC of proteins, mainly on ion exchange and size exclusion columns [37, 38]. However, those systems were either not commercially available or had a low capacity. With proper choice of eluent and pore size, octyl and octadecyl silica could be used for high-resolution reverse-phase HPLC of both peptides and proteins. Accordingly, with *n*-propanol as eluent, the use of LiChrosorb RP-8 (octyl silica) columns for protein fractionation was a major factor in the success of the purification (Fig. 5A,C,D). In addition, LiChrosorb Diol, which is chemically similar to glycophase resins that have been used for exclusion chromatography of proteins, was introduced as a support for normal partition chromatography of proteins (Fig. 5B). High recoveries of interferon activity were obtained in each chromatographic step, a requirement when small amounts of initial starting material are present. Although the initial experiments were performed with leukocytes from normal donors [7, 8], it was found that leukocytes from patients with chronic myelogenous leukemia (CML) who were undergoing leukapheresis to lower their peripheral white blood cell counts were a rich source of interferon that appeared to be essentially identical

**Table 2** Specific Activities of Representative Purified Human Interferons

| Interferon | Source | Specific activity (units/mg) | Assay cells | Relative titers MDBK/WISH | Relative titers MDBK/AG-1732 | Ref. |
|---|---|---|---|---|---|---|
| IFN-$\alpha$ ($\gamma_2$) | Leukocytes | 4.0 × $10^8$ | MDBK | — | — | 7–9 |
| IFN-$\alpha$ ($\alpha_2$) | Leukocytes | 4.0 × $10^8$ | MDBK | — | 1.3 | 9 |
| IFN-$\alpha$ (b3) | KG-1 cells | 4.0 × $10^8$ | MDBK | — | 1.5 | 39 |
| IFN-$\alpha$ (Ly) | Namalwa cells | 2.5 × $10^8$ | Human fibroblasts | — | — | 15 |
| IFN-$\alpha$ A | *E. coli* | 3.0 × $10^8$ | MBDK | 1.7 | 1.6 | 40, 41 |
| IFN-$\beta$ | Fibroblasts | 2-10 × $10^8$ | GM-258 | — | — | 12, 13 |
| IFN-$\beta$ | Fibroblasts | 4.0 × $10^8$ | AG-1732 | — | — | 11 |
| IFN-$\beta$ | Fibroblasts | 3.2 × $10^8$ | AG-1732 | — | — | 10 |
| IFN-$\beta$ | *E. coli* | 9.4 × $10^7$ | WISH | — | — | 42 |
| [Ser$^{17}$]IFN-$\beta$ | *E. coli* | 1.2 × $10^8$ | GM-2504 | — | — | 43 |
| IFN-$\gamma$ | Leukocytes | 5.9 × $10^7$ | WISH | — | — | 44, 45 |
| IFN-$\gamma$ | *E. coli* | 1.0 × $10^7$ | WISH | — | — | 46 |

to the human leukocyte interferon purified from leukocytes from normal donors [30]. As with HPLC of interferon from normal leukocytes on the Diol column (Fig. 5B), three major peaks of activity, labeled $\alpha$, $\beta$, and $\gamma$,* were observed with interferon prepared from CML cells. Although the protein profiles were almost identical, the activity profiles showed that the amount of activity under peak $\gamma$ was lower in preparations from leukemic cells compared to normal leukocytes [8, 30]. However, even from normal leukocytes, the ratio of peaks $\alpha$, $\beta$, and $\gamma$ varied from one preparation to another. Human lymphoblastoid interferon produced by suspension cultures of Namalva cells was purified by a combination of immunoaffinity chromatography and other methods by Zoon et al. [15]. The amino acid composition of human leukocyte interferon purified by HPLC as described above [8] shows similarity with human lymphoblastoid interferon [15] and one of the types of mouse interferon [14].

## C. Multiple Species of Leukocyte Interferon

During the purification of leukocyte interferon, it became evident that multiple species existed (Figs. 4, 5). Human leukocyte interferon is heterogeneous, and several bands containing antiviral activity ranging in MW from 15,000 to 21,000 are observed on SDS-polyacrylamide gel electrophoresis [47]. Heterogeneity of human leukocyte interferon has also been observed by isoelectric focusing [48] and several types of chromatographic procedures [9, 49–52]. As noted above, our initial work with HPLC revealed three major groups of interferon species, which were labeled $\alpha$, $\beta$, and $\gamma$ according to their order of elution from a LiChrosorb Diol (polar-bonded phase) column [8, 9]. These groups were further resolved into several homogeneous components. Although others had reported heterogeneity in crude human leukocyte interferon preparations [49–52], this was not thought to be due to amino acid sequence heterogeneity. In fact, it had been reported by a number of groups that leukocyte interferon contained carbohydrate and that heterogeneity was due to differences in carbohydrate content of the protein [48, 53–55]. Thus, the well-established heterogeneity of human leukocyte interferon was attributed to differences in the degree of glycosylation. However, five purified species of leukocyte interferon examined contained no detectable carbohydrate [9]: the amino sugar content of each species analyzed ($\alpha$, $\beta 1$, $\beta 2$, $\beta 3$, and $\gamma 3$) was determined to be much less than one residue of either glucosamine

*The natural interferons isolated from the mixture present in leukocyte interferon by HPLC [5–7] were then designated $\alpha 1$, $\alpha 2$, $\beta 1$, $\beta 2$, $\beta 3$, $\gamma 1$, $\gamma 2$, $\gamma 3$, $\gamma 4$, $\gamma 5$, and $\delta$. Unfortunately, the same terminology was later applied to designate leukocyte, fibroblast, and immune interferons, respectively as $\alpha$, $\beta$, $\gamma$.

or galactosamine per molecule of interferon [9]. Allen and Fantes [16] also found no carbohydrate on the species of leukocyte interferon they purified. We therefore concluded that, contrary to the prevailing dogma, human leukocyte interferon is largely devoid of carbohydrate. Furthermore, because peptide mapping and sequencing revealed significant structural differences among the species, we concluded that leukocyte interferon represents a family of homologous proteins. By analogous procedures, additional leukocyte interferon species were isolated from cultured myeloblasts [39, 56]. Since our initial purification, other reports [16, 18, 19, 57] have also described multiple species of leukocyte interferon.

## D. Amino Acid Sequences of Leukocyte Interferons

Since only relatively small amounts of each species were isolated in these early experiments, it was difficult to obtain information about their amino acid sequence. Determinations of the amino acid sequences of the amino-terminal end of human IFN-$\alpha$ were reported [58, 59], as was that of IFN-$\beta$ [10, 11, 17, 60]. It was clear that all the amino acid sequences obtained for human fibroblast interferon were identical and that we had all purified and sequenced the same protein. At the time, it was comforting to know that the new microsequencing procedures were dependable. However, it was striking that the amino-terminal sequences of individual species of human leukocyte interferon were different [58, 59]. The differences confirmed that the leukocyte interferons consisted of a family of closely related proteins. We subsequently isolated a human interferon DNA recombinant [5, 61], the coding sequence of which was virtually identical to the sequence of our pure proteins.

Thereafter, Levy et al. [62] and Shively et al. [63] reported amino acid sequences of three species of human leukocyte interferon. So far, the sequences of two leukocyte interferons were determined almost completely (Fig. 6). Additional sequences were reported by Zoon [57]. Allen and Fantes [16] reported the sequences of tryptic fragments obtained from a mixture of several leukocyte interferon species. All these sequences are sufficiently different to establish very clearly the concept of a family of closely related proteins. As described above [5, 61], the first clone of human leukocyte interferon isolated in our laboratory was almost identical in sequence to human leukocyte interferons $\alpha 2$ and $\beta$ species, which were, however, 10 amino acids shorter than expected from the DNA sequence. It should be noted that during this time several groups [14, 20, 64–67] reported the purification of mouse interferons, and some amino acid sequences were reported [68].

## E. Carbohydrate Content

The carbohydrate content of the species of human IFN-$\alpha$ derived from patients with chronic myelogenous leukemia (CML) and from normal donors

1 10 20
CYS ASP LEU PRO GLN THR HIS SER LEU GLY SER ARG ARG THR LEU MET LEU LEU ALA GLN

21 30 40
MET ARG LYS ILE SER LEU PHE SER CYS LEU LYS ASP ARG HIS ASP PHE GLY PHE PRO GLN

41 50 60
GLU GLU PHE GLY ASN GLN PHE GLN LYS ALA GLU THR ILE PRO VAL LEU HIS GLU MET ILE

61 70 80
GLN GLN ILE PHE ASN LEU PHE SER THR LYS ASP SER SER ALA ALA TRP ASP GLU THR LEU

81 90 100
LEU ASP LYS PHE TYR THR GLU LEU TYR GLN GLN LEU ASN ASP LEU GLU ALA CYS VAL ILE

101 110 120
GLN GLY VAL GLY VAL THR GLU THR PRO LEU MET LYS GLU ASP SER ILE LEU ALA VAL ARG

121 130 140
LYS TYR PHE GLN ARG ILE THR LEU TYR LEU LYS GLU LYS LYS TYR SER PRO CYS ALA TRP

141 150 155
GLU VAL VAL ARG ALA GLU ILE MET ARG SER PHE SER LEU SER THR

**Fig. 6** Sequence of human leukocyte interferons $\alpha 2$ and $\beta$. The bars under the sequence represent the tryptic peptides isolated and sequenced. Solid bars represent the sequence determined by Edman degradation of the peptides. Unfilled bars represent sequences that were consistent with the composition of the peptides and/or sequence assignments derived from the DNA of the corresponding recombinant. Details of these experiments have been reported [62, 63]. The molecular weight of the protein as shown is 18,056.

was determined [69, 70]. Amino sugar content was measured by HPLC and fluorescamine detection of acid hydrolysates of each sample [69]. O-linked glycosylation was also detected by a combination of HPLC, enzymatic analysis, and SDS-polyacrylamide gel electrophoresis [70]. Two species showed significant amounts of glucosamine [69]. Most of the purified species of leukocyte interferon from a myeloblast cell line were also tested, and two species were found to contain sugar residues. These forms also differed from the CML interferons in that they revealed the presence of greater amounts of glactosamine. The apparent lack of carbohydrate in some of the higher molecular weight species of interferon implicated factors other than glycosylation in the molecular weight differences. The results indicated that some species of IFN-$\alpha$ are glycosylated to various degrees.

## III. ISOLATION OF RECOMBINANTS

Because recombinant DNA technology offered an opportunity to produce large amounts of Hu-IFNs economically, many scientific teams set out to clone them in bacteria. Several groups achieved the isolation of recombinants for several Hu-IFN-$\alpha$ species [61, 71] and for IFN-$\beta$ [61, 72–75], achieving their goals by somewhat different but analogous approaches. The cloning and expression of Hu-IFN-$\alpha$ as an illustration of these procedures is described.

Isolating Hu-IFN DNA sequences was a formidable task since it meant preparing DNA recombinants from cellular mRNA that was present at a low level. This task had never been accomplished previously using a protein whose structure was unknown. In addition, in order to reconstruct DNA recombinants that would express natural IFN, it is useful to know the partial amino acid sequence of the proteins, particularly at the $NH_2$- and COOH-terminal ends. Without this information, synthesis of natural Hu-IFN in bacterial cells would not have been possible. Thus, purification of the Hu-IFNs and determination of their structure [7–9, 15, 16, 39, 60, 62, 63] assisted us and others in these efforts.

To isolate recombinants containing the human DNA corresponding to IFN-$\alpha$, we used a number of procedures. First, it was necessary to isolate and measure the IFN mRNA. This was accomplished several years earlier when IFN mRNA was translated in cell-free extracts (Fig. 7) [76, 77] and

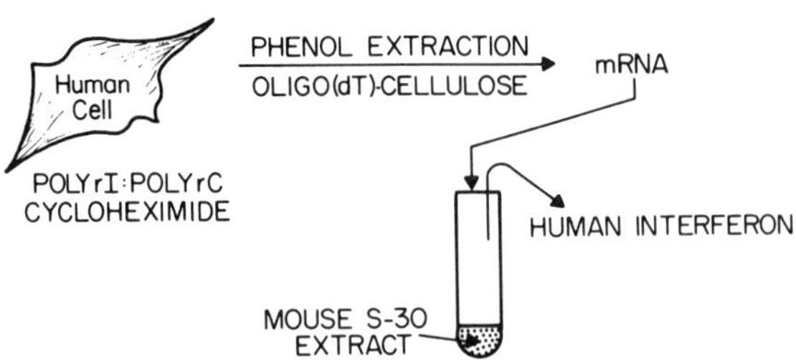


**Fig. 7** IFN synthesis in a cell-free system. Human fibroblasts were stimulated to produce IFN by treatment with the inducer poly(I):poly(C). The total RNA present was extracted 4 hours later from the cell with phenol, and the fraction enriched in mRNA was selected on an oligo(dT)-cellulose column. An S-30 supernatant translation fraction was prepared from mouse cells. This was able to translate the various mRNA species, including that for IFN-$\beta$, into the corresponding proteins. The IFN formed was detected in a standard antiviral assay. In this way, biologically active Hu-IFN was synthesized in the test tube for the first time. By injecting the mRNA into intact frog oocytes, the mRNA could be measured at 1/100 to 1/1000 the levels that could be detected in the cell-free extracts [5].

in frog oocytes [78–81]. The next step was to prepare sufficient mRNA from cells synthesizing IFN, and this was accomplished with both fibroblasts and leukocytes [82, 83].

A library of complementary DNA (cDNA) was prepared from a template of partially purified mRNA isolated from human leukocytes synthesizing IFN (Fig. 8). The dC-tailed double-stranded (ds) DNA obtained was hybridized to dG-tailed DNA from plasmid pBR322, which had been cleaved at the *Pst*I restriction nuclease site and introduced into *Escherichia coli* by transformation. About 14,000 tetracycline-resistant and ampicillin-sensitive transformants were obtained. This provided a large group of cDNA recombinants with DNA copies of all the mRNAs extracted from the leukocytes. The next and the hardest part of the procedure was to find in this vast library of recombinant plasmids those that contained DNA encoding IFN. If we had been able to begin with pure IFN mRNA, this would have been a simple task. However, we did not have pure IFN mRNA. We began with a mixture of mRNA molecules, and only relatively few were IFN-specific. We could show their presence by translating the RNA and assaying the products for IFN activity (Fig. 7). In this situation, we had to devise an indirect two-stage procedure. In the first stage, we screened all the bacterial colonies to find those with cDNA made from the RNA of induced cells; among these there might have been some carrying IFN cDNA. We therefore screened all the recombinants for their ability to bind to mRNA from cells synthesizing IFN (induced cells), but not to mRNA from uninduced cells (those not producing IFN) (Fig. 9). To do this, individual transformant colonies were screened by colony hybridization for the presence of induced-specific sequences with $^{32}$P-labeled IFN mRNA (mRNA from induced cells) as probe. In the presence of excess mRNA from uninduced cells (Fig. 9), recombinants that were representative of mRNA sequences existing only in induced cells should be evident on hybridization. This screening procedure allowed us to discard about 90% of the colonies; since their plasmids carried no induced cDNA, these could not encode IFN [61, 84].

In the second stage, we had to identify those recombinants containing the IFN DNA sequences among the remaining 10%. To do this, we pooled the recombinant plasmids in groups of 10 and examined these for the presence of IFN-specific sequences by an assay that depends upon hybridization of IFN mRNA to plasmid DNA [61, 85]. Plasmid DNA from 10 recombinants was isolated and covalently bound to diazobenzloxymethyl (DBM) paper (Fig. 10). The mRNA from induced cells was hybridized to each filter. Unhybridized mRNA was removed by washing. After the specifically hybridized mRNA was eluted, both fractions were translated in *Xenopus laevis* oocytes. Once a positive group had been found (one in which the specifically hybridized mRNA yielded IFN after microinjection into frog oocytes), it

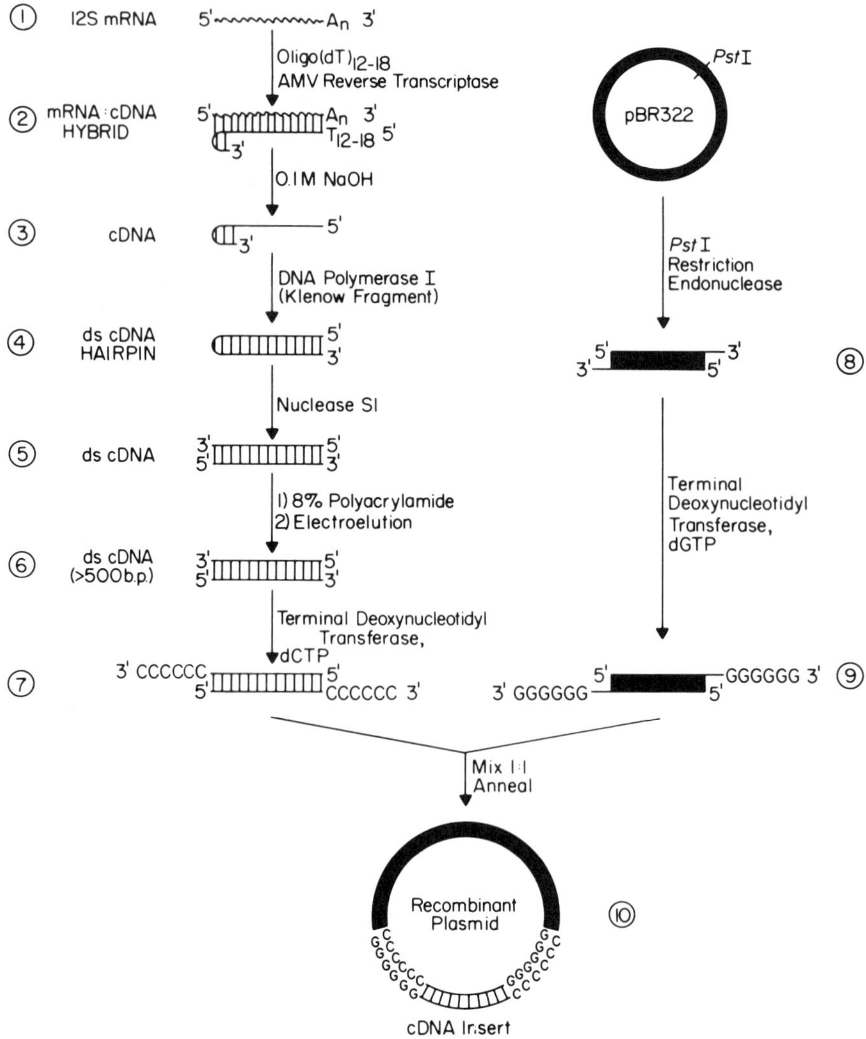


**Fig. 8** Preparation of IFN DNA recombinants from mRNA. Step 1: A human leukocyte suspension was induced to form IFN by stimulation with Sendai virus. An extract was made 6 hours later from which mRNA was prepared that was enriched in 12S mRNA by differential centrifugation. Step 2: The mRNA fraction was used as a template with AMV reverse transcriptase in the presence of all four deoxynucleotide triphosphates and oligo(dT)$_{12\text{-}18}$ as a primer to generate a DNA stand complementary to the mRNA (cDNA) forming mRNA:cDNA hybrids. Step 3: Treatment with 0.1 M NaOH digested away the RNA, leaving a cDNA fragment with a self-annealed 3′ end. Step 4: Extension of the chain with DNA polymerase (Klenow fragment) produced as ds-cDNA containing a hairpin loop. Step 5: Treatment with nuclease S1 opened the hairpin loop. Step 6: The ds-cDNA was sized on an 8% polyacrylamide gel followed

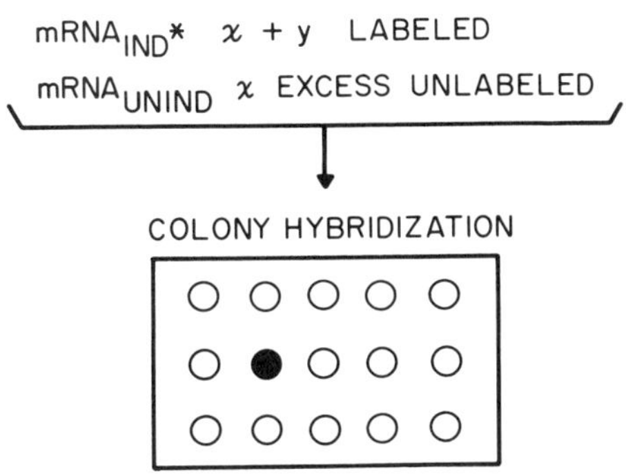


**Fig. 9** Schematic outline of hybridization procedure. *E. coli* cells were transformed with the recombinant plasmids generated as described in Figure 8. Colonies derived from individual transformed bacterial cells were transfered to filter paper, fixed and probed with a $^{32}$P-labeled mRNA preparation from cells producing IFN, and, therefore, enriched in IFN mRNA (x + y). The hybridization was performed in the presence of excess unlabeled mRNA from uninduced cells (x). This procedure identified bacterial colonies containing DNA coding for the protein specifically formed in induced leukocytes, including IFN. The induced-specific sequences (y) include IFN sequences as well as others that are induced concomitantly with IFN [5, 86].

was necessary to identify the specific clone or clones containing IFN cDNA. The 10 individual colonies were grown, the plasmid DNAs were prepared, and each individual DNA was examined by mRNA hybridization as above (Fig. 10). By these procedures a recombinant, plasmid 104 (p104), containing most of the coding sequence for a Hu-IFN-$\alpha$ was identified [61]. The DNA sequence was determined and found to correspond to what was then known of the amino acid sequence of purified Hu-IFN-$\alpha$ [60, 62]. The cDNA insert in p104 contains the sequence corresponding to more than 80% of the amino acids in IFN-$\alpha$, but not for those at its amino-terminal end. It was

---

by electroelution to give a fraction containing at least 500 base pairs. Step 7: Treatment with terminal deoxynucleotidyl transferase in the presence of dCTP added cytosine homopolymer tails at the 3′ ends of each strand. Step 8: The plasmid pBR322 was cleaved (linearized) at the *Pst*I site with *Pst*I restriction endonuclease. Step 9: Homopolymer tails of oligodeoxyguanylate were added to the 3′ ends of the linearized plasmid DNA with terminal deoxynucleotidyl transferase in the presence of dGTP. Step 10: The two fragments with complementary ends were mixed in equal proportions and annealed to yield a recombinant plasmid. A larger number of similar plasmids not containing IFN genetic information were also formed during this procedure. This cDNA library contained copies of all the mRNA in these cells including IFN-specific mRNA.

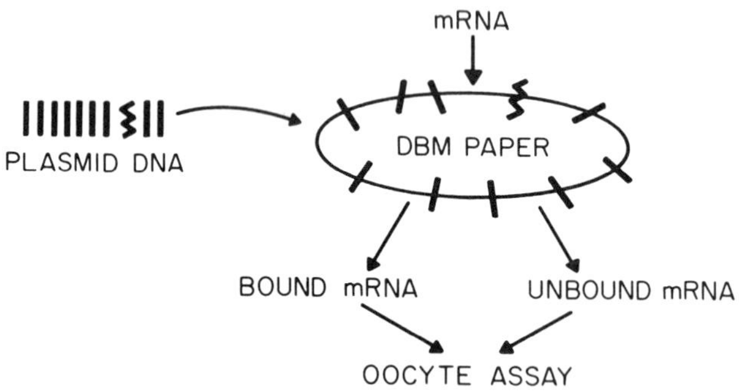


**Fig. 10** Schematic illustration of screening of recombinants with DBM paper. Plasmid DNA was isolated from a pool of colonies, e.g., 10 colonies as shown in the figure, and bound covalently to DBM paper. To detect a recombinant containing an IFN sequence (shown as a zigzag in the illustration), mRNA prepared from cells synthesizing IFN was hybridized to the bound DNA. After unhybridized mRNA had been removed by washing, the specifically hybridized mRNA was eluted and translated in *Xenopus laevis* oocytes. By this procedure, those pools of clones in which at least one recombinant contained an IFN sequence were identified. Thereafter, individual clones in each pool were separately screened by the same procedure. Unbound mRNA was microinjected into oocytes as well as a control to ascertain that the mRNA was not destroyed by the manipulations.

therefore used as a probe for finding a full-length copy of the IFN cDNA sequence which could be used for expression of Hu-IFN-$\alpha$ in *E. coli.* In addition, p104 DNA was used to isolate DNA sequences corresponding to other IFN-$\alpha$ species directly from a human gene bank.

Examination of the coding regions of the IFN-$\alpha$ genes that have been isolated in our laboratory and others has shown that these correspond to a family of homologous proteins, the IFN-$\alpha$ species [5, 86], which are closely related to each other and yet each unique in amino acid sequence. Thus, the previously discovered heterogeneity in Hu-IFN-$\alpha$ was shown to be at least in part the result of distinct genes representing each expressed Hu-IFN-$\alpha$ sequence. The cloned Hu-IFN-$\alpha$A, which was the first one we isolated, corresponds to the natural Hu-IFN-$\alpha$s which we purified from the mixture present in IFN-$\alpha$ by HPLC and termed $\alpha2$ and $\beta$. The $\alpha2$ and $\beta$ indicated here refer to two different IFN-$\alpha$ fractions.

By similar procedures to those described for 104, p101 was shown to contain the sequence for Hu-IFN-$\beta$. Thus, the nucleotide sequences coding for Hu-IFN-$\alpha$ and -$\beta$ were identified.

# IV. CONSTRUCTION OF EXPRESSION VECTORS

## A. Expression of Hu-IFN-$\alpha$ in *E. coli*

As noted above, p104 contained most of the sequence for a Hu-IFN-$\alpha$, but did not contain the sequence coding for the amino terminus of the protein. Accordingly, p104 was used to screen additional cDNA recombinants, and a number of cDNA recombinants which hybridized to its unique IFN-coding sequence were identified [1, 5, 87]. Most contained IFN DNA sequences of sufficient size to code for an entire IFN-$\alpha$ protein.

Our first full-length recombinant isolated corresponded to IFN-$\alpha$A [61, 87], and its entire *Pst*I insert was sequenced. Existing knowledge about IFN protein sequences permitted us to determine the correct translational reading frame and, hence, to predict the entire amino acid sequence for the IFN species encoded by this recombinant. The mature IFN-$\alpha$A was expressed directly by reconstruction of the recombinant [87]. The leader sequence of the protein was removed, and an ATG translation-initiation codon was placed immediately preceding the codon for the first amino acid of mature IFN-$\alpha$. Next, a 300-base-pair *Eco*RI fragment of *E. coli* DNA was constructed, containing the tryptophan (trp) promoter-operator and the trp leader ribosome-binding site, but stopping short of the ATG sequence needed to initiate translation of the leader peptide of the trp regulatory region. This DNA fragment was attached to the reconstructed Hu-IFN-$\alpha$ in front of the ATG codon (Fig. 11). Inserted into *E. coli*, the recombinant yielded high levels of activity, about $2 \times 10^8$ units (about 1 mg) of IFN per liter of culture. The IFN protein produced in *E. coli* behaves similarly to IFN-$\alpha$ formed directly by human leukocytes: it is stable to acid treatment, is neutralized by antiserum to Hu-IFN-$\alpha$, and binds to monoclonal antibodies specific for Hu-IFN-$\alpha$. It can be purified to homogeneity with the use of monoclonal antibodies [40, 41]. With improvements in fermentation and in the bacterial strains, high levels of Hu-IFN-$\alpha$ ($1 \times 10^{10}$ units/L, 50 mg/L) can be obtained in large-scale cultures. Similar high levels have been produced with other IFNs and other eukaryotic proteins.

## B. Expression of Hu-IFN-$\beta$ in *E. coli*

As already mentioned, a bacterial clone containing IFN-$\beta$ DNA was identified [61, 75]. In contrast to the multiple species of IFN-$\alpha$, experiments have indicated that there is only a single Hu-IFN-$\beta$ gene that corresponds to this recombinant. To express mature Hu-IFN-$\beta$ directly in *E. coli*, a series of plasmids that placed the synthesis of the 166-amino-acid polypeptide under trp promoter control (Fig. 11) were constructed. The IFN-$\beta$ produced in bacteria is similar to that formed by human fibroblasts by several criteria. It contains the same amino acid sequences, has the same relative antiviral

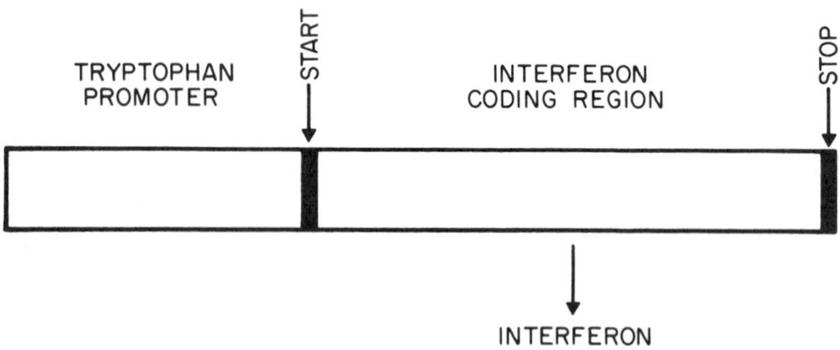


**Fig. 11** Regulation of IFN expression in *E. coli*. A 300-base-pair fragment of *E. coli* DNA was prepared with the restriction endonuclease *Eco*RI. This contained the trp promoter-operator and ribosome-binding site. The complete DNA sequence coding for IFN-αA was prepared, and an ATG codon (which is the signal for the initiation of translation of the mRNA into a protein) was placed immediately in front of the codon for the first amino acid of the mature protein. The *Eco*RI trp promoter-operator fragment was ligated distal to this ATG condon and inserted into plasmids. Bacteria transformed with a plasmid containing this control region and the IFN-coding sequence formed IFN in large amounts in the absence of trp. Leukocyte IFN-αA expression was thus regulated by the trp promoter-operator [5].

activity on human and bovine cells, and is neutralized by rabbit antibodies to IFN-β but not by antibodies to Hu-IFN-α. However, IFN-β made in bacteria is not glycosylated, whereas that made by human cells contains carbohydrate [11, 12].

## C. Other Expression Vectors

Although *E. coli* has been the predominant host used for the production of recombinant proteins, other host-vector systems have been studied and may be used more in the future. For example, the Hu-IFNs have been expressed in yeast vectors [88, 89]. In addition, the regulatory regions of eukaryotic viruses have been utilized to obtain expression of IFNs [90–95]. Furthermore, by direct transformation of cells with the Hu-IFN-β gene together with the gene for dihydrofolate reductase resistance, the Hu-IFN-β gene has been amplified in Chinese hamster cells [96]. With the use of such eukaryotic vectors, glycosylated Hu-IFN-β has been produced at high levels.

## V. PURIFICATION OF RECOMBINANT HUMAN LEUKOCYTE INTERFERON

Monoclonal antibodies to the human leukocyte interferons were used to purify recombinant human leukocyte A interferon (IFN-$\alpha$A) produced in bacteria [40, 41]. *E. coli* containing the human leukocyte interferon, IFN-$\alpha$A, were broken. Unbroken cells and cellular debris were removed by centrifugation. The IFN-$\alpha$A and soluble bacterial proteins remain in the cell lysate. Nucleic acids (DNA and RNA) that make the lysate viscous and thus difficult to handle easily are precipitated by combination with polymin P. The soluble proteins remaining in the lysate can be concentrated, or without concentration, passed directly through a column containing a monoclonal antibody to human leukocyte interferon (Fig. 12). The antibodies bind only the interferon; all the other components and proteins pass through the column. After washing the column, the IFN-$\alpha$A bound to the column is removed by elution with an acidic solution [40, 41]. A virtually pure interferon solution is eluted from the monoclonal antibody column (Figs. 13, 14). The column is then washed and neutralized so that it can be used repeatedly. The interferon solution is concentrated by passage over a column of carboxymethyl-cellulose [40, 41]. The activity of the purified interferon made in bacteria is very similar to that of the same human leukocyte interferon species synthesized by human cells.

Since repeated use of the monoclonal antibody columns is possible, these affinity columns provide a convenient method for preparing homogeneous human leukocyte interferon from bacterial fermentations. Interferon prepared by modifications of these procedures is now being used in clinical trials in humans. Several biological activities of this purified recombinant interferon have been determined. The recombinant IFN-$\alpha$A exhibits antiviral activity and antiproliferative activity comparable to those of crude and purified natural leukocyte interferons [98]. IFN-$\alpha$A also stimulates natural killer cell activity [99] as do the natural species of human leukocyte interferon [100]. With the eventual availability of large amounts of homogeneous IFN-$\alpha$A, extensive clinical trials, biological studies, and determination of its three-dimensional structure are achievable.

Rapid advances in recombinant DNA technology have made it possible to produce virtually an unlimited supply of interferon. As noted by McGregor and Ramel [101], worldwide demand for interferon as a therapeutic agent will likely be in the kilograms but not in the tons as for antibiotics.

Expression of interferon in bacterial cells and subsequent purification with the use of immobilized monoclonal antibodies as shown above is essentially a one-step purification scheme. When combined with high expression

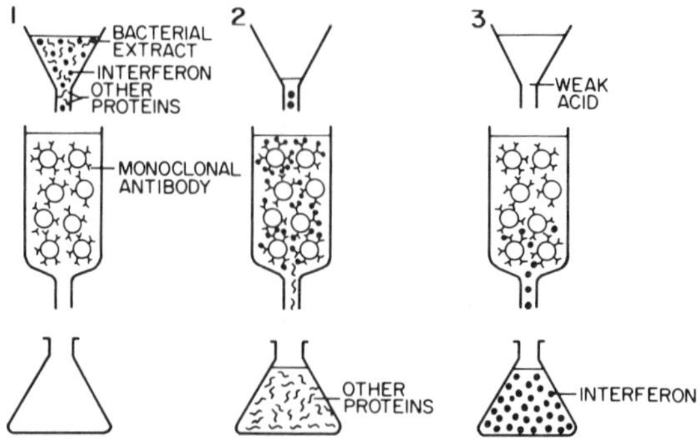


**Fig. 12** Schematic illustration of purification of interferon-$\alpha$ with monoclonal antibodies. Monoclonal antibody is attached covalently to a solid support. For the purification of IFN-$\alpha$A, monoclonal antibody LI-8 was coupled to Affi-gel [40, 41]. The bacterial extract containing IFN-$\alpha$A is passed through the monoclonal antibody column (#1). IFN-$\alpha$A, but not other proteins, bind to the column, which is exhaustively washed to remove other contaminating proteins (#2). Purified IFN-$\alpha$A is then eluted by adjusting the elution buffer to pH 2.5 with acetic acid (#3).

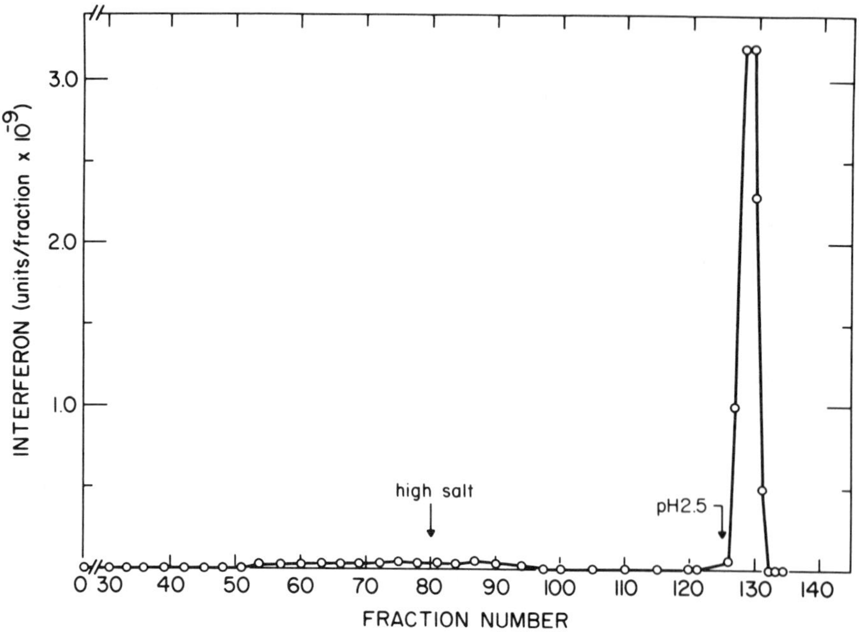


**Fig. 13** Purification of interferon by monoclonal antibody immunoadsorbent column chromatography. Experimental details are summarized in the text and given elsewhere [40, 41]. The column consisting of monoclonal antibody LI-8 attached to Affi-gel 10 was washed sequentially with several buffers. Fractions 127–130 containing interferon activity were eluted with 0.2 N acetic acid, 0.15 M NaCl, 0.1% Triton X-100, pH 2.5. Almost all of the protein appeared in the flowthrough fraction of the column. Interferon was measured by radioimmunoassay [97].

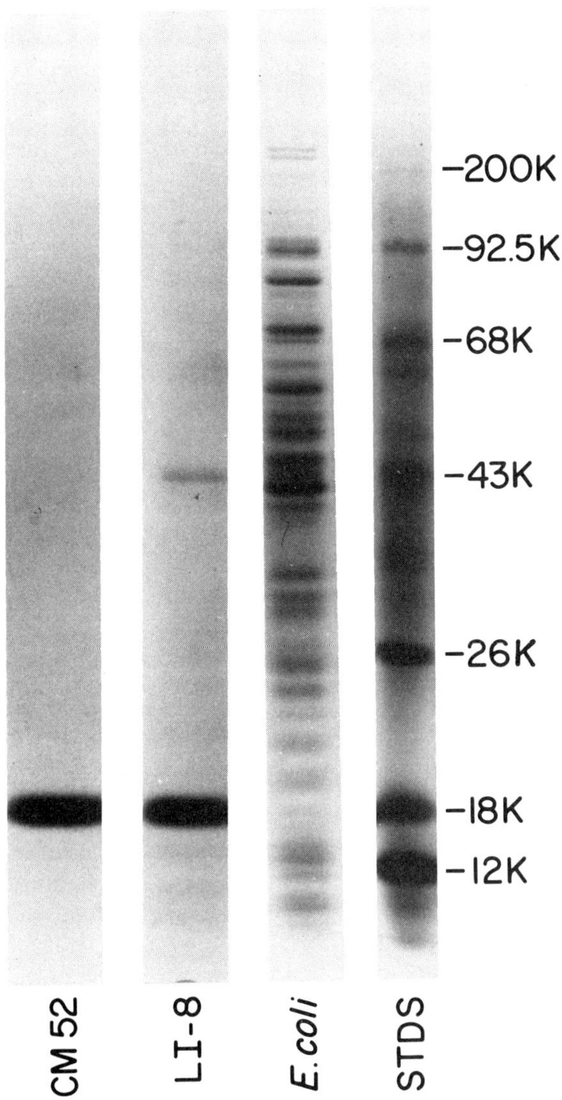


**Fig. 14** Sodium dodecyl-sulfate polyacrylamide gel electrophoresis (SDS-PAGE) of purified interferon. The gel was stained with 2.5% Coomassie Brilliant Blue. Approximately 20 μg of interferon purified by monoclonal antibody column LI-8 was subjected to electrophoresis. Stds, the standard molecular weight markers; *E. coli*, total proteins from *Escherichia coli* S30; LI-8, the fraction after passage through the monoclonal antibody column; CM-52, the purified interferon after passage through the CM-52 column [40, 41].

in bacteria, this procedure provides high recoveries and low cost of the interferon. A scaled-up purification of recombinant leukocyte A interferon with immobilized monoclonal antibodies is described in the following section. This purified material is being used clinically as an antiviral and/or antitumor agent [102].

## VI. LARGE-SCALE IMMUNOAFFINITY CHROMATOGRAPHY

### A. General Principles

McGregor and Ramel [101], Tarnowski [104], and Dunnill [105] have considered the large-scale recovery and containment of recombinant proteins destined for clinical application. In our goal to obtain a pure homogeneous product, purification procedures were developed that would minimize steps and provide a high yield and purity. In principle, immunoaffinity chromatography as described above on the laboratory scale can be used. Simply, the antibodies or antigens are chemically coupled to an inert solid matrix and subsequently crude samples containing the antigen or antibody to be purified are passed over a column of the immobilized protein. Other components of the crude sample can be washed free from the column and the absorbed antigens or antibodies subsequently recovered by elution with a suitable dissociating agent. The greater the specificity of the immobilized component (the monoclonal antibody), the greater the likelihood of developing a rapid and convenient purification.

Eveleigh [106] has noted that the general acceptance of immunoaffinity chromatography has been rather slow and that the potential of the technique has yet to be fully realized. Recently, however, immunoaffinity techniques have been gaining popularity [107–110]. Zoon et al. [15] utilized antibody affinity chromatography in their multistep procedure to purify human leukocyte interferon from Namalva lymphoblastoid cells. Berg et al. [6, 19] isolated 13 species of leukocyte interferon in essentially one step by immunoaffinity chromatography with polyclonal antibodies to human leukocyte interferon.

As noted above, Staehelin et al. [40, 41, 111, 112] used hybridoma techniques for production of monoclonal antibodies that were subsequently immobilized and used to purify IFN-$\alpha$A from bacterial cells. They had identified 13 hybridomas secreting monoclonal antibodies against human leukocyte interferon. These hybridomas were subsequently grown in mice, and large amounts of monoclonal antibodies were recovered from acidic fluid. One of the hybridomas, designated LI-8, was a particularly stable cell line and was used for routine production of monoclonal antibodies. Subsequently, the monoclonal antibodies were purified and immobilized on activated cross-linked agarose, Affi-gel 10 [40, 41]. Relatively crude *E. coli* extracts containing IFN-$\alpha$A were passed over a column of immobilized LI-8 monoclonal antibody after which desorption with dilute acetic acid resulted in a 1200-fold purification with at least 95% recovery. With the exception of a small amount of dimeric IFN-$\alpha$A, the interferon appeared homogeneous when analyzed on denaturing gel electrophoresis.

Establishing stable hybridomas that secrete monoclonal antibody can be a very tedious and expensive undertaking. However, once hybridoma cell cultures are established, monoclonal antibodies offer certain advantages over serum antibodies. They are monospecific; they provide a homogeneous interaction with the antigen; they can be chosen for unique properties such as stability in certain reagents or for low affinity to make elution of the antigen more efficient; hybridomas can produce homogeneous antibodies reproducibly; and in general the yield of monoclonal antibodies is much greater than polyclonal antibodies obtained from serum. Even with these important advantages, the use of monoclonal antibodies for the large-scale purification of proteins presents a serious supply problem. This problem was recognized by Eveleigh [106]. One solution is to automate the purification process. Anderson et al. [113] designed a preparative immunoaffinity system which was programmed by mechanical switches. With the advent of commercial microprocessors, it is relatively convenient to automate immunoaffinity chromatography for the purification of IFN-$\alpha$A with the use of electronic controls. Basically, the procedure includes a column of immunobilized LI-8 monoclonal antibody interfaced with a time-based microprocessor controlling solution absorption, washing, and elution from the column. Control with a time-based microprocessor is economical and versatile.

## B. Examples

Specific procedures for large-scale fermentations, cell extraction, and preparation of the immunoabsorbent gel have been described by Tarnowski and Liptak [114] and Tarnowski et al. [115]. Briefly, bacteria were harvested during logarithmic growth by centrifugation and the bacterial cell pellets were stored at $-20°C$ until used. All fermentations carrying the plasmid pIFN-$\alpha$A and procedures in the purification were performed in accordance with the NIH Guidelines for Recombinant DNA Research. Frozen cell pellets were suspended in lysis buffer and passed twice through a Manton-Gaulin homogenizer at 7000 p.s.i. [40, 41]. Polyethyleneimine (Polymin P) at pH 7.9 was added to the crude lysate to a final concentration of 0.35% (w/v) to facilitate nucleic acid and cell debris removal. The lysate was then centrifuged and the supernatant subsequently obtained was reduced to approximately one-half to one-fourth volume by ultrafiltration on a Millipore Pellicon unit equipped with 50 $ft^2$ of PTGC membrane (10,000 mwco, Millipore Corporation, Bedford, MA) [114]. Alternatively, cells could be extracted directly with 2 M guanidine hydrochloride as described by Tarnowski et al. [115].

As noted above, Affi-gel 10 was utilized for the laboratory scale purification of IFN-$\alpha$A. However, insufficient availability of Affi-gel 10 for production scale applications prompted development of an alternative gel which afforded the same performance. Nishikawa and Bailon [116] synthesized the aminopropyl derivative of Sepharose 4B (Pharmacia Fine Chemicals, Piscataway, NJ) and extended the ligand structure by succinylation of amino groups to produce agarose bearing N-acyloxysuccinimido groups (P. Bailon and A. H. Nishikawa, personal communication). The coupling reaction was carried out producing an antibody density of 11–13 mg of protein per ml of gel [114]. Although the density of this gel was only about half that reported by Staehelin et al. [40, 41], it did not affect the performance of the column. The binding capacity of interferon on this immunoadsorbent was approximately 1 mg of IFN-$\alpha$A per ml of gel.

The IFN-$\alpha$A purification steps were essentially as described above [40, 41], however, modifications for practical considerations in scale-up were implemented [115, 117]. Ion exchange chromatography of the immunoabsorbent-purified IFN-$\alpha$A was performed on carboxymethylcellulose (CM-52, Whatman, Inc., Clifton, NJ) as described [40, 41]. This step was essential for the removal of the nonionic detergent Triton X-100.

Table 3 summarizes the purification of IFN-$\alpha$A after 15 cumulative elutions of the antibody column. At each cycle, sufficient concentrated *E. coli* extract was loaded onto the column to achieve complete saturation with IFN-$\alpha$A. Recovery was 73% with a specific activity of $2 \times 10^8$ units/mg of protein. The IFN-$\alpha$A was purified approximately 160-fold and appeared to be homogeneous when analyzed by SDS-polyacrylamide gel electrophoresis as above. The difference in purification level (157- vs. 1200-fold) between these data [114] and that reported by Staehelin et al. [40, 41] reflects improvements both in expression and in the fermentation process. Specific activity of the purified IFN-$\alpha$A in comparison to other leukocyte interferon species is given in Table 2.

**Table 3** Summary of Large-Scale Purification of IFN-$\alpha$A

| Step | Volume (L) | Total units | Total protein (g) | Specific activity (units/mg) | Recovery (%) | Purification factor |
|---|---|---|---|---|---|---|
| Polyethyleneimine supernatant | 137 | $2.6 \times 10^{12}$ | 1863 | $1.4 \times 10^6$ | 100 | 1.0 |
| Antibody eluate | 16.5 | $1.9 \times 10^{12}$ | 8.7 | $2.2 \times 10^8$ | 73 | 157 |

*Source*: Adapted from Ref. 114.

## C. Aspects of Immunoaffinity Chromatography

Purification of human leukocyte interferon synthesized in bacteria was accomplished by employing these immobilized monoclonal antibodies. Utilization of this essentially, one-step purification procedure provided the first pure human interferon for clinical evaluation, and on January 15, 1981, material produced at Hoffmann-La Roche Inc. was used in a patient for the first time. The development of technology from the laboratory level to a prototype operation for commercial production was essential to provide sufficient material for continued large-scale clinical trials. Since sufficient antibody supplies were a limiting factor, it was imperative to develop a system whereby a column of immobilized monoclonal antibody could be used repeatedly and the longevity evaluated. After several hundred cycles, the capacity of the column for interferon was not diminished. There were, however, detectable levels of mouse immunoglobulin in each antibody column elution, which was removed below detectable levels in the subsequent purification steps [115]. Several thousand column cycles would be required before a decrease in IFN-$\alpha$A yield would be observed through loss of antibody. The use of dilute acetic acid as an eluting agent does not appear to be particularly denaturing to the immobilized antibody. Contamination with *E. coli* proteins does not appear to be a serious problem. Success with the immunoaffinity purification of IFN-$\alpha$A has prompted the extension of similar purification procedures to other proteins and other affinity chromatography procedures. Nevertheless, nonimmunoaffinity procedures have also been successful. The use of a series of chromatographic procedures without immunoaffinity chromatography to purify IFN-$\alpha$2 produced in *E. coli* was described by Thatcher and Panayotatos [118].

Immunosorbents made by covalently coupling monoclonal antibodies to agarose gels have high specificities and therefore are powerful tools for the purification of proteins. Specificity was demonstrated in the case of IFN-$\alpha$A: crude extracts of *E. coli* are passed over a column of immunoabsorbent gel and IFN-$\alpha$A is purified in essentially one step. Recovery yields are high after this step, but the formation of IFN-$\alpha$A oligomers via intermolecular disulfide bonds [119] requires additional steps in the purification scheme to obtain purified monomers [115]. The lower specific activity of oligomers and the possibility they might cause adverse reactions in human clinical trials make it desirable to obtain a monomer preparation.

The monomer preparation contains at least two molecular forms, slow-moving monomer (SMM) and fast-moving monomer (FMM). Ten monomer forms are predicted if all the possible combinations of disulfide bonds and free sulfhydryl forms are considered. Radiolabeling the preparation with the alkylating agent N-ethyl maleimide showed that SMM contained free sulfhydryl groups but FMM did not [115]. The free -SH in SMM potentially could give rise to oligomers on storage. It is assumed that FMM contains two disulfide bonds. Separation of these two species is desirable to obtain a stable product form. Bodo and Fogy [120] isolated at least seven monomer forms of IFN-$\alpha$2C(Arg) (identical to [Arg$^{23}$Arg$^{34}$]IFN-$\alpha$A) by affinity purification and reverse-phase chromatography. Subsequent characterization of these component monomers showed that disulfide bonds were partially and completely reduced, scrambled, and correctly formed between cysteine residues 1–98 and 29–138. They concluded, as we have, that these various species may arise from the reduced monomer.

The formation and removal of IFN-$\alpha$A oligomers adversely impacts on the overall recovery of the purification process. Since most oligomers are disulfide linked, and pH-dependent polymerizations can be controlled, conversion to fully active monomer has been demonstrated with reduction-oxidation systems [115, 121]. Incorporation of a redox system into the purification scheme could make the process one of extraordinary yield.

The high homology among the leukocyte interferon $\alpha$ subtypes engenders an epitope on many that is recognized by monoclonal antibody LI-8. Consequently, other recombinant interferons, IFN-$\alpha$A/D (Bg/II), IFN-$\alpha$C, IFN-$\alpha$D, IFN-$\alpha$I, IFN-$\alpha$J, IFN-$\alpha$K, and IFN-$\alpha$2 have been purified by procedures similar to the process described here.

Despite initial skepticism, monoclonal antibody immunosorbent chromatography has proven to be a viable procedure for the purification of proteins for pharmaceutical applications. The ability to reuse the same column hundreds of times makes these columns practical because the quantity of monoclonal antibody required is reasonable and readily obtainable without heroic efforts. Accordingly, the commercial manufacture of protein therapeutics by immobilized monoclonal antibodies for purification should be considered when planning the research and development of these pharmaceuticals.

## VII. PURIFICATION OF HUMAN FIBROBLAST INTERFERON

Several laboratories reported the purification and partial structural analysis of human fibroblast interferon with the use of SDS-polyacrylamide gel electrophoresis as the last step in purification [12, 13]. To obtain a product free of salt and solvent, we developed a simple two-step purification of fibroblast interferon [10]. The first step in the purification from the crude interferon-containing medium involved Blue-Sepharose chromatography, a procedure described previously [51, 59]. The second step involved HPLC on octyl silica. The amino acid composition and 19 residues of the amino-terminal sequence of human fibroblast interferon were determined [10]. The sequence was identical to the first 13 residues reported by Knight et al. [59] and Okamura et al. [17] and the first 10 residues reported by Friesen et al. [11].

The Blue-Sepharose step (Fig. 15) provides a high purification factor, but results in a dilute solution of interferon in 50% ethylene glycol. The final product is then obtained in concentrated form free of ethylene glycol and buffer salts by HPLC (Fig. 16). Because only volatile eluents are used, the interferon may be recovered salt- and solvent-free simply by evaporation. The specific activity of the purified protein is $3 \times 10^8$ units/mg of protein (Table 2), similar to that of the purified human leukocyte interferon species. Representative specific activities of various purified natural and recombinant IFN-$\beta$ preparations are summarized in Table 2. It should be noted that the last step in the purification employed by Knight [12] and Berthold et al. [13] consisted of SDS-polyacrylamide gel electrophoresis.

By analogous procedures, IFN-$\beta$ produced in *E. coli* has been purified [42]. *E. coli* cells were broken with a Manton-Gaulin homogenizer. Most of the IFN-$\beta$ was associated with the sedimentable cell debris, which was extracted with 7 M guanidine hydrochloride. Blue-Sepharose chromatography was then employed to purify IFN-$\beta$ as described above.

Purification of [Ser[17]]IFN-$\beta$ from *E. coli* producing this analog of IFN-$\beta$ was accomplished by sonication of cells followed by extraction of cellular

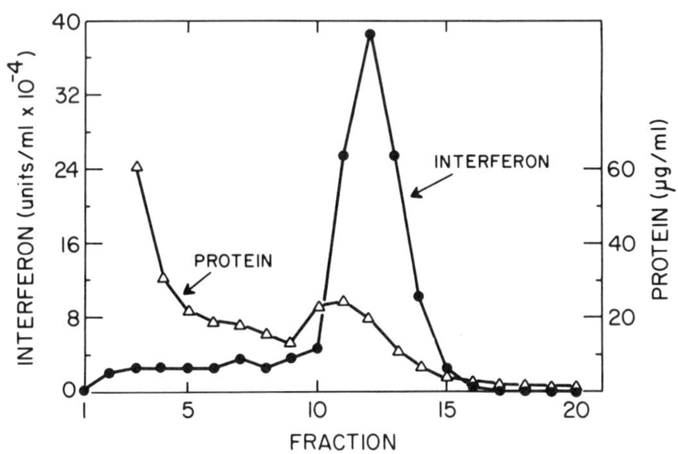


**Fig. 15** Blue-Sepharose chromatography of crude human fibroblast interferon (IFN-$\beta$). Fractions 1–9 are eluted with 30% ethylene glycol, whereas the remaining fractions are eluted with 50% ethylene glycol [10]. The volume per fraction was 25 ml. Solid circles represent interferon activity, solid triangles represent protein concentration.

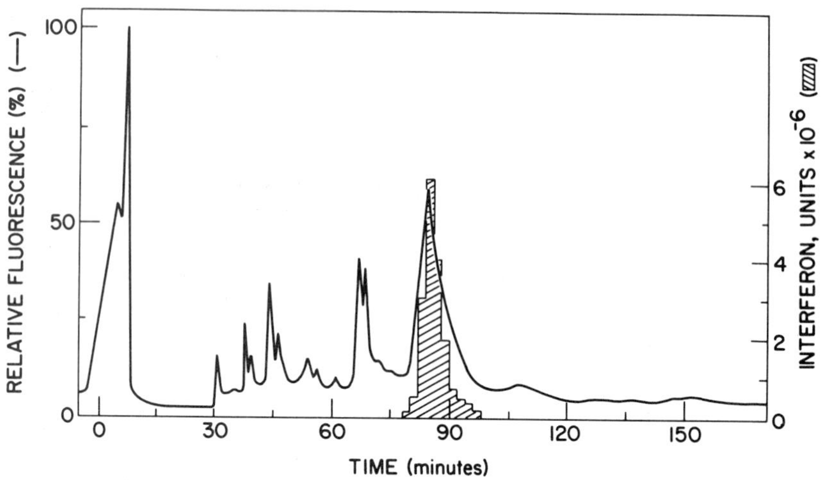


**Fig. 16** HPLC of human fibroblast interferon (IFN-$\beta$). About $10^6$ units of interferon were applied to an RP-8 column. A step gradient of increasing *n*-propanol at pH 4.2 was pumped at 22 ml/h. Interferon was eluted in a broad peak toward the end of the 32% *n*-propanol step. A portion (3%) of the column effluent was monitored with fluorescamine for determination of protein [10].

| | S1–S10 | S20 | S23 | 1–10 | 20 | 30 | 40 | 50 | 60 | 70 |
|---|---|---|---|---|---|---|---|---|---|---|
| IFN-α consensus | MALSFSLLMA | VLVLSYKSIC | SLG | CDLPQTHSLG | NRRALILLAQ | MGRISPFSCL | KDRHDFGFPQ | EEFDGNQFQK | AQAISVLHEM | IQQTFNLFST |
| IFN-αK (α6) | ...P.A.... | LV...C..S. | ..D | .......... | H..TMM.... | .R...L.... | ......R... | .......... | .E.......V | .......... |
| IFN-α5 (αG) | ...P.V.... | LV..NC.... | ... | .........S | ...T.MIM.. | .......... | .......... | .......... | .......... | .......... |
| IFN-αA (α2) | ...T.A..V. | L....C..S. | .V. | .......... | S..T.M.... | .RK..L.... | .......... | ...-...... | .ET.P..... | ...I...... |
| IFN-αD (α1) | ..SP.A...V | LV...C..S. | ... | ....E....D | ...T.M.... | .S....S... | M......... | .......... | .P.......L | ...I....T. |
| IFN-αH1 (αH2) | ...P...M.. | LV...C..S. | ... | .N.S.....N | ...T.M.M.. | .R........ | ......E... | .......... | .......... | M......... |
| IFN-αB2 (α8) | ...T.Y..V. | LV......FS | ... | .......... | .......... | .R........ | ......E... | ....DK.... | .......... | .......... |
| IFN-αB | ...T.Y.MV. | LV......FS | ... | .......... | .......... | .R........ | ......E... | ....DK.... | .......... | .......... |
| IFN-α4b | .......... | .......... | ... | .......... | .......... | .....H.... | .........E | .....H.... | T......... | .......... |
| IFN-αC | .......... | .......... | ... | .......... | ........G. | .......... | ......RI.. | .......... | .......... | .......... |
| IFN-αL (ψα10) | .......... | .........* | ... | .......T.R | ........G. | .......... | ......RI.. | .......... | .......... | .......... |
| IFN-αJ1 (α7) | ..R......V | .......... | ... | .........R | .......... | .......... | ....E.R..E | .....H.... | T......... | .......... |
| IFN-αJ2 | ..R......V | .......... | ... | .........R | .......... | .......... | ....E.R..E | .....H.... | T......... | .......... |
| IFN-αI | .......... | .......... | ... | .......... | .......... | .......... | ...P...L.. | .......... | T......... | .......... |
| IFN-αF | .......... | .......... | ... | .......... | .......... | .......... | .......... | .......... | .......... | .......... |
| IFN-αWA | .......... | .......... | ... | .......... | .......... | .....H.... | ...Y...... | .V........ | .....AF... | .......... |
| IFN-αGx-1 | ...P...M.. | LV...C..S. | ... | .N.S.....N | ...T.MIM.. | .......... | .......... | .......... | .......... | .......... |
| IFN-α76 | .......... | .......... | ... | .......... | .......... | .....H.... | .........E | .....H.... | .......... | .......... |
| IFN-α88 | | ....... | ... | .......... | .......... | .......... | .......L.. | .......... | T......... | .......... |

| | 80 | 90 | 100 | 110 | 120 | 130 | 140 | 150 | 160 | 166 |
|---|---|---|---|---|---|---|---|---|---|---|
| IFN-α consensus | KDSSAAWDES | LLEKFSTELY | QQLNDLEACV | IQEVGVEETP | LMNEDSILAV | RKYFQRITLY | LTEKKYSPCA | WEVVRAEIMR | SFSFSTNLQK | RLRRKD |
| IFN-αK (α6) | ....V....R | ..D.LY.... | .......... | M...W.GG.. | .......... | .......... | .......... | .......... | ...S.R...E | .....E |
| IFN-αG (α5) | .....T...T | ..D..Y.... | .........M | M......D.. | ...V....T. | .......... | .......... | .......... | ...L.A...E | .....E |
| IFN-αA (α2) | .........T | ..D..Y.... | .......... | ..G...T... | ..K....... | .......... | .K........ | .......... | ...L.....E | S..S.E |
| IFN-αD (α1) | .........D | ..D..C.... | .......... | M..ER.G... | ...V...... | K...R..... | .......... | .......... | .L.L.....E | .....E |
| IFN-αH1 (αH2) | .N.......T | .....YI..F | ..M....... | .......... | .......... | K......... | .M........ | .......... | .......... | ...... |
| IFN-αB2 (α8) | ......L..T | ..DE.YI..D | .......S.. | M.....I.S. | ..Y....... | .......... | .......S.. | .......... | ...L.I.... | ..KS.E |
| IFN-αB | ......L..T | ..DE.YI..D | .......VLC | D.....I.S. | ..Y....... | .......... | .......S.. | .......... | ...L.I.... | ..KS.E |
| IFN-α4b | E......EQ. | .......... | .......... | .......... | ...V...... | .......... | .......... | .......... | .L........ | ...... |
| IFN-αC | E......EQ. | .......... | .......... | .......... | .......... | .......... | .I.R...... | .......... | .L........ | ...... |
| IFN-αL (ψα10) | E......EQ. | ........I. | .......... | .......... | .......... | .......... | .I.R...... | .......... | .L........ | ...... |
| IFN-αJ1 (α7) | E......EQ. | .......... | .......... | .......... | .....F.... | .......... | .M........ | .......... | ........K. | G..... |
| IFN-αJ2 | E......EQ. | .......... | .......... | .......... | .....F.... | .......... | .M........ | .......... | .......... | ...... |
| IFN-αI | E......EQ. | .......... | ....N..... | .....M.... | .......... | .......... | .......... | .......... | .L........ | I..... |
| IFN-αF | .....T.EQ. | .........N | .....M.... | .......... | ...V...... | K......... | .......... | .......... | ...L.KIF.E | .....E |
| IFN-αWA | .........T | ..D..YI..F | .......... | T.......IA | .......... | .......... | .MG....... | .......... | .......... | G..... |
| IFN-αGx-1 | .....T...T | ..D..Y.... | .........M | M......D.. | ...V....T. | .......... | .......... | .......... | ...L.A...E | .....E |
| IFN-α76 | E......EQ. | .......... | .......... | .......... | .......... | .......... | .......... | .......... | .L........ | ...... |
| IFN-α88 | E......EQ | .......... | ....N..... | .....M.... | .......... | .......... | .......... | .......... | .L........ | ...... |

**Fig. 17** The amino acid sequences of human leukocyte interferon (IFN-$\alpha$) species derived from cDNA or genomic DNA sequences. Sequences, including the signal peptide (S1-S23), are present in comparison with a consensus sequence. Correspond-

debris with 2% SDS [43]. The [Ser$^{17}$]IFN-$\beta$ is the purified by successive steps of extraction with 2-butanol, acid precipitation, and gel filtration (Sephacryl S-200 and Sephadex G-75 chromatography).

Unlike human leukocyte interferon, which has been isolated as several different species [8, 9, 16, 18, 19, 30, 39, 56], only a single fibroblast interferon (IFN-$\beta$) species has so far been isolated. Human fibroblast and leukocyte interferons appear to bind to the same cell receptor [1, 122] and have similar activities. Some homology is evident from comparison of the DNA sequences coding for these interferons.

---

ing residues are presented only when they differ from the consensus sequence. Residues common to all listed sequences are underlined in the consensus sequence. Sequences A-L are from the laboratories of Pestka, Goeddel, and colleagues [61, 87, 134], whereas sequences with numeric designations are from the laboratory of Weissmann and colleagues [133]. Closely related sequences are listed together [135]. Sequences are listed as two classes (Class I: $\alpha$K, $\alpha$5, $\alpha$A, and $\alpha$D; Class II: $\alpha$4b, $\alpha$C, $\alpha$L, $\alpha$J1, $\alpha$J2, $\alpha$I, and $\alpha$F) and an intermediate class ($\alpha$H1, $\alpha$H2, $\alpha$B2, and $\alpha$B). Within each class, order is determined according to increasing difference from the consensus sequence. The $\alpha$5 sequence is complete, whereas the G sequence begins at residue 34, since only a partial length clone was isolated; identity of G and $\alpha$5 is proposed on the basis of the extant sequences. The cloned L ($\Psi\alpha$10) sequence has a termination codon within the signal sequence (indicated by an asterisk) and may therefore represent a pseudogene; however, since the coding region for the mature protein is otherwise normal, it is possible that in vivo suppression might lead to the production of a normal protein with this sequence. Indeed, it has been shown IFN-$\alpha$L exhibits antiviral activity when expressed in *E. coli* without the signal peptide [136] or with a modified signal peptide [137]. The clone IFN-$\alpha$WA is from Torczynski et al. [138, 139]. The interferons IFN-$\alpha$Gx-1 [140] and IFN-$\alpha$76 [141] appear to represent recombinants between, respectively, IFN-$\alpha$H1(1–16) and IFN-$\alpha$G(17–166) on the one hand and between IFN-$\alpha$4(1–50)/IFN-$\alpha$C(51–131)/IFN-$\alpha$4b(132–166) on the other. The signal peptide of IFN-$\alpha$Gx-1 may be as shown in this figure rather than as reported: the codon at position S1 was reproted as AAT (Asn or N) rather than ATG (Met or M) as in all other IFN-$\alpha$ genes. Interferons reported by Meyer [142] appear to be similar to those listed in the figure, although there are some minor differences of one amino acid in some cases. The following interferons are of identical amino acid sequence: $\alpha$K = $\alpha$6; $\alpha$J = $\alpha$7; $\alpha$B2 = $\alpha$8; $\alpha$L = $\Psi\alpha$10. The following interferons are identical except for the residues shown in parentheses: IFN-$\alpha$A (Lys$^{23}$), IFN-$\alpha$2 (Arg$^{23}$); IFN-$\alpha$D (Val$^{114}$), IFN-$\alpha$1 (Ala$^{114}$); IFN-$\alpha$J (Lys$^{159}$ Gly$^{161}$), IFN-$\alpha$J1 (Gln$^{159}$ Arg$^{161}$), IFN-$\alpha$7 (Lys$^{159}$ Gly$^{161}$); IFN-$\alpha$H1 (Phe$^{152}$), IFN-$\alpha$H2 (Leu$^{152}$). A gap was introduced at position #44 in IFN-$\alpha$A to provide for maximum alignment with the other species. Gaps are indicated by dashes. In several positions, alternative amino acids could be chosen for the consensus sequence: #S11, V or L; #78, D or E; #79, E or Q; #80, S or T; #83, D or E; #86, S or Y; #154, F or L; #166, D or E.

## VIII. PURIFICATION OF IMMUNE INTERFERON, IFN-$\gamma$

Natural IFN-$\gamma$ was purified by several groups with the use of similar procedures [1, 44, 45, 123–129]. The use of controlled-pore glass, concanavalin A–Sepharose, and gel filtration were generally used by most laboratories. The procedures vary from laboratory to laboratory as described in detail in the above reports. Natural IFN-$\gamma$ is glycosylated [45, 126, 127]. Specific activity of the purified IFN-$\gamma$ was about $6 \times 10^7$ units/mg (Table 2).

Although IFN-$\gamma$ appears as monomers of MW 20,000 and 25,000 on SDS-polyacrylamide gel electrophoresis [124, 126, 127], the functional unit of IFN-$\gamma$ appears to have a target size equivalent to the tetramer [130].

Recombinant IFN-$\gamma$ produced in *E. coli* could be extracted from cells by sonication or directly with 7 M guanidine hydrochloride. This extract, after absorption and elution from silica, was then chromatographed on a column containing a monoclonal antibody reacting with the carboxy-terminal end of IFN-$\gamma$ [46]. The specific activity of the purified product was $1 \times 10^7$ units/mg, comparable to that of the purified natural protein (Table 2). Similar procedures could be used for natural IFN-$\gamma$. Although the monomer of IFN-$\gamma$ produced in *E. coli* has a MW of about 17,000 [4, 46], the target size of the functional unit also appears to be a tetramer [130].

## IX. PURIFICATION OF ANIMAL INTERFERONS

This review does not summarize the extensive work carried out on many animal interferons from mammalian species as well as avian species. For the production and purification of these interferons, the reader should consult reviews noted above as well as specific articles describing these [1–6, 131, 132].

## X. SEQUENCES OF INTERFERONS

The sequences of human IFN-$\alpha$ species have been determined from a combination of protein and nucleic acid sequencing. Most of the sequences of the proteins have been deduced from the nucleic acid sequence of genomic or cDNA clones (see Refs. 1, 5, 133, 134 for further details and references). A summary of the known human IFN-$\alpha$ sequences in given in Figure 17. The sequences of IFN-$\beta$ and IFN-$\gamma$ from several animal species are given in Figures 18 and 19, respectively.

## XI. CONCLUDING COMMENTS

Although purification of the interferons to homogeneiety remained elusive for about two decades after their discovery, they are now available in purified

| | S10 | S20 | S21 | 10 | 20 | 30 | 40 | 50 | 60 | 70 |
|---|---|---|---|---|---|---|---|---|---|---|
| IFN-β consensus | MTxRCLLQxA | LLLCFSTTAL | S | xSYxLLxFQQ | RxSxxxCQKL | LxQLxxxxxx | CLxxRMDFxx | PEEMKQxQQF | QKEDAALxIY | EMLQNIFxIF |
| Hu-IFN-β | ..NK....I. | .......... | . | M..N..G.L. | .S.NFQ.... | .W..NGRLEY | ..KD..N.DI | ...I..L... | .......T.. | .......A.. |
| Mo-IFN-β | ..NK....I. | .......... | . | M..N..G.L. | .S.SFQ.... | .W..NGSLEY | ..KD..N.DI | ...I..P... | .......T.. | .......A.. |
| Bo-IFN-β1 | ..Y.....MV | .......... | . | R..S..R... | .Q.LKE.... | .G..PSTSQH | ..EA....QM | ......E... | .....I.VM. | .V..H..G.L |
| Bo-IFN-β2 | ..H.....MV | .......... | . | R..S..R... | .R.LAL.... | .R..PSTPQH | ..EA....QM | ......A... | .....I.V.. | ....Q..N.L |
| Bo-IFN-β3 | ..Y....PMV | .......... | . | R..S..R... | .R.AEV.... | .G..HSTPQH | ..EAK...QV | ....N.A... | R....I.V.. | ....Q..N.L |
| Mu-IFN-β | .NN.WI.HA. | F......... | . | IN.KQ.QL.E | .TNIRK..E. | .E..NGKI-- | N.TY.A..KI | ....TE-KM- | ..SYT.FA.Q | .....V.LV. |

| | 80 | 90 | 100 | 110 | 120 | 130 | 140 | 150 | 160 | 166 |
|---|---|---|---|---|---|---|---|---|---|---|
| IFN-β consensus | RxDFSSTGWN | ETIVExLLxE | LYxQxNxLKT | VLEEKxEKEN | xTxGxxMSS--L | HLKxYYxRxx | xYLKxKEYxx | CAWTVVRVEI | LRNFxFIxRL | TGYLRN |
| Hu-IFN-β | .Q.S...... | .....N..AN | V.H.I.H... | .....L...D | F.R.KL...--. | ...R..G.IL | H...A...SH | ....I..... | ....Y..N.. | ...... |
| Mo-IFN-β | .Q.L...... | .....K..AN | V.H.IDH... | I....L...D | F.R.KF...--. | ...R..G.IL | H...A...SH | ....I..... | ....F..NK. | ...... |
| Bo-IFN-β1 | TR.......S | ...I.D..K. | ..W.M.R.QP | IQK.IMQ.Q. | S.TEDTIV---P | ..GK..FNLM | Q..ES...DR | ......Q.Q. | .T.VS.LM.. | ...V.D |
| Bo-IFN-β2 | TR.......S | ...I.D..E. | ..E.M.H.EP | IQK.IMQ.Q. | S.M.DTTV---. | ..RK..FNLV | Q...S...NR | ........Q. | ....S.LT.. | .....E |
| Bo-IFN-β3 | TR.......S | ...I.D..V. | ..G.M.R.QP | IQK.IMQEQ. | F.M.DTTV---. | ...K..FNLV | Q..ES...NR | ........Q. | .T..S.LM.. | .AS..D |
| Mu-IFN-β | .NN....... | ....VR..D. | .HQ.TVF... | .....Q.-.R | L.WE--...TA. | ...S..W.VQ | R...LMK.NS | Y..M...A.. | F...LI.R.. | .RNFQ. |

**Fig. 18** Comparison of amino acid sequences of IFN-β from several sources. The amino acid sequences predicted from DNA sequences for IFN-β from human [61, 72–75, 143], bovine [144], murine [145], and monkey [134, 146] genes are presented as they differ from a consensus sequence. Numbering is according to the human sequence. Amino acids of the consensus sequence which are common to all the sequences are underlined. Positions where no clear consensus exists are indicated in the consensus sequence by "x." To accommodate the murine sequence, a gap of two residues (indicated by hyphens) was introduced in the consensus (and other) sequences between residues 119 and 120; other gaps have been introduced into the murine sequence to facilitate alignment.

```
                      S1            S10                  S20    S23
Hu-IFN-γ              M K Y T S Y I L A F   Q L C I V L G S L G   C Y C
Bo-IFN-γ              . . . . . . F . . L   L . . G L . . F S .   S . G
Mu-IFN-γ              . N A . H C . . . L   . . F L M A V . - .   . . .
Ra-IFN-γ              . S A . R R V . V L   . . . L M A L . - .   . . .

                      1                10                   20                   30
Hu-IFN-γ              Q D P Y V K E A E N   L K K Y F N A G H S   D V A D N G T L F L
Hu-IFN-γ (protein)    e . . . . . . . . .   . . . . . . . . . .   . . . . . . . . . .
Bo-IFN-γ              . G Q F F R . I . .   . . E . . . . S S P   . . . K G . P . . S
Mu-IFN-γ              H G T V I E S L . S   . N N . . . S S G I   . . - E E K S . . .
Ra-IFN-γ              . G T L I E S L . S   . . N . . . S S S M   . A M E G K S . L .

                                       40                   50                   60
Hu-IFN-γ              G I L K N W K E E S   D R K I M Q S Q I V   S F Y F K L F K N F
Hu-IFN-γ (protein)    . . . . . . . . . .   . . . . . . . . . .   . . . . . . . . . .
Bo-IFN-γ              D . . . . . . D . .   . K . . I . . . . .   . . . . . . . E . L
Mu-IFN-γ              D . W R . . Q K D G   . M . . L . . . . I   . . . L R . . E V L
Ra-IFN-γ              D . W R . . Q K D G   N T . . L E . . . I   . . . L R . . E V L

                                       70                   80                   90
Hu-IFN-γ              K D D Q S I Q K S V   E T I K E D M N V K   F F N S N K K K R D
Hu-IFN-γ (protein)    . . . . . . . . . .   . . . . . . . . . .   . . . . . . . . . .
Bo-IFN-γ              . . N . V . . R . M   D I . . Q . . F Q .   . L . G S S E . L E
Mu-IFN-γ              . . N . A . S N N I   S V . E S H L I T T   . . S N S . A . K .
Ra-IFN-γ              . . N . A . S N N I   S V . E S H L I T N   . . S N S . A . K .

                                      100                  110                  120
Hu-IFN-γ              D F E K L T N Y S V   T D L N V Q R K A I   H E L I Q V M A E L
Hu-IFN-γ (protein)    . . . . . . . . . .   . . . . . . . . . .   . . . . . . . . . .
Bo-IFN-γ              . . K . . I Q I P .   D . . Q I . . . . .   N . . . K . . N D .
Mu-IFN-γ              A . M S I A K F E .   N N P Q . . . Q . F   N . . . R . V H Q .
Ra-IFN-α1             A . M S I A K F E .   N N P Q I . H . . V   N . . . R . I H Q .

                                      130                  140    143
Hu-IFN-γ              S P A A K T G K R K   R S Q M L F R G R R   A S Q
Hu-IFN-γ (protein)    . . . . . . † † † †   † † † †
Bo-IFN-γ              . . K S N L R . . .   . . . N . . . . . .   . . M
Mu-IFN-γ              L . E S S L R . . .   . . R C*
Ra-IFN-γ              . . E S S L R . . .   . . R C*
```

**Fig. 19** Comparison of amino acid sequences of IFN-γ from several sources. The amino acid sequences predicted from the DNA sequences of human [92, 147], murine [148], rat [149, 150], and bovine [151] IFN-γ have been aligned. The structure derived by direct amino acid sequencing of natural IFN-γ is denoted as "Hu-IFN-γ (protein)" [127]. The first residue of this protein is pyroglutamate, indicated as "e." Various residues which were found as the COOH terminus of the isolated protein are indicated by "†." Only differences from the human sequence are indicated for the bovine, murine, and rat molecules. Gaps (indicated by hyphens) in the mouse sequence were introduced to allow alignment. The end of the murine and rat sequences are indicated by an asterisk.

form in many laboratories. The largest amounts available are the species produced in *E. coli*. For purification, immunoaffinity chromatography has proven to be generally useful both on a laboratory as well as a commercial scale. Nevertheless, techniques other than immunoaffinity chromatography have proven to be successful as well. The availability of these proteins for laboratory and clinical studies has already catalyzed extensive new developments with these agents. The interferons are approved therapeutic agents worldwide. In the years ahead, it is likely our understanding and use of these agents will be even more extensive and provide new insights into their actions. Conceivably, we may begin to understand the physiological roles of the interferons as well.

## ACKNOWLEDGMENTS

For the work done in my laboratory discussed in this review, I thank my many colleagues who have carried out the studies cited. Work discussed was supported by Hoffmann-La Roche, Inc. while I was at the Roche Institute of Molecular Biology. Work accomplished since 1986 was carried out at UMDNJ-Robert Wood Johnson Medical School and supported by grants awarded to SP from the National Institutes of Health: RO1-CA46465 and UO1-AI25914. I thank Eleanor Kells for her expert assistance in the preparation of this manuscript.

## REFERENCES

1. S. Pestka, J. A. Langer, K. C. Zoon, and C. E. Samuel, *Am. Rev. Biochem. 56*, 727 (1987).
2. S. Pestka, in *Meth. Enzymol.* (S. Pestka, ed.), Vol. 78, Academic Press, New York, 1981, 1-632.
3. S. Pestka, in *Meth. Enzymol.* (S. Pestka, ed.), Vol. 79, Academic Press, New York, 1981, 1-677.
4. S. Pestka, in *Meth. Enzymol.* (S. Pestka, ed.), Vol. 119, Academic Press, New York, 1986, p. 1.
5. S. Pestka, *Arch. Biochem. Biophys. 221*, 1 (1983).
6. K. Berg, *Acta Path. Microbiol. Scand. 279* (Suppl.) 1 (1982).
7. M. Rubinstein, S. Rubinstein, P. C. Familletti, M. S. Gross, R. S. Miller, A. A. Waldman, and S. Pestka, *Science 202*, 1289 (1978).
8. M. Rubinstein, S. Rubinstein, P. C. Familletti, R. S. Miller, A. A. Waldman, and S. Pestka, *Proc. Natl. Acad. Sci. USA 76*, 640 (1979).
9. M. Rubinstein, W. P. Levy, J. A. Moschera, C.-Y. Lai, R. D. Hershberg, R. T. Bartlett, and S. Pestka, *Arch. Biochem. Biophys. 210*, 307 (1981).
10. S. Stein, C. Kenny, H.-J. Friesen, J. Shively, U. Del Valle, and S. Pestka, *Proc. Natl. Acad. Sci. USA 77*, 5716 (1980).

11. H.-J. Friesen, S. Stein, M. Evinger, P. C. Familletti, J. Moschera, J. Meienhofer, J. Shively, and S. Pestka, *Arch. Biochem. Biophys. 206*, 432 (1981).
12. E. Knight, Jr., *Proc. Natl. Acad. Sci. USA 73*, 520 (1976).
13. W. Berthold, C. Tan, Y. H. Tan, *J. Biol. Chem. 253*, 5206 (1978).
14. B. Cabrer, H. Taira, R. J. Broeze, T. D. Kempe, K. Williams, W. H. Slattery, W. H. Konigsberg, and P. Lengyel, *J. Biol. Chem. 254*, 3681 (1979).
15. K. C. Zoon, M. E. Smith, P. J. Bridgen, D. Zur Nedden, and C. B. Anfinsen, *Proc. Natl. Acad. Sci. USA 76*, 5601 (1979).
16. G. Allen and F. H. Fantes, *Nature* (London) *287*, 408 (1980).
17. H. Okamura, W. Berthold, L. Hood, M. Hunakpiller, M. Inoue, H. Smith-Johannsen, and Y. H. Tan, *Biochemistry 19*, 3831 (1981).
18. K. C. Zoon, in *Meth. Enzymol.* (S. Pestka, ed.), Vol. 78, Academic Press, New York, 1981, 457.
19. K. Berg and I. Heron, in *Meth. Enzymol.* (S. Pestka, ed.), Vol. 78, Academic Press, New York, 1981, 487.
20. Y. Kawade, J. Fujisawa, S. Yonehara, Y. Iwakura, and Y. Yamamoto, in *Meth. Enzymol.* (S. Pestka, ed.), Vol. 78, Academic Press, New York, 1981, 522.
21. E. Knight, Jr. and D. Fahey, *J. Interferon Res. 2*, 421 (1982).
22. P. C. Familletti and S. Pestka, *Antimicrob. Agents Chemother. 20*, 1 (1980).
23. P. C. Familletti, R. McCandliss, and S. Pestka, *Antimicrob. Agents Chemother. 20*, 5 (1981).
24. A. A. Waldman, R. S. Miller, P. C. Familletti, S. Rubinstein, and S. Pestka, in *Meth. Enzymol.* (S. Pestka, ed.), Vol. 78, Academic Press, New York, 1981, p. 39.
25. R. D. Hershberg, E. G. Gusciora, P. C. Familletti, S. Rubinstein, C. A. Rose, and S. Pestka, in *Meth. Enzymol.* (S. Pestka, ed.), Vol. 78, Academic Press, New York, 1981, p. 45.
26. K. Cantell and D. R. Tovell, *Appl. Microbiol. 22*, 625 (1971).
27. E. F. Wheelock, *J. Bacteriol. 92*, 1415 (1966).
28. S. H. S. Lee, C. E. Van Rooyen, and R. L. Ozere, *Cancer Res. 29*, 645 (1969).
29. G. Y. Hadhazy, L. Gergely, F. E. Toth, and G. Y. Szegedi, *Acta Microbiol. Acad. Sci. Hung. 14*, 391 (1967).
30. M. Rubinstein, S. Rubinstein, P. C. Familletti, L. D. Brink, R. D. Hershberg, J. Gutterman, J. Hester, and S. Pestka, in *Peptides: Structure and Biological Function* (E. Gross and J. Meienhofer, eds.), Pierce Chemical Company, Rockford, IL, 1979, p. 99.
31. P. C. Familletti, S. Rubinstein, and S. Pestka, in *Meth. Enzymol.* (S. Pestka, ed.), Vol. 78, Academic Press, New York, 1981, p. 387.
32. S. Rubinstein, P. C. Familletti, and S. Pestka, *J. Virol. 37*, 755 (1981).
33. S. Udenfriend, S. Stein, P. Bohlen, W. Dairman, W. Leimgruber, and M. Weigele, *Science 178*, 871 (1972).
34. S. Stein, P. Bohlen, J. Stone, W. Dairman, and S. Udenfriend, *Arch. Biochem. Biophys. 155*, 203 (1973).
35. P. Bohlen, S. Stein, J. Stone, and S. Udenfriend, *Anal. Biochem. 67*, 438 (1975).
36. M. Rubinstein and S. Pestka, in *Meth. Enzymol.* (S. Pestka, ed.), Vol. 78, Academic Press, New York, 1981, p. 464.

37. F. E. Regnier and R. Noel, *J. Chromatogr. Sci. 14*, 316 (1976).
38. S.-H. Chang, R. Noel, and F. E. Regnier, *Anal. Chem. 48*, 1839 (1976).
39. D. S. Hobbs and S. Pestka, *J. Biol. Chem. 257*, 4071 (1982).
40. T. Staehelin, D. S. Hobbs, H.-F. Kung, and S. Pestka, *J. Biol. Chem. 256*, 9750 (1981).
41. T. Staehelin, D. S. Hobbs, H.-F. Kung, and S. Pestka, in *Meth. Enzymol.* (S. Pestka, ed.), Vol. 78, Academic Press, New York, 1981, p. 505.
42. J. A. Moschera, D. Woehle, K. P. Tsai, C.-H. Chen, and S. J. Tarnowski, in *Meth. Enzymol.* (S. Pestka, ed.), Vol. 119, Academic Press, New York, 1986, p. 177.
43. L. S. Lin, R. Yamamoto, and R. J. Drummond, in *Meth. Enzymol.* (S. Pestka, ed.), Vol. 119, Academic Press, New York, 1986, p. 183.
44. I. A. Braude, *Prep. Biochem. 13*, 177 (1983).
45. I. A. Braude, *Biochemistry 23*, 5603 (1984).
46. H.-F. Kung, Y.-C. E. Pan, J. Moschera, K. Tsai, E. Bekesi, M. Chang, H. Sugino, in *Meth. Enzymol.* (S. Pestka, ed.), Vol. 119, Academic Press, New York, 1986, p. 204.
47. W. E. Stewart, II, *Virology 61*, 80 (1974).
48. W. E. Stewart, II, L. S. Lin, M. Wiranowska-Stewart, and K. Cantell, *Proc. Natl. Acad. Sci. USA 74*, 4200 (1977).
49. E. T. Torma and K. Paucker, *J. Biol. Chem. 251*, 4810 (1976).
50. J. K. Chen, W. J. Jankowski, J. A. O'Malley, E. Sulkowski, and W. A. Carter, *J. Virol. 19*, 425 (1976).
51. W. J. Jankowski, W. Von Muenchhausen, E. Sulkowski, and W. A. Carter, *Biochemistry 15*, 5182 (1976).
52. P. M. Grob and K. C. Chadha, *Biochemistry 18*, 5782 (1979).
53. S. Bose, D. Gurari-Rotman, U. Th. Ruegg, K. Corley, and C. B. Anfinsen, *J. Biol. Chem. 251*, 1659 (1976).
54. S. Bose and J. Hickman, *J. Biol. Chem. 252*, 8336 (1977).
55. P. J. Bridgen, C. B. Anfinsen, L. Corley, S. Bose, K. C. Zoon, U. Th. Ruegg, and C. E. Buckler, *J. Biol. Chem. 252*, 6585 (1977).
56. D. S. Hobbs, J. Moschera, W. P. Levy, and S. Pestka, in *Meth. Enzymol.* (S. Pestka, ed.), Vol. 78, Academic Press, New York, 1981, p. 472.
57. K. C. Zoon, in *The Biology of the Interferon System* (E. De Maeyer, G. Galasso, and H. Schellekens, eds.), Elsevier/North Holland, Amsterdam, 1981, p. 47.
58. K. C. Zoon, M. E. Smith, P. J. Bridgen, C. B. Anfinsen, M. W. Hunkapiller, and L. E. Hood, *Science 207*, 527 (1980).
59. W. P. Levy, J. Shively, M. Rubinstein, U. Del Valle, and S. Pestka, *Proc. Natl. Acad. Sci. USA 77*, 5102 (1980).
60. E. Knight, Jr., M. W. Hunkapiller, B. D. Korant, R. W. F. Hardy, and L. E. Hood, *Science 207*, 525 (1980).
61. S. Maeda, R. McCandliss, M. Gross, A. Sloma, P. C. Familletti, J. M. Tabor, M. Evinger, W. P. Levy, and S. Pestka, *Proc. Natl. Acad. Sci. USA 77*, 7010 (1980); *78*, 4648 (1981).
62. W. P. Levy, M. Rubinstein, J. Shively, U. Del Valle, C.-Y. Lai, J. Moschera, L. Brink, L. Gerber, S. Stein, and S. Pestka, *Proc. Natl. Acad. Sci. USA 78*, 6186 (1981).

63. J. E. Shively, U. Del Valle, R. Blacher, D. Hawke, W. P. Levy, M. Rubinstein, S. Stein, W. C. McGregor, J. Tarnowski, R. Barlett, D. Lee, and S. Pestka, *Anal. Biochem. 126*, 318 (1982).
64. Y. Iwakura, S. Yonehara, and Y. Kawade, *J. Biol. Chem. 253*, 5074 (1978).
65. M. Kawakita, B. Cabrer, H. Taira, M. Rebello, E. Slattery, H. Weideli, and P. Lengyel, *J. Biol. Chem. 253*, 598 (1978).
66. J. De. Maeyer-Guignard, M. G. Tovey, I. Gresser, and E. De Maeyer, *Nature* (London) *27*, 622 (1978).
67. J. De Maeyer-Guignard, in *Meth. Enzymol.* (S. Pestka, ed.), Vol. 78, Academic Press, New York, 1981, p. 513.
68. H. Taira, R. J. Broeze, B. M. Jayaram, P. Lengyel, M. W. Hunkapiller, and L. E. Hood, *Science 207*, 528 (1980).
69. J. E. Labdon, K. D. Gibson, S. Sun, and S. Pestka, *Arch. Biochem. Biophys. 232*, 422 (1984).
70. G. R. Adolf, I. Kalsner, H. Ahorn, I. Maurer-Fogy, and K. Cantell, *Biochem. J. 276*, 511 (1991).
71. S. Nagata, H. Taira, A. Hall, L. Johnsrud, M. Streuli, J. Ecsodi, W. Boll, K. Cantell, and C. Weissmann, *Nature* (London) *284*, 316 (1980).
72. T. Taniguchi, S. Ohno, Y. Fujii-Kuriyama, and M. Muramatsu, *Gene 10*, 11 (1980).
73. R. Derynck, J. Content, E. De Clercq, G. Volckaert, J. Tavernier, R. Devos, and W. Fiers, *Nature* (London) *285*, 542 (1980).
74. M. Houghton, A. G. Steward, S. M. Doel, J. S. Emtage, M. A. W. Eaton, J. S. Smith, T. P. Patel, H. M. Lewis, A. G. Porter, J. R. Birch, T. Cartwright, and N. H. Carey, *Nucleic Acids Res. 8*, 1913 (1980).
75. D. V. Goeddel, H. M. Sheppard, E. Yelverton, D. Leung, R. Crea, A. Sloma, and S. Pestka, *Nucleic Acids Res. 8*, 4057 (1980).
76. S. Pestka, J. McInnes, E. A. Havell, and J. Vilcek, *Proc. Natl. Acad. Sci. USA 72*, 3898 (1975).
77. M. N. Thang, D. C. Thang, E. De Maeyer, and L. Montagnier, *Proc. Natl. Acad. Sci. USA 72*, 3975 (1975).
78. F. H. Reynolds, Jr., E. Premkumar, and P. M. Pitha, *Proc. Natl. Acad. Sci. USA 72*, 4881 (1975).
79. R. L. Cavalieri, E. A. Havell, J. Vilcek, and S. Pestka, *Proc. Natl. Acad. Sci. USA 74*, 3287 (1977).
80. R. L. Cavalieri, E. A. Havell, J. Vilcek, and S. Pestka, *Proc. Natl. Acad. Sci. USA 74*, 4415 (1977).
81. R. L. Cavalieri and S. Pestka, *Tex. Rep. Biol. Med. 35*, 117 (1977).
82. R. McCandliss, A. Sloma, and S. Pestka, in *Meth. Enzymol.* (S. Pestka, ed.), Vol. 79, Academic Press, New York, 1981, p. 51.
83. P. C. Familletti, R. McCandliss, and S. Pestka, *Antimicrob. Agents Chemother. 20*, 5 (1981).
84. S. Maeda, M. Gross, and S. Pestka, in *Meth. Enzymol.* (S. Pestka, ed.), Vol. 79, Academic Press, New York, 1981, p. 613.
85. R. McCandliss, A. Sloma, and S. Pestka, in *Meth. Enzymol.* (S. Pestka, ed.), Vol. 79, Academic Press, New York, 1981, p. 618.

86. S. Pestka, *Sci. Am. 249*(2), 36 (1983).
87. D. V. Goeddel, E. Yelverton, A. Ullrich, H. L. Heyneker, G. Miozzari, W. Holmes, P. H. Seeburg, T. Dull, L. May, N. Stebbing, R. Crea, S. Maeda, R. McCandliss, A. Sloma, J. M. Tabor, M. Gross, P. C. Familletti, and S. Pestka, *Nature* (London) *287*, 411 (1980).
88. M. D. Schaber, T. M. DeChiara, and R. A. Kramer, in *Meth. Enzymol.* (S. Pestka, ed.), Vol. 119, Academic Press, New York, 1986, p. 416.
89. R. A. Hitzeman, D. W. Leung, L. J. Perry, W. J. Kohr, H. L. Levine, and D. V. Goeddel, *Science 219*, 620 (1983).
90. K. Zinn, P. Mellon, M. Ptashne, and T. Maniatis, *Proc. Natl. Acad. Sci. USA 79*, 4897 (1982).
91. D. Canaani and P. Berg, *Proc. Natl. Acad. Sci. USA 79*, 5166 (1982).
92. R. Devos, H. Cheroutre, Y. Taya, W. Degrave, H. Van Heuverswyn, and W. Fiers, *Nucleic Acids Res. 10*, 2487 (1982).
93. R. Derynck, P. W. Gray, E. Yelverton, D. W. Leung, H. M. Shepard, R. M. Lawn, A. Najarian, D. Pennica, F. E. Hagle, R. A. Hitzeman, P. J. Sherwood, A. D. Levinson, and D. V. Goeddel, in *From Genes to Protein: Translation into Biotechnology* (F. Ahmad, J. Schultz, E. E. Smith, and W. J. Whelan, eds.), Academic Press, New York, 1982, p. 249–262.
94. L. Mulcahy, M. Kann, B. Kelder, E. Rehberg, S. Pestka, and D. W. Stacey, in *Meth. Enzymol.* (S. Pestka, ed.), Vol. 119, Academic Press, New York, 1986, p. 383.
95. E. Remaut, P. Stanssens, G. Simons, and W. Fiers, in *Meth. Enzymol.* (S. Pestka, ed.), Vol. 119, Academic Press, New York, 1980, p. 366.
96. M. A. Innis and F. McCormic, in *Meth. Enzymol.* (S. Pestka, ed.), Vol. 119, Academic Press, New York, 1986, p. 397.
97. T. Staehelin, C. Stahli, D. S. Hobbs, and S. Pestka, in *Meth. Enzymol.* (S. Pestka, ed.), Vol. 79, Academic Press, New York, 1981, p. 589.
98. M. Evinger, S. Maeda, and S. Pestka, *J. Biol. Chem. 256*, 2113 (1981).
99. J. R. Ortaldo, A. Mason, E. Rehberg, J. Moschera, B. Kelder, S. Pestka, and R. B. Herberman, *J. Biol. Chem. 258*, 15011 (1983).
100. J. R. Ortaldo, A. Mantovani, D. Hobbs, M. Rubinstein, S. Pestka, and R. B. Hebberman, *Int. J. Cancer 31*, 285 (1983).
101. W. C. McGregor and A. H. Ramel, in *Recombinant DNA Products: Insulin-Interferon-Growth Hormone* (A. P. Bollon, ed.), Chemical Rubber Co., Boca Raton, FL, 1984, p. 129.
102. G. Realdi, G. Diodati, P. Bonetti, S. Scaccabarozzi, A. Alberti, and A. Ruol, *J. Hepatol. 11* (Suppl 1), 68 (1990).
103. J. U. Gutterman, S. Fine, J. Quesada, S. J. Hornings, J. F. Levine, R. Alexanian, L. Berhardt, M. Kramer, H. Spiegel, W. Colburn, P. Trown, T. Merigan, and Z. Dziewanowska, *Ann. Intern. Med. 96*, 549 (1982).
104. S. J. Tarnowski, *Pharmac. Tech. 7*, 70 (1983).
105. P. Dunnill, *Chem. Indust. 22*, 877 (1982).
106. J. W. Eveleigh, in *Affinity Chromatography and Related Techniques* (T. C. J. Gribnau, J. Visser, and R. J. F. Nivard, eds.), Elsevier, New York, 1982, p. 293.
107. M. Maze and G. M. Gray, *Biochemistry 19*, 2351 (1975).

108. J. P. Chen and H. M. Shurley, *Thromb. Res. 7*, 425 (1975).
109. K. H. Brooks and T. L. Feldbrush, *J. Immunol. 127*, 963 (1981).
110. C. D. Benjamin, A. Miller, E. E. Serarz, and M. A. Harvey, *J. Immunol. 125*, 1017 (1980).
111. T. Staehelin, B. Durrer, J. Schmidt, B. Takacs, J. Stocker, V. Miggiano, C. Stahli, M. Rubinstein, W. P. Levy, R. Hershberg, and S. Pestka, *Proc. Natl. Acad. Sci. USA 78*, 1848 (1981).
112. T. Staehelin, B. Durrer, J. Schmidt, B. Takacs, J. Stocker, V. Miggiano, C. Stahli, H.-F. Kung, D. S. Hobbs, W. P. Levy, J. A. Moschera, and S. Pestka, *Tex. Rep. Biol. Med. 41*, 198 (1982).
113. N. G. Anderson, D. D. Willis, D. W. Holladay, J. E. Caton, J. W. Holleman, J. W. Eveleigh, J. E. Attrill, F. L. Ball, and N. L. Anderson, *Anal. Biochem. 66*, 159 (1975).
114. S. J. Tarnowski and R. A. Liptak, Jr., *Adv. Biol. Processes 2*, 271 (1983).
115. S. J. Tarnowski, S. K. Roy, R. A. Liptak, D. K. Lee, and R. Y. Ning, in *Meth. Enzymol.* (S. Pestka, ed.), Vol. 119, Academic Press, New York, 1986, p. 153.
116. A. H. Nishikawa and P. Bailon, *J. Solid-Phase Biochem. 1*, 33 (1986).
117. S. Pestka and S. J. Tarnowski, *Pharmacol. Ther. 29*, 299 (1985).
118. D. R. Thatcher and N. Panayotatos, in *Meth. Enzymol.* (S. Pestka, ed.), Vol. 119, Academic Press, New York, 1986, p. 166.
119. S. Pestka, B. Kelder, D. K. Tarnowski, and S. J. Tarnowski, *Anal. Biochem. 132*, 328 (1983).
120. G. Bodo and I. Fogy, in *The Biology of the Interferon System* (H. Kirchner and H. Schellekens, eds.), Elsevier Science Publishers B.V., Amsterdam, 1985, p. 23.
121. J. A. Langer and S. Pestka, in *Meth. Enzymol.* (S. Pestka, ed.), Vol. 119, Academic Press, New York, 1986, p. 248.
122. J. A. Langer and S. Pestka, *Immunol. Today 9*, 393 (1988).
123. Y. K. Yip, R. H. L. Pang, C. Urban, and J. Vilcek, *Proc. Natl. Acad. Sci. USA 78*, 1601 (1981).
124. Y. K. Yip, B. S. Barrowclough, C. Urban, and J. Vilcek, *Proc. Natl. Acad. Sci. USA 79*, 1820 (1982).
125. Y. K. Yip, B. S. Barrowclough, C. Urban, and J. Vilcek, *Science 215*, 411 (1982).
126. I. A. Braude, in *Meth. Enzymol.* (S. Pestka, ed.), Vol. 119, Academic Press, New York, 1986, p. 193.
127. E. Rinderknecht, B. H. O'Connor, and H. Rodriguez, *J. Biol. Chem. 259*, 6790 (1984).
128. M. P. Langford, J. A. Georgiades, G. J. Stanton, F. Dianzani, and H. M. Johnson, *Infect. Immun. 26*, 36 (1979).
129. M. DeLey, J. Van Damme, H. Claeys, H. Weening, J. W. Heine, A. Billiau, C. Vermylen, and P. DeSomer, *Eur. J. Immunol. 10*, 877 (1980).
130. S. Pestka, B. Kelder, P. C. Familletti, J. A. Moschera, R. Crowl, and E. S. Kempner, *J. Biol. Chem. 228*, 9706 (1983).
131. S. Baron, F. Dianzani, and G. J. Stanton, *Tex. Rep. Biol. Med. 41*, 1 (1982).
132. S. Baron, F. Dianzani, and G. J. Stanton, *Tex. Rep. Biol. Med. 41*, 411 (1982).

133. K. Henco, J. Brosius, A. Fujisawa, J.-I. Fujisawa, J. R. Haynes, J. Hockstadt, T. Kovacic, M. Pasek, A. Schamböck, J. Schmid, K. Todokoro, M. Wälchli, S. Nagata, and C. Weissmann, *J. Mol. Biol. 185*, 227 (1985).
134. S. Pestka, in *Methods Enzymol.* (S. Pestka, ed.), Vol. 119, Academic Press, New York, 1986, p. 1.
135. J. A. Langer and S. Pestka, *Pharmacol. Ther. 27*, 371 (1985).
136. X.-Y. Liu, V. Jung, X.-X. Zhao, R. S. Bhatt, S. Maeda, and S. Pestka, *J. Interferon Res. 7*, 641 (1987).
137. M. Fuke, L. C. Hendrix, and A. P. Bollon, *Gene 32*, 135 (1984).
138. R. M. Torczynski, M. Fuke, and A. P. Bollon, *Proc. Natl. Acad. Sci. USA 81*, 6451 (1984).
139. A. P. Bollon, M. Fuke, and R. M. Torczynski, in *Meth. Enzymol.* (S. Pestka, ed.), Vol. 119, Academic Press, New York, 1986, p. 359.
140. A. Sloma, European Patent Application 83102893.1 (1983).
141. M. A. Innis, International Patent Application PCT/USA83/00032 (1983).
142. F. Meyer, European Patent Application 82109094.1 (1983).
143. S. Maeda, R. McCandliss, T.-R. Chiang, L. Costello, W. P. Levy, N. T. Chang, and S. Pestka, in *Developmental Biology Using Purified Genes* (D. D. Brown, ed.), Academic Press, New York, 1981, p. 85.
144. D. W. Leung, D. J. Capon, and D. V. Goeddel, *Biotechnology 2*, 458 (1984).
145. Y. Higashi, Y. Sokawa, Y. Watanabe, Y. Kawade, S. Ohno, C. Takaoka, and T. Taniguchi, *J. Biol. Chem. 258*, 9522 (1983).
146. P. Gold and S. Pestka, *Fed. Proc., Fed. Am. Soc. Exp. Biol. 44*, 1613 (1985).
147. P. W. Gray, D. W. Leung, D. Pennica, E. Yelverton, R. Najarian, C. C. Simonsen, R. Derynck, P. J. Sherwood, D. M. Wallace, S. L. Berger, A. D. Levinson, and D. V. Goeddel, *Nature* (London) *295*, 503 (1982).
148. P. W. Gray and D. V. Goeddel, *Proc. Natl. Acad. Sci. USA 80*, 5842 (1983).
149. R. Dijkema, P. H. van der Meide, M. Dubbeld, M. Caspers, J. Wubben, and H. Schellekens, in *Meth. Enzymol.* (S. Pestka, ed.), Vol. 119, Academic Press, New York, 1986, p. 453.
150. R. Dijkema, P. H. van der Meide, P. H. Pouwels, M. Caspers, M. Dubbeld, and H. Schellekens, *EMBO J. 4*, 761 (1985).
151. R. Derynck, in *Interferon* (I. Gresser, ed.), Vol. 5, Academic Press, New York, 1984, p. 181.

# II
# GROWTH FACTORS

# 9
# Transforming Growth Factor-$\alpha$ and Related Growth Factors

**James T. Elder**
*University of Michigan*
*Ann Arbor, Michigan*

## I. INTRODUCTION

### A. Historical Perspectives

Epidermal growth factor (EGF) and its receptor hold a special place in the history of growth factor research. The separation of EGF from nerve growth–promoting substance by Stanley Cohen in 1960 [1] led to the recognition that tissue-specific factors were central to the process of tissue growth and repair. In 1962, Cohen demonstrated that injection of purified EGF into newborn mice resulted in precocious eyelid opening and eruption of incisor teeth [2], demonstrating its relevance to the intimately linked processes of epidermal proliferation and differentiation [3]. Moreover, the discovery that urogastrone, now recognized as the human homolog of EGF, could also inhibit gastric acid secretion [4], demonstrated that growth factors were also important for the regulation of ongoing physiological process.

The purification of EGF made possible the identification and eventual purification of its receptor and the characterization of its EGF-binding properties [5]. These advances in turn made possible the identification of an EGF receptor-binding activity in sarcoma growth factor (SGF), a partially purified substance isolated from tumors and transformed cells capable of supporting anchorage-independent growth [6, 7]. SGF was later resolved into two structurally unrelated components, termed transforming growth factors (TGF)-$\alpha$ and -$\beta$ [8]. Purified TGF-$\alpha$ was shown to compete specifically with EGF for

EGF receptor binding [9], although it is structurally [10] and antigenically [7] distinct from EGF. Initially, TGF-$\alpha$ was assumed to be expressed specifically by oncogenically transformed cells; however, subsequent studies revealed that it is expressed by many normal adult cells and tissues and during embryonic development [11, 12].

Within the past few years, there has been an increasing realization that EGF and TGF-$\alpha$ are not the only growth factors capable of acting through the EGF receptor. At present at least eight structurally defined peptides have been shown to elicit functional cellular responses via the EGF receptor (reviewed below). Thus, 30 years after the discovery of EGF, a picture of increasing complexity but undiminished interest continues to evolve.

### B. Objectives

The principal objective of this chapter will be to familiarize the reader with the expanding family of EGF-like growth factors in terms of structure, expression, and biological actions, including evidence for involvement of EGF-like growth factors in human skin disease states, including psoriasis, other inflammatory skin diseases, and skin cancer. However, a discussion of these actions would be incomplete without consideration of the receptor itself and the postreceptor mechanisms involved in EGF receptor signal transduction. Therefore, an attempt will be made to summarize the large body of knowledge in this area.

## II. THE EGF/TGF-$\alpha$ GENE FAMILY

Since cutaneous wound healing and psoriasis are processes that involve increased epidermal proliferation and yet are confined largely to the skin, it would be predicted that local (autocrine) production of EGF would occur if interactions of EGF with its receptor are important in this process [13]. However, early studies by Byyny et al. in 1972 failed to document expression of EGF in mouse skin [14]. This paradox appeared to be answered by the discovery that TGF-$\alpha$ was structurally and functionally related to EGF [10–12] and was expressed in human [15] and murine [16] keratinocytes as well as normal human skin [15, 17, 18]. However, like many other gene families, this explanation has proven to be too simplistic, as the EGF-like family of growth factors continues to grow. At this time, at least eight factors that bind to the EGF receptor and/or display EGF-like biological activity have been structurally characterized (Table 1). These can be divided into cellular and virally derived products and subdivided into heparin-binding and nonbinding subsets. In addition, an ever-increasing number of proteins are being identified which display homology to EGF but do not bind to the receptor with high affinity (for reviews, see Refs. 19, 20). After discussing the com-

**Table 1** EGF Protein Family

| Protein | Function | Ref. |
|---|---|---|
| Factors with EGF-like biological activity | | |
| EGF | growth factor | 5 |
| TGF-$\alpha$ | growth factor | 11 |
| Amphiregulin | growth factor | 21–23 |
| Heparin-binding EGF | growth factor | 24 |
| Schwannoma-derived growth factor | growth factor | 25 |
| Vaccinia virus growth factor | growth factor | 26 |
| Shope fibroma virus growth factor | growth factor | 27 |
| Myxoma virus growth factor | growth factor | 28 |
| Cripto | growth factor (?) | 29 |
| Factors without known EGF-like biological activity | | |
| Pfs (*Plasmodium falciparum*) | unknown | 30 |
| Notch (*Drosophila*) | adhesion/neurogenesis | 31 |
| Delta (*Drosophila*) | adhesion/neurogenesis | 31 |
| Crumbs (*Drosophila*) | cell polarity | 31 |
| Slit (*Drosophila*) | adhesion/neurogenesis | 32 |
| Serrate (*Drosophila*) | ectodermal development | 33 |
| Lin-12 (*Caenorhabditis elegans*) | adhesion | 34 |
| uEGF1 (*Strongylocentrotus purpuratus*) | gastrulation | 35 |
| SpEGF2 (*Strongylocentrotus purpuratus*) | gastrulation | 35 |
| Urokinase | serine protease | 36 |
| Tissue plasminogen activator | serine protease | 37 |
| Clotting factors (VII, IX, X, XII) | blood clotting | 38 |
| Protein S | blood clotting | 39 |
| Protein C | blood clotting | 40 |
| Thrombomodulin | blood clotting | 41 |
| Low-density lipoprotein (LDL) receptor | LDL uptake | 42 |
| Laminin $\beta$1 chain | extracellular matrix protein | 19 |
| Thrombospondin | extracellular matrix protein | 19 |
| Tenascin (cytotactin) | extracellular matrix protein | 19 |
| Nidogen | extracellular matrix protein | 43 |
| Human proteoglycan core protein | extracellular matrix protein | 44 |
| Clr, Cls | complement | 45 |

*Source*: Adapted from Ref. 12.

mon structural features of all the EGF-like growth factors, we will focus on TGF-$\alpha$ and amphiregulin (AR), two factors whose expression and function in the skin and in cultured keratinocytes have been established [11, 15–18, 21–23]. Future reviews will undoubtedly need to address the cutaneous roles of heparin-binding EGF-like growth factors [24, 25], proteoglycan-derived EGF-like growth factor(s) [44], and a variety of novel EGF-like factors yet to be discovered, not to mention proteins such as amphiregulin-associated protein [46], which may modulate the activity of the associated growth factor(s). For purposes of this review, EGF-like growth factors are defined as a subset of these proteins characterized by high-affinity binding for the EGF receptor and the capability to either stimulate or inhibit the growth of EGF-responsive cells.

## A. Common Structural Features

The common structural features of the EGF-like family of proteins and growth factors have been the subject of numerous studies [47–58]. Several of these soluble growth factors have been isolated in multiple different molecular weight forms, generated by differential proteolysis and/or glycosylation, as shown for TGF-$\alpha$ in Figure 1. The most fully processed (mature) forms

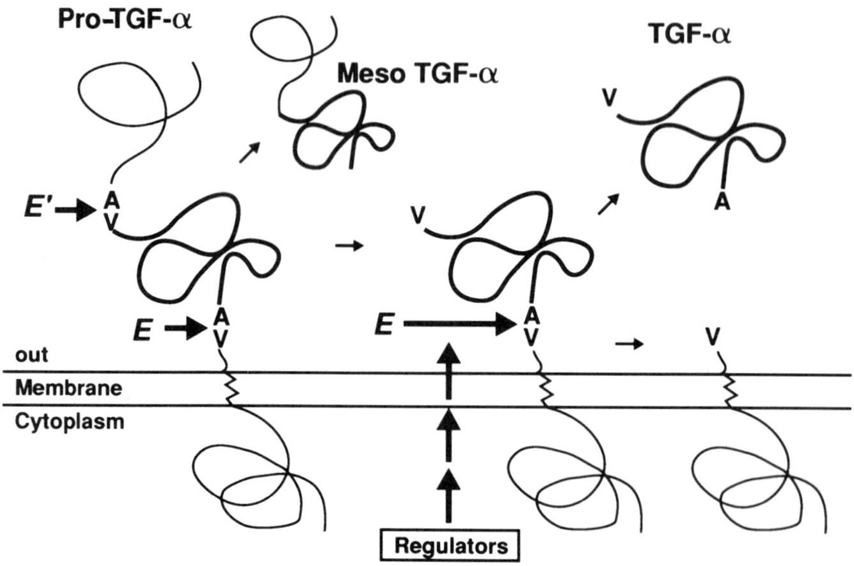


**Fig. 1** Model for cleavage of the membrane-anchored TGF-$\alpha$ precursor. Soon after newly synthesized pro-TGF-$\alpha$ reaches the cell surface, it is rapidly cleaved (by enzyme E′) at an Ala-Val (AV) cleavage site located at the N terminus of the mature TGF-$\alpha$ sequence. In a second step, which is very slow under basal conditions, cleavage (by enzyme E) occurs at the C terminus of the mature TGF-$\alpha$ sequence and results in the release of soluble TGF-$\alpha$. This step can be rapidly accelerated by activation of enzyme E in response to PKC-dependent and -independent mechanisms. In some cell types, meso-TGF-$\alpha$ may be released by C-terminal cleavage prior to N-terminal cleavage. (Adapted from Ref. 154.)

are approximately 50–60 amino acids long and contain six highly-conserved half-cystine residues (Fig. 2). The consensus organization for these cystines is $X_nCX_7CX_{2\text{-}3}GXCX_{10\text{-}13}CXCX_3YXGXRCX_4LX_n$, where X is any amino acid [54]. The fact that all of the cysteine residues must be present and disulfide-bonded to a specific partner for full biological activity [55] suggested the general structure shown for four members of the family in Figure 2 [56]. Interestingly, this motif of six cysteine residues is conserved in the several cell surface and extracellular proteins, which do not bind to the EGF receptor or display EGF-like biological activity display (Table 1). As it has recently been shown that extracellular matrix (ECM) molecules are capable of activating tyrosine kinases in target cells [57], it is possible that under appropriate

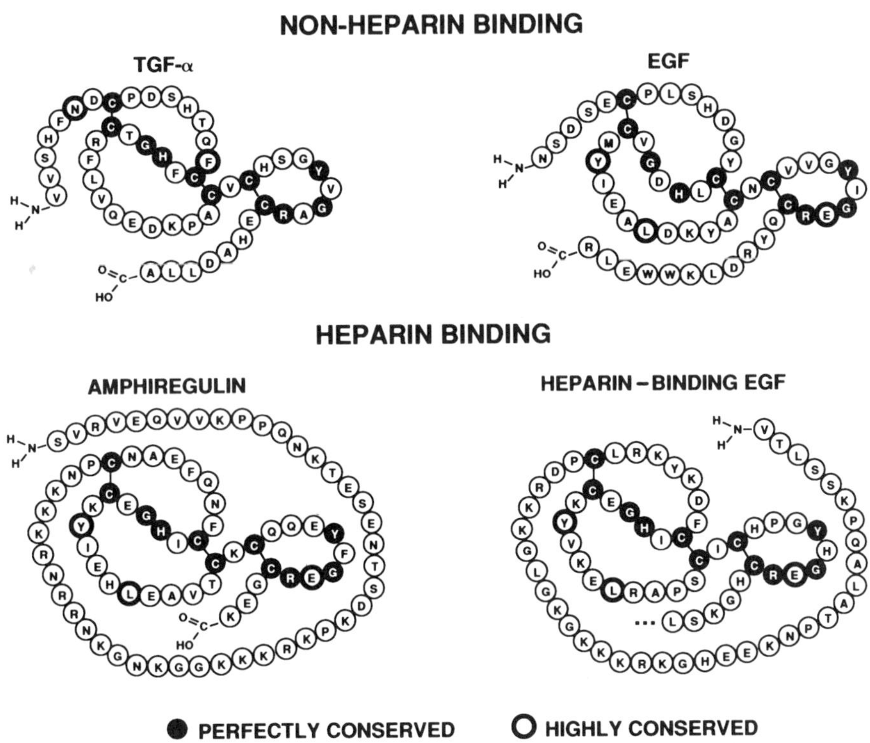


**Fig. 2** Common structural features of EGF-like growth factors. Amino acid residues conserved in at least three of the four polypeptides shown are depicted as bold circles, and those conserved in all four as solid circles. The 3′ terminus of heparin-binding EGF has not been determined, as indicated by the dotted line. (Adapted from Ref. 21.)

conditions, some of these EGF-like domains may mediate cell activation via the EGF receptor or related receptors. Moreover, recent evidence has indicated that the membrane-bound precursors of both TGF-$\alpha$ and EGF are capable of inducing signal transduction on neighboring cells, a mechanism called juxtracrine stimulation [73]. This may be a general feature of EGF-like growth factors, since several EGF-like proteins are expressed on the cell surface and display multiple EGF-like repeats (Fig. 3). It is possible that EGF-like structural domains may function as receptors for as-yet-undefined ligands, whether in soluble form, bound to (or as a component of) the extracellular matrix, or on the surface of adjacent cells [73]. Given the prominent role of such molecules in *Drosophila* [31–33] and *C. elegans* [34] morphogenesis, it is likely that such mechanisms are of general importance in development.

Although no X-ray crystallographic structures have been reported to date, the solution structures of both EGF [48, 49] and TGF-$\alpha$ [50–52] have been analyzed by nuclear magnetic resonance techniques. Both molecules display two domains of antiparallel beta-sheet structure, with the larger domain located near the N terminus, and the smaller toward the C terminus. Given these similarities in structure, it is not surprising that both molecules bind the EGF receptor with similar affinity [9] and display similar biological activities [11]. However, despite these similarities, recent analysis of the structural dynamics of these two molecules by circular dichroism and infrared spectroscopy/deuterium exchange [53] revealed that TGF-$\alpha$ is a much more flexible molecule than EGF. It is possible that these subtle structural differences may account for the differences in competition for receptor binding with anti-EGF receptor antibodies [59], intracellular processing [58], and biological activities [11, 58] displayed by EGF and TGF-$\alpha$.

## B. Members of the Family

### *1. Epidermal Growth Factor (EGF)*

The history of purification, structure and function of EGF has been reviewed extensively [5, 54, 60–62] and will not be discussed in detail here. As discussed by Carpenter and Cohen [54], one of the most interesting recent developments involving EGF is the discovery of eight EGF-like domains in the EGF precursor, the function of which are unknown (Fig. 3). In terms of skin function, the apparently limited tissue distribution of EGF (kidney, salivary gland, parietal region of the stomach, and in macrophages) coupled with the absence of detectable expression in the skin [14, 18] suggest that EGF is not a major determinant of epidermal growth. However, reports of EGF expression

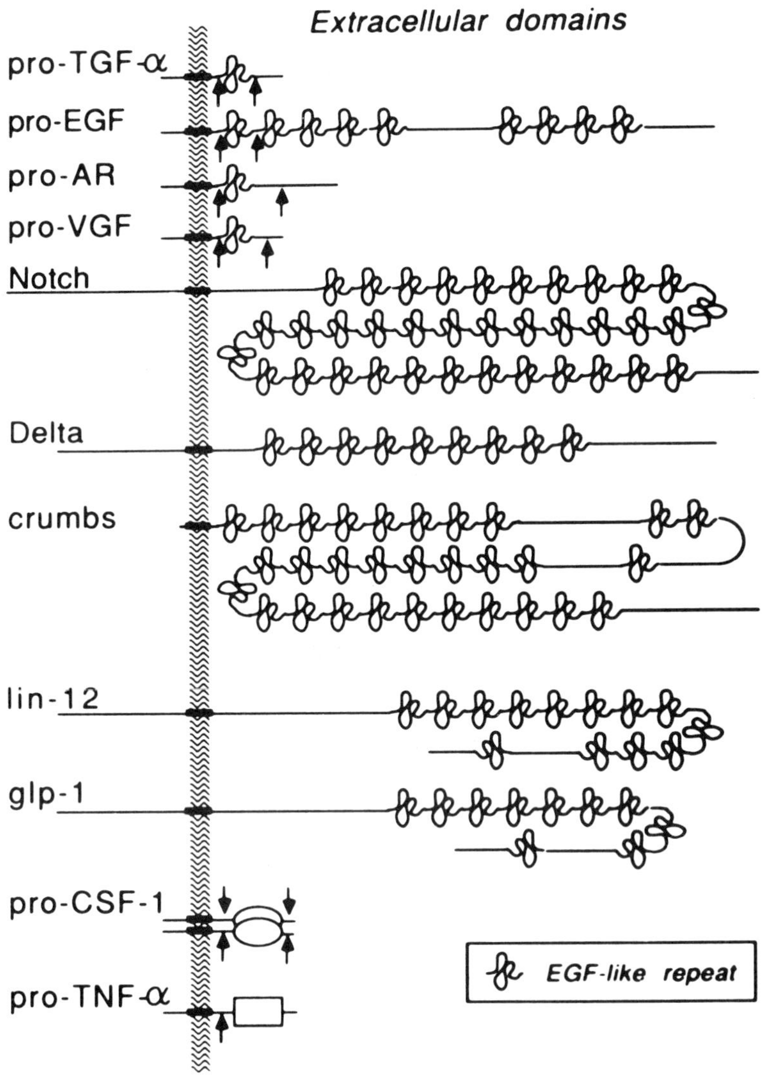


**Fig. 3** Membrane-anchored growth factors and related molecules. The cell membrane is indicated by the vertical shaded line. Known sites of proteolytic cleavage are shown by arrows. AR, amphiregulin; VGF, vaccinia virus growth factor; CSF-1, colony-stimulating factor-1; TNF, tumor necrosis factor. (From Ref. 154.)

in macrophages [63, 64] coupled with the presence of cells of this lineage in many inflammatory skin diseases including psoriasis [65] demonstrate that a role for EGF in inflammatory epidermal hyperplasia cannot be ruled out.

### 2. *Transforming Growth Factor-α (TGF-α)*

Purification [9, 10, 66], molecular cloning [67], and the development of specific antibodies to TGF-α [17, 18] allowed further characterization of its interactions with the EGF receptor [9, 10, 59] and facilitated studies of its expression in normal as well as tumor cells. These early studies, which have been the subject of several excellent reviews [8, 11, 12, 60–62], demonstrated that TGF-α is structurally related to EGF and binds to the EGF receptor with high affinity. Multiple secreted forms of TGF-α, ranging in size from 5 to 20 kd, result from alternative patterns of cleavage, glycosylation, and phosphorylation of a 160 kd membrane-associated precursor (Fig. 1).

The skin has been the focus of numerous investigations involving TGF-α. In fact, the first reported finding of TGF-α expression in normal human tissue was in neonatal foreskins [15]. TGF-α expression is markedly increased in healing skin wounds [68] and in several benign and malignant skin diseases characterized by epidermal hyperplasia [17, 18, 69, 70]. Taken together with evidence for positive autoregulation of TGF-α expression and for the mitogenicity of TGF-α in cultured keratinocytes (reviewed below), these observations have led to the hypothesis that TGF-α is a major autocrine mitogen in the epidermis [15, 17, 18]. However, our laboratory has found that antibodies or antisense oligonucleotides directed against TGF-α are ineffective in inhibiting the growth of normal keratinocytes (J.T.E., unpublished observations). In contrast, antibodies against the EGF receptor are highly effective inhibitors of keratinocyte growth [71, 72]. It seems likely that this apparent paradox will be resolved when more is known about the complete repertoire of EGF-like mitogens capable of being expressed by keratinocytes (see below). Alternatively, it is possible that growth stimulation by TGF-α in these cultures occurs via a "juxtacrine" pathway [73] inaccessible to available antibodies.

### 3. *Amphiregulin (AR)*

AR was so named because it either stimulates or inhibits growth in various cell lines [21, 74, 75]. AR was originally purified from MCF-7 breast cancer cells [74]; however, its expression is highly variable in other tumor cell lines [21, 23, 77]. Its expression in normal cells and tissues is not yet completely characterized; however, it is expressed in at least some normal tissues including breast, placenta, ovary, gut, and skin [21, 23, 77]. AR is not detectable in cultured fibroblasts and melanocytes [22] but is overexpressed in many carcinomas [23, 77], suggesting that its expression may be specific for cells of epithelial origin. The AR gene has been characterized and found to contain six exons spanning 10.2 kb of genomic DNA, which correspond to extracellular, transmembrane, and cytoplasmic domains [21]. Like EGF and TGF-α, soluble AR is produced by proteolytic cleavage of a glycosylated membrane precursor (Fig. 1). Moreover, the intron-exon structure of all three genes is similar [21], demonstrating that all three have a common, if ancient, evolutionary origin. In contrast, other proteins (such as coagulation factor IX and thrombospondin) that have EGF-like domains but do not appear to bind to or activate the EGF receptor (Table 1) have a different exon-intron structure, suggesting an even earlier divergence.

Under appropriate experimental conditions (density greater than $3 \times 10^3$ cells/cm$^2$), keratinocytes are capable of robust proliferation in the absence of exogenous growth factors [72]; this behavior is not observed under clonal growth conditions. However, conditioned medium (CM) from high-density keratinocytes is able to support clonal keratinocyte growth [72], suggesting that the autocrine growth pattern observed at higher cell densities is mediated by soluble secreted factors. Heparin partially inhibited CM-stimulated clonal growth, suggesting that at least some of the soluble autocrine factors were heparin-sensitive [72]. Pursuing these results, the soluble factor was purified by heparin-Sepharose, ion-exchange, and reverse-phase chromatography and called KAF (keratinocyte autocrine factor) [22]. On the basis of N-terminal amino acid sequence, immunological cross-reactivity, biochemical, and biological properties, KAF was found to be similar or identical to AR [22]. KAF/AR was shown to be abundantly expressed in keratinocytes by RNA blot hybridization [22, 76] and to be secreted into the medium in biologically active form by these cells [22]. The relatively abundant expression of a second EGF-like autocrine growth factor may explain why human keratinocytes appear to be refractory to growth inhibition by antisense oligonucleotides and antibodies directed against TGF-α (J.T.E., unpublished data).

Recently, Cook et al. reported [23] and our laboratory has confirmed [76] that AR mRNA is markedly overexpressed in psoriatic lesions. While these preliminary results will require confirmation at the level of immunoreactive protein and biological activity, they do suggest that epidermal hyperproliferation in vivo is associated with the expression of more than one EGF-like growth factor. Because AR is produced by and strongly mitogenic for keratinocytes [22, 76] but only weakly mitogenic for other cell types [74], it is likely that AR will prove to be an important autocrine regulator of epidermal proliferation.

### 4. *Heparin-Binding EGF (HB-EGF)*

In the course of screening macrophage-like U937 cells for the production of heparin-binding growth factors, Klagsbrun and coworkers purified a soluble, secreted, heparin-binding factor which stimulated the growth of 3T3 indicator fibroblasts [24]. The derived amino acid sequence of a cDNA clone isolated using degenerate oligonucleotides displayed marked homologies to EGF. Heparin-binding EGF (HB-EGF), as it was called, competed with EGF for EGF receptor binding in a radioreceptor assay and stimulated the growth of EGF-responsive target cells [24]. To date, expression of HB-EGF in the skin has not been reported. By analogy with TGF-$\alpha$ and AR, however, it can be predicted that this factor is likely to be expressed in cultured keratinocytes and overexpressed in psoriasis. The observation that both AR and HB-EGF interact directly with heparin and that heparin modulates their effects on target cells [21, 24] suggests that these factors, their receptors, or both may interact with glycosaminoglycan-containing extracellular matrix elements such as hyaluronic acid (mucin, ground substance), proteoglycans, and complex glycosphingolipids at the interface of the cell surface and extracellular matrix in vivo.

#### 5. *Schwannoma-Derived Growth Factor (SDGF)*

In the course of screening various rat cell lines for secreted glial cell mitogens, SDGF was purified by Kimura et al. [25]. N-terminal sequencing followed by synthesis of degenerate oligonucleotides and cDNA library screening revealed that SDGF is 76% homologous to mature human AR and 69% homologous to its precursor. However, the Mr of mature SDGF is about 10,000 da greater than AR, and unlike AR, SDGF has no inhibitory effect on A431 cell growth [25]. It remains to be determined whether SDGF is the rat homolog of human AR, or whether both species express SDGF in addition to AR. There is at present no information regarding SDGF expression in the skin.

#### 6. *Cripto*

Cripto was isolated fortuitously during the course of screening for full-length glucose-6-phosphate cDNA, as similarities to the EGF/TGF-$\alpha$ gene family were noted after sequencing a candidate cDNA [29]. Transfection and expression of cripto in NIH 3T3 fibroblasts or NOG-8 mouse mammary epithelial cells leads to morphological transformation in vitro [78], but not in vivo [29]. Very similar results are seen after transfection of TGF-$\alpha$ (see Sec. III.B), suggesting that cripto has TGF-$\alpha$–like biological activity. Cripto appears to be expressed primarily in embryonic cells [78]; however, its expression in the skin has not been studied. Given the structural similarity of EGF and related growth factors to the products of the *notch, delta, crumbs, slit,* and *serrate* loci in *Drosophila* and the *lin*-12 locus in *C. elegans*, each of which is important during embryogenesis [31–34], it seems likely that other EGF-like growth factors such as cripto, which are expressed primarily during embryonic development, will be identified.

*7. Vaccinia Growth Factor (VGF) and Related Growth Factors*

The similarity of a vaccinia poxvirus early gene product to rat TGF-α was noted by Blomquist et al. in 1984 [79] and by Todaro and coworkers in 1985 [26]. Shortly afterwards, EGF was shown to inhibit vaccinia virus infection by occupying the EGF receptor [80], and a 25 kd protein was isolated from vaccinia virus–infected cells and shown to have EGF-like biological activity [81]. More recently, an EGF-like factor encoded by the Shope rabbit fibroma virus has been characterized by DNA sequencing [27] and shown to have biological activity [82], and a similar sequence has been identified in the myxoma poxvirus [28]. Sequences homologous to EGF, TGF-α, and VGF are also present at similar positions in the early region of molluscum contagiosum virus [83]. Deletion of the VGF gene reduces viral virulence [84] and reduces host cell proliferation [85], suggesting that the viral life cycle makes use of activation of cellular signal transduction mechanisms activated by the EGF receptor. Consistent with the notion that viral infection induces epidermal hyperplasia, it is notable that marked epidermal thickening accompanies several poxvirus infections, including orf, milker's nodules, and molluscum contagiosum [86].

## III. CUTANEOUS BIOLOGICAL ACTIVITIES OF EGF-LIKE GROWTH FACTORS

### A. Normal Epidermal Growth and Differentiation

Ever since the initial descriptions of the biological activities of EGF by Cohen some 30 years ago, it has been clear that the effects of EGF on epidermal proliferation and differentiation are intimately linked [1–3]. Although still poorly understood, this interrelationship continues to characterize the cutaneous biological activities of the entire family of EGF-like growth factors, as will be evident from the various systems discussed below.

*1. In Vitro Studies*

*Cell Culture.* In the pioneering studies of Rheinwald and Green [87] on the serial cultivation of human keratinocytes in 1977, EGF was found to markedly increase the culture lifespan by inhibiting the onset of senescence in vitro. During the subsequent development of serum-free growth media, which allowed keratinocyte growth in the absence of feeder layers [88, 89], it was recognized that EGF was also needed for optimal growth, especially under clonal growth conditions [90]. Like EGF, TGF-α is also potently mitogenic for human [91–92] and murine [16] keratinocytes. However, TGF-α was slightly more potent than EGF in stimulating the growth and migration of normal human skin keratinocytes in the presence of a feeder cell layer [91].

Despite the evidence for a role for EGF/TGF-$\alpha$ in the growth of keratinocytes at clonal density, it has been the experience of our laboratory and others that the growth factor requirements for keratinocytes become obscure under conditions of higher density growth. Recently, careful analysis of this phenomenon [72] (reviewed above) revealed that the major requirement for exogenous EGF or TGF-$\alpha$ under serum-free conditions occurs at clonal cell density, at the time of cell plating. When tested after attachment in complete medium at higher cell densities [72], and in our hands, after colony establishment at clonal density [93], EGF and/or TGF-$\alpha$ are largely dispensable. This autocrine growth was shown to be due to the secretion of soluble keratinocyte growth factors, including AR [22], whose proliferative effects could be markedly inhibited by heparin [72]. In contrast, growth stimulation by TGF-$\alpha$ was poorly inhibited by heparin, suggesting that it was not the only autocrine growth factor in keratinocyte conditioned medium.

*Organ Cultures/Organotypic Culture Systems.* Kondo and coworkers have shown that EGF increases the rate of epidermal proliferation in organ cultures of rabbit skin, under conditions in which viability is preserved for as long as 12 weeks [94]. Similar proliferative effects of TGF-$\alpha$ have been reported by Fuchs and coworkers in raft cultures of human epidermal cells grown on collagen lattices [95], along with an increase in invasiveness (see Sec. III.B). The commercial availability of organotypic culture systems with well-defined epidermal differentiation characteristics [96] and the demonstration that human skin biopsy specimens can be successfully maintained in organ culture for prolonged periods [97] are developments likely to accelerate the pace of future research in this area.

### 2. *In Vivo Studies*

*Transgenic Mice.* Several recent studies of TGF-$\alpha$ overexpression in transgenic mice under the direction of metallothionein and murine mammary tumor virus promoters revealed marked alterations in breast, liver, and pancreatic tissues [98–100] and in sebaceous glands [101]; however, no effects on interfollicular epidermis were observed. In contrast, marked epidermal hyperplasia was observed when overexpression of TGF-$\alpha$ was targeted to the skin through the use of keratin promoters [102, 103]. Vassar and Fuchs [102] prepared rat TGF-$\alpha$ constructs driven by human keratin 14 promoter, which is normally expressed in basal epidermal cells. Roop and coworkers engineered expression of human TGF-$\alpha$ cDNA from the human keratin 1 promoter, normally expressed only in suprabasal epidermal cells [103]. Interestingly, both studies found that transgenic animals developed thickened, flaky skin, sparse hair, and reduced body weight in the neonatal period, despite the fact that overexpression of TGF-$\alpha$ would be expected in different subsets of epidermal cells as a function of the promoter used. As the animals aged, however, scaliness and epidermal thickness were reduced and hair density was increased, leaving residual epidermal hyperplasia only in regions normally relatively devoid of hair. Similar results were reported by Cohen and coworkers, who found that adult mouse skin was unresponsive to subcutaneously administered EGF [3]. Paralleling this reduction in hyperplasia, a redistribution of EGF receptors from a suprabasilar plus basilar to an exclusively basilar location was observed as the animals aged [102], as observed previously for normal mice [104]. This reduction in EGF receptors is likely to account for the reduction in epidermal hyperplasia in postnatal transgenic mice. These important experiments demonstrated that overexpression of TGF-α can lead to epidermal hyperplasia when expressed in the skin. However, TGF-α overexpression alone appears to be insufficient to explain the phenotype of hyperproliferative skin diseases such as psoriasis (see below).

*Psoriasis.* There is general agreement that TGF-α is overexpressed in the involved skin of psoriatic lesions [17, 18]. However, to date, demonstration that TGF-α is the proximate cause of psoriatic epidermal hyperplasia has proven elusive. The transgenic mouse studies discussed above revealed no evidence of inflammation in the more generalized hyperplastic skin lesions characteristic of younger animals [102, 103]. In older animals, hyperplasia developed only at sites characterized by persistent overexpression of TGF-α and intercurrent epidermal injury and/or infection. In these areas, patchy leukocytic infiltration and loss of the epidermal granular layer were observed, reminiscent of psoriatic lesions [102]. Consistent with these observations, cyclosporin A (CsA), an immunosuppressant that is highly effective in psoriasis [105] and is relatively specific for helper T cells, has little or no effect on keratinocyte responses to cytokine stimuli [106, 107]. Taken together, these results strongly suggest that one or more immune system–derived stimuli, in addition to overexpression of EGF-like growth factors by keratinocytes, is required for the development of psoriatic lesions.

Unambiguous assignment of a causal link between TGF-α overexpression and epidermal hyperplasia is further complicated by the fact that AR is also markedly overexpressed in psoriasis and highly expressed by rapidly growing keratinocytes in vitro [22, 23, 76]. Moreover, Turbitt et al. [69] and Finzi et al. [70] have demonstrated marked expression of TGF-α mRNA and protein in the suprabasal layers of psoriatic epidermis, at sites in which mitotic activity is reduced or absent. Despite these caveats, the pronounced biological effects of EGF and TGF-α on keratinocytes in vivo and in vitro strongly suggest that overexpression of one or more EGF-like growth factors will prove highly relevant to the pathophysiology of psoriatic epidermal hyperplasia.

*Appendageal Structures.* In addition to the marked suprabasal overexpression of TGF-$\alpha$ in psoriatic lesions, Finzi et al. observed marked expression of TGF-$\alpha$ in normal skin in several differentiated appendageal structures, including the outer root sheath of the hair follicle, sebaceous glands, and apocrine glands [70]. Curiously, however, no TGF-$\alpha$ expression was seen in the rapidly proliferating hair bulb [70]. Taken together with the prior identification of the EGF receptor in these differentiated, largely postmitotic appendageal structures [108] and in postmitotic suprabasal keratinocytes of psoriatic lesions [109], these results support the concept arising from Cohen's original observations [3] that TGF-$\alpha$/EGF receptor interactions may play an important role in directing epidermal differentiation, as well as proliferation [70, 71]. In this regard, it has been noted that precocious induction of epidermal differentiation markers is a characteristic feature of psoriatic lesions [110].

*Wound Healing.* EGF and/or TGF-$\alpha$ have both been shown to significantly accelerate the healing of cutaneous wounds in several species [111, 112], including humans [113]. However, reepithelialization of wounds is a complex process that involves early epidermal cell spreading of nonproliferative keratinocytes, generally considered to be an accelerated differentiation response [114]. Moreover, TGF-$\alpha$ is potently angiogenic in the hamster cheek pouch model [115] and has been shown to increase the number of dermal fibroblasts and granulation tissue [111]. Therefore, it is not simple to associate the beneficial effects of EGF/TGF-$\alpha$ in wound healing with direct effects on epidermal proliferation alone. In general, these studies have found rather limited, albeit highly significant improvements over placebo controls; this is likely to be due to the fact that EGF-like [116] and multiple other growth factors are present normally in the milleu of the healing wound. Multiple cellular sources of TGF-$\alpha$ have been identified in the healing wound environment [108], including activated macrophages, mast cells, and eosinophils [117] in addition to keratinocytes. Although these studies suggest that native exogenous growth factors may have rather limited practical value in wound healing, they do underscore the importance of EGF-like factors as normal mediators of epidermal proliferation, and suggest avenues for development of genetically engineered wound healing factors with improved selectivity, potency, and/or stability in the wound environment.

## B. Transformation/Neoplastic Growth

### 1. *Autocrine Transformation*

The concept that inappropriate autocrine production of growth factors may be an important mechanism in tumorigenesis is not a new one, having been proposed by Temin in 1966 [118]. A comprehensive review of this subject has been published recently [119]. Here, we will focus on the role of autocrine overexpression of TGF-$\alpha$ in the development of the malignant phenotype.

There are numerous studies documenting the overexpression of TGF-$\alpha$ by transformed epithelial cells of epidermal as well as nonepidermal origin [120–123]. However, as in psoriasis, a direct cause-and-effect relationship between TGF-$\alpha$ overexpression and transformation has been difficult to establish. Although transfection of constructs encoding mature rat and human TGF-$\alpha$ resulted in transformation of certain rat [124, 125] and human [126] cell types, high-level expression of TGF-$\alpha$ in mouse NIH 3T3 cells [127] or normal human keratinocytes or fibroblasts [128] did not. To address this issue in the context of the cutaneous environment, Finzi et al. engineered massive overexpression of biologically active secreted TGF-$\alpha$ in nontransformed BALB/MK mouse keratinocytes or papilloma-derived SP-1 cells, followed by grafting back onto isogenic recipients [129]. Although TGF-$\alpha$ is potently mitogenic for these cells in culture [16], autocrine overexpression of TGF-$\alpha$ in BALB/MK cells did not result in epidermal hyperplasia of either the transfected cells or the surrounding normal skin. In contrast, overexpression of TGF-$\alpha$ in SP-1 papilloma cells resulted in marked enhancement in papilloma size after grafting, as did mixing of of normal cells overexpressing TGF-$\alpha$ with nontransfected SP-1 cells [129]. These results indicate that overexpression of TGF-$\alpha$ is insufficient for the development of epidermal hyperplasia or malignant transformation of normal keratinocytes in vivo, but do imply that papilloma cells, which are thought to be intermediates in the pathway to complete neoplastic transformation, are abnormally responsive to the proliferative effects of TGF-$\alpha$ in vivo.

It seems likely that the variable results reported by different laboratories regarding the neoplastic consequences of TGF-$\alpha$ overexpression will ultimately be reconciled by elucidation of differences in the number of EGF receptors and/or the postreceptor signal transduction mechanisms employed by the target cells. For example, neoplastic transformation of NIH 3T3 cells takes place following concomitant overexpression of TGF-$\alpha$ and the EGF receptor, but not after overexpression of either one alone [130]. As another example, co-transfection of v-ras and v-fos is sufficient for malignant transformation of primary mouse keratinocytes, whereas transfection of v-Ha-ras alone is insufficient [131, 132]. Finally, differences in the in vivo host environment may be important, as skin wounding has long been known to increase papilloma frequency in tumor promotion models [133], and tumor incidence can be reduced by co-inoculation of nontransformed cells [134].

### 2. *Motility/Invasiveness*

Irrespective of the molecular mechanisms involved, there is evidence that interfering with autocrine stimulation of the EGF receptor can inhibit tumor growth in vivo. Thus, treatment with monoclonal anti-TGF-α antibodies resulted in significant reduction of ovarian carcinoma growth in vivo [120]. Therefore, further examination of the EGF receptor-dependent molecular mechanisms of tumor invasion and metastasis is clearly warranted. Recently, Fuchs and coworkers have shown that TGF-α treatment of human epidermal keratinocyte raft cultures grown on a dermal equivalent composed of collagen and fibroblasts leads not only to a marked increase in keratinocyte proliferation, but also to invasion of the collagen matrix by basaloid epidermal cells, preceded by induction of type I collagenase and gelatinase [95]. However, these changes were transient, suggesting that additional alterations in ligand responsiveness underlie the malignant phenotype in EGF-responsive tumors.

Aggressive squamous cell carcinomas frequently assume a spindled phenotype [135] and are known to frequently overexpress TGF-α [17]. Thus, it is of interest that rat NBT-II bladder carcinoma cells can be induced to display a spindled phenotype characterized by enhanced migration in vitro after transfection with TGF-α [136]. In addition, transgenic keratinocytes overexpressing TGF-α assumed an elongated, apparently hypermotile phenotype [102]. Although these effects may not be specific to TGF-α and/or other EGF receptor ligands, and have yet to be correlated with tumorigenicity in vivo, they do reinforce the concept that TGF-α overexpression can contribute to the tumorigenic phenotype in the appropriate cellular background.

## IV. REGULATION OF TGF-α AND AR GENE EXPRESSION IN KERATINOCYTES

Under appropriate conditions, treatment of murine and human keratinocytes with either EGF or TGF-α induces the expression of TGF-α (but not EGF) mRNA and protein [15, 71]. This phenomenon has been called autoinduction [15] and is a property observed for several other peptide growth factors [11]. Because TGF-α is mitogenic for keratinocytes and has been suggested as an important autocrine mitogen in the skin (see above), it is worthwhile to focus on the mechanisms by which expression of TGF-α may be regulated in keratinocytes. Therefore, after describing TGF-α autoinduction in human keratinocytes, we will summarize what is known of the structure and regulation of the TGF-α and AR promoters and consider the role of mRNA stabilization in regulation of AR and TGF-α mRNA levels in these cells.

### A. Autoinduction of TGF-α

Since the manifestations of psoriasis are largely confined to the skin, it is attractive to hypothesize that autocrine overproduction of TGF-α by keratinocytes could be an important pathogenetic mechanism in psoriasis. Unfortunately, no perfect experimental system exists for replicating the environment experienced by epidermal keratinocytes in vivo. Most studies of TGF-α autoregulation in keratinocytes have made use of low-calcium, serum-free MCDB153 medium modified for high-density keratinocyte growth [88–90]. Under these conditions, keratinocytes grow as a monolayer with a basaloid phenotype, do not stratify effectively, and undergo density-dependent irreversible arrest of growth [90]. However, because keratinocytes are capable of vigorous autocrine growth under appropriate conditions, and because at least two of these autocrine growth factors (TGF-α and AR) are known to activate the EGF receptor, it is very important to define conditions under which autocrine stimulation of the EGF receptor is minimized. Empirically, it has been determined that depletion of all growth factors for 48 hours, beginning when the cells are 40–50% confluent, minimizes endogenous TGF-α production and renders the cells maximally sensitive to addition of exogenous EGF or TGF-α [15, 71, 92]. Under these conditions, addition of EGF or TGF-α (2–200 ng/ml) induces a four- to sixfold increase in TGF-α mRNA, which is maximal within 4 to 6 hours, followed by a corresponding increase in secreted TGF-α protein [15, 71, 92]. This effect is clearly mediated through the EGF receptor (see Sec. V.E), as induction is not observed with polypeptide growth factors other than EGF or TGF-α, can be blocked by anti-EGF receptor monoclonal antibodies, and is inhibited by the tyrphostin RG50864, a specific inhibitor of EGF receptor tyrosine kinase [71]. Although TGF-α can also be induced by phorbol esters in keratinocytes [92], evidence reviewed in Section V.E suggests that PKC is not a downstream mediator of the autoinductive process.

## B. Transcriptional Regulation

The 5′ regulatory regions of the human [137, 138] and rat [139] TGF-α genes have been cloned and sequenced and subjected to limited functional analysis by means of reporter gene and in vitro transcription assays. Apparently the two promoters differ in that transcription is initiated from two major and a number of minor sites in the rat [139], but only from a single site in humans [137]. The two promoters display a high degree of homology, and highly GC-rich regions (70–76%) are present in both promoters within 600 bp upstream of the transcription start site(s). The GC-rich regions both direct transcription of the chloramphenicol acetyltransferase (CAT) gene in reporter assays, albeit rather weakly relative to the control, pSV2-CAT [137–139]. Interestingly, longer fragments (600–1900 bp) of the promoter display much weaker promoter activity, suggesting the presence of inhibitory sites in the distal upstream regions. Several consensus SP1 sites and TCCC elements are found in the proximal 600 bp region, but both promoters lack canonical

CCAAT or TATAA sequences. These features are characteristic of several other "TATAA-less" promoters, including the EGF receptor, $\alpha_2$1 collagen, and immunoglobulin $V_H$ genes [137]. However, the exact nature of the trans-acting factors which confer EGF responsiveness upon the TGF-$\alpha$ promoter have not been determined. Merchant et al. have identified a GC-rich EGF-response element, GGGGCGGGGTGGGGGG, in the regulatory region of the gastrin gene [140]. This element interacts specifically with a novel DNA binding protein distinct from other transcription factors, such as Sp1, which are known to bind GC-rich regions. Whether this or related factors proves to be relevant to transcriptional regulation of TGF-$\alpha$ in keratinocytes remains to be determined.

TGF-$\alpha$ expression in keratinocytes can also be regulated by members of the steroid receptor superfamily of ligand-dependent enhancer factors [138, 141]. Thus, retinoic acid (RA) increases TGF-$\alpha$ mRNA levels approximately three- to fourfold [141], and hydrocortisone inhibited the induction of TGF-$\alpha$ mRNA by exogenous IL-1$\alpha$ by approximately 50% [142]. Interestingly, the TGF-$\alpha$ promoter displays a region (around −400 bp) with high homology (20/26 nucleotides) to the core element which controls hormonal responsiveness of the EGF receptor gene [138]. However, the exact mechanisms by which steroid receptor–like transcription factors regulate TGF-$\alpha$ expression and the role of such regulation in epidermal physiology remain to be determined.

The promoter region of the human AR gene has been sequenced and subjected to limited functional analysis by Plowman et al. [21]. Similar to the TGF-$\alpha$ promoter, a GC-rich region of about 150 bp is located upstream of the transcription start site, and no consensus CCAAT box is present. Unlike TGF-$\alpha$, however, the AR promoter contains a consensus TATA sequence 28 bp upstream of the major RNA start site. Despite the fact that both TGF-$\alpha$ and AR genes are inducible by tetradecanoyl phorbol acetate (TPA) in epithelial cells [21, 92], no consensus TPA-response element [TGA(G/C)TCA] is found in the cognate promoters. This suggests that the mechanism of stimulation of transcription of AR and TGF-$\alpha$ by TPA may be indirect. Consistent with this concept, the early induction of TGF-$\alpha$ by phorbol ester occurs at the transcriptional level in transformed rat liver epithelial cells [143]. However, early accumulation of TGF-$\alpha$ mRNA after phorbol ester treatment was blocked by cycloheximide, suggesting a requirement for synthesis of one or more regulatory protein(s).

Direct analysis of transcription rates by nuclear runoff assays has proven difficult in normal human keratinocytes, and more work is needed to define experimental conditions suitable for this type of analysis in this cell type. Recently, Coffey and coworkers were unable to detect transcriptional regulation of the TGF-$\alpha$ gene by TGF-$\alpha$ in normal human keratinocytes [144].

However, as reviewed below, there are already indications that transcriptional regulation is not the only mechanism active in dictating TGF-$\alpha$ or AR mRNA levels in keratinocytes.

### C. Control of mRNA Stability

Until very recently, there have been no published reports on the effect of TGF-$\alpha$ or EGF treatment on the stability of TGF-$\alpha$ mRNA in keratinocytes. However, our laboratory (unpublished observations) and Coffey et al. [144] have found that treatment of growth factor–depleted normal human keratinocytes with EGF or TGF-$\alpha$ increases the half-life of TGF-$\alpha$ measured after actinomycin D treatment. Even more dramatic results were seen when the effects of EGF/TGF-$\alpha$ on AR mRNA were studied [76]. TGF-$\alpha$ treatment increased the measured half-life of AR mRNA from about 2 hours to over 6 hours. These results may reflect a more general effect of EGF receptor activation on mRNA stability, as EGF treatment has been shown to increase the stability of EGF receptor, $\beta$-tubulin and $\beta$-actin mRNAs in KB epidermoid carcinoma cells [145]. Similarly, EGF and TGF-$\alpha$ have been shown to increase the stability, but not the transcription rate, of IL-1$\alpha$, IL-1$\beta$, and IL-6 mRNAs in thymic epithelial cells in vitro [146]. In our studies and those of Jinno et al. [76, 145 and J.T.E., unpublished data], TPA treatment did not increase the stability of TGF-$\alpha$, AR, or EGF receptor mRNAs. Moreover, TGF-$\beta$ did not alter the half-life of TGF-$\alpha$ mRNA in bovine anterior pituitary cells [147]. Although the exact mechanism(s) responsible for mRNA stabilization require further elucidation, there are indications that the presence of AUUUA and related sequence motifs in the 3′ untranslated region may serve either to up- or downregulate the stability of various mRNAs [148]. Interestingly, several AUUUA motifs are present in the 3′ untranslated regions of human AR mRNA [21]. The recent discovery of a protein capable of specific binding to the AUUUA determinant [149] may help to elucidate the mechanism of mRNA stabilization. Taken together, these results suggest that mRNA stabilization may be the predominant mechanism by which EGF/TGF-$\alpha$ treatment influences steady-state transcript levels in keratinocytes.

## V. EGF RECEPTOR

The discovery that EGF receptors could be solubilized without loss of EGF-stimulated kinase activity [150] allowed its biochemical purification [5] and development of specific antibodies [7]. The discovery of strong similarities to the v-erbB oncogene led to the eventual cloning of EGF receptor cDNA and deduction of its complete amino acid sequence [151]. The availability of specific antibodies and ligand binding assays allowed demonstration of EGF receptors in the skin (reviewed in Ref. 150). As one of the first growth factor receptors subjected to purification and biochemical characterization, an extensive and complex literature has developed regarding the structure and function of the EGF receptor. Although a complete review of this literature is beyond the scope of this chapter, the interested reader is referred to several recent, cogent, and comprehensive reviews [54, 60, 150, 152, 153]. Here, we will review the basics of EGF receptor structure and function, briefly discuss emerging concepts in EGF receptor signal transduction, and consider what is known of EGF receptor function in normal epidermal keratinocytes.

## A. EGF Receptor Structure

The mature human EGF receptor is composed of a single polypeptide chain of Mr 170,000 da made up of 1186 amino acids and about 40,000 da of carbohydrate in the form of 10–11 N-linked oligosaccharide chains [54]. The extracellular, ligand-binding domain contains two clusters of cysteine residues flanking the putative ligand-binding domain. The extracellular domain is connected via a single hydrophobic membrane anchor to the cytoplasmic domain containing the tyrosine kinase activity (see below). The C terminus contains a cluster of tyrosine residues, which may be involved in interactions with other cellular components and/or in autoregulation of tyrosine kinase activity. The EGF receptor gene is also known as c-erbB, due to its extensive similarity to the v-erb gene of avian erythroblastosis virus. Several different v-erbB oncogenes have been isolated and studied in avian systems, and the truncation of the extracellular domain appears to be the common feature essential for oncogenicity (reviewed in Ref. 152).

## B. EGF Receptor Gene Family

The EGF receptor gene family in man is composed of at least three members: the canonical EGF receptor (c-erbB), c-erbB2/HER-2/ERBB2 [155, 156] (in the rat, also known as *neu*) [157], and the recently described ERBB3, also known as HER3 [158, 159]. All three forms are expressed in human skin and/or cultured keratinocytes [159, 160]. EGF and TGF-$\alpha$ do not bind efficiently to c-erbB2 [161], and until recently, no ligands for these receptors had been described. Recently, however, two potential ERBB2 ligands have been isolated: a 30 kd glycoprotein, which binds to both the EGF receptor and ERBB2, and a 75 kd protein, which binds specifically to ERBB2 [162]. EGF receptors are extensively conserved in evolution, as are most other protooncogenes. Thus, the chicken receptor is about 75% identical, and the *Drosophila* receptor about 50% identical to the human EGF receptor [152]. However, the extent to which the three related forms of the receptor are conserved in evolution remains to be worked out. These receptors are more distantly related to other membrane-spanning, ligand-binding tyrosine kinases, including the insulin and PDGF receptors. The general phylogeny of the eukaryotic protein kinases has been elegantly reviewed [163].

## C. EGF Receptor Expression

EGF receptors are expressed on most human cell types, with the possible exception of mature hematopoietic cells, at a level of 20,000–200,000 receptors/cell [152]. In nontransformed cells, EGF receptor expression generally appears to be regulated within rather narrow intervals. In normal and transformed human keratinocytes, EGF receptor expression is regulated at the levels of transcription, mRNA stability, translation, and posttranslational modification [164]. However, in certain tumor cell lines such as A431 epidermoid carcinoma, EGF receptor mRNA and protein levels are markedly increased as a result of amplification of the EGF receptor gene [165], resulting in approximately $10^6$ receptors per cell. Although EGF receptor expression can be modulated by EGF/TGF-α itself [145, 166], other cytokines and growth factors such as interferon-γ and TGF-β [167], and members of the steroid receptor superfamily including retinoic acid [166] and thyroid hormone [168] are also effective in this regard. EGF receptor gene regulation is obviously a complex process, as evidenced by the variability of cytokine and growth factor effects depending on cell type [167, 169], and even on the position in the cell cycle [170]. Some insights into this process are emerging with the detailed analysis of the EGF receptor promoter region [171, 172]. This promoter belongs to the class of "TATA-less" promoters with high G+C content, characteristic of several "housekeeping" genes, and contains binding sites for at least eight transcription factors in A431 cells, three of which have been characterized. To date, however, little work has been reported on the regulation of EGF receptor transcription in normal keratinocytes.

## D. EGF Receptor Signal Transduction

### *1. Ligand Binding/Receptor Dimerization*

As mentioned earlier, TGF-α is somewhat more potent than EGF in stimulating certain biological responses [11, 58]. While many explanations are possible (see below), one is that subtle differences in EGF receptor binding exist. Thus, monoclonal antibodies that block binding of TGF-α to the EGF receptor but have no effect of the affinity of EGF have been described [173]. However, to date there is no evidence for more than one binding site per receptor molecule. Ligand binding triggers a process of dimerization and perhaps oligomerization of receptors, as has been shown by chemical cross-linking experiments [174]. This dimerization is accompanied by intermolecular tyrosine phosphorylation, as demonstrated by a combination of biochemical and molecular biological approaches [175].

### 2. *Tyrosine Phosphorylation*

Elegant experiments involving mutagenesis of the acceptor site for ATP at Lys 721 of the EGF receptor molecule clearly demonstrated that the tyrosine kinase activity of the receptor is required for all known effects of EGF [176, 177]. Tyrosine autophosphorylation is a very early event after ligand binding and receptor dimerization; however, the precise requirements for tyrosine kinase activation are not known. Five sites of tyrosine autophosphorylation are known, and four of these cluster near the C-terminus of the receptor [152, 178]. In addition, several serine and threonine residues of the intracellular domain are targets for phosphorylation by other cellular kinases, some of which display autoregulatory activity (see below). The EGF receptor tyrosine kinase is certainly capable of ligand-dependent tyrosine phosphorylation of other substrates, such as angiotensin [176] and lipocortin I [179, 180] in broken cell systems. However, the physiological substrates for EGF-stimulated tyrosine phosphorylation other than the receptor itself appear to be limited, at least in normal human keratinocytes [71]. EGF-dependent phosphorylation of lipocortin has been observed in intact A431 cells [181]; however, this has been suggested to occur within endosomes and not at the cell surface.

### 3. *Postreceptor Signal Transduction Mechanisms*

The molecular events that direct cellular responses after activation of the EGF receptor tyrosine kinase continue to be the target of intense experimental scrutiny, from which few hard-and-fast conclusions have emerged (for reviews, see Refs. 153, 182). Several downstream signal transduction pathways have been proposed, including activation of phospholipases A2 [183] and multiple forms of phospholipase C [184, 185], adenylate cyclase [186], phosphoinositol (PI) kinases [187], the proto-oncogene *ras* [188], and microtubule-associated protein (MAP) kinase [189]. Particular attention has been focused on phosphoinositol-bisphosphate ($PIP_2$)-specific phospholipase C, because its activation has been proposed to trigger two important intracellular processes (Fig. 4): (a) an increase in intracellular calcium as a result of release from intracellular stores in response to $IP_3$, and (b) activation of protein kinase C in response to DAG. In A431 cells, there is solid experimental evidence that one isoform of PLC, PLC-$\gamma$, can be phosphorylated on tyrosine by the EGF receptor, resulting in increased $IP_3$ production [190]. However, it is not clear whether this represents an increase in intrinsic enzymatic activity or a shift in subcellular localization of the enzyme to a membranous environment [191]. (In this regard, there are several reports of

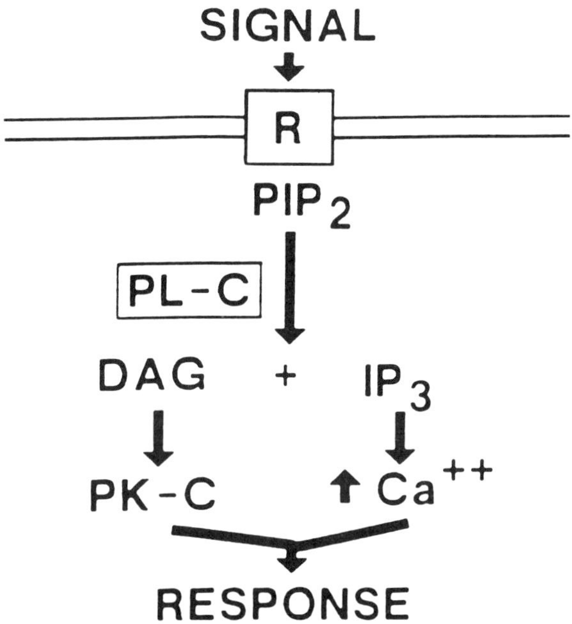


**Fig. 4** Model for signal transduction coupling of phospholipase-C and protein kinase C. Activation of $PIP_2$-specific phospholipase C by ligand binding to cell surface receptors results in formation of 1,2-diacylglycerol (DAG) and inositol 1,4,5-tris-phosphate ($IP_3$), which in turn leads to activation of protein kinase C (PK-C) and release of $Ca^{2+}$ from intracellular stores. (Adapted from Ref. 182.)

specific stimulation of EGF receptor tyrosine kinase activity by membrane glycolipids, including ceramides [192], sphingolipids [193], and gangliosides [194].) It has been even more difficult to demonstrate activation of PKC in response to PI-derived DAG (reviewed in Ref. 71). In cell types in which EGF-stimulated DAG is detectable, the DAG appears to be derived from phosphatidyl choline (PC) via a PC-specific PLC [185]. Adding to the complexity of this situation is the fact that the various pathways outlined above appear to be active to different extents in different cell types. It is important to emphasize that none of these intracellular pathways are thought to be exclusively coupled to the EGF receptor. Moreover, there is substantial evidence for "cross-talk" and feedback inhibition between the various pathways, as reviewed recently [182].

One of the most useful recent discoveries in this area has been the identification of src homology (SH) domains (reviewed in Ref. 195). SH domains are regions approximately 100 amino acids long which appear to mediate the physical association of proteins in a manner that depends on tyrosine phosphorylation. Importantly, only the proximal molecule in the signal transduction pathway need undergo tyrosine phosphorylation, obviating a requirement for trans-phosphorylation on tyrosine in this process [196]. This suggests that altered patterns of association between different cellular components, rather than phosphorylation of specific target proteins, may be the key determinant of signal transduction. Consistent with this notion, SH2 domains have been identified in molecules of diverse biochemical function, including c-src and related intracellular tyrosine kinases, PLC-gamma, GAP (GTPase-activating protein), and the p85 subunit of PI-3-kinase [195]. Note that with the exception of the src-like tyrosine kinases, each of these proteins has been implicated in EGF receptor signal transduction. While many questions remain, the discovery of SH2 domains has provided a new conceptual framework for the understanding of signal transduction.

The ultimate target of signal transduction is the nucleus, the site of new transcription and DNA replication. For several years, a small but persistent community of researchers has been pursuing the concept that polypeptide growth factors and/or their receptors may undergo direct trafficking to the nucleus, where they might interact directly with target genes [197, 198]. While this mechanism must still be considered as speculative, the recent localization of AR sequences to the nucleus of ovarian epithelial cells [199] suggests that nuclear binding should be given serious consideration as a component of the EGF receptor signal transduction mechanism.

#### 4. Attenuation of Receptor Activity

As discussed earlier (Sec. III.B), overexpression of otherwise normal EGF receptors can result in transformation; therefore, mechanisms are required to limit signal transduction through the receptor when appropriate. Three major mechanisms of attenuation have thus far been identified: (a) inhibition of the EGF receptor tyrosine kinase activity, (b) receptor internalization, and (c) protein tyrosine phosphatase activity. Although somewhat controversial, it is interesting that reduction in ligand affinity has not been identified as a major mechanism of attenutation [200]. The major mechanism of attenuation of the receptor kinase activity involves phosphorylation of $Ser^{654}$ by protein kinase C [200]. Another regulatory site is $Thr^{669}$, which is phosphorylated by two cellular kinases, MAP kinase and a 46 kd protein called ERT (EGF receptor threonine) kinase [201]. In contrast to $Ser^{654}$, phosphorylation of $Thr^{669}$ leads to a reduction in receptor affinity as well as impaired receptor interalization [202].

Receptor internalization is a multistep process triggered by ligand binding and which depends upon receptor tyrosine kinase activity [203]. Within minutes after ligand binding, receptors become bound to coated pits, followed by trafficking to the multivesicular body (MVB) [204]. From the MVB, receptors are targeted either to the lysosomal compartment for degradation or recycled to the surface, a process that also requires the receptor tyrosine kinase activity [205]. Interestingly, EGF and TGF-α differ markedly in their ability to be internalized by the EGF receptor [58], offering another plausible explanation for the different biological potencies of EGF and TGF-α. Many epithelial tumors are characterized by surface overexpression of the EGF receptor in the absence of gene amplification or apparent overexpression of EGF receptor mRNA [206]. It is possible that defects in the internalization mechanism may underlie these abnormalities. Thus, internalization-defective mutants of the EGF receptor confer hypersensitivity to EGF and result in ligand-dependent transformation of NIH-3T3 cells [207].

Protein tyrosine phosphatases (PTPases) are ubiquitous and have been suggested to participate in a variety of cell regulatory processes, including T-cell activation [208]. PTPase activity has been identified in normal human [209] and mouse [210] skin, and PTPase activity is increased in psoriatic lesions [209]. To date, little is known about the molecular nature of epidermal PTPases, especially those which may reverse tyrosine phosphorylation by the EGF receptor; however, PTP-1B, a cytosolic PTPase, has recently been shown to be expressed in human epidermis and cultured keratinocytes [211].

## E. EGF Receptor System in Normal and Diseased Skin

### *1. Regulation of EGF Receptor Signal Transduction in Normal Keratinocytes*

Most studies of EGF receptor function in epithelial cells have involved transformed cell lines overexpressing EGF receptors, such as A431. We have suggested [18, 71] that defective negative regulation of the EGF receptor in psoriasis (see below) could create a "positive feedback loop" leading to overexpression of TGF-α and epidermal hyperplasia (Fig. 5). In pursuit of this hypothesis, we have investigated several aspects of EGF receptor signal transduction in normal human epidermal keratinocytes [71] as well as dermal fibroblasts [212] in vitro. EGF and TGF-α markedly stimulated tyrosine phosphorylation of the EGF receptor in both cell types, and the growth of keratinocytes could be blocked by anti-EGF receptor monoclonal antibodies. However, unlike A431 cells, no evidence for $IP_3$ hydrolysis in response to EGF or TGF-α was observed in either cell type. EGF and TGF-α stimulated DAG formation and phosphorylation of MARCKS protein (a specific cellular substrate for PKC) in fibroblasts, but not in keratinocytes. However, PC, and not PI, was the source of DAG formation. Inhibition of over 90% of cellular PKC activity with bryostatin failed to inhibit or potentiate the in-

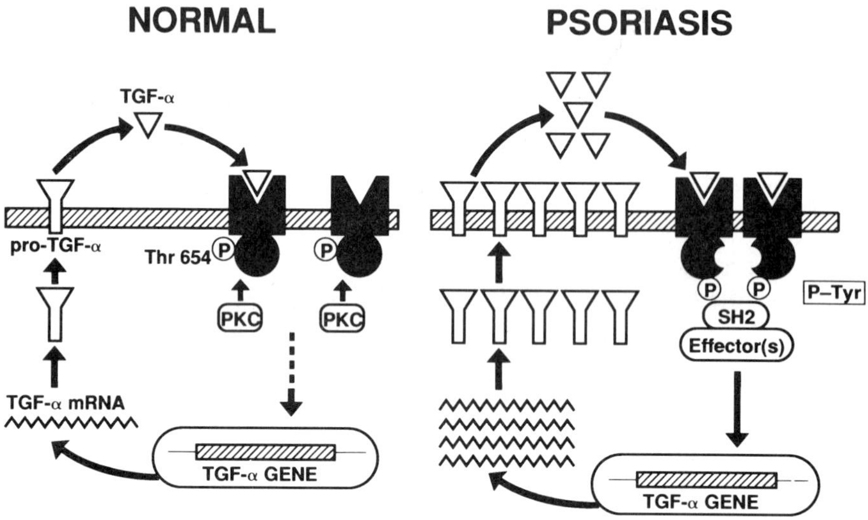


**Fig. 5** Model for regulation of TGF-$\alpha$ autoinduction by protein kinase C in psoriasis. Phosphorylation of [654]Thr of the EGF receptor (solid black) by protein kinase C results in inhibition of receptor tyrosine kinase activity. Reduced levels of protein kinase C in psoriatic lesions [182] allows derepression of the tyrosine kinase activity, and trans-phosphorylation of EGF receptor dimers results. One or more effector molecules bearing SH2 domains (e.g., phospholipase C, ras, src, etc.) then become associated with the receptor, leading to signal transduction and increased expression of the TGF-$\alpha$ gene. Increased translation, cell surface expression, and cleavage of TGF-$\alpha$ results in increased EGF receptor binding and activation and formation of a positive feedback loop.

duction of TGF-$\alpha$ mRNA by EGF or TGF-$\alpha$, a downstream event that was shown to depend specifically upon EGF receptor tyrosine kinase activation. Taken together with the DAG and MARCKS phosphorylation data, these results strongly suggest that PKC activation is not a major downstream mediator of EGF action in keratinocytes. Moreover, the lack of potentiation of TGF-$\alpha$ after inhibition of PKC activity indicates that protein kinase C does not act in a tonic fashion to downregulate EGF receptor tyrosine kinase activity in these cells. These results argue against the hypothesis (Fig. 5) that altered regulation of TGF-$\alpha$ autoinduction by PKC might be an important determinant of psoriatic epidermal hyperplasia. However, they do demonstrate the importance of the EGF receptor in the growth control of normal, nontransformed cells, reveal interesting cell-type–specific differences in postreceptor mechanisms, and suggest that alterations in these mechanisms may be concomitants of malignant conversion.

### 2. *EGF Receptors in Skin Disease*

The experimental evidence for the roles of EGF receptor number and autocrine production of EGF-like growth factors in neoplastic transformation was discussed in Section III.B. However, systematic studies of EGF receptor/ligand expression in actual human skin tumors have been rather limited. To date, one biochemical and four immunohistochemical studies of EGF receptor expression in various epidermal tumors have appeared (reviewed in Ref. 213). Although not all studies are in agreement [214, 215], several groups found reduced EGF receptor expression in basal cell carcinoma relative to normal skin, and prominent but patchy expression in squamous cell carcinomas. Recently, our laboratory has compared EGF receptor mRNA levels in normal skin, basal cell, and squamous cell carcinoma (G. Majmudar, T. Johnson, and J. T. Elder, unpublished data). EGF receptor mRNA levels were normal in 10 of 10 nonmetastatic SCC and 11 of 11 BCC; however, marked overexpression was observed in one of two metastatic SCC of primary cutaneous origin. Groves et al. [213] observed cytoplasmic redstribution of EGF receptors at the invasive margins of SCCs. It is possible, therefore, that factors affecting the intracellular trafficking of EGF receptors, rather than overexpression at the gene level, is characteristic of most primary cutaneous SCCs, with gene amplification occurring in the course of progression of highly malignant, metastatic tumors. This interpretation would be consistent with the observation that the E5 gene product of the oncogenic human papillomavirus HPV 16, like its bovine homolog, can interfere with normal cellular trafficking of EGF receptors [216, 217]. Curiously, however, EGF receptors were undetectable in common viral verrucae [218].

The expression of EGF receptors in normal and psoriatic skin has been extensively characterized at the levels of ligand binding and immunoreactivity by King and coworkers [108, 109], and at the level of mRNA by our laboratory [219] and others [220]. Although there is a persistence of EGF receptor in the upper suprabasal cell layers in psoriasis, no increased expression of the EGF receptor gene was observed. These observations again support an important role for altered intracellular trafficking, rather than overexpression, of EGF receptors in psoriasis.

## VI. CONCLUSIONS

We have attempted here to summarize a very large body of information regarding the EGF family of growth factors and their cognate receptor. Any such summary is of necessity incomplete, and it has not been possible to comprehensively cite all of the important work done in this field. To summarize, all available data strongly point to the importance of autocrine production of multiple EGF-like growth factors in the cutaneous environment and to the importance of the regulation the expression and function of their receptors at multiple levels (e.g., gene expression, tyrosine kinase activity, and intracellular trafficking) in cutaneous homeostasis. Despite the apparent complexity of this system, it is very clear that continued definition of the molecules that regulate the expression and function of the EGF-like growth factors and their receptors in the skin will dramatically expand our understanding of the regulation of epidermal growth and differentiation.

## REFERENCES


1. S. Cohen, *Proc. Natl. Acad. USA 46*, 30 (1960).
2. S. Cohen, *J. Biol. Chem. 237*, 1555 (1962).
3. S. Cohen and G. A. Elliott, *J. Invest. Dermatol. 40*, 1 (1963).
4. H. Gregory, *Nature 257*, 325 (1975).
5. G. Carpenter and S. Cohen, *Ann. Rev. Biochem. 48*, 193 (1979).
6. J. E. DeLarco and G. J. Todaro, *Proc. Natl. Acad. USA 75*, 4001 (1978).
7. G. C. Carpenter, C. M. Stoscheck, Y. A. Preston, and J. E. DeLarco, *Proc. Natl. Acad. USA 800*, 5627 (1983).
8. A. B. Roberts, C. A. Frolik, M. A. Anzano, and M. B. Sporn, *Fed. Proc. 42*, 2621 (1983).
9. J. Massaque, *J. Biol. Chem. 258*, 13614 (1983).
10. H. Marquardt, M. W. Hunkapiller, L. E. Hood, D. R. Twardzik, J. E. DeLarco, J. R. Stephenson, and G. J. Todaro, *Proc. Natl. Acad. Sci. USA 80*, 4684 (1983).
11. R. Derynck, *Cell 54*, 593 (1988).
12. D. S. Salomon, N. Kim, T. Saeki, and F. Ciardiello, *Cancer Cells 2*, 389 (1990).
13. J. T. Elder, in *Encyclopedia of Human Biology* (R. Dulbecco, ed.), Vol. 3, Academic Press, La Jolla, CA, 1991, p. 445.
14. R. L. Byyny, D. N. Orth, and S. Cohen, *Endocrinology 90*, 1261 (1972).
15. R. J. Coffey, Jr., R. Derynck, J. N. Wilcox, T. S. Bringman, A. S. Groustin, H. L. Moses, and M. R. Pittelkow, *Nature* (London) 328, 817 (1987).
16. R. Coffey, N. Sipes, C. Bascom, R. Graves-Deal, C. Pennington, B. Weissman, and H. Moses, *Cancer Res. 48*, 1596 (1988).
17. A. Gottlieb, C. Chang, D. Posnett, B. Fanelli, and J. Tam, *J. Exp. Med. 167*, 670 (1988).
18. J. Elder, G. Fisher, P. Lindquist, G. Bennett, M. Pittelkow, E. Coffey, Jr., L. Ellingsworth, R. Derynck, and J. Voorhees, *Science 243*, 811 (1989).
19. J. Engel, *FEBS Lett. 251*, 1 (1989).
20. E. Appella, I. T. Webber, and F. Blasi, *FEBS Lett. 231*, 1 (1988).
21. G. D. Plowman, J. M. Green, V. L. McDonald, M. G. Neubauer, C. M. Disteche, G. J. Todaro, and M. Shoyab, *Mol. Cell. Biol. 10*, 1969 (1990).
22. P. W. Cook, P. A. Mattox, W. W. Keeble, M. R. Pittelkow, G. D. Plowman, M. Shoyab, J. P. Adelman, and G. D. Shipley, *Mol. Cell. Biol. 11*, 2547 (1991).
23. P. W. Cook, M. R. Pittelkow, W. W. Keeble, R. Graves-Deal, R. J. Coffey, Jr., and G. D. Shipley, *Cancer Res. 52*, 3224 (1992).
24. S. Higashiyama, J. A. Abraham, J. Miller, J. C. Fiddes, and M. Klagsbrun, *Science 251*, 936 (1990).

25. H. Kimura, W. H. Fischer, and D. Schubert, *Nature 348*, 257 (1990).
26. J. P. Brown, D. R. Twardzik, H. Marquardt, and G. J. Todaro, *Nature 313*, 491 (1985).
27. W. Chang, C. Upton, S. L. Hu, A. F. Purchio, and G. McFadden, *Mol. Cell. Biol. 7*, 535 (1987).
28. C. Upton, J. L. Macen, and G. McFadden, *J. Virol. 61*, 1271 (1987).
29. F. Ciardiello, R. Dono, N. Kim, M. G. Persico, and D. S. Salomon, *Cancer Res. 51*, 1051 (1991).
30. D. C. Kaslow, I. A. Quakyi, C. Syin, M. G. Raum, D. B. Keister, J. E. Coligan, T. F. McCutchan, and L. H. Miller, *Nature 333*, 74 (1988).
31. I. Rebay, R. J. Fleming, R. G. Fehon, L. Cherbas, P. Cherbas, and S. Artavanis-Tsakonas, *Cell 67*, 687 (1991).
32. J. M. Rothberg, J. R. Jacobs, C. S. Goodman, and A. Artavanis-Tsakonas, *Genes Devel. 4*, 2169 (1990).
33. R. J. Fleming, T. N. Scottgale, R. J. Diederich, and S. Artavanis-Tsakonas, *Genes Devel. 4*, 2188 (1990).
34. I. Greenwald, *Cell 43*, 583 (1985).
35. Q. Yang, L. M. Angerer, and R. C. Angerer, *Science 246*, 806 (1989).
36. C. T. Przysiecki, J. E. Staggers, H. G. Ramjit, D. G. Musson, A. M. Stern, C. D. Bennett, and P. A. Friedman, *Proc. Natl. Acad. Sci. USA 84*, 7856 (1987).
37. V. V. Novakhatny, K. C. Ingham, and L. V. Medved, *J. Biol. Chem. 266*, 12994 (1991).
38. P. A. Handford, M. Mayhew, M. Baron, P. R. Winship, I. D. Campbell, and G. G. Brownlee, *Nature 351*, 164 (1991).
39. J. Stenflo, A. Lundwall, and B. Dahlback, *Proc. Natl. Acad. Sci. USA 84*, 368 (1987).
40. A. K. Ohlin, G. Landes, P. Bourdon, C. Oppenheimer, R. Wydro, and J. Stenflo, *J. Biol. Chem. 263*, 19240 (1988).
41. M. Zushi, M. Gomi, S. Yamamoto, I. Maruyama, T. Hayashi, and K. Suzuki, *J. Biol. Chem. 264*, 10351 (1989).
42. T. Yamomoto, R. W. Bishop, M. S. Brown, J. L. Goldstein, and D. W. Russell, *Science 232*, 1230 (1986).
43. K. Mann, R. Deutzmann, M. Aumailley, R. Timpl, L. Raimondi, Y. Yamada, T. C. Pabn, D. Conway, and M. L. Chu, *Embo J. 8*, 65 (1989).
44. C. T. Baldwin, A. M. Reginato, and D. J. Prockop, *J. Biol. Chem. 264*, 15747 (1989).
45. N. M. Thielens, A. Van-Dorsselaer, J. Gagnon, and G. J. Arlaud, *Biochemistry 29*, 3570 (1990).
46. M. Shoyab, V. L. McDonald, K. Dick, B. Modrell, N. Malik, and G. D. Plowman, *Biochem. Biophys. Res. Comm. 179*, 572 (1991).
47. P. A. Handford, M. Mayhew, M. Baron, P. R. Winship, I. D. Campbell, and G. G. Brownlee, *Nature 351*, 164 (1991).
48. R. M. Cooke, A. J. Wilkinson, M. Baron, A. Pastore, M. J. Tappin, I. D. Campbell, H. Gregory, and B. Sheard, *Nature 327*, 339 (1987).
49. G. T. Montelione, J. Winthrich, E. C. Nice, A. W. Burgess, and H. A. Scheraga, *Proc. Natl. Acad. Sci. USA 84*, 5526 (1987).

50. G. T. Montelione, M. E. Winkler, L. E. Burton, E. Rinderknecht, M. B. Sporn, G. Wagner, *Proc. Natl. Acad. Sci. USA 86*, 1519 (1989).
51. M. J. Tappin, R. M. Cooke, J. E. Fitton, and I. D. Campbell, *Eur. J. Biochem. 179*, 629 (1989).
52. D. Kohda, I. Shimda, T. Miijake, T. Fuwa, and F. Inagaki, *Biochem. 28*, 953 (1989).
53. S. J. Prestrelski, T. Arakawa, C.-S. C. Wu, K. D. O'Neil, K. R. Westcott, and L. O. Narhi, *J. Biol. Chem. 267*, 319 (1992).
54. G. Carpenter and S. Cohen, *J. Biol. Chem. 265*, 7709 (1990).
55. J. M. Taylor, W. M. Mitchell, and S. Cohen, *J. Biol. Chem. 247*, 5928 (1972).
56. C. R. Savage, J. H. Hash, S. Cohen, *J. Biol. Chem. 260*, 5205 (1973).
57. L. Kornberg and R. L. Juliano, *Trends Pharm. Sci. 13*, 93 (1992).
58. R. Ebner and R. Derynck, *Cell Reg. 2*, 599 (1991).
59. M. E. Winkler, L. O'Connor, M. Winget, and B. Fendly, *Biochem. 28*, 6373 (1989).
60. L. E. King, C. M. Stoscheck, R. E. Gates, and L. B. Nanney, in *Physiology, Biochemistry, and Molecular Biology of the Skin* (L. A. Goldsmith, ed.), 2d ed., Oxford University Press, New York, 1991, p. 329.
61. R. A. Yates, L. B. Nanney, R. E. Gates, and L. E. King, Jr., *Int. J. Dermatol. 30*, 687 (1991).
62. C. A. Browne, *Bailliers Clin. Endocrin. Metabol. 5*, 553 (1991).
63. D. K. Madtes, E. W. Raines, K. S. Sakariassen, R. K. Assoian, M. B. Sporn, G. I. Bell, and R. Ross, *Cell 53*, 285 (1988).
64. D. A. Rappolee, D. Mark, M. J. Banda, Z. Werb, *Science 241*, 708 (1988).
65. O. Baadsgaard, A. K. Gupta, R. S. Taylor, C. N. Ellis, J. J. Voorhees, and K. D. Cooper, *J. Invest. Dermatol. 92*, 190 (1989).
66. H. Marquardt, M. W. Hunkapiller, and G. J. Todaro, *Nature* (London) *223*, 1079 (1984).
67. R. Derynck, A. B. Roberts, M. E. Winkler, E. Y. Chen, and D. V. Goedde, *Cell 38*, 287 (1984).
68. D. Murphy, B. Smoller, A. B. Gottlieb, A. Hsu, D. M. Carter, and J. G. Krueger, *J. Invest. Dermatol. 94*, 557 (1990).
69. M. L. Turbitt, R. J. Akhurst, S. I. White, and R. M. MacKie, *J. Invest. Dermatol. 95*, 229 (1990).
70. E. Finzi, R. Harkins, and T. Horn, *J. Invest. Dermatol. 96*, 328 (1991).
71. S. B. Klein, G. J. Fisher, T. C. Jensen, J. Mendelsohn, J. J. Voorhees, and J. T. Elder, *J. Cell. Physiol. 151*, 326 (1992).
72. P. W. Cook, M. R. Pittelkow, and G. D. Shipley, *J. Cell. Physiol. 146*, 277 (1991).
73. S. T. Wong, L. F. Mitchell, B. K. McCune, H. S. Earp, J. Texido, J. Massague, B. Herman, and D. C. Lee, *Cell 56*, 495 (1989).
74. M. Shoyab, V. L. McDonald, J. G. Bradley, and G. J. Todaro, *Proc. Natl. Acad. Sci. USA 85*, 6528 (1988).
75. M. Shoyab, G. D. Plowman, V. L. McDonald, J. G. Bradley, and G. J. Todaro, *Science 243*, 1074 (1989).
76. B. Hardas, Q. Yang, and J. T. Elder, *Clin. Res. 40*, 187A (1992).

77. F. Ciardiello, N. Kim, T. Saiki, R. Dono, M. G. Persico, G. D. Plowman, J. Garrigues, S. Radke, G. J. Todaro, and D. S. Salomon, *Proc. Natl. Acad. Sci. USA 88*, 7792 (1991).
78. A. Ciccodicola, R. Dono, S. Cinci, A. Simeone, M. Zollo, and M. G. Persico, *EMBO J. 8*, 1987 (1989).
79. M. C. Blomquist, L. T. Hunt, and W. C. Barker, *Proc. Natl. Acad. Sci. USA 81*, 7363 (1984).
80. D. A. Eppstein, Y. V. Marsh, A. B. Schreiber, S. R. Newman, G. J. Todaro, and J. J. Nestor, Jr., *Nature 318*, 663 (1985).
81. D. R. Twardzik, J. P. Brown, J. E. Ranchalis, G. J. Todaro, and B. Moss, *Proc. Natl. Acad. Sci. USA 82*, 5300 (1985).
82. D. S. Strayer and J. L. Leibowitz, *Am. J. Pathol. 128*, 203 (1987).
83. C. D. Porter and L. C. Archard, *J. Gen. Virol. 3*, 673 (1987).
84. R. M. Buller, S. Chakrabarti, J. A. Cooper, D. R. Twardzik, and B. Moss, *J. Virol. 62*, 866 (1988).
85. R. M. Buller, S. Chakrabarti, B. Moss, and T. Fredrickson, *Virology 164*, 182 (1988).
86. W. F. Lever and G. Schaumburg-Lever, in *Histopathology of the Skin*, J. B. Lippincott Co., Philadelphia, PA, 1988, p. 399.
87. J. R. Rheinwald and H. Green, *Nature 265*, 421 (1977).
88. M. C. Tsao, B. J. Walthall, and R. G. Ham, *J. Cell. Physiol. 110*, 219 (1982).
89. S. T. Boyce and R. G. Ham, in *In Vitro Models for Cancer Research* (M. M. Webber and L. I. Sekely, eds.), Vol. III, CRC Press, Boca Raton, FL, 1983, p. 245.
90. J. J. Wille, Jr., M. R. Pittelkow, and G. R. Shipley, *J. Cell. Physiol. 121*, 31 (1984).
91. Y. Barrandon and H. Green, *Cell 50*, 1131 (1987).
92. M. R. Pittelkow, P. B. Lingquist, R. T. Abraham, R. Graves-Deal, R. Derynck, and R. J. Coffey, Jr., *J. Biol. Chem. 264*, 5164 (1989).
93. J. T. Elder, S. B. Klein, and J. J. Voorhees, *J. Invest. Dermatol. 92*, 424A (1989).
94. S. Kondo, Y. Hozumi, and K. Aso, *J. Invest. Dermatol. 95*, 397 (1990).
95. K. Turksen, Y. Choi, and E. Fuchs, *Cell Reg. 2*, 613 (1991).
96. J. T. Elder, A. Astrom, U. Pettersson, A. Tavakkol, C. E. M. Griffiths, A. Krust, P. Kastner, P. Chambon, and J. J. Voorhees, *J. Invest. Dermatol. 98*, 673 (1992).
97. S. Kondo, Y. Hozumi, and K. Aso, *J. Invest. Dermatol. 98*, 753 (1992).
98. Y. Matsui, S. A. Halter, J. T. Holt, B. L. M. Hogan, and R. J. Coffey, Cell 61, 1147 (1990).
99. C. Jhappan, C. Stahle, R. N. Harkins, N. Fausto, G. H. Smith, and G. T. Merlino, *Cell 61*, 1137 (1990).
100. E. P. Sandgren, N. C. Luetteke, R. D. Palmiter, R. L. Brinster, and D. C. Lee, *Cell 61*, 1121 (1990).
101. S. A. Halter, P. Dempsey, Y. Matsui, M. K. Stokes, R. Graves-Deal, B. L. M. Hogan, and R. J. Coffey, *Am. J. Pathol. 140*, 1131 (1992).
102. R. Vassar and E. Fuchs, *Genes Devel. 5*, 714 (1991).

103. A. M. Dominey, D. Bundman, J. A. Rothnagel, and D. R. Roop, *J. Invest. Dermatol. 98*, 564A (1992).
104. M. R. Green, D. A. Basketter, J. R. Couchman, and D. A. Rees, *Dev. Biol. 100*, 506 (1983).
105. C. N. Ellis, D. C. Gorsulowsky, T. A. Hamilton, J. K. Billings, M. D. Brown, J. T. Headington, K. D. Cooper, O. Baadsgaard, E. A. Duell, T. M. Annesley, J. G. Turcotte, and J. J. Voorhees, *JAMA 256*, 3310 (1986).
106. A. B. Gottlieb, R. M. Grossman, L. Khandke, D. M. Carter, P. B. Sehgal, S. M. Fu, A. Granelli-Piperno, M. Rivas, L. Barazani, and J. G. Krueger, *J. Invest. Dermatol. 98*, 302 (1992).
107. T. Kojima, M. A. Cromie, S. Benrazavi, G. Majmudar, G. J. Fisher, J. J. Voorhees, and J. T. Elder, *J. Invest. Dermatol. 98*, 564A (1992).
108. L. B. Nanney, C. M. Stoscheck, and L. E. King, Jr., *J. Invest. Dermatol. 83*, 385 (1984).
109. L. B. Nanney, C. M. Stoscheck, M. Magid, and L. E. King, *J. Invest. Dermatol. 86*, 260 (1986).
110. B. A. Bernard, D. Asselineau, L. Shaffar-Deshayes, and M. Y. Darmon, *J. Invest. Dermatol. 90*, 801 (1988).
111. L. B. Nanney, *J. Invest. Dermatol. 94*, 624 (1990).
112. G. Schultz, D. S. Rotatori, and W. Clark, *J. Cell. Biochem. 45*, 346 (1991).
113. G. L. Brown, L. B. Nanney, J. Griffen, A. B. Cramer, J. M. Yancey, L. J. Curtsinger, L. Holtzin, G. S. Schultz, M. J. Jurkiewicz, and J. B. Lynch, *N. Engl. J. Med. 321*, 76 (1989).
114. P. A. Hebda, *J. Invest. Dermatol. 91*, 440 (1988).
115. A. Schreiber, M. E. Winkler, and R. Derynck, *Science 232*, 1250 (1986).
116. G. R. Grotendorst, Y. Soma, K. Takehara, and M. Charette, *J. Cell. Physiol. 139*, 617 (1989).
117. R. Todd, B. R. Donoff, T. Chiang, M. Y. Chow, A. Elovic, G. T. Gallagher, and D. T. Wong, *J. Cell. Biochem. 45*, 346 (1991).
118. H. M. Temin, *J. Natl. Cancer. Inst. 32*, 167 (1966).
119. R. A. Lang and A. W. Burgess, *Immunol. Today 11*, 244 (1990).
120. H. Kurachi, K.-I. Morishig, K. Amemiya, H. Adachi, K. Hirota, A. Miyake, and O. Tanizawa, *Cancer Res. 51*, 5956 (1991).
121. K. Stromberg, T. J. Collins, IV, A. W. Gordon, C. L. Jackson, and G. R. Johnson, *Cancer Res. 52*, 341 (1992).
122. M. Reiss, E. B. Stash, V. F. Vellucci, and Z.-L. Zhou, *Cancer Res. 51*, 6254 (1991).
123. K.-I. Morishige, H. Kurachi, K. Amemiya, H. Adachi, M. Inoue, A. Miyake, O. Tanizawa, and Y. Sakoyama, *Cancer Res. 51*, 5951 (1991).
124. S. Watanabe, E. Lazar, and M. B. Sporn, *Proc. Natl. Acad. Sci. USA 84*, 1258 (1987).
125. A. Rosenthal, P. B. Lindquist, T. S. Bringman, D. W. Goeddel, and R. Derynck, *Cell 46*, 301 (1986).
126. V. Shankar, F. Ciardiello, N. Kim, R. Derynck, D. S. Liscia, G. Merlo, B. C. Langton, D. Sheer, R. Callahan, R. H. Bassin, M. E. Lippman, N. Hynes, D. S. Salomon, *Mol. Carcinogen. 2*, 1 (1989).

127. E. Finzi, T. Fleming, O. Segatto, C. Y. Pennington, T. S. Bringman, R. Derynck, and S. A. Aaronson, *Proc. Natl. Acad. Sci. USA 84*, 3733 (1987).
128. E. Finzi, T. Fleming, and J. H. Pierce, *J. Invest. Dermatol. 95*, 382 (1990).
129. E. Finzi, A. Kilkenny, J. E. Strickland, M. Balaschak, T. Bringman, R. Cerynck, S. Aaronson, and S. H. Yuspa, *Mol. Carcinogen. 1*, 7 (1988).
130. E. Di Marco, J. H. Pierce, T. P. Fleming, M. H. Kraus, C. J. Molloy, S. A. Aaronson, and P. P. Di Fiore, *Oncogene 4*, 831 (1989).
131. D. A. Greenhalgh, D. J. Welty, A. Player, and S. H. Yuspa, *Proc. Natl. Acad. Sci. USA 87*, 643 (1990).
132. D. R. Roop, D. R. Lowy, P. E. Tambourin, J. Strickland, J. R. Harper, M. Balaschak, E. F. Spangler, and S. H. Yuspa, *Nature 323*, 822 (1986).
133. M. H. Sieweke, A. W. Stoker, and M. J. Bissell, *Cancer Res. 49*, 6419 (1989).
134. G. P. Dotto, R. A. Weinberg, and A. Ariza, *Proc. Natl. Acad. Sci. USA 85*, 6389 (1988).
135. W. F. Lever and G. Schaumburg-Lever, in *Histopathology of the Skin*, J. B. Lippincott Company, Philadelphia, PA, 1989, p. 552.
136. J. Gavrilovic, G. Moens, J. P. Thiery, and J. Jouanneau, *Cell Reg. 1*, 1003 (1990).
137. E. B. Jakobovits, U. Schlokat, J. L. Vannice, R. Derynck, and A. D. Levinson, *Mol. Cell. Biol. 8*, 5549 (1988).
138. R. H. Raja, A. J. Paterson, T. H. Shin, and J. E. Kudlow, *Mol. Endocrin. 5*, 514 (1991).
139. A. J. Blasband, K. T. Rogers, X. Chen, J. C. Azizkhan, and D. C. Lee, *Mol. Cell. Biol. 10*, 2111 (1990).
140. J. L. Merchant, B. Demediuk, and S. J. Brand, *Mol. Cell. Biol. 11*, 2686 (1991).
141. J. T. Elder, G. J. Fisher, Q.-Y. Zhang, D. Eisen, A. Krust, P. Kastner, P. Chambon, and J. J. Voorhees, *J. Invest. Dermatol. 96*, 425 (1991).
142. S. W. Lee, V. B. Morhenn, M. Ilnicka, E. M. Eugui, and A. C. Allison, *J. Invest. Dermatol. 97*, 106 (1991).
143. V. W. Raymond, D. C. Lee, J. W. Grisham, and H. S. Earp, *Cancer Res. 49*, 3608 (1989).
144. R. J. Coffey, Jr., R. Graves-Deal, P. J. Dempsey, R. H. Whitehead, and M. R. Pittelkow, *Cell Growth Diff. 3*, 347 (1992).
145. Y. Jinno, G. T. Merlino, and I. Pastan, *Nucl. Acids Res. 16*, 49 (1988).
146. P. T. Le, S. Lazorick, L. P. Whichard, B. F. Haynes, and K. H. Singer, *J. Exp. Med. 174*, 1147 (1991).
147. S. G. Mueller and J. E. Kudlow, *Mol. Endocrinol. 5*, 1439 (1991).
148. J. A. Atwater, R. Wisdom, and I. M. Verma, *Annu. Rev. Genet. 24*, 519 (1990).
149. J. S. Malter, *Science 246*, 664 (1989).
150. L. E. King, Jr., R. E. Gates, C. M. Stoscheck, and L. B. Nanney, *J. Invest. Dermatol. 94*, 164S (1990).
151. A. Ullrich, L. Coussens, J. S. Hayflick, T. J. Dull, A. Gray, A. W. Tam, J. Lee, Y. Yarden, T. A. Libermann, J. Schlessinger, J. Downward, E. L. V. Mayes, N. Whittle, M. D. Waterfield, and P. H. Seeburg, *Nature 309*, 418 (1984).

152. T. J. Velu, *Mol. Cell. Endocrinol. 70*, 205 (1990).
153. S. Iwashita, M. Kobayashi, *Cell. Signal. 4*, 123 (1992).
154. J. Massague, *J. Biol. Chem. 265*, 21393 (1990).
155. T. Yamamoto, S. Ikawa, T. Akiyama, K. Semba, N. Nomura, N. Miyajima, T. Saito, and K. Toyoshima, *Nature 319*, 230 (1986).
156. L. Coussens, T. L. Yang-Feng, Y.-C. Liao, E. Chen, A. Gray, J. McGrath, P. H. Seeburg, T. A. Liberman, J. Schlessinger, U. Francke, A. Levinson, and A. Ullrich, *Science 230*, 1132 (1985).
157. D. F. Stern, P. A. Heffernan, and R. A. Weinberg, *Mol. Cell. Biol. 6*, 1729 (1986).
158. M. H. Kraus, W. Issing, T. Miki, N. C. Popescu, and S. A. Aaronson, *Proc. Natl. Acad. Sci. USA 86*, 9193 (1989).
159. G. D. Plowman, G. S. Witney, M. G. Neubauer, J. M. Green, V. L. McDonald, G. J. Todaro, and M. Shoyab, *Proc. Natl. Acad. Sci. USA 87*, 4905 (1990).
160. H. C. Maguire, Jr., C. Jaworsky, J. A. Cohen, M. Hellman, D. B. Weiner, and M. I. Greene, *J. Invest. Dermatol. 89*, 786 (1989).
161. A. L. Schechter, M. C. Hung, L. Vaidyanathan, R. A. Weinberg, T. L. Yang-Feng, U. Francke, A. Ullrich, and L. Coussens, *Science 229*, 976 (1985).
162. R. Lupu, R. Colomer, B. Kannan, and M. E. Lippman, *Proc. Natl. Acad. Sci. USA 89*, 2287 (1992).
163. S. K. Hanks, A. M. Quinn, and T. Hunter, *Science 241*, 42 (1988).
164. M. F. W. te Pas, P. M. P. van Bergen en Henegouwen, J. Boonstra, and M. Ponec, *Arch. Dermatol. Res. 283*, 125 (1991).
165. G. T. Merlino, Y.-H. Xu, S. Ishii, A. J. L. Clark, K. Semba, K. Toyoshima, T. Yamamoto, and I. Pastan, *Science 224*, 117 (1984).
166. K. L. Thompson and M. R. Rosner, *J. Biol. Chem. 264*, 3230 (1989).
167. B. Nickoloff and R. Mitra, *J. Invest. Dermatol. 93*, 799 (1989).
168. P. Kesavan, S. Mukhopadhayay, S. Murphy, M. Rengaraju, M. A. Lazar, and M. Das, *J. Biol. Chem. 266*, 10282 (1991).
169. K. L. Thompson, R. Assoian, M. R. Rosner, *J. Biol. Chem. 263*, 19519 (1988).
170. B. O. Fanger, R. A. Currie, and J. A. Cidlowski, *Arch. Biochem. Biophys. 249*, 116 (1986).
171. R. Kageyama, G. T. Merlino, and I. Pastan, *Proc. Natl. Acad. Sci. USA 85*, 5016 (1988).
172. L. G. Hudson, K. L. Thompson, J. Xu, G. N. Gill, *Proc. Natl. Acad. Sci. USA 87*, 7536 (1990).
173. M. E. Winkler, L. O'Connor, M. Winget, and B. Fendly, *Biochem. 28*, 6373 (1989).
174. B. O. Fanger, J. E. Stephens, and J. V. Staros, *FASEB J. 3*, 71 (1989).
175. A. M. Honegger, A. Schmidt, A. Ullrich, and J. Schlessinger, *Mol. Cell. Biol. 10*, 4035 (1990).
176. W. S. Chen, C. S. Lazar, M. Poenie, R. Y. Tsien, G. N. Gill, and M. G. Rosenfeld, *Nature 328*, 818 (1987).
177. A. Honegger, T. Dull, S. Felder, E. Van Obberghen, F. Bellot, D. Szaparu, A. Schmidt, A. Ullrich, and J. Schlessinger, *Cell 51*, 199 (1987).

178. Q. C. Vega, C. Cochet, O. Filhol, C.-P. Chang, S. G. Rhee, and G. N. Gill, *Mol. Cell. Biol. 12*, 128 (1992).
179. R. B. Peinsky and L. K. Sinclair, *Nature 321*, 81 (1986).
180. M. Abdel-Ghany, H. K. Kole, M. A. E. Saad, and E. Racker, *Proc. Natl. Acad. Sci. USA 86*, 6072 (1989).
181. S. T. Sawyer and S. Cohen, *J. Biol. Chem. 260*, 8233 (1985).
182. J. T. Elder, G. J. Fisher, E. A. Duell, K. Kragballe, J. J. Voorhees, in *Physiology, Biochemistry, and Molecular Biology of the Skin* (L. A. Goldsmith, ed.), 2d ed., Oxford University Press, New York, 1991, p. 266.
183. M. P. Peppelenbosch, L. G. J. Tertoolen, J. den Hertog, and S. W. de Laat, *Cell 69*, 295 (1992).
184. S. Nishibe, M. Wahl, P. Wedegaertner, J. Kim, S. Rhee, S. Carpenter, *Proc. Natl. Acad. Sci. USA 87*, 424 (1990).
185. T. M. Wright, H. S. Shin, and D. M. Raben, *Biochem. J. 267*, 501 (1990).
186. B. G. Nair, H. M. Rashed, and T. B. Patel, *Biochem. J. 264*, 563 (1989).
187. C. Cochet, O. Filhol, B. Payrastre, T. Hunter, and G. N. Gill, *J. Biol. Chem. 266*, 637 (1991).
188. L. C. Cantley, K. R. Auger, C. Carpenter, B. Duckworth, A. Graziani, R. Kapeller, and S. Soltoff, *Cell 64*, 281 (1991).
189. G. Thomas, *Cell 68*, 3 (1992).
190. S. Nishibe, M. I. Whal, S. M. T. Hernandez-Sotomayor, N. K. Tonks, S. G. Rhee, and G. Carpenter, *Science 250*, 1253 (1990).
191. G. Todderud, M. I. Whal, S. G. Rhee, and G. Carpenter, *Science 249*, 296 (1990).
192. T. Goldkorn, K. A. Dressler, J. Juindi, N. S. Radin, J. Mendelsohn, D. Menaldino, D. Liotta, and R. N. Kolesnick, *J. Biol. Chem. 266*, 16092 (1991).
193. Y. Igarashi, K. Kitamura, T. Toyokuni, B. Dean, B. Fenderson, T. Ogawa, and S.-I. Hakomori, *J. Biol. Chem. 265*, 5385 (1990).
194. N. Hanai, T. Dohi, G. A. Nores, and S.-I. Hakomori, *J. Biol. Chem. 263*, 6296 (1988).
195. C. A. Koch, D. Anderson, M. F. Moran, C. Ellis, and T. Pawson, *Science 252*, 668 (1991).
196. B. Margolis, N. Li, A. Koch, M. Mohammadi, D. R. Hurwitz, A. Zilberstein, A. Ullrich, T. Pawson, and J. Schlessinger, *EMBO J. 9*, 4375 (1990).
197. S. J. Burwen and A. L. Jones, *TIBS 12*, 159 (1987).
198. A. Logan, *J. Endocrinol. 125*, 339 (1990).
199. G. R. Johnson, T. Saeki, N. Auersperg, A. W. Gordon, M. Shoyab, D. S. Salomon, and K. Stromberg, *Biochem. Biophys. Res. Commun. 180*, 481 (1991).
200. R. J. Davis, *J. Biol. Chem. 263*, 9462 (1988).
201. I. C. Northwood, F. A. Gonzalez, M. Wartmann, D. L. Raden, and R. J. Davis, *J. Biol. Chem. 266*, 15266 (1991).
202. G. J. Heisermann, H. S. Wiley, B. J. Walsh, H. A. Ingraham, C. J. Fiol, and G. N. Gill, *J. Biol. Chem. 165*, 12820 (1990).
203. H. S. Wiley, J. J. Herbst, B. J. Walsh, D. A. Lauffenburger, M. G. Rosenfeld, and G. N. Gill, *J. Biol. Chem. 266*, 11083 (1991).

204. C. R. Hopkins, A. Gibson, M. Shipman, and K. Miller, *Nature 346*, 335 (1990).
205. S. Felder, K. Miller, G. Moehren, A. Ullrich, J. Schlessinger, and C. R. Hopkins, *Cell 61*, 623 (1990).
206. J. Ro, S. M. North, G. E. Gallick, G. N. Hortobagyi, J. U. Gutterman, and M. Blick, *Cancer Res. 48*, 161 (1988).
207. A. Wells, J. B. Welsh, C. S. Lazar, H. S. Wiley, G. N. Gill, and M. G. Rosenfeld, *Science 247*, 962 (1989).
208. T. Hunter, *Cell 58*, 1013 (1989).
209. S. Gentleman, T. M. Martenson, J. J. Digiovanna, and G. J. Chader, *Biochem. Biophys. Acta 798*, 53 (1984).
210. C. M. Stoscheck, D. B. Friedman, L. E. King, Jr., *J. Invest. Dermatol. 92*, 12 (1989).
211. P. Gunaratne, C. M. Stroscheck, R. D. Strough, R. E. Gates, G. P. Stricklin, and L. E. King, Jr., *Clin. Res. 40*, 490A (1992).
212. N. J. Reynolds, J. J. Baldassare, P. A. Henderson, J. T. Elder, J. J. Voorhees, and G. J. Fisher, *J. Invest. Dermatol. 98*, 564A (1992).
213. R. W. Groves, M. H. Allen, and D. M. MacDonald, *J. Cutan. Pathol. 19*, 66 1991).
214. A. Kikuchi, M. Amagai, K. Hayakawa, M. Ueda, S. Hirohashi, N. Shimizu, and T. Nishikawa, *Br. J. Dermatol. 123*, 49 (1990).
215. A. P. M. Lavrijsen, L. M. Tieben, M. Ponce, J. G. van der Schroeff, and G. N. P. van Muijen, *Arch. Dermatol. Res. 281*, 83 (1989).
216. D. Pim, M. Collins, and L. Banks, *Oncogene 7*, 27 (1992).
217. P. Martin, W. C. Vass, J. T. Schiller, D. R. Lowy, and T. J. Velu, *Cell 59*, 21 (1989).
218. L. B. Nanney, D. L. Ellis, J. Levine, and L. E. King, *Am. J. Pathol. 140*, 915 (1992).
219. J. T. Elder, A. Tavakkol, S. B. Klein, M. E. Zeigler, M. Wicha, and J. J. Voorhees, *J. Invest. Dermatol. 94*, 19 (1990).
220. H. Kobayashi, H. Yasuda, H. Matsue, A. Ohkawara, Y. Ogiso, and N. Kuzumaki, *J. Dermatol. 17*, 104 (1990).

# 10
# Regulation of Tissue Inflammation, Repair, and Fibrosis by Transforming Growth Factor Beta

**Sharon M. Wahl**
*National Institute of Dental Research*
*National Institutes of Health*
*Bethesda, Maryland*

## I. INTRODUCTION

Transforming growth factor beta (TGF-$\beta$) is a 25 kd peptide involved in many fundamental biological processes including growth, differentiation, and morphogenesis [1, 2]. Originally designated as a growth factor because of its ability to influence cell growth patterns in vitro, TGF-$\beta$ has subsequently been shown to be a multifunctional signaling molecule, the production and regulation of which is pivotal to the outcome of numerous physiological and pathological events. Based on the ability of TGF-$\beta$ to regulate cell growth, extracellular matrix deposition and degradation, and inflammatory responses [1–4], TGF-$\beta$ most certainly plays an important role in the immunobiology of many tissues including the skin.

TGF-$\beta$ represents a highly homologous family of at least five homodimeric polypeptides, which share many biological activities and are part of a much larger superfamily [1, 2]. The human TGF-$\beta$ isoforms (TGF-$\beta$1, $\beta$2, and $\beta$3) are encoded as precursors of 390–412 amino acids with a hydrophobic signal sequence of 20–23 amino acids at the N-terminus [5]. After signal peptidase and proteolytic cleavage, TGF-$\beta$ is processed to the 112 residue form (12.5 kd), which dimerizes to generate mature TGF-$\beta$ (25 kd). Secreted TGF-$\beta$ exists as a biologically inactive or latent complex due to its association with a 75 kd glycosylated latency-associated protein (LAP), which may be covalently linked to a 135 kd binding protein [1, 6]. Cellular or tissue localization and persistence may be facilitated by the fibronectin cellular recognition (RGD) sequence found within the LAP of TGF-$\beta$1 and TGF-$\beta$3, but absent in TGF-$\beta$2 [7]. Activation of the latent complex must precede receptor binding and appears to involve a multistep process requiring protease activity and/or acidic conditions [6, 8]. Once activated, TGF-$\beta$ may bind to cellular receptors, reassociate with LAP, bind to extracellular matrix proteins, or interact with one of several binding proteins for maintenance or clearance. Thus, latency confers stability, target cell specificity, and a means for extracellular control of the diverse activities of this ubiquitous molecule.

## II. INFLAMMATION

### A. Leukocyte Recruitment

An injury to the skin, whether due to trauma, infection or antigen deposition, initiates an inflammatory response. One of the earliest occurences in this complex process is the aggregation and activation of platelets (Fig. 1). Among the numerous mediators and factors released by activated platelets is TGF-$\beta$, which is stored in abundance in the $\alpha$ granules [9]. Once released and activated, TGF-$\beta$ functions at femtomolar concentrations as a chemoattractant for monocytes, neutrophils, and T lymphocytes [10–13], all of which are essential to inflammation and the host response to immunological challenge (Fig. 1). Moreover, the recruitment potential of TGF-$\beta$ has been confirmed in situ following subcutaneous injection [14] or local injections into other tissues [15, 16].

At the site of inflammation, circulating leukocytes must exit from the vessels by adhering to and traversing the vascular wall including the basement membrane, a barrier of type IV collagen, laminin, and fibronectin. One mechanism whereby TGF-$\beta$ may promote these leukocyte-endothelial cell and leukocyte-matrix interactions is by enhancing cell surface integrin expression. Integrins are heterodimers composed of an $\alpha$ and $\beta$ subunit, which serve as transmembrane links between the extracellular matrix and the cellular cytoskeletal elements [17, 18]. Functionally, the $\beta_2$ heterodimers mediate cell-cell interactions, whereas the $\beta_1$ integrins, referred to as very late antigens (VLA), can foster cell-matrix and possibly cell-cell binding. In response to picomolar levels of TGF-$\beta$, VLA-3 ($\alpha_3\beta_1$) receptors which interact with laminin, collagen, and fibronectin cell binding domains increase on circulating monocytes, as do VLA-5 receptors which uniquely recognize the RGDS (Arg-Gly-Asp-Ser) sequence in the central region of fibronectin [19]. Augmentation of integrin receptor expression by TGF-$\beta$ or other cytokines is reflected by increased mononuclear phagocyte adhesiveness to structural

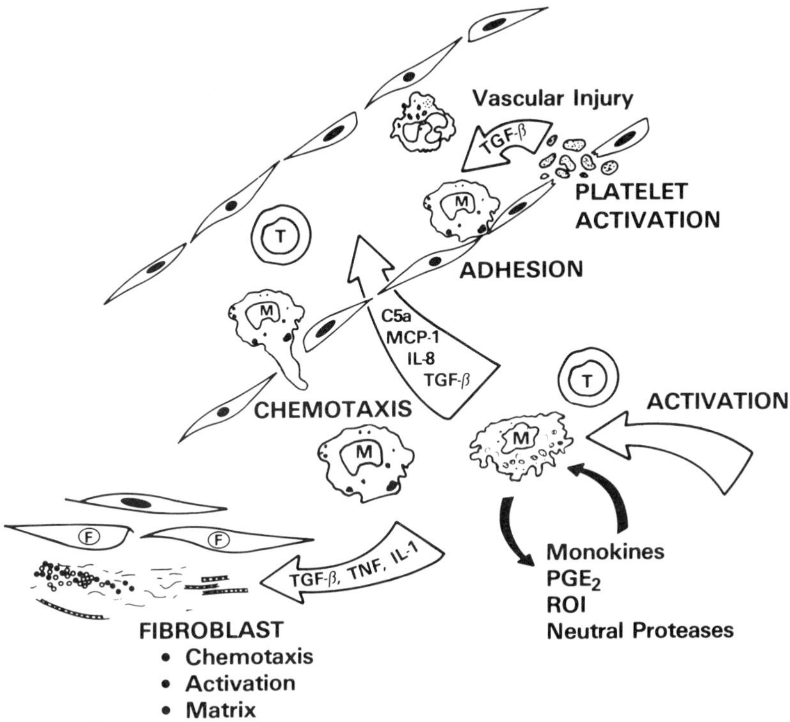


**Fig. 1** TGF-β regulates inflammation and repair. Platelet activation results in release of TGF-β, which promotes adhesion and chemotaxis of leukocytes to the site of inflammation. Within the tissues, higher levels of TGF-β stimulate T cells and monocytes with the release of inflammatory mediators and cytokines. As the lymphocytes and macrophages undergo activation and differentiate, they become susceptible to inhibition by TGF-β and immune suppression occurs. TGF-β promotes the repair process directly by regulating fibroblast chemotaxis, growth, and matrix generation and indirectly by stimulating inflammatory cells to secrete growth- and matrix-inducing cytokines.

matrix substrates and may be critically important in the homing and positioning of these cells at sites of inflammation.

Having adhered to basement membrane components, leukocytes need to digest these structural proteins in order to traverse this barrier. TGF-β contributes to this process by stimulating augmented levels of the 92 and 72 kd gelatinase/type IV collagenases in monocytes [19]. Based on these and other data, it appears that the rapid release of TGF-β, first by platelets and then by inflammatory cells themselves [1, 3, 4, 9], promotes leukocyte recruitment by mediating integrin expression, attachment, and collagenolytic activity essential to leukocyte margination, diapedesis, movement across the basement membrane, and extravascular directed migration (Fig. 1).

## B. Leukocyte Activation

Once within an inflammatory site, the increase in integrin expression and the ability of TGF-$\beta$ to induce receptors for IgG (Fc$\gamma$RIII, CD16) on newly recruited monocytes [20], promotes their phagocytic and microbicidal activities [21, 22], which are important in host defense. Several types of cells are capable of producing TGF-$\beta$ including activated lymphocytes, macrophages, and neutrophils [23–27] contributing to the high levels of this peptide identified within inflammatory sites [21, 28]. Moreover, TGF-$\beta$ has been shown to augment its own secretion in many cells through specific AP-1 sites on its own promoter [29], setting in motion both autocrine and paracrine circuits of potentially cyclic release. Consequently, expression of TGF-$\beta$ mRNA appears most abundant during active inflammation and cell-mediated immune reactions [30].

Apart from its capacity to promote cell recruitment, TGF-$\beta$ is a potent regulator of many other critical cell functions (Fig. 1). At picomolar concentrations, TGF-$\beta$ stimulates circulating monocytes, but not macrophages, to generate several inflammatory cytokines including interleukin 1 (IL-1), tumor necrosis factor (TNF-$\alpha$), platelet-derived growth factor (PDGF), basic fibroblast growth factor (bFGF), and IL-6 [10, 15, 25, 31–33]. Thus, one of the principal actions of TGF-$\beta$ may be to transiently control monocyte gene transcription for a series of biologically active molecules that control many of the subsequent events in the inflammatory process.

TGF-$\beta$ also influences lymphocyte functions by regulating antibody production and by augmenting proliferation, which is triggered through the T-cell receptor/CD3 complex of relatively undifferentiated T cells [4, 34]. By inducing conversion of putative precursors to mature T-helper (TH1) CD4+ cells [34, 35], the accumulation of TGF-$\beta$ at sites of immunological challenge may foster the generation of such a population essential to the evolution of delayed-type hypersensitivity and antigenic memory.

## C. Reversal of Inflammation

As the host sequesters and/or eliminates the injurious or immunological challenge, mechanisms for termination of an inflammatory response are invoked to prevent pathological tissue damage. Although TGF-$\beta$ has many pro-inflammatory activities, it appears that this cytokine is also crucial in suppressing inflammatory events. This apparent paradox may be resolved by accumulating evidence that indicates that the ability of TGF-$\beta$ to promote or suppress the functions of any particular cell population is critically dependent on the state of differentiation or activation of that cell. This is perhaps nowhere more evident than in the regulation of mononuclear cell functions in inflammatory and immune events. For example, nonactivated circulating monocytes are exquisitely sensitive to recruitment and activation by TGF-$\beta$, whereas once these cells become activated, as would occur within an inflammatory lesion, their TGF-$\beta$ receptors are downregulated, preventing further TGF-$\beta$ activation [4, 36]. Differentiated macrophages are functionally suppressed by TGF-$\beta$ [37], emphasizing that the effects of any given cytokine must be considered within the context of the environment in which it is generated or delivered. Similarly, immature T lymphocytes are induced to differentiate into TH1 cells in the presence of TGF-$\beta$ [34, 35], whereas activated T cells which, in contrast to activated macrophages, exhibit increased TGF-$\beta$ receptors, are inhibited by TGF-$\beta$ [27]. Thus, the differential expression of TGF-$\beta$ receptors during different stages of effector cell activation may be crucial to the ability of TGF-$\beta$ to reverse inflammatory events.

In contrast to suppression of mature CD4+ T-cell growth, TGF-$\beta$ is less inhibitory to CD8+ cells, which have further immunosuppressive effects [38, 39]. Additional mechanisms of TGF-$\beta$ immunosuppression include inhibition of IL-1 receptor expression [40] and the induction of transcription and translation of the IL-1 receptor antagonist (IL-1ra) [41, 42]. IL-1ra is a 22 kd protein which binds to the IL-1 receptor but has no agonist properties and therefore blocks IL-1 binding and signal transduction, aborting IL-1–dependent responses [43]. Numerous other cell-specific pathways of suppression by TGF-$\beta$ may also contribute to the ability of TGF-$\beta$ to terminate immune and inflammatory events [4].

## D. Tissue Repair

As the inflammatory response subsides, TGF-$\beta$ plays a critical role in tissue repair and fibrosis. The concerted actions of TGF-$\beta$ with other inflammatory mediators and with matrix components contribute to the regulation of fibroblast chemotaxis, proliferation, and controlled synthesis and degradation of extracellular matrix necessary for tissue repair (Fig. 1). Fibroblasts are recruited by TGF-$\beta$ [15, 44] and express an increased repertoire of integrins [2], which facilitate cell-cell and cell-matrix interactions. Although TGF-$\beta$ does not directly stimulate fibroblasts to proliferate, this peptide indirectly triggers fibroblast proliferation through the induction of PDGF-A chain and PDGF$\alpha$-receptors [45, 46] and by enhancement of cellular receptors for and sensitivity to epidermal growth factor (EGF) [47]. By promoting both recruitment and growth of fibroblasts, TGF-$\beta$ contributes to local expansion of this matrix-synthesizing population.

When injected subcutaneously into newborn mice, TGF-β caused a rapid fibrotic and angiogenic response [14], prompting studies to define the mechanisms whereby this potent growth factor so dramatically influenced the formation of granulation tissue and matrix accumulation. Subsequently, TGF-β was shown to directly regulate transcription and translation of certain matrix components by mesenchymal cells (Fig. 2). Following receptor-ligand interaction, TGF-β enhances the nuclear factor 1–collagen promoter interaction to increase collagen mRNA expression [48]. Not only are types I, III, VI, and X collagens upregulated by TGF-β, but other matrix components are also synthesized in response to this peptide, including fibronectin and glycosaminoglycans [48–53]. Moreover, many of the effects of TGF-β on connective tissue regeneration and neovascularization [14, 15] may well be secondary to TGF-β–induced cytokine release by the infiltrating mononuclear phagocytes.

Compounding the TGF-β–mediated matrix-regenerating potential of these cells is the ability of the cytokine to enhance the generation of protease inhibitors while suppressing production of proteolytic enzymes [54–56] (Fig. 2). Although TGF-β did not independently induce fibroblasts to syn-

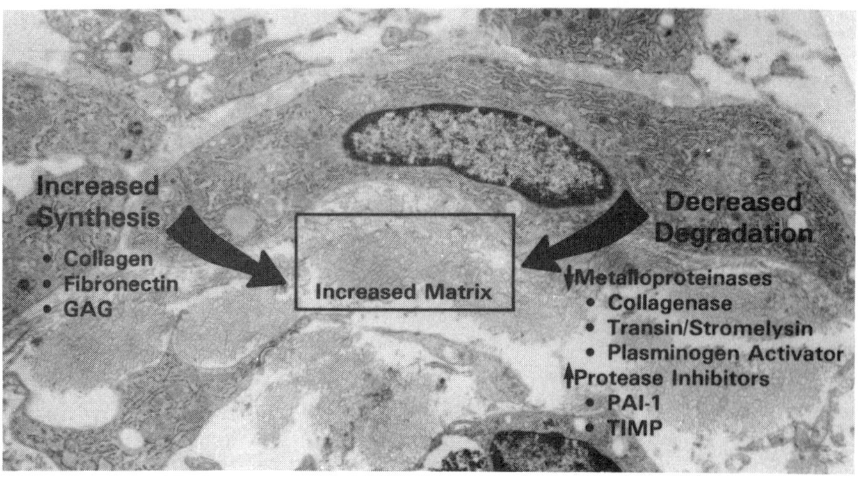


**Fig. 2** Regulation of matrix production by TGF-β. Electron micrograph of synovial fibroblasts after intraarticular injection of TGF-β. TGF-β promotes the accumulation of extracellular matrix by stimulating increased transcription and translation of collagen, fibronectin, and GAG and by inhibiting their degradation. The net effect of inhibiting metalloproteinases and augmenting protease inhibitors is to minimize degradation of the increased matrix proteins in the presence of TGF-β.

thesize tissue inhibitor of metalloproteinases (TIMP) or plasminogen activator inhibitor (PAI), the peptide synergistically induced these inhibitors in the presence of other growth factors [55]. Similarly, TGF-$\beta$ transcriptionally suppresses collagenase, stromelysin, and elastase production stimulated by basic FGF or EGF [54, 55]. Nonetheless, the overall effect of this differential regulation of matrix proteins, enzymes, and enzyme inhibitors is the accumulation of extracellular matrix and scar formation. In deficiencies of healing, TGF-$\beta$ may be useful clinically to promote wound healing [57, 58].

## III. FIBROPROLIFERATIVE DISORDERS

### A. Role of TGF-$\beta$ in Fibrosis

In addition to its physiological role in inflammation and scar formation and its ability to promote deficient healing, aberrations in persistence, production, or regulation of TGF-$\beta$, leading to increased local concentrations, may promote excessive matrix generation and fibrosis. TGF-$\beta$ apparently must be present at controlled levels, since insufficient amounts of the peptide may impede inflammatory and healing processes, and excess TGF-$\beta$ may potentiate chronic inflammatory and fibrotic lesions. By virtue of its ability to upregulate collagen gene expression, TGF-$\beta$ is a candidate for playing a significant role in the pathogenesis of certain fibrotic diseases. Excessive concentrations of TGF-$\beta$ have been identified within fibrotic skin lesions [59, 60] and in other fibrotic inflammatory conditions occurring in the liver, lung, eye, and synovium [28, 39, 61–64], consistent with a role for overexpression of the molecule in pathological processes. Whether this abundance of TGF-$\beta$ is the consequence of increased synthesis or absence of regulation is unclear.

### B. Scleroderma

Progressive systemic sclerosis (scleroderma), a generalized connective tissue disorder that involves the skin and often internal organs, is a prototypic fibrotic disease [65]. The precise mechanisms leading to activation of collagen expression and abnormal accumulation of matrix are poorly understood. However, one of the earliest events appears to be vascular damage leading to platelet activation and mononuclear cell infiltration. Identification of factors capable of coordinately directing these responses, their cellular sources, and targets is important to defining the pathogenesis of scleroderma and other fibrotic diseases. If platelets are viewed as early participants in this process [65], then the various mediators abundant in platelets, including

TGF-$\beta$, become prime candidates as initiators of the subsequent pathogenic events (Table 1).

TGF-$\beta$ has been identified within sclerodermal lesions, especially around inflamed blood vessels [59], where it may function to recruit the monocytes and lymphocytes found in the area. This increase in cellularity may be mediated by mechanisms in addition to direct chemotaxis, perhaps including regulation of adhesion molecules. Furthermore, the spatial association between inflammatory cells and cells producing increased collagen implicates the mononuclear cell infiltrate in the regulation of the connective tissue abnormalities. Beyond the close proximity of the inflammatory cells and the matrix-generating fibroblast populations, the identification of the associated TGF-$\beta$ suggests that this peptide provides a venue for intercellular communication. In vitro, TGF-$\beta$ has been shown to increase collagen and glycosaminoglycan (GAG) synthesis by cultures of scleroderma fibroblasts more effectively than in cultures of normal dermal fibroblasts [53]. GAG are prominently identified in the vessel walls of patients with early disease [53]. Moreover, by in situ hybridization, the TGF-$\beta$2 gene was found to colocalize with collagen type I using the pro $\alpha$1(I) collagen chain probe [59]. This observation establishes a link between this peptide and abnormal matrix deposition and is consistent with other reports of a selective expression of TGF-$\beta$2 at sites of active fibrosis [64], although both TGF-$\beta$1 and $\beta$2 have

**Table 1** Potential Sites of TGF-$\beta$ Action in Scleroderma

| |
|---|
| Endothelial cell damage |
| Platelet activation |
|   Release of TGF-$\beta$ |
|   Activation of latent TGF-$\beta$ |
| Mononuclear cell infiltration |
|   Chemotaxis |
|   Increased integrins |
|   Type IV collagenase |
|   T-cell and monocyte activation and cytokine release |
| Fibroblast activation |
|   Chemotaxis |
|   Increased PDGF and PDGF-R |
|   Increased collagen, fibronectin, and GAG |
|   Stimulation of IL-1 and TNF |
| Fibrosis |
|   Increased matrix synthesis |
|   Decreased matrix degradation |

been reported [60, 66]. Furthermore, the presence of TGF-$\beta$2, although highly homologous with TGF-$\beta$1, implicates inflammatory cells as the primary source of the peptide as human platelets and fibroblasts apparently do not express TGF-$\beta$2 [59], although their secretion of TGF-$\beta$1 may induce TGF-$\beta$2 in adjacent inflammatory cells. Scleroderma fibroblasts have not been reported to synthesize significantly increased amounts of TGF-$\beta$ compared with normal fibroblast [53, 67]. In summary, overexpression of and/or increased responsiveness to TGF-$\beta$ are clearly associated with increased matrix accumulation, the most prominent clinical manifestation of scleroderma.

### C. Inhibition of TGF-$\beta$ and Fibrosis

Confirmation of TGF-$\beta$ gene expression and peptide within scleroderma lesions, and in other chronic inflammatory and fibrotic sites, offers a rationale for attempting to antagonize the biological activity of this potent cytokine. This approach has both therapeutic and pathogenetic implications. Recent studies have utilized neutralizing antibodies to block TGF-$\beta$ activity, resulting in significant reductions in pathology. Administration of antibodies to TGF-$\beta$ alleviated inflammation and connective tissue changes in both experimental glomerulonephritis and erosive polyarthritis [68, 69], establishing that TGF-$\beta$ has a direct causal role in these events. Additionally, IFN-$\gamma$ and TNF have been recently identified as TGF-$\beta$ antagonists by virtue of their ability to counteract the pro-fibrotic activity of TGF-$\beta$ in vitro [70]. Taking this observation to the next level, patients with chronic active hepatitis due to hepatitis C virus who received IFN-$\alpha$ therapy showed both decreased liver TGF-$\beta$1 mRNA and procollagen type 1 mRNA [71]. Whereas TGF-$\beta$ is important to normal inflammation and tissue repair, its uncontrolled production or activity appears to lead to chronic destructive and fibrotic disease.

## IV. CONCLUSIONS

TGF-$\beta$ has emerged as a signaling molecule with a central regulatory role in a diverse spectrum of fundamental biological processes. Numerous checks and balances are normally in place to control the potent activity of this cytokine including its latent status, different isoforms, target cell type, natural inhibitors and, perhaps most important, the state of differentiation or activation of the target cell. Moreover, the presence of other synergistic and antagonistic cytokines and growth factors and the influence of extracellular matrix constituents must all be factored into the determination of the effects of TGF-$\beta$ within a given biological response. As this complex story continues to be unraveled, one of the most interesting new arenas to be explored is the identification of specific, nontoxic TGF-$\beta$ antagonists. The use of

TGF-$\beta$ antagonists is important to establishing cause and effect of the polypeptide and also suggests pathways amenable to therapeutic intervention.

## REFERENCES


1. A. B. Roberts and M. B. Sporn, *Handb. Exp. Pharm. 95*, 419 (1990).
2. J. Massagué, *Annu. Rev. Cell Biol. 6*, 597 (1990).
3. S. M. Wahl, N. McCartney-Francis, and S. E. Mergenhagen, *Immunol. Today 10*, 258 (1989).
4. S. M. Wahl, *J. Clin. Immunol. 12*, 1 (1992).
5. R. Derynck, J. A. Jarett, E. Y. Chen, D. H. Eaton, J. R. Bell, K. Assoian, A. B. Roberts, M. B. Sporn, and D. V. Goeddel, *Nature 3162*, 701 (1985).
6. L. M. Wakefield, D. M. Smith, K. C. Flanders, and M. B. Sporn, *J. Biol. Chem. 263*, 7646 (1988).
7. E. Ruoslahti and M. D. Pierschbacher, *Cell 44*, 517 (1986).
8. L. M. Wakefield, D. M. Smith, T. Masui, C. C. Harris, and M. B. Sporn, *J. Cell Biol. 105*, 965 (1987).
9. R. K. Assoian, A. Komoriya, C. A. Meyers, D. M. Miller, and M. B. Sporn, *J. Biol. Chem. 258*, 7155 (1983).
10. S. M. Wahl, D. A. Hunt, L. Wakefield, N. McCartney-Francis, L. M. Wahl, A. B. Roberts, and M. B. Sporn, *Proc. Natl. Acad. Sci. 84*, 5788 (1987).
11. M. E. Brandes, U. E. H. Mai, K. Ohura, and S. M. Wahl, *J. Immunol. 147*, 1600 (1991).
12. J. Reibman, S. Meisler, T. C. Lee, L. I. Gold, B. N. Cronstein, K. A. Haines, S. L. Kolasinski, and G. W. Weissmann, *Proc. Natl. Acad. Sci. 85*, 6805 (1991).
13. D. H. Adams, M. Hathaway, J. Shaw, D. Burnett, E. Elias, and A. J. Strain, *J. Immunol. 147*, 609 (1991).
14. A. B. Roberts, M. B. Sporn, R. K. Assoian, J. M. Smith, N. S. Roche, L. M. Wakefield, U. I. Heine, L. A. Liotta, V. Falanga, and J. H. Kehrl, *Proc. Natl. Acad. Sci. 83*, 4167 (1986).
15. J. B. Allen, C. L. Manthey, A. Hand, K. Ohura, L. Ellingsworth, and S. M. Wahl, *J. Exp. Med. 171*, 231 (1990).
16. R. A. Fava, N. J. Olsen, A. E. Postlethwaite, K. N. Broadley, J. M. Davidson, L. B. Nanney, C. Lucas, and A. S. Townes, *J. Exp. Med. 173*, 1121 (1991).
17. E. Ruoslahti, *J. Clin. Invest. 81*, 1 (1991).
18. T. A. Springer, *Nature 346*, 425 (1990).
19. S. M. Wahl, J. B. Allen, B. S. Weeks, H. L. Wong, and P. E. Klotman, *Proc. Natl. Acad. Sci. 90*, In press (1993).
20. G. Welch, H. Wong, and S. M. Wahl, *J. Immunol. 1244*, 344 (1990).
21. S. M. Wahl, J. B. Allen, G. Welch, and H. Wong, *J. Immunol. 148*, 485 (1992).
22. J. B. Allen, H. L. Wong, P. Guyre, G. Simon, and S. M. Wahl, *J. Clin. Invest. 87*, 1773 (1991).
23. R. K. Assoian, B. E. Fleurdelys, H. C. Stevenson, P. J. Miller, D. K. Madtes, E. W. Raines, R. Ross, and M. B. Sporn, *Proc. Natl. Acad. Sci. 84*, 6020 (1987).

24. S. M. Wahl, N. McCartney-Francis, J. B. Allen, E. B. Dougherty, and S. F. Dougherty, *Ann. N.Y. Acad. Sci. 593*, 188 (1990).
25. N. McCartney-Francis, D. Mizel, H. Wong, L. M. Wahl, and S. M. Wahl, *Growth Factors 4*, 27 (1990).
26. G. R. Grotendorst, G. Smale, and D. Pencev, *J. Cell Physiol. 140*, 396 (1989).
27. J. H. Kehrl, L. M. Wakefield, A. B. Roberts, S. Jakowlew, M. Alvarez-Mon, R. Derynck, M. B. Sporn, and A. S. Fauci, *J. Exp. Med. 163*, 1037 (1986).
28. S. M. Wahl, J. B. Allen, H. L. Wong, S. F. Dougherty, and L. R. Ellingsworth, *J. Immunol. 145*, 2514 (1990).
29. S. J. Kim, K. T. Jeang, A. Glick, M. B. Sporn, and A. B. Roberts, *J. Biol. Chem. 264*, 7041 (1989).
30. M. Yamamura, K. Uyemura, R. J. Deans, K. Weinberg, T. H. Rea, B. R. Bloom, and R. L. Modlin, *Science 254*, 277 (1991).
31. D. M. Wiseman, P. J. Polverini, D. W. Kamp, and S. J. Leibovich, *Biochem. Biophys. Res. Commun. 157*, 793 (1988).
32. D. Chantry, M. Turner, E. Abney, and M. Feldmann, *J. Immunol. 142*, 4295 (1989).
33. M. Turner, D. Chantry, and M. Feldmann, *Cytokine 2*, 211 (1990).
34. H. M. Lee and S. Rich, *J. Immunol. 147*, 1127 (1991).
35. S. L. Swain, G. Huston, S. Tonkonogy, and A. Weinberg, *J. Immunol. 147*, 2991 (1991).
36. M. E. Brandes, L. M. Wakefield, and S. M. Wahl, *J. Biol. Chem. 266*, 19697 (1991).
37. A. Ding, C. F. Nathan, J. Graycar, R. Derynck, D. L. Stuehr, and S. Srimal, *J. Immunol. 145*, 940 (1990).
38. P. Salgame, J. S. Abrams, C. Clayberger, and H. Goldstein, J. Convit, R. L. Modlin, and B. R. Bloom, *Science 254*, 279 (1991).
39. M. Lotz, J. Kekow, and D. A. Carson, *J. Immunol. 144*, 4189 (1990).
40. C. M. Dubois, F. W. Ruscetti, E. W. Palaszynski, L. A. Falk, J. J. Oppenheim, and J. R. Keller, *J. Exp. Med. 172*, 737 (1990).
41. M. Turner, D. Chantry, P. Katsikis, A. Berger, G. M. Brennan, M. Feldmann, *J. Immunol. 21*, 1635 (1991).
42. S. M. Wahl, G. Costa, M. Corcoran, L. M. Wahl, and A. E. Berger, *J. Immunol.* In press (1993).
43. D. J. Dripps, B. J. Brandhuber, R. C. Thompson, and S. P. Eisenberg, *J. Biol. Chem. 266*, 10331 (1991).
44. A. E. Postlethwaite, J. Keski-Oja, H. L. Moses, and A. H. Kang, *J. Exp. Med. 165*, 251 (1987).
45. E. B. Leof, J. A. Proper, A. S. Goustin, G. D. Shipley, P. E. DiCorleto, and H. C. Moses, *Proc. Natl. Acad. Sci. 83*, 2453 (1986).
46. O. Ishikawa, E. C. LeRoy, and M. Trojanowska, *J. Cell Physiol. 145*, 181 (1990).
47. R. K. Assoian, C. A. Frolick, A. B. Roberts, D. M. Miller, and M. B. Sporn, *Cell 36*, 35 (1984).
48. P. Rossi, A. B. Roberts, N. S. Roche, B. Karsenty, M. B. Sporn, and B. de Crombrugghe, *Cell 52*, 405 (1988).
49. R. A. Ignotz, T. Endo, and J. Massagué, *J. Biol. Chem. 262*, 6443 (1987).

50. R. A. Ignotz and J. Massagué, *J. Biol. Chem. 261*, 4337 (1986).
51. J. Varga, J. Rosenbloom, and S. A. Jimenez, *Biochem. J. 247*, 597 (1987).
52. A. Bassols and J. Massagué, *J. Biol. Chem. 263*, 3039 (1988).
53. V. Falanga, S. L. Tiegs, S. P. Alstadt, A. B. Roberts, and M. B. Sporn, *J. Invest Dermatol. 89*, 100 (1987).
54. C. M. Overall, J. L. Wrana, and J. Sodek, *J. Biol. Chem. 264*, 1860 (1989).
55. D. R. Edwards, G. Murphy, J. J. Reynolds, S. E. Whitman, A. J. P. Docherty, P. Angel, and J. K. Heath, *EMBO J. 6*, 1899 (1987).
56. M. Laiho, O. Saksela, P. A. Andreasen, and J. Keski-Oja, *J. Cell Biol. 103*, 2403 (1986).
57. T. A. Mustoe, G. F. Pierce, A. Thomason, P. Gramates, M. B. Sporn, and T. F. Deuel, *Science 237*, 1333 (1987).
58. W. E. Smiddy, B. M. Glaser, R. Green, T. B. Connor, A. B. Roberts, and M. B. Sporn, *Arch. Opthalmol. 107*, 577 (1989).
59. M. Kulozik, A. Hogg, B. Lankat-Buttgereit, and T. Kreig, *J. Clin. Invest. 86*, 917 (1990).
60. J. Peltonen, L. Kahari, S. Jaakkola, V. M. Kahari, J. Varga, J. Uitto, and S. A. Jimenez, *J. Invest. Dermatol. 94*, 365 (1990).
61. C. L. Manthey, J. B. Allen, L. R. Ellingsworth, and S. M. Wahl, *Growth Factors 4*, 17 (1990).
62. N. Khalil, O. Bereznay, M. Sporn, and A. H. Greenberg, *J. Exp. Med. 170*, 727 (1989).
63. E. A. Perkett, R. M. Lyons, H. L. Moses, K. L. Brigham, and B. Meyrick, *J. Clin. Invest. 86*, 1459 (1990).
64. T. B. Connor, A. B. Roberts, M. B. Sporn, D. Danielpour, L. L. Dart, R. G. Michels, S. de Bustros, C. Enger, H. Kato, M. Lansing, H. Hayashi, and B. M. Glaser, *J. Clin. Invest. 83*, 1661 (1989).
65. E. A. Smith and E. C. Leroy, *J. Invest. Dermatol. 95*, 1255 (1990).
66. M. Grushwitz, P. D. Nuller, N. Sepp, E. Hofer, A. Fontana, and G. Wick, *J. Invest. Dermatol. 94*, 197 (1990).
67. B. W. Needleman, J. Choi, A. Burrows-Mezu, J. A. Fontana, *Arthritis Rheum. 33*, 650 (1990).
68. W. A. Border, S. Okuda, L. R. Languino, M. B. Sporn, and E. Ruoslahti, *Nature 346*, 6282 (1990).
69. S. M. Wahl, J. B. Allen, H. Wong, and J. Dasch, *J. Exp. Med. 177*, 225 (1993).
70. V. M. Kahari, Y. Q. Chen, M. W. Su, F. Ramirez, and J. Uitto, *J. Clin. Invest 86*, 1489 (1990).
71. A. Castilla, J. Prieto, and N. Fausto, *N. Engl. J. Med. 324*, 933 (1991).

# 11
# Platelet-Derived Growth Factor

**John C. Ansel and Cheryl A. Armstrong**
*Veterans Affairs Medical Center and*
*Oregon Health Sciences University*
*Portland, Oregon*

**Charles E. Hart**
*ZymoGenetics Inc.*
*Seattle, Washington*

## I. INTRODUCTION

Platelet-derived growth factor (PDGF) is a ubiquitous peptide regulatory factor for mesenchymal derived cells. Originally isolated from platelets, PDGF can be synthesized and secreted by a variety of cell types including many neoplastic cells, endothelial cells, fibroblasts, smooth muscle cells, macrophages, monocytes, astrocytes, glial cells, and most recently keratinocytes. Although primarily a growth factor for mesenchymal-derived cells, PDGF acts on other target cells including some types of epithelial cells, endothelial cells, and even leukocytes. Experimental studies indicate that PDGF may have an important role in regulating certain aspects of normal growth and development, rheumatoid arthritis, pulmonary fibrosis, atherosclerosis, neoplasia, wound healing, tissue repair, and certain skin diseases.

This chapter will review the present knowledge concerning the nature of the (a) PDGF molecule, (b) PDGF receptor, (c) biological activities of PDGF, (d) cells that secrete PDGF, (e) the effects of PDGF in various biological responses, and (f) role of PDGF in the skin.

## II. PDGF MOLECULE

PDGF was first isolated from human platelets and consists of two peptide chains denoted A and B with a molecular weight of approximately 16,000 and 14,000, respectively [1–7]. Three PDGF isoforms are possible: the heterodimer PDGF-AB and the homodimers PDGF-AA and PDGF-BB. There is approximately 60% amino acid homology between the A and B chains [8–11]. Each PDGF chain has multiple intra- and interchain disulfide bonds, which are important for maintaining bioactivity [4, 12]. Some cells produce multiple isomers of PDGF, whereas others produce only a single isoform. Platelets, which are a major reservoir of PDGF, contain all three PDGF isoforms in approximately equal amounts [13, 14]. PDGF is a highly cationic molecule with a pI of 9.8–10.0 and a hydrophobic leader sequence, which allows the transport and secretion through cellular membranes [15–17]. The PDGF molecule and its receptor appear to be highly conserved through evolution. Significant structural homology of the PDGF receptor exists for all chordates, and a PDGF-like molecule has been identified even in primitive coelenterates [18–20].

PDGF-A and PDGF-B are encoded from genes containing seven exons, which span approximately 24 kb of genomic DNA. It is likely that the two PDGF genes were derived from a common ancestral gene [21–25]. The A chain gene is located on the proximal long arm of chromosome 7 and codes for three mRNA transcripts with sizes of 1.9, 2.3, and 2.8 kb [24, 26–28], and the PDGF-B chain gene is located on human chromosome 22 and is transcribed into a prominent 3.5–3.7 kb mRNA band and minor 2.6–2.7 kb and 1.3 kb mRNA bands [29–31]. The B chain is encoded by the c-*sis* proto-oncogene, which is the homolog of the simian sarcoma virus oncogene [6, 7, 21, 32–36]. The expression of human PDGF-B gene is regulated by cell type regulatory elements in the first intron [37]. The different sizes of PDGF-A and PDGF-B mRNAs are thought to be due to differential mRNA splicing [22, 24, 27, 28, 31, 38–40].

Significant differences occur in the secretion and processing of the two different PDGF chains [5–7]. Each PDGF chain is synthesized as a large precursor molecule, which is processed intracellularly into smaller molecules. The differences in cellular localization of PDGF-A and PDGF-B appear to reflect variations in peptide processing and are not due to different rates of synthesis [41]. Processing of PDGF does not seem to be necessary for biological activity [42]. PDGF-B is predominately cell membrane associated, whereas PDGF-A is freely secreted [43, 44]. Although PDGF is produced in low or undetectable levels in normal cells, its expression is augmented in response to tissue culture conditions such as cell substrate and confluency [45]. Increased cellular PDGF production is also induced by factors released at the site of injury including transforming growth factor $\beta$ (TGF-$\beta$), tumor necrosis factor $\alpha$ (TNF-$\alpha$), thrombin, epidermal growth factor (EGF), PDGF, and interleukin 1 (IL-1) [46–55]. These agents can differentially regulate the cellular production of the PDGF-A and PDGF-B chains. There are multiple levels of control of cellular PDGF production, including transcription, alternative mRNA synthesis, peptide dimer composition and processing, storage pools, interaction of PDGF with binding proteins and/or matrix, proteolytic cleavage, and specificity of PDGF receptor distribution and expression on target cells.

## III. PDGF RECEPTOR

PDGF activates target cells after binding to high affinity receptors. This initiates a number of intracellular events, including the activation of tyrosine kinase, mobilization of intracellular calcium, phosphorylation of specific intracellular molecules, and ultimately DNA synthesis and cell division. The availability of recombinant PDGF isoforms has made it possible to study the binding of each of these specific molecules to the PDGF receptor. PDGF receptors are found on mesenchymal cells, including fibroblasts, osteoblasts, chondroblasts, smooth muscle cells, glial cells, and some leukocytes and endothelial cells. A wide range of neoplastic cells also express the PDGF receptor.

Mature high affinity PDGF receptors consist of two peptides termed $\alpha$ and $\beta$ receptor subunits [56]. The $\alpha$ and $\beta$ receptor subunits are similar in size and have a relative molecular mass from 170 to 190 kd [57–60]. The $\alpha$ receptor subunit has approximately 40% homology with the $\beta$ subunit [61, 62]. The structure of the two receptor subunits are highly homologous in several regions, particularly the transmembrane region and the split tyrosine kinase region [61]. PDGF receptors contain a large ligand-binding domain in the extracellular portion. This region of the receptor contains five immunoglobulinlike domains indicating that the PDGF receptor is a member of the immunoglobulin superfamily [63]. PDGF receptors remain on the cell surface and have a half-life of approximately 3–4 hours [60, 64]. After ligand binding and receptor aggregation, the half-life decreases to approximately 30 minutes [64–66]. Receptor ligand aggregates disappear from the surface of the cell within 1–2 minutes and are found in endosomes within the cell and subsequently in lysosomes, where both the receptor and PDGF are degraded [64–66].

The binding of PDGF to its receptor has been the topic of a number of recent publications [56, 60, 67–70]. Experimental studies indicate that dimers of the PDGF $\alpha$ and $\beta$ receptor subunits are required for high affinity ligand binding. Exposure of the target cell to the various isoforms of PDGF (AA,AB,BB) recruits and dimerizes the appropriate combination of $\alpha$ or $\beta$ subunits in the cell membrane [68, 71]. There is variable binding specificity by PDGF A and B chains for the two PDGF receptor subunits. PDGF-A binds only to the $\alpha$ subunit, whereas PDGF-B can bind to either the $\alpha$ or the

$\beta$ receptor subunits. Thus PDGF-BB can bind to any one of three receptor subunit combinations ($\alpha\alpha$,$\alpha\beta$,$\beta\beta$); PDGF-AB can bind either to the $\alpha\alpha$ receptor or to the $\alpha\beta$ receptor; and PDGF-AA can bind only to the $\alpha\alpha$ receptor [68]. There can be significant differences in the number of $\alpha$ versus $\beta$ PDGF subunits on different cell types [68]. The response of a given cell type to the different dimeric forms of PDGF is dependent upon both the specific isoforms of PDGF to which they are exposed as well as the number of $\alpha$- and $\beta$-receptor subunits present on the cells [67, 68]. For example, human dermal fibroblasts respond poorly to PDGF-AA, but are highly responsive to PDGF-BB because they express 10 times more $\beta$-receptor subunits compared to the $\alpha$-subunit. In contrast, other cell types such as murine 3T3 cells contain approximately equal amounts of $\alpha$- and $\beta$-receptor subunits and are equally responsive to PDGF-AA and PDGF-BB [68]. Thus the receptor subunit composition on the responding cells as well as amount and type of PDGF ligand will co-determine the capacity of PDGF to be mitogenic and to exert its numerous biological responses.

The dimerization of the $\alpha$ and $\beta$ PDGF receptor subunits by the PDGF isoforms seems to be necessary for signal transmission [71, 72]. Signal transduction by the PDGF receptor is causally associated with a conformational change of the receptor protein in the carboxyl-terminal region of the molecule. The transmembrane region of the PDGF receptor is responsible for transmitting this signal and thus functions as more than a membrane anchor for the molecule [73, 74]. The intracellular portion of the receptor contains a split tyrosine kinase domain. Phosphorylation of several tyrosine molecules in the intracellular domain occurs after PDGF binding to its receptor and appears to be critical for intracellular signaling [75–82]. These signaling molecules include tyrosine and serine kinases [83, 84], phospholipase C-$\gamma$ [85–88], GTPase-activating proteins (GAP) [78, 80, 89], and phosphatidlyinositol 3-kinase (PI3-kinase) [90]. When the PDGF receptor binds to its ligand, the receptor physically associates with the phosphatidylinositol kinase that leads to the production of novel inositol phosphate second messengers [88, 91, 92]. A recent study indicated that the phospholipase C–mediated hydrolysis of phosphatidlycholine is a key step in PDGF-stimulated DNA synthesis [93]. Although the tyrosine kinase activity of the receptor is important for most of the cellular responses to PDGF including mitogenesis, it is not required for ligand-induced receptor downregulation. The intracellular link between tyrosine kinase and the increased expression of PDGF-regulated genes has not yet been identified. The receptor kinase insert domain is important for the specific mitogenic action of PDGF; however, a kinase insert deletion mutant indicates that phosphoinositol turnover, pH change, and increase in cellular calcium are not sufficient to mediate the mitogenic action of PDGF. Future studies on the PDGF receptor and related molecules should provide a more complete picture of the structural changes and intermolecular associations that occur when a ligand binds to its receptor.

In humans, the gene for the $\beta$-receptor chain is located on the long arm of human chromosome 5, close to the site of the gene for the colony-stimulating factor (CSF-1) receptor [94]. The PDGF $\beta$ receptor and the CSF-1 receptors are co-expressed during monocyte differentiation [95]. The PDGF $\alpha$-receptor gene has been mapped to chromosome 4 adjacent to the gene coding for c-kit [96]. The localization of the genes on chromosomes 4 and 5 is an example of gene duplication as both sets of the genes code for receptors containing split tyrosine kinase domains. Both the $\alpha$- and $\beta$-receptor PDGF genes contain a consensus ATP-binding site as well as several ATTTA sequences in the 3′ untranslated region of the gene. This motif has been implicated in regulating the stability of transcripts for several other growth factors and receptors including c-fos and granulocyte-macrophage colony-stimulating factor (GM-CSF).

It is apparent that cells can regulate both PDGF ligand and receptor expression, thus presenting a new level of complexity to the roles of PDGF in vivo. In addition to being able to regulate the form of PDGF made and secreted by a cell, the same cell can also regulate the receptor phenotype by modulating the receptor subunit expression, thus modulating the responsiveness to the secreted PDGF. Therefore, the individual cells would have variable responses to PDGF depending on both the dimer form of PDGF and upon the regulation of its receptor phenotype.

## IV. BIOLOGICAL ACTIVITIES OF PDGF

PDGF has a direct mitogenic effect on most mesenchymal-derived cells as well as some cells of epithelial and endothelial origin [97–102]. As previously indicated, the response of these target cells is dependent on both the PDGF isotype and receptor dimer expressed on the target cell. PDGF may also have an indirect mitogenic effect on target cells by inducing the target cell to produce a second factor that is mitogenic for the cells. For example, PDGF stimulates fibroblasts and smooth muscle cells to secrete somatomedin C, which itself is mitogenic for these cells [103, 104]. A significant amount of the PDGF mitogenic effect on these cells can be inhibited by anti–somatomedin C antisera. PDGF also can induce fibroblasts to secrete PDGF, which could further amplify its mitogenic effect [49].

In addition to mitogenesis, other biological properties of PDGF include cell-directed migration, modification of cellular matrix constituents, and vasoconstriction. PDGF is chemotactic for mesenchymal cells, fibroblasts, smooth muscle cells, and possibly monocytes and neutrophils [105–111] and was recently reported to modulate the production of T-cell cytokines

[112]. PDGF also activates mesenchymal cells to secrete both collagen and collagenase, thus mediating processes such as wound healing and tissue repair [113–116]. It has been reported that PDGF also can stimulate the contraction of some arterial vessels [117].

## V. CELLS THAT SECRETE PDGF

PDGF is expressed and secreted by both normal and transformed cells of connective tissue, muscle, nervous tissue, epithelial tissue, and cells of hematopoietic origin. In normal diploid cells the production of PDGF appears to be tightly regulated.

### A. PDGF Production by Normal Cells

Platelets are anucleate circulating blood cells derived from megakaryocytes in the bone marrow. Platelets are released by the megakaryocyte and have a half-life of 10 days. PDGF in the platelet is formed and packaged in $\alpha$-granules of the megakaryocyte [8]. Platelets appear to be a storage vehicle for active mitogens such as PDGF, which are released upon exposure of platelets to agents such as thrombin, collagen, and ADP. In case of vascular injury, the exposed connective tissue quickly loses its thrombogenic properties and decreased platelet deposition occurs. Thus, although PDGF and other platelet mitogens are widely accessible to a number of tissues, the release of these mitogens is dependent on the thrombogenic properties of the site of injury. There are approximately 0.06 ng of PDGF per $10^6$ human platelets. PDGF is responsible for about 50% of platelet-derived cellular mitogenic activity of serum with the remaining due to EGF and TGF$\beta$. All three isoforms of PDGF (AA,AB,BB) have been detected in platelet extracts [13, 14].

Mononuclear cells are derived from the bone marrow, circulating in the blood as monocytes, and differentiate into macrophages in tissues such as liver, lung, spleen, lymph node, and skin, where they reside for several months. Little PDGF is detected in resting monocytes. When activated by agents such as LPS and immune complexes, cultured macrophages and monocytes express increased PDGF-A and PDGF-B mRNA [109, 118, 119]. They do not store significant amounts of PDGF and thus must synthesize this factor de novo.

Cultured vascular endothelial cells release growth-promoting activity into the culture medium [120]. A significant amount of this activity is due to PDGF [25, 120–122]. Freshly isolated bovine and human umbilical vein endothelial cells express only low levels of PDGF-B mRNA, whereas cultured cells express both PDGF-A and PDGF-B mRNA [122]. Likewise, microvascular endothelial cells can be induced by PMA, thrombin, TGF-$\beta$, and TNF-$\alpha$ to express both PDGF-B and PDGF-A mRNA [46, 123]. Coagulation system components such as thrombin and factor Xa also induce endothelial PDGF production [51, 52].

Vascular smooth muscle cells (SMC) secrete PDGF and respond to PDGF. Thus PDGF may be an autocrine growth factor for these cells. There is evidence that developmentally regulated production of PDGF by vascular smooth muscle cells contributes to the autocrine stimulation of SMC proliferation and biosynthetic activity in the growing rat aorta [124]. Production of PDGF by cultured rat SMC appears to be increased if the SMC have been stimulated to proliferate in vivo as is the case in tissue injury [125]. PDGF-A and PDGF-B mRNA are differentially regulated in aortic smooth muscle cells. Smooth muscle cells from diseased human arteries produce increased quantities of PDGF-AA, which is highly mitogenic for these cells and may contribute to the lesions typical of atherosclerosis.

Normal astrocytes are capable of producing PDGF, which has been proposed to be crucial for the control of myelination in the developing CNS [126]. PDGF is detected throughout brain and posterior pituitary [127] and may act as a neuronal regulatory agent contributing to nerve regeneration and to glial proliferation that leads to gliosis and scarring [127, 128].

Some epithelial cells also are capable of producing PDGF. It has been reported that African green monkey kidney cells and porcine epidermal cells can produce PDGF [129, 130]. Most recently human keratinocytes have been reported to constitutively express PDGF-A mRNA [131–133]. After induction with TGF-$\beta$, both PDGF-A and PDGF-B mRNA are expressed in human keratinocytes. Likewise, significant amounts of PDGF-A are secreted by these cells, whereas PDGF-B is mostly cell associated. Keratinocytes do not express PDGF receptors and thus do not respond to PDGF.

Embryonic cytotrophoblasts have also been reported to be produce both PDGF-A and PDGF-B [134].

## B. PDGF Production by Transformed Cells

There are a variety of transformed cells that are capable of expressing PDGF mRNA and secreting PDGF protein. Some of these transformed cell lines also respond mitogenically to PDGF, whereas others lack PDGF receptors and thus do not respond to this factor. A number of cell-transforming agents and viruses result in increased cellular PDGF production. Cells derived from a wide range of human tumors can express and secrete PDGF, including hepatomas, bladder carcinomas, colon carcinomas, gastric carcinomas, mammary carcinomas, melanomas, mesotheliomas, osteocarcinomas, gliomas, and simian sarcoma virus–transformed cells [8].

## VI. THE EFFECTS OF PDGF IN BIOLOGICAL RESPONSES

### A. Embryogenesis and Development

Embryogenesis and development involve cell proliferation, cell migration, matrix production, and extensive tissue modeling. PDGF is capable of mediating all of these cellular activities, leading investigators to propose that developmentally regulated production of PDGF and its receptors contributes to autocrine stimulation of proliferation in embryogenesis [134–138]. This hypothesis is supported by the demonstration of PDGF-A and PDGF-B mRNA in first and second trimester placentas. In addition, PDGF and PDGF receptors are expressed in developing embryonic endoderm, smooth muscle cells, and cytotrophoblasts.

### B. Atherosclerosis

There is much evidence that PDGF may play a role in the pathogenesis of atherosclerosis [139–141]. The hallmark of this disease process is the marked proliferation of intimal smooth muscle cells and connective tissue in the luminal atherosclerotic plaques [142–144]. These cell types are highly responsive to PDGF. There are several local sources of PDGF in a developing atherosclerotic lesion. Platelets adhere to the luminal surface of the diseased blood vessel and release PDGF [145]. Increased PDGF is also produced in macrophages, endothelial cells, and smooth muscle cells of the atherosclerotic plaques [45, 146–151]. It has been proposed that this local production of PDGF could mediate many of the changes characteristic of atherosclerosis. Supporting this possibility is a recent study in which a polyclonal antibody to PDGF inhibited neointimal smooth muscle accumulation following balloon angioplasty in a rat model of vascular restenosis [140].

### C. Rheumatoid Arthritis

The joint changes in rheumatoid arthritis (RA) are characterized by the proliferation of joint synovial cells, which results in pannus formation, joint fibrosis, bony changes, and a crippling arthritis. Increased PDGF and PDGF receptors have been detected in the synovial tissue and synovial fluid of patients with RA, thus implicating this factor in the pathogenesis of RA [152, 153].

## D. Fibrosis

Fibrosis occurs in a number of pathological disease processes [154]. One such disease group characterized by fibrosis is interstitial pulmonary fibrosis, which is a heterogeneous group of disorders of the lower respiratory tract with alveolar inflammation and fibrosis [155]. The PDGF-secreting pulmonary macrophage appears to be the predominant cell type mediating the inflammatory changes in interstitial pulmonary fibrosis [109, 118, 156, 157].

Fibrosis of the bone marrow may arise as the result of a number of infectious, inflammatory, and neoplastic processes [158]. A common feature is the excess of megakaryocytes and monocytes/macrophages in the bone marrow of patients with these disease processes [158]. These cells are rich sources of PDGF, which is capable of mediating bone marrow inflammatory/fibrotic changes.

Scleroderma is a systemic disease characterized by the proliferation of connective tissue surrounding the blood vessels of the skin and other target tissues. The sera of scleroderma patients have increased mitogenic activity for fibroblasts compared to normal sera [159]. It was found that 70% of this mitogenic activity is due to PDGF. In another study increased PDGF was detected in skin biopsies of scleroderma patients [160]. Thus PDGF may be an important mediating factor in this fibrotic disease.

## E. Neoplasia

There has been much interest in the role of PDGF in neoplasia since the observation that simian sarcoma virus (SSV)–transformed cells secrete a protein p28sis, which is coded for by the oncogene v-sis [6, 7, 35]. This oncogene is 93% homologous with the B-chain of PDGF. Transformation of cells by this oncogene appears to be limited to connective tissue cells that express receptors for PDGF [42]. The transformed phenotype induced by v-sis could be inhibited or blocked by antibodies to PDGF-B or its receptor on the cell surface [161–163]. All of these observations are consistent with the role of PDGF-B in transformation of these cells. The addition of exogenous PDGF to SSV-infected cells will elicit the transformed phenotype in soft agar [164].

Many human tumors express PDGF mRNA and secrete PDGF. It is not clear if the production of PDGF is associated with the initial transformation event or occurs subsequent to initiation of transformation. Likewise, the role of PDGF in the growth and progression of these tumors is not known. A number of the neoplasms that produce PDGF have no receptors for this factor. Thus, PDGF may have an indirect effect on the progression of these tumors by the modulation of the surrounding stroma. Other tumors both produce and respond to PDGF, which may give them a selective advantage in their growth and development. Thus, PDGF may have an autocrine and/or paracrine effect on different human neoplasms.

## F. Wound Healing

PDGF appears to play a major role in normal wound healing. Many of the cells involved in repairing tissue injury are known to either produce and/or respond to PDGF. Tissue injury initiates a sequence of biological responses that have been well characterized in terms of morphological changes that occur at the wound site over time [165–167]. Initially, platelet aggregation to collagen and platelet degranulation initiate clot formation by activation of the coagulation cascade. Activated platelets also release a number of factors including PDGF that are chemotactic for mesenchymal-derived cells and leukocytes [3, 168, 169]. The initial tissue infiltrate of neutrophils, monocytes, and lymphocytes that occurs in the first 1–2 days after injury may be mediated, at least in part, by the local production of leukocyte chemotactic factors. Monocytes differentiate into tissue macrophages and are a major source of growth factors implicated in wound healing including EGF, fibroblast growth factor (FGF), TGF-$\beta$, and PDGF. Macrophages appear to be a key inflammatory cell type in wound healing. In experiments designed to block macrophage influx into a wound site, there is a decrease in the accummulation of fibroblasts and of collagen synthesis [170–172]. Early in the process of wound healing, an extracellular matrix is formed which is largely fibrin and fibronectin. This extracellular matrix acts as the framework for cell migration into the wound. In vitro studies indicate that PDGF stimulates the synthesis of fibronectin and hyalurionic acid [173, 174]. Thrombin and factor Xa produced by the coagulation cascade also induce PDGF secretion by cultured endothelial cells and by microvascular endothelial cells [51, 52]. Locally secreted PDGF is chemotactic and mitogenic for fibroblasts, which migrate into the wound after 48–72 hours and synthesize collagen, elastin, and proteoglycans during the next phase of granulation tissue formation over the next 2–3 weeks [105, 108, 165]. Fibroblasts have also been reported to secrete PDGF after induction by exogenous PDGF [49]. Moreover, there is evidence that microvascular endothelial cells express PDGF receptors, suggesting a role for this factor in wound angiogenesis, which is another prominent feature of this stage of tissue repair [175]. Finally, the late stage of repair consists of remodeling of the wound from 2 weeks to 1 year after injury. PDGF stimulates collagenase, which is required for collagen turnover and tissue repair [114, 176].

Recently, several in vivo studies have directly evaluated the presence of PDGF in wounded skin. PDGF activity was detected in wound fluid that accumulated in subcutaneously implanted stainless steel mesh chambers in vivo [177]. In another study, experimentally induced partial thickness wounds in diabetic human volunteers were biopsied at various times after tissue injury and analyzed by immunohistochemistry for the appearance and location of PDGF-A chain, PDGF-B chain, and PDGF-$\beta$ receptor [178]. PDGF-A chain was detected in the fibrin matrix of early wounds but not in the granulation tissue of later wounds. Additionally, epithelially derived tissue as well as smooth muscle and blood vessels stained positively for PDGF-A. PDGF-B chain was also detected in the epidermis including the migrating tongue of epidermis of early wounds. PDGF-$\beta$ receptor appeared in the granulation tissue of wounds greater than 7 days old but not in epithelial structures. This study provides in vivo evidence that the epidermis is a source of both PDGF-A and -B chains during the process of tissue repair. Another immunohistochemical analysis of normal human skin and chronic human wounds again demonstrated no epidermal staining for PDGF-$\beta$ receptor [179]. In wounds, there was increased staining of dermal fibroblasts and blood vessels for PDGF-$\beta$ receptor compared to normal skin. As in in vitro experiments, the absence of PDGF-$\beta$ receptor on epidermis implies that epidermally derived PDGF functions in a paracrine rather than autocrine manner.

With the availability of recombinant human PDGF, several wound models have been utilized to evaluate the effect of exogenous PDGF on tissue repair. A single application of PDGF-BB to experimental wounds in both rat and rabbit skin was reported to accelerate the recruitment and activation of macrophages and fibroblasts, the deposition of matrix, and the development of wound strength, but did not alter the normal sequence of tissue repair [180–182]. Because healthy animals have intact wound-healing responses, it has been proposed that improvement in wound repair from exogenously added growth factors may be relatively subtle [183]. The use of genetically diabetic mice (db/db) that exhibit impaired healing has shown that treatment with human recombinant PDGF-BB for 5–14 days caused a statistically significant increase in closure of experimentally induced full thickness wounds [183]. PDGF was also reported to restore a normal healing response as measured in subcutaneous wound chambers in drug-induced diabetic mice [184]. Chronic lower extremity ulcerations in humans that represent abnormal healing states have been treated with the topical application of an autologous platelet preparation containing a combination of platelet-derived growth factors and other mediators including PDGF [185, 186]. This treatment led to rapid formation of granulation tissue followed by reepithelialization in a significant number of patients with previously nonhealing wounds.

## VII. CONCLUSION

A large body of research indicates that PDGF is a ubiquitous cytokine that mediates a wide range of normal and pathological conditions including embryogenesis and development, atherosclerosis, rheumatoid arthritis, fibrotic diseases, neoplasia, and wound healing. PDGF is produced by a wide range of normal and neoplastic cell types. It was recently appreciated that keratinocytes located in the epidermis are capable of producing PDGF, thus providing another source of this factor in wound healing, inflammation, and tissue repair in the skin. PDGF production and target cell activation is a complex series of events, which is controlled at many different levels. Understanding the regulation of PDGF production and activity will allow intervention strategies to either inhibit or augment production in certain clinical states. For example, inhibition of PDGF may be useful in rheumatoid arthritis or atherosclerosis, whereas increased PDGF may be helpful in wound healing. Like other cytokines and growth factors, PDGF does not act in isolation but acts on target cells in concert with other soluble factors, thus adding to the complexity of defining the precise role of PDGF in vivo. Future studies will lead to a new understanding of the importance of this ubiquitous growth factor in health and disease.

## REFERENCES

1. H. N. Antoniades, *Proc. Natl. Acad. Sci. USA 78*, 7314 (1981).
2. C.-H. Heldin, B. Westermark, and A. Wasteson, *Biochem. J. 193*, 907 (1981).
3. T. F. Deuel, J. S. Huang, R. T. Proffitt, J. U. Baenziger, D. Chang, and B. B. Kennedy, *J. Biol. Chem. 256*, 8896 (1981).
4. E. W. Raines and R. Ross, *J. Biol. Chem. 257*, 5154 (1982).
5. H. N. Antoniades and M. W. Humkapiller, *Science 220*, 963 (1983).
6. M. D. Waterfield, G. T. Scrace, N. Whittle, P. Stroobant, A. Johnsson, A. Wasteson, B. Westermark, C.-H. Heldin, J. S. Huang, and T. F. Deuel, *Nature 304*, 35 (1983).
7. A. Johnsson, C.-H. Heldin, A. Wasteson, B. Westermark, T. F. Deuel, J. S. Huang, P. H. Seeburg, A. Gray, A. Ullrich, G. Scrace, P. Stroobant, and M. D. Waterfield, *EMBO J. 3*, 921 (1984).
8. R. Ross, E. W. Raines, and D. F. Bowen-Pope, *Cell 46*, 155 (1986).
9. T. F. Deuel, *Ann. Rev. Cell. Biol. 3*, 443 (1987).
10. C. D. Stiles, *Cell 33*, 653 (1983).
11. B. Westermark, C.-H. Heldin, B. Ek, et al., in *Growth and Maturation Factors* (G. Guroff, ed.), Wiley and Sons, Philadelphia, PA, 1983, p. 73.
12. C.-H. Heldin, B. Westermark, and A. Wasteson, *Proc. Natl. Acad. Sci. USA 76*, 3722 (1979).
13. A. Hammacher, U. Helllman, A. Johnsson, A. Ostman, K. Gunnarsson, B. Westermark, A. Wasteson, and C.-H. Heldin, *J. Biol. Chem. 263*, 16493 (1988).

14. C. E. Hart, M. Bailey, D. A. Curtis, S. Osborn, E. W. Raines, R. Ross, and J. W. Forstrom, *Biochemistry 29*, 166 (1990).
15. C.-H. Heldin, A. Wasteson, and B. Westermark, *Exp. Cell. Res. 109*, 429 (1977).
16. R. Ross, A. Vogel, P. Davies, E. Raines, B. Kariya, M. J. Rivest, C. Gustafson, and J. Glomset, in *Hormones in Cell Culture. Cold Spring Harbor Conferences on Cell Proliferation*, Vol. 6, Cold Spring Harbor, New York, 1979, p. 27.
17. H. N. Antoniades, C. D. Scher, and C. D. Stiles, *Proc. Natl. Acad. Sci. USA 76*, 1809 (1979).
18. J. P. Singh, M. A. Chaikin, and C. D. Stiles, *J. Cell. Biol. 95*, 667 (1982).
19. E. W. Raines and R. Ross, *Methods Enzymol. 109*, 749 (1985).
20. H. A. Andersen, H. Flodgaard, H. Klenow, and V. Leick, *Biochim. Biophys. Acta 782*, 437 (1984).
21. I.-M. Chiu, E. P. Reddy, D. Givol, K. C. Robbins, S. R. Tronick, and S. A. Aaronson, *Cell 37*, 123 (1984).
22. T. Collins, D. Ginsburg, J. M. Boss, S. H. Orkin, and J. S. Pober, *Nature 31*, 748 (1985).
23. C. D. Rao, H. Igarashi, I.-M. Chiu, K. C. Robbins, and S. A. Aaronson, *Proc. Natl. Acad. Sci. USA 83*, 2392 (1986).
24. C. Betscholtz, A. Johnsson, C.-H. Heldin, B. Westermark, P. Lind, M. S. Urdea, R. Eddy, T. B. Shows, K. Philpott, A. L. Mellor, T. J. Knott, and J. Scott, *Nature 323*, 226 (1986).
25. T. Collins, D. Ginsburg, J. M. Boss, S. H. Orkin, and J. S. Pober, *Nature 316*, 748 (1985).
26. C. Betsholtz, J. Bergh, M. Bywater, M. Pettersson, A. Johnsson, C.-H. Heldin, R. Ohlsson, T. J. Knott, J. Scott, G. I. Bell, and B. Westermark, *Int. J. Cancer 39*, 502 (1987).
27. D. T. Bonthron, C. C. Morton, S. H. Orkin, and T. Collins, *Proc. Natl. Acad. Sci. USA 85*, 1492 (1988).
28. B. Matoskova, F. Rorsman, V. Svensson, and C. Betsholtz, *Mol. Cell. Biol. 9*, 3148 (1989).
29. R. Dalla Favera, R. C. Gallo, A. Giallongo, and C. M. Croce, *Science 218*, 686 (1982).
30. D. C. Swan, O. W. McBride, K. C. Robbins, D. A. Keithley, E. P. Reddy, and S. A. Aaronson, *Proc. Natl. Acad. Sci. USA 79*, 4691 (1982).
31. T. B. Barrett, C. M. Gajdusek, S. M. Schwartz, J. K. McDougall, and E. P. Benditt, *Proc. Natl. Acad. Sci. USA 81*, 6772 (1984).
32. E. P. Gelmann, F. Wong-Staal, R. A. Kramer, and R. C. Gallo, *Proc. Natl. Acad. Sci. USA 78*, 3373 (1981).
33. P. Besmer, H. W. Snyder, J. E. Murphy, W. D. Hardy, Jr., and A. Parodi, *J. Virol. 46*, 606 (1983).
34. S. G. Devare, E. P. Reddy, D. J. Law, K. C. Robbins, and S. A. Aaronson, *Proc. Natl. Acad. Sci. USA 80*, 731 (1983).
35. R. F. Doolittle, M. W. Hunkapiller, L. E. Hood, S. G. Devare, K. C. Robbins, S. A. Aaronson, and H. N. Antoniades, *Science 221*, 275 (1983).
36. S. F. Josephs, C. Guo, L. Ratner, and F. Wong-Staal, *Science 223*, 487 (1984).

37. G. C. Franklin, M. Donovan, G. I. R. Adam, L. Holmgren, S. Pfeifer-Ohlsson, and R. Ohlsson, *EMBO J. 10*, 1365 (1991).
38. T. Collins, J. S. Pober, M. A. Gimbrone, Jr., A. Hammacher, C. Betsholtz, B. Westermark, and C.-H. Heldin, *Am. J. Pathol. 127*, 7 (1987).
39. B. D. Tong, D. E. Auer, M. Jaye, J. M. Kaplow, G. Ricca, E. McConathy, W. Drohan, and T. F. Deuel, *Nature 328*, 619 (1987).
40. F. Rorsman, M. Bywater, T. J. Knott, J. Scott, and C. Betsholtz, *Mol. Cell. Biol. 8*, 571 (1988).
41. M. Bywater, F. Rorsman, E. Bongcam-Rudloff, G. Mark, A. Hammacher, C.-H. Heldin, B. Westermark, and C. Betsholtz, *Mol. Cell. Biol. 8*, 2753 (1988).
42. F. Leal, L. T. Williams, K. C. Robbins, and S. A. Aaronson, *Science 230*, 327 (1985).
43. K. C. Robbins, F. Leal, J. A. Pierce, and S. A. Aaronson, *EMBO J. 4*, 1783 (1985).
44. M. P. Beckmann, C. Betsholtz, C.-H. Heldin, B. Westermark, E. DiMarco, P. P. DiFiore, K. C. Robbins, and S. A. Aaronson, *Science 241*, 1346 (1988).
45. M. Sjolund, U. Hedin, T. Sejersen, C.-H. Heldin, and J. Thyberg, *J. Cell. Biol. 106*, 403 (1988).
46. W. M. Kavanaugh, G. R. Harsh, N. F. Starksen, C. M. Rocco, and L. T. Williams, *J. Biol. Chem. 263*, 8470 (1988).
47. N. F. Starksen, G. R. Harsh, V. C. Gibbs, and L. T. Williams, *J. Biol. Chem. 262*, 14381 (1987).
48. K. A. Hajjar, D. P. Hajjar, R. L. Silverstein, and R. L. Nachman, *J. Exp. Med. 166*, 235 (1987).
49. Y. Paulsson, A. Hammacher, C.-H. Heldin, and B. Westermark, *Nature 328*, 715 (1987).
50. E. W. Raines, S. K. Dower, and R. Ross, *Science 243*, 393 (1989).
51. J. M. Harlan, P. J. Thompson, R. Ross, and D. F. Bowen-Pope, *J. Cell. Biol. 103*, 1129 (1986).
52. C. Gajdusek, S. Carbon, R. Ross, P. Nawroth, and D. Stern, *J. Cell. Biol. 103*, 419 (1986).
53. T. O. Daniels and Z. Fen, *J. Biol. Chem. 263*, 19815 (1988).
54. E. B. Leof, J. A. Proper, A. S. Goustin, G. D. Shipley, P. E. DiCorleto, and H. L. Moses, *Proc. Natl. Acad. Sci. USA 83*, 2453 (1986).
55. E. J. Battegay, E. W. Raines, R. A. Siefert, D. F. Bowen-Pope, and R. Ross, *Cell 63*, 515 (1990).
56. D. F. Bowen-Pope, C. E. Hart, and R. A. Seifert, *J. Biol. Chem. 264*, 2502 (1989).
57. K. Glenn, D. F. Bowen-Pope, and R. Ross, *J. Biol. Chem. 257*, 5172 (1982).
58. C.-H. Heldin, B. Ek, and L. Ronnstrand, *J. Biol. Chem. 258*, 10054 (1983).
59. L. T. Williams, P. M. Tremble, M. F. Lavin, and M. E. Sunday, *J. Biol. Chem. 259*, 5287 (1984).
60. C. E. Hart, R. A. Seifert, R. Ross, and D. F. Bowen-Pope, *J. Biol. Chem. 262*, 10780 (1987).
61. T. Matsui, M. Heidaran, T. Miki, N. Popescu, W. LaRochelle, M. Kraus, J. Pierce, and S. Aaronson, *Science 243*, 800 (1989).

62. L. Claesson-Welsh, A. Eriksson, B. Westermark, and C.-H. Heldin, *Proc. Natl. Acad. Sci. USA 86*, 4917 (1989).
63. L. Claesson-Welsh, A. Eriksson, A. Moren, L. Severinsson, B. Ek, A. Ostman, C. Betsholtz, and C.-H. Heldin, *Mol. Cell. Biol. 8*, 3476 (1988).
64. S. S. Huang and J. S. Huang, *J. Biol. Chem. 263*, 12608 (1988).
65. C. E. Hart, J. W. Forstrom, J. D. Kelly, R. A. Smith, R. Ross, M. J. Murray, and D. F. Bowen-Pope, in *Growth Factors and their Receptors: Genetic Control and Rational Applications*, Vol. 102, Liss, New York, 1989, p. 297.
66. M. T. Keating and L. T. Williams, *Science 239*, 914 (1988).
67. C. E. Hart, J. W. Forstrom, J. D. Kelly, R. A. Seifert, R. A. Smith, R. Ross, M. J. Murray, and D. F. Bowen-Pope, *Science 240*, 1529 (1988).
68. R. A. Seifert, C. E. Hart, P. E. Phillips, J. W. Forstrom, R. Ross, M. J. Murray, and D. F. Bowen-Pope, *J. Biol. Chem. 264*, 8771 (1988).
69. C. E. Hart and D. F. Bowen-Pope, *J. Invest. Dermatol. 94*, 53 (1990).
70. C.-H. Heldin, G. Backstrom, A. Ostman, A. Hammacher, L. Ronnstrand, K. Rubin, M. Nister, and B. Westermark, *EMBO J. 7*, 1387 (1988).
71. C.-H. Heldin, A. Ernlund, C. Rorsman, and L. Ronnstrand, *J. Biol. Chem. 264*, 8905 (1989).
72. W. Li and J. Schlessinger, *Mol. Cell. Biol. 11*, 3756 (1991).
73. L. T. Williams, *Science 243*, 1564 (1989).
74. J. A. Escobedo, P. J. Barr, and L. T. Williams, *Mol. Cell. Biol. 8*, 5126 (1988).
75. B. Ek and C.-H. Heldin, *J. Biol. Chem. 257*, 10486 (1982).
76. J. Nishimura, J. S. Huang, and T. F. Deuel, *Proc. Natl. Acad. Sci. USA 79*, 4303 (1982).
77. L. J. Pike, D. Bowen-Pope, R. Ross, and E. G. Krebs, *J. Biol. Chem. 258*, 9383 (1983).
78. A. Kazlauskas, C. Ellis, T. Pawson, and J. A. Cooper, *J. Biol. Chem. 263*, 12805 (1988).
79. E. B. Pasquale, P. A. Maher, and S. J. Singer, *J. Cell. Physiol. 137*, 146 (1988).
80. C. J. Molloy, D. P. Bottaro, T. P. Fleming, M. S. Marshall, J. B. Gibbs, and S. A. Aaronson, *Eur. J. Biochem. 191*, 761 (1989).
81. A. Kazlauskas and J. A. Cooper, *Cell 58*, 1121 (1989).
82. K. L. Gould and T. Hunter, *Mol. Cell. Biol. 8*, 3345 (1988).
83. R. M. Kypta, Y. Goldberg, E. T. Ulug, and S. A. Courtneidge, *Cell 62*, 481 (1990).
84. D. K. Morrison, D. R. Kaplan, J. A. Escobedo, U. R. Rapp, T. M. Roberts, and L. T. Williams, *Cell 58*, 649 (1989).
85. D. A. Kumjian, M. I. Wahl, S. G. Rhee, and T. O. Daniel, *Proc. Natl. Acad. Sci. USA 86*, 8232 (1989).
86. J. Meisenhelder, P.-G. Suh, S. G. Rhee, and T. Hunter, *Cell 57*, 1109 (1989).
87. D. K. Morrison, D. R. Kaplan, S. G. Rhee, and L. T. Williams, *Mol. Cell. Biol. 10*, 2359 (1990).
88. M. I. Wahl, N. E. Olashaw, S. Nishibe, S. G. Rhee, W. J. Pleger, and G. Carpenter, *Mol. Cell. Biol. 9*, 2934 (1989).
89. D. R. Kaplan, D. K. Morrison, G. Wong, F. McCormick, and L. T. Williams, *Cell 61*, 125 (1990).

90. S. R. Coughlin, J. A. Escobedo, and L. T. Williams, *Science 243*, 1191 (1989).
91. D. A. Kumjian, M. I. Wahl, S. G. Rhee, and T. O. Daniel, *Proc. Natl. Acad. Sci. USA 86*, 8232 (1989).
92. B. Margolis, A. Zilberstein, C. Franks, S. Felder, S. Kremer, A. Ullrich, S. G. Rhee, K. Skorecki, and J. Schlessinger, *Science 248*, 607 (1990).
93. P. Larrodera, M. E. Cornet, M. T. Diaz-Meco, M. Lopez-Barahona, I. Diaz-Laviada, P. H. Guddal, T. Johansen, and J. Moscat, *Cell 61*, 1113 (1990).
94. W. M. Roberts, A. T. Look, M. F. Roussel, and C. J. Sherr, *Cell 55*, 655 (1988).
95. P. Pantazis, S. Kharbanda, A. S. Goustin, T. Galanopoulos, and D. Kufe, *Proc. Natl. Acad. Sci. USA 88*, 2481 (1991).
96. T. Matsui, M. Heidaran, T. Miki, N. Popescu, W. La Rochelle, M. Kraus, J. Pierce, and S. Aaronson, *Science 243*, 800 (1989).
97. N. Kohler and A. Lipton, *Exp. Cell Res. 87*, 297 (1974).
98. R. Ross, J. A. Glomset, B. Kariya, and L. Harker, *Proc. Natl. Acad. Sci. USA 71*, 1207 (1974).
99. R. B. Rutherford and R. Ross, J. Cell. Biol. 69, 196 (1976).
100. C. Busch, A. Wasteson, and B. Westermark, *Thromb. Res. 8*, 493 (1976).
101. B. Westermark and A. Wasteson, *Exp. Cell. Res. 98*, 170 (1976).
102. B. Brewitt and J. I. Clark, *Science 242*, 777 (1988).
103. D. R. Clemmons, L. E. Underwood, and J. J. Van Wyk, *J. Clin. Invest. 67*, 10 (1981).
104. D. R. Clemmons and J. J. Van Wyk, *J. Clin. Invest. 75*, 1914 (1985).
105. H. Seppa, G. Grotendorst, S. Seppa, E. Schiffmann, and G. R. Martin, *J. Cell. Biol. 92*, 584 (1982).
106. G. Grotendorst, H. E. J. Seppa, H. K. Kleimnan, and G. Martin, *Proc. Natl. Acad. Sci. USA 78*, 3669 (1981).
107. G. R. Grotendorst, T. Chang, H. E. J. Seppa. H. K. Kleinman, and G. R. Martin, *J. Cell. Physiol. 113*, 261 (1982).
108. G. Grotendorst, *Cell 36*, 279 (1984).
109. Y. Martinet, P. B. Bitterman, J.-F. Mornex, G. R. Grotendorst, G. R. Martin, and R. G. Crystal, *Nature 319*, 158 (1986).
110. T. F. Deuel, R. M. Senior, J. S. Huang, and G. L. Griffin, *J. Clin. Invest. 69*, 1046 (1982).
111. L. T. Williams, H. N. Antoniades, and E. J. Goetzl, *J. Clin. Invest. 72*, 1759 (1983).
112. R. A. Raymond, A. Daynes, T. Dowell, and B. A. Araneo, *J. Exp. Med. 174*, 1323 (1991).
113. E. Canalis, *Metabolism 30*, 970 (1981).
114. C. C. Chua, D. E. Geiman, G. H. Keller, and R. L. Ladda, *J. Biol. Chem. 260*, 5213 (1985).
115. A. S. Narayanan and R. C. Page, *J. Biol. Chem. 258*, 11694 (1983).
116. A. J. Owen, R. P. Geyer, and H. N. Antoniades, *Proc. Natl. Acad. Sci. USA 79*, 3203 (1982).
117. B. C. Berk, R. W. Alexander, T. A. Brock, M. A. Gimbrone, and C. R. Webb, *Science 232*, 87 (1986).

118. K. Shimokado, E. W. Raines, D. K. Madtes, T. B. Barrett, E. P. Benditt, and R. Ross, *Cell 43*, 277 (1985).
119. J.-F. Mornex, Y. Martinet, K. Yamauchi, P. B. Bitterman, G. R. Grotendorst, A. Chytil-Weir, G. R. Martin, and R. G. Crystal, *J. Clin. Invest. 78*, 61 (1986).
120. P. E. DiCorleto and D. F. Bowen-Pope, *Proc. Natl. Acad. Sci. USA 80*, 1919 (1983).
121. M. Jaye, E. McConathy, W. Droham, B. Tong, T. Deuel, and T. Maciag, *Science 228*, 882 (1984).
122. T. B. Barrett, C. M. Gajdusek, S. M. Schwartz, J. K. McDougall, and E. P. Benditt, *Proc. Natl. Acad. Sci. USA 81*, 6772 (1984).
123. T. O. Daniel, V. C. Gibbs, D. F. Milfay, M. R. Garovoy, and L. T. Williams, *J. Biol. Chem. 261*, 9579 (1986).
124. R. A. Seifert, S. M. Schwartz, and D. F. Bowen-Pope, *Nature 311*, 669 (1984).
125. L. N. Walker, D. F. Bowen-Pope, R. Ross, and M. A. Reidy, *Proc. Natl. Acad. Sci. USA 83*, 7311 (1986).
126. W. D. Richardson, N. Pringle, M. J. Mosley, B. Westermark, and M. Dubois-Dalcq, *Cell 53*, 309 (1988).
127. M. Sasahara, J. W. U. Fries, E. W. Raines, A. M. Gown, L. E. Westrum, M. P. Frosch, D. T. Bonthron, R. Ross, and T. Collins, *Cell 64*, 217 (1991).
128. H. J. Yeh, K. G. Ruit, Y. X. Wang, W. C. Parks, W. D. Snider, and T. F. Deuel, *Cell 64*, 109 (1991).
129. S. Kartha, D. M. Bradham, G. R. Grotendorst, and F. G. Toback, *Am. J. Physiol. 255*, F800 (1988).
130. H. N. Antoniades, T. Galanopoulos, J. Neville-Golden, C. P. Kiritsy, and S. E. Lynch, *Proc. Natl. Acad. Sci. USA 88*, 565 (1991).
131. D. C. Damm, G. D. Shipley, C. E. Hart, and J. C. Ansel, in *Molecular and Cellular Biology of Cytokines* (J. Oppenheim, M. C. Powanda, M. J. Kluger, C. Dinarello, eds.), Wiley-Liss, New York, 1990, p. 111.
132. J. C. Ansel, D. C. Tara, J. Krueger, J. Olerud, C. Hart, *J. Invest. Dermatol. 98*, 565 (1992).
133. J. Ansel, P. Perry, J. Brown, D. Damm, T. Phan, C. Hart, T. Luger, and S. Hefeneider, *J. Invest. Dermatol. 94*, 101S (1990).
134. A. S. Goustin, C. Betsholtz, S. Pfeiffer-Ohlsson, H. Persson, J. Rydnert, M. Bywater, G. Holmgren, C.-H. Heldin, B. Westermark, and R. Ohlsson, *Cell 41*, 301 (1985).
135. R. N. Taylor and L. T. Williams, *Mol. Endocrinol. 2*, 627 (1988).
136. B. H. Cochran, J. Zullo, I. M. Verma, C. D. Stiles, *Science 226*, 1080 (1984).
137. M. Mercola, D. A. Melton, and C. D. Stiles, *Science 241*, 1223 (1988).
138. D. A. Rappolee, C. A. Brenner, R. Schultz, D. Mark, and Z. Werb, *Science 241*, 1823 (1988).
139. M. A. Golden, Y. P. Tina Au, T. R. Kirkman, J. N. Wilcox, E. W. Raines, R. Ross, A. W. Clowes, *J. Clin. Invest. 87*, 406 (1991).
140. G. A. A. Ferns, E. W. Raines, K. H. Sprugel, A. S. Motani, M. A. Reidy, R. Ross, *Science 253*, 1129 (1991).
141. T. A. McCaffrey, A. C. Nicholson, P. E. Szasbo, M. E. Weksler, and B. B. Weksler, *J. Exp. Med. 167*, 163 (1988).

142. R. Ross and J. A. Glomset, *Science 180*, 1332 (1973).
143. R. Ross and J. A. Glomset, *N. Engl. J. Med. 295*, 369 (1976).
144. R. Ross, *N. Engl. J. Med. 314*, 488 (1986).
145. S. R. Hanson and L. A. Harker, *Proc. Natl. Acad. Sci. USA 85*, 3184 (1988).
146. P. Libby, S. J. C. Warner, R. N. Salomon, and L. K. Birinyi, *N. Engl. J. Med. 318*, 1493 (1988).
147. J. N. Wilcox, K. M. Smith, L. T. Williams, S. M. Schwartz, and D. Gordon, *J. Clin. Invest. 82*, 1134 (1988).
148. T. B. Barrett and E. P. Benditt, *Proc. Natl. Acad. Sci. USA 84*, 1099 (1987).
149. T. Sejersen, C. Betsholtz, M. Sjolund, C.-H. Heldin, B. Westermark, and J. Thyberg, *Proc. Natl. Acad. Sci. 83*, 6844 (1986).
150. M. W. Majesky, E. P. Benditt, and S. M. Schwartz, *Proc. Natl. Acad. Sci. 85*, 1524 (1988).
151. P. Jin, M. Rahm, L. Claesson-Welsh, C.-H. Heldin, and T. Sejersen, *J. Cell Biol. 110*, 1665 (1990).
152. K. Rubin, L. Terracio, L. Ronnstrand, C.-H. Heldin, and L. Klareskog, *Scand. J. Immunol. 27*, 285 (1988).
153. D. Hamerman, S. Taylor, I. Kirschenbaum, M. Klagsbrun, E. W. Raines, R. Ross, and K. A. Thomas, *Proc. Soc. Exp. Biol. Med. 186*, 384 (1987).
154. T. F. Deuel and R. M. Senior, *N. Engl. J. Med. 317*, 236 (1987).
155. A. R. Brody and J. E. Craighead, *Virchows Arch. 372*, 39 (1976).
156. Y. Martinet, W. N. Rom, G. R. Grotendorst, G. R. Martin, and R. G. Crystal, *N. Engl. J. Med. 317*, 202 (1987).
157. I. Nagaoka, B. C. Trapnell, and R. G. Crystal, *J. Clin. Invest. 85*, 2023 (1990).
158. H. S. Gilbert, in *Myelofibrosis and the Biology of Connective Tissue* (P. D. Berk, H. Castro-Malaspina, and L. R. Wasserman, eds.), Liss, New York, 1984, p. 3.
159. K. Takehara, G. R. Grotendorst, R. Silver, and E. C. LeRoy, *Arteriosclerosis 7*, 152 (1987).
160. S. Gay, R. E. Jones, G. Huang, R. E. Gay, *J. Invest. Dermatol. 92*, 301 (1989).
161. J. S. Garrett, S. R. Coughlin, H. L. Niman, P. M. Tremble, G. M. Giels, and L. T. Williams, *Cell Biol. 81*, 7466 (1984).
162. J. S. Huang, S. S. Huang, and T. F. Deuel, *Proc. Natl. Acad. Sci. USA 81*, 342 (1984).
163. A. Johnsson, C. Betsholtz, K. von der Helm, C.-H. Heldin, and B. Westermark, *Proc. Natl. Acad. Sci. USA 82*, 1721 (1985).
164. R. K. Assoian, G. R. Grotendorst, D. M. Miller, and M. B. Sporn, *Nature 309*, 804 (1984).
165. V. Falanga, J. A. Zitelli, and W. H. Eaglstein, *J. Am. Acad. Dermatol. 19*, 559 (1988).
166. R. Ross, *Biol. Rev. 43*, 51 (1968).
167. R. A. Clark, *Curr. Opin. Cell Biol. 1*, 1000 (1989).
168. S. M. Wahl, D. A. Hunt, L. M. Wakefield, N. McCartney-Francis, L. M. Wahl, A. B. Roberts, and M. B. Sporn, *Proc. Natl. Acad. Sci. USA 84*, 5788 (1987).

169. R. M. Senior, G. L. Griffin, J. S. Huang, D. A. Walz, and T. F. Deuel, *J. Cell. Biol. 96*, 382 (1983).
170. S. J. Liebovich and R. Ross, *Am. J. Pathol. 78*, 71 (1975).
171. G. F. Pierce, T. A. Mustoe, J. Lingelbach, V. R. Masakowski, P. Gramates, and T. F. Deuel, *Proc. Natl. Acad. Sci. USA 86*, 2229 (1989).
172. T. A. Mustoe, J. Purdy, P. Gramates, T. F. Deuel, A. Thomason, and G. F. Pierce, *Am. J. Surg. 158*, 345 (1989).
173. S. P. Blatti, D. N. Foster, G. Ranganathan, H. L. Moses, and M. J. Getz, *Proc. Natl. Acad. Sci. USA 85*, 1119 (1988).
174. P. Heldin, T. C. Laurent, and C.-H. Heldin, *Biochem. J. 258*, 919 (1989).
175. M. Hermansson, M. Nister, C. Betsholtz, C.-H. Heldin, B. Westermark, and K. Funa, *Proc. Natl. Acad. Sci. USA 85*, 7748 (1988).
176. E. A. Bauer, T. W. Cooper, J. S. Huang, J. Altman, T. F. Deuel, *Proc. Natl. Acad. Sci. USA 82*, 4132 (1985).
177. G. R. Grotendorst, C. A. Grotendorst, and T. Gilman, in *Growth Factors and Other Aspects of Wound Healing: Biological and Clinical Implications*, Liss, New York, 1988, p. 47.
178. J. E. Olerud, M. L. Usui, and C. E. Hart, *J. Invest. Dermatol. 96*, 563 (1991).
179. J. F. Krane, D. P. Murphy, A. B. Gottlieb, D. M. Carter, C. E. Hart, and J. G. Krueger, *J. Invest. Dermatol. 96*, 983 (1991).
180. G. F. Pierce, T. A. Mustoe, R. M. Senior, J. Reed, G. L. Griffin, A. Thomason, and T. F. Deuel, *J. Exp. Med. 167*, 974 (1988).
181. T. A. Mustoe, G. F. Pierce, C. Morishima, and T. F. Deuel, *J. Clin. Invest. 87*, 694 (1991).
182. G. F. Pierce, J. Vande Berg, R. Rudolph, J. Tarpley, and T. A. Mustoe, *Am. J. Path. 138*, 629 (1991).
183. D. G. Greenhalgh, K. H. Sprugel, M. J. Murray, and R. Ross, *Am. J. Path. 136*, 1235 (1990).
184. G. R. Grotendorst, G. R. Martin, D. Pencev, J. Sodeck, and A. K. Harvey, *J. Clin. Invest. 76*, 2323 (1985).
185. D. R. Knighton, M. Doucette, V. D. Fiegel, K. Ciresi, E. Butler, and L. Austin, in *Growth Factors and Other Aspects of Wound Healing: Biological and Clinical Implications*, Liss, New York, 1988, p. 319.
186. D. R. Knighton, K. F. Ciresi, V. D. Fiegel, L. L. Austin, and E. L. Butler, *Ann. Surg. 204*, 322 (1986).

# 12

# Fibroblast Growth Factors

**Ruth Halaban and Gisela Moellmann**
*Yale University School of Medicine*
*New Haven, Connecticut*

## I. INTRODUCTION

Fibroblast growth factors (FGFs) are heparin-binding peptides with multifunctional regulatory properties. Seven members of this growth factor family are known and share significant sequence identity (up to 55%). They are acidic FGF (aFGF), basic FGF (bFGF), Int-2, K-FGF/Hst-1, FGF-5, FGF-6/Hst-2, and keratinocyte growth factor (KGF) [1–9]. These have recently been renamed FGF-1 through FGF-7, respectively [10]. Four are putative oncogene products (FGF-3, FGF-4, FGF-5, and FGF-6) [3, 5–8, 11, 12].

Acidic and basic FGF were the first identified and are still the best characterized members of the FGF family. Their three-dimensional structure was determined by x-ray crystallography and shows homology to interleukin 1$\beta$ (IL-1$\beta$) [13–15]. These two FGFs are different from the others in that they lack a signal peptide that would allow them to be secreted through the classic secretory pathway [1–9]. Even so, both aFGF and bFGF are present in extracellular matrix [16–19].

The in vitro effects of aFGF and bFGF appear to be similar and very complex. These two peptides are mitogenic toward cells of mesenchymal, neuronal, and epidermal origin (reviewed in Refs. 10, 20–21). They promote survival and differentiation of specific classes of neurons [22–24], are potently angiogenic [25], and enhance the migration and invasion properties of endothelial [26, 27] and epithelial cells [28]. Other functions of bFGF include induction of mesoderm in early *Xenopus* development [29–31], prevention of differentiation of skeletal myoblasts [32], and support of early hematopoiesis [33]. Acidic FGF induces the formation of organoid neovascular structures [34]. Basic FGF is widely distributed, localized in basement membranes and in cells of mesodermal and neuroectodermal origin of various organs such as adrenal glands, testes and ovaries, both in embryos and adults [17–21]. Acidic FGF is found in the synovium of patients with rheumatoid arthritis [35], and bFGF is released from endothelial cells on wounding [36]. These widespread distributions and diverse biological effects suggest that aFGF and bFGF function not only in development, but also in inflammation and wound healing.

FGFs in the skin are of importance because they stimulate the proliferation of keratinocytes, fibroblasts, melanocytes, and endothelial cells [25, 37–41] and have implicit impact on abnormal as well as normal cutaneous processes. In pig skin, a single application of human recombinant bFGF at the time of injury accelerates the rate of epithelialization by 20%, suggesting the potential for application of this growth factor in clinical medicine [42]. In this review we focus on the role of FGFs in melanocyte proliferation, differentiation, and malignant transformation and summarize the latest developments in the identification of receptors and intermediate substrates in the FGF signal transduction pathway.

## II. MELANOCYTE PROLIFERATION

In order to proliferate in vitro, normal human melanocytes need at least two mutually synergistic factors in addition to the common growth factors required by all mammalian cells. FGFs mitogenic for melanocytes are bFGF, aFGF, K-FGF/Hst-1, FGF-5, and FGF-6 [38, 41, 43–45]. Factors identified to act in synergy with FGF are those that raise intracellular levels of cAMP (cyclic adenosine monophosphate) to activate protein kinase A (e.g., dibutyryl cAMP), TPA (12-*O*-tetradecanoyl phorbol-13-acetate), which activates protein kinase C, and hepatocyte growth factor (HGF), which activates Met, a receptor protein tyrosine kinase [38, 41, 43–47] (Fig. 1).

Basic FGF appears to play a central role in melanocyte biology. In situ, the peptide is provided by basal keratinocytes [48, 49]. Unlike other cells that respond to bFGF, normal melanocytes do not produce this peptide on their own. Basic FGF is expressed neither at the mRNA nor at the protein level [41, 44, 50]. In fact, melanocytes do not produce any mitogen that stimulates their own growth (our unpublished results), which is the reason for their failure to proliferate in media suitable for other cell types, including metastatic melanoma cells. In contrast, proliferating fibroblasts and keratinocytes produce bFGF and, in co-culture with melanocytes, maintain melanocyte viability (Fig. 2) [51, 52]. Like purified bFGF and other melanocyte growth factors, the melanocyte mitogens that are present in whole-cell extract of fibroblasts and keratinocytes depend on at least one of the above-

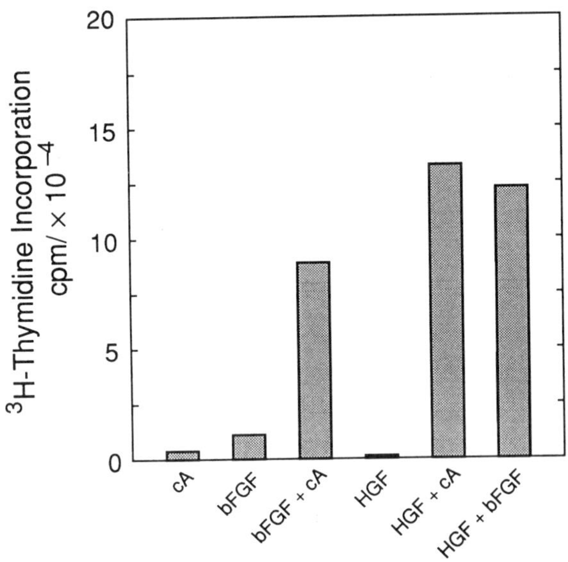


**Figure 1** Synergy among melanocyte growth factors. Normal human neonatal melanocytes were incubated in PC-1 defined medium with different combinations of melanocyte-growth factor for 24 h, and DNA synthesis was determined during the last 3 h by $^3$H-thymidine incorporation. Additions were basic fibroblast growth factor (bFGF, 1 ng/ml), hepatocyte growth factor (HGF, 20 ng/ml), and dibutyryl cyclic AMP (cA, 1.0 mM), as indicated.

cited synergistic factors. Among cultured skin cells, dermal fibroblasts contain the highest melanocyte-directed mitogenic activity, five times as much as proliferating keratinocytes [51] (Table 1 and Fig. 3). Irradiation of proliferating keratinocytes with ultraviolet B (UVB) doubles the level of their activity. Stratifying keratinocytes possess by far the lowest concentration of melanocyte mitogen. Neutralizing anti-bFGF antibodies inhibit the melanocyte mitogen is stratifying keratinocytes and proliferating keratinocytes by 95% [140]. Failure to abolish 100% of the activity with doses of antibodies sufficient to inhibit similar activity of pure bFGF suggests that proliferating keratinocytes contain additional melanocyte mitogens. Indeed, we have recently identified mast cell growth factor (MGF), known also as Kit-ligand, steel-ligand, and stem cell growth factor [53–57], as a melanocyte mitogen [58], demonstrated production of MGF by proliferating keratinocytes, and detected MGF-mRNA in the epidermis [141]. These findings suggest that, in vivo, melanocytes are regulated by keratinocyte-derived mito-

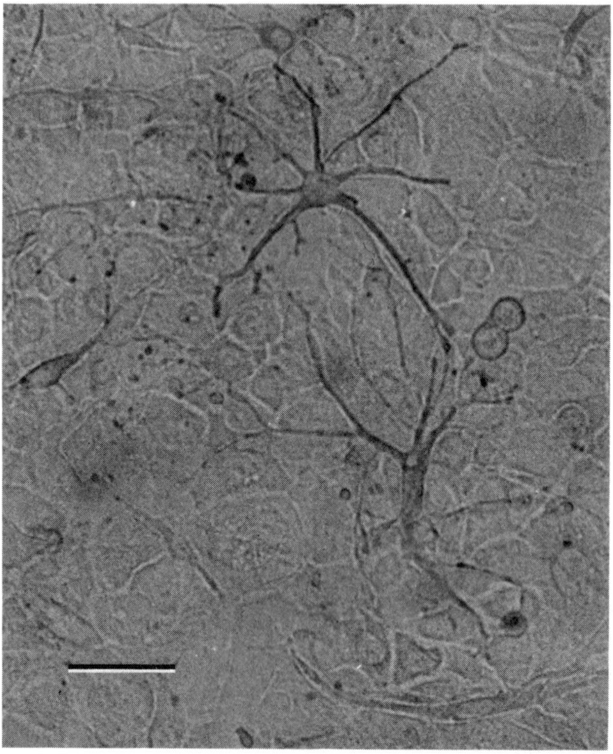

**Figure 2** Phase micrograph of melanocytes co-cultured with keratinocytes in keratinocyte growth medium containing low calcium and pituitary extract. Note the dendritic morphology of the melanocytes induced by contact with proliferating keratinocytes. This morphology was not observed in the absence of keratinocytes. The small black dots are packages of melanin granules, transferred into keratinocytes from the tips of the melanocytic dendrites. (See Ref. 51 for more experimental details.) Scale bar, approx 50 $\mu$m.

gens, the abundance of which is augmented by at least one agent that also induces pigmentation, namely UVB.

The demonstration that, in vitro, rapidly proliferating keratinocytes produce much higher levels of bFGF than do stratifying keratinocytes is in agreement with the preferred location and/or activity of melanocytes in intact skin, i.e., at the bottom of deep epidermal ridges. This location correlates with the site of highest $^3$H-thymidine uptake (80%) by normal human and simian palmar epidermis [59]. It is thus likely that proliferating keratinocytes stimulate neighboring melanocytes to divide and/or produce more

**Table 1** Relative Levels of Melanocyte Mitogen in Cells Derived from Skin

| Cell type | Dose needed to obtain 50% mitogenic response in human melanocytes ($\mu$g protein/ml) |
|---|---|
| Keratinocytes, stratifying | >160 |
| Keratinocytes, proliferating | 10 |
| Keratinocytes, proliferating, after UVB | 5 |
| Fibroblasts | 2 |

Mitogenic response of human melanocytes to extracts of human keratinocytes and fibroblasts. Neonatal melanocytes were incubated with increasing doses of extract, and DNA synthesis was determined 24 h later as for Figure 1. Cell extracts were added in PC-1 defined medium plus 1 mM dibutyryl cyclic AMP. UVB dose, 150 mJ/cm$^2$. Numbers indicate amount of protein required to elicit 50% of maximum $^3$H-thymidine incorporation. (See also Fig. 3. For more details see Ref. 51.)

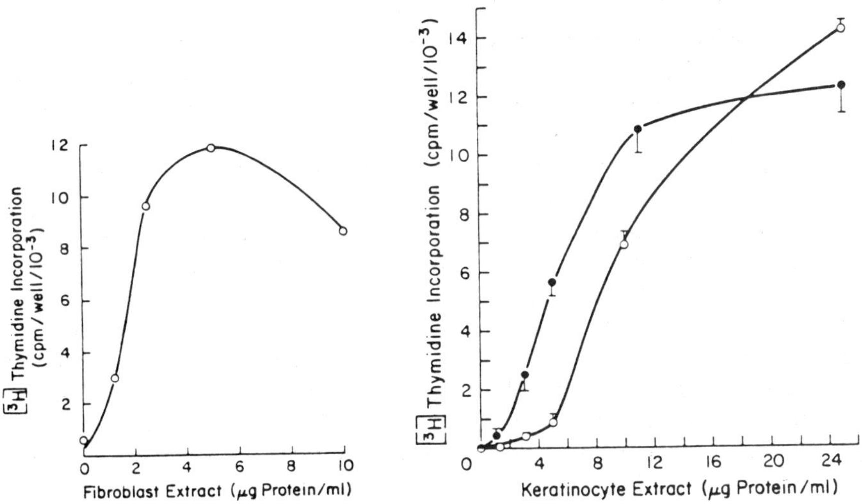


**Figure 3** Mitogenic stimulation of human melanocytes by extracts of human dermal fibroblasts (left) and keratinocytes (right). Extracts were added to melanocyte cultures in PC-1 defined medium plus 1 mM dibutyryl cAMP. The cells were incubated for 24 h and DNA synthesis was determined as for Figure 1. Keratinocytes were harvested after UVB irradiation (●), or without irradiation (○). (Other details as in Table 1 and Ref. 51.)

melanin. Another well-known site of growth-associated, cyclic melanocyte activity is in the anagen hair follicle, where melanocytes come to lie in close proximity to the rapidly proliferating keratinocytes that constitute the cellular bulb matrix. Anagen hair bulbs from rats, like bFGF, are highly angiogenic [60], hair bulbs of sheep produce bFGF [61], and in mice UVB irradiation causes a correlative increase in the mitotic index of both melanocytes and basal keratinocytes [62].

## III. MELANOCYTE DIFFERENTIATION

Exogenous bFGF promotes not only melanocyte proliferation but also differentiation. As shown with embryonic quail dorsal root ganglia [63], stimulation of expression of the melanocytic phenotype by bFGF is fully effective only in the presence of TPA, indicating that differentiation, too, requires a synergistic factor. In vivo, this second factor might be MGF.

Continuous stimulation of human postnatal cutaneous melanocytes in vitro with exogenous bFGF or MGF plus dbcAMP or TPA maintains the differentiated phenotype (our unpublished results). In fact, any substance that stimulates the proliferation of normal or malignant melanocytes on addition to the culture medium also stimulates the production of melanocyte-specific mRNAs, the enzyme tyrosinase, and the final product, melanin [64–66]. Therefore, signal transduction from exogenous growth factors triggers a cascade of events leading to proliferation and expression of melanocytic differentiated functions.

Signal transduction from endogenous growth factors appears to be more restricted. The introduction of bFGF cDNA into the murine melanocyte line L-B10.BR via a recombinant retrovirus conferred, as expected, autonomous growth in culture [67]. Not necessarily expected was the loss of all differentiated functions, including pigmentation, expression of tyrosinase (the key enzyme in melanin synthesis), synthesis of melanosomes (the subcellular organelles in which melanin is normally deposited), and formation of dendrites. The bFGF-transformed melanocyte no longer resembles its original counterpart but rather appears like a fibroblast or endothelial cell [67]. Though independent of exogenous growth factor in vitro, the transformants were not fully malignant in that they failed to grow as tumors in syngeneic or nude mice. Instead, in vivo, they regained their differentiated functions, including the ability to produce melanin, and behaved in all respects like normal melanocytes. These observations suggest that differentiation of melanocytes is dependent on continuous stimulation at the cell surface and, possibly, endocytosis. The endogenous bFGF produced in transfected melanocytes appears to activate a pathway that maintains only proliferation but not differentiation. Whether this pathway is the same as the one that is part of the transduction cascade after external stimulation is not known. As mentioned before, bFGF does not have a signal peptide and is probably not transported by the same subcellular route as the membrane-bound glycoprotein receptors that circulate to and from the cell surface.

## IV. SURFACE RECEPTORS AND SIGNAL TRANSDUCTION

Both high- and low-affinity classes of receptor for basic and acidic FGF have been identified and their cDNAs cloned. The high affinity receptors (bFGF-R and aFGF-R) are tyrosine-protein kinases of 125 and 145 kd [68–91]. There are at least four different genes encoding variants of FGF-R. They are designated FGF-R1, FGF-R2 (formerly *flg* and *bek*), FGF-R3, and FGF-R4 [73–90]. The amino acid sequences deduced from the respective cDNAs show that all four receptors belong to the immunoglobulin superfamily of proteins. Receptor isoforms with two or three immunoglobulinlike extracellular loops, translated from alternatively spliced mRNAs, have been identified. Human bFGF-R isoforms 1 and 2 (encoded by *flg* and *bek*, respectively) bind basic and acidic FGF with similar affinity [76], and possibly K-FGF/Hst-1 [82], and activate the same signal transduction pathway. The murine FGF-R2 homolog, with two Ig-like domains, binds KGF and aFGF with high affinity and bFGF with approximately 20 times less affinity [84, 86]. On the other hand, the FGF-R2 that contains three Ig-like domains can bind both aFGF and bFGF, with a slightly higher affinity for aFGF [80]. FGF-R3 also appears to bind both ligands [89], and FGF-R4 binds only aFGF [87].

The significance of the FGF-R variants is not clear, but perhaps the isoforms play a role in different tissues or during different developmental stages, as shown already for FGF-R1 and FGF-R4 [87, 90]. In addition, an mRNA species encoding only the extracellular domain of the FGF receptor has been cloned [76, 86], suggesting the existence of a soluble FGF-binding protein.

The low-affinity receptor was shown to be a membrane-bound heparan-sulfate proteoglycan (HSPG) [91], and the suggestion was made that binding of bFGF to cell surface HSPG was obligatory for binding to high-affinity receptors, because a CHO cell mutant expressing high- but not low-affinity receptors did not bind bFGF unless heparan sulfate was included in the binding medium [92]. Indeed, direct involvement of surface heparan sulfate was demonstrated in fibroblast growth and myoblast differentiation by treatment with agents that remove heparan sulfate or block sulfation, such as heparitinase and sodium chlorate, respectively [93]. However, the significance of high- versus low-affinity FGF receptors is clearly not fully established, since an HSPG with high affinity to aFGF has recently been identified in a rat parathyroid cell line [94].

The integral membrane high-affinity glycoprotein FGF-Rs are tyrosine kinases [95], which undergo autophosphorylation and induce a cascade of activation phosphorylations of target proteins. Binding of bFGF and aFGF to NIH 3T3 cells induces autophosphorylation of 125- and 145-kd receptor proteins and phosphorylation of additional proteins of 145, 90, 46, and 42 kD [69–72]. The additional 145-kd phosphoprotein was identified as phospholipase C$\gamma$ [71, 96, 97]. This enzyme hydrolyzes the membrane phospholipid phosphatidylinositol-4,5-bisphosphate $(PIP)_2$ to form two second messengers: 1,2-diacylglycerol (DG), which activates protein kinase C, and inositol triphosphate, which causes release of calcium from internal stores [98]. Stimulation of protein kinase C by treatment with bFGF was demonstrated in bovine aortic endothelial cells [99].

The 42-kd phosphoprotein was identified as microtubule-associated protein 2-kinase or extracellular signal-regulated kinase 2 (MAP-2-kinase/ERK), a common intermediate in signal transduction that has been identified in other cellular systems for other receptors [100]. MAP-2 kinase is a serine/threonine kinase that, in turn, phosphorylates and activates S6 kinase, thereby leading to phosphorylation of ribosomal protein S6 and concomitant acceleration of protein synthesis. Therefore, activation of the FGF-R tyrosine kinase leads to stimulation of at least one serine/threonine kinase, a pattern observed also with other receptor-tyrosine kinases (reviewed in Ref. 101).

In melanocytes, the same phosphorylated intermediates may be operative in the phosphorylation cascade, because bFGF elicits the appearance of 125- and 42-kd phosphoproteins and causes an increase in MAP-2 kinase activity [142].

The role of exogenous FGFs may not be restricted to activation of the FGF receptors at the cell surface. Both bFGF and aFGF have been localized in the nucleus [102–104]. Two synthetic aFGF gene products, each with a mutation at the nuclear targeting domain that abolishes nuclear localization, were unable to initiate cell proliferation and DNA synthesis in NIH 3T3 fibroblasts, even though they were able to bind to the FGF receptor, stimulate the phosphorylation of membrane-bound and cytosolic proteins, and induce c-*fos* expression, an early response of endothelial cells to aFGF [104]. On the other hand, a six-amino-acid deletion in the amino acid sequence similar to that proposed to target aFGF to the nucleus did not affect the mitogenic activity of bFGF toward several cell types, including NIH 3T3 fibroblasts, but reduced by two orders of magnitude the ability of the peptide to stimulate the production of plasminogen activator in endothelial cells [105]. In this experiment, the cellular localization of the bFGF was not determined, but others have shown that the various natural forms of bFGF, all fully mitogenic, have different subcellular localization, the smallest form occurring predominantly in the cytosol, while the larger ones, with molecular weights of 22, 22.5, and 24 kd, are associated with the nucleus (reviewed in Ref. 106). The nuclear localization signal of the higher molecular weight forms resides in an $NH_2$-terminal extension [106]. Thus, the detailed molecular pathways by which FGFs stimulate their target cells is not entirely elucidated. Knowledge of these pathways is, however, important for learning the reason why bFGF, aberrantly produced intracellularly by bFGF-transfected melanocytes or metastatic melanoma cells (see below), causes extinction of differentiated functions, whereas when supplied extracellularly, it induces and maintains the melanocytic phenotype.

## V. FGFs AND MALIGNANT TRANSFORMATION

Basic FGF is probably the principal factor that stimulates growth of melanocytes in melanocytic lesions. Messenger RNA for bFGF can be detected in dysplastic and dermal nevi, as well as in primary and metastatic melanomas, by in situ hybridization with a bFGF riboprobe [48]. Mitogenic activity toward normal human melanocytes was verified in freshly excised dermal nevi (our unpublished results) and in cultures of advanced primary and metastatic melanoma cells [38, 41, 107–109]. Melanoma cells that proliferate in culture autonomously depend on intrinsic bFGF, because internalized neutralizing anti-bFGF antibodies [41] and antisense, but not sense, a oligodeoxynucleotides targeted against human bFGF mRNA [110] inhibit their growth. Antisense oligodeoxynucleotides to nerve growth factor mRNA and insulinlike growth factor-I mRNA [110] are not inhibitory, suggesting that the respective peptides, which are produced by melanoma cells [110], do not give autocrine growth advantage to melanomas in vitro.

Intrinsic bFGF appears to stimulate melanoma cells through an internal loop, because bFGF-neutralizing antibodies inhibit melanoma growth only when injected into the cells but not by simple addition to the culture medium [41]. As mentioned above, expression of intrinsic bFGF alone was insufficient to confer the malignant phenotype on melanocytes in vivo [67]. Likewise, the melanocytes in dysplastic nevi that express bFGF mRNA [48] are not malignant. People with the dysplastic nevus syndrome, who may have hundreds of dysplastic nevi, develop at best only a small number of primaries [111]. The spontaneous expression of bFGF in melanomas is probably due to gene activation rather than amplification or rearrangement [112, 113]. The gene for bFGF has been mapped to human chromosome region 4q26-q27 [114, 115], but chromosome 4 is not among those known to be affected in melanomas [116–119].

Basic FGF-R kinase activity is critical for the proliferation of melanomas, because synthetic bFGF peptides that span the receptor's ligand-binding domain and act as bFGF antagonists inhibit melanoma cell growth [41].

Sequences from nonrelevant domains do not have this effect [41]. Likewise, internalized antiphosphotyrosine antibodies inhibit melanoma cell growth [41], again suggesting growth inhibition via abrogation of receptor activity. In agreement with the importance of bFGF-R activity in melanoma growth is our recent finding that the bFGF-R is constitutively phosphorylated in a metastatic human melanoma cell line [113]. In this case, the receptor appeared to be encoded by a *flg*-related gene, resulting in a 125-kd protein compatible with the two-loop form of receptor [113]. FGF-R1 and FGF-R2 genes (*bek* and *flg*) are not amplified or rearranged in nine metastatic melanomas so tested [113], and receptor protein is not expressed at abnormally high levels (our unpublished results). Taken together, the data indicate that melanoma growth is due to intrinsic, intracellular activation and not overexpression of bFGF-R.

Southern blot analysis of other genes from the FGF family has shown that 2 of the 15 melanomas tested contained amplification of the linked FGF-related oncogenes *int*-2 and *K-FGF/hst* [113, 120]. However, in one such melanoma, YU SIT1, with 12-fold amplification of the *int-2* and *K-FGF* genes, both known to encode secreted factors [3, 5, 6], there was no mitogenic activity in the culture medium toward normal human melanocytes [45, 113], and the corresponding mRNAs were not detectable on Northern blot. The cell-associated mitogenic activity toward melanocytes in this melanoma was neutralized by antibodies specific for bFGF (45, 113). These results suggest that the amplification of the *int-2* and *K-FGF/hst* genes was of no consequence to the viability of the melanoma cells. More recently, the polymerase chain reaction (PCR) was used to detect low levels of transcripts for several growth factors in 19 melanoma and 14 normal pigment cell lines [50]. This study confirmed the reports, discussed above, on the pattern of expression of mRNAs for bFGF and K-KGF/Hst. Furthermore, it showed that mRNAs for aFGF and FGF-5 were present in 15 and 25%, respectively, of the melanoma cell lines tested but not in normal melanocytes, whereas mRNA for KGF, a peptide not mitogenic for normal melanocytes, was expressed in almost all of the normal and malignant melanocyte lines [50].

## IV. OTHER GROWTH FACTORS FOR MELANOCYTES AND THEIR RELATIONSHIP TO THE FGF FAMILY OF PEPTIDES

Because a single growth factor is not sufficient to sustain melanocyte proliferation, and because activation of FGF-Rs by internal bFGF is not sufficient to confer tumorigenicity, it is likely that, in vivo, additional receptor-kinases play a synergistic role. MGF and HGF, the two melanocyte mitogens not related to the FGFs, stimulate the tyrosine-kinase receptors known as c-Kit and Met, respectively. C-Kit, like the FGF-Rs, is a member of the immunoglobulin superfamily of genes [121–124], and Met is a member of the insulin growth factor receptor family [125, 126].

MGF and its receptor are known to be important for optimal melanoblast viability. Mice with mutations at the dominant white spotting (*W*) and steel (*Sl*) loci, encoding c-Kit and MGF, respectively [54, 57, 121–124, 127, 128], have a deficiency either in the receptor-tyrosine kinase or its ligand [129–134]. In addition to the white spots, *W* and *Sl* mutations in mice cause anemia and sterility by reducing the proliferation and differentiation of hematopoietic and germ cells [129–134]. Human melanocytes are also dependent on c-Kit kinase for normal distribution. A mutation at codon 664 in c-*kit*, which causes substitution of glycine with arginine in the kinase domain, was observed in a proband with classic, autosomal dominant piebaldism [135].

V-*kit*, the oncogenic form of c-*kit*, induces sarcomas in cats [122,123], and a chimeric molecule, composed of the extracellular portion of EGF-R and the transmembrane and cytoplasmic domain of c-Kit, confers an EGF-dependent transformed phenotype on NIH-3T3 cells [136]. *Met* has been identified as an oncogene by transfection of NIH-3T3 cells with DNA from a carcinogen-treated human osteosarcoma cell line [137]. It was, therefore, of particular interest to determine the role of *kit* and *met* gene products in melanomas.

We found that c-Kit, activated by MGF, is one of the most abundant tyrosine-phosphorylated proteins in normal human melanocytes. MGF triggers the tyrosine-phosphorylation of several proteins, the most prominent being c-Kit itself. Among the Kit-kinase substrates and intermediates identified so far in normal human melanocytes is MAP-2 kinase [58]. Several metastatic melanoma cell lines, however, were not stimulated by MGF, and in these, c-*kit* was expressed only at low levels or not at all, on both the mRNA- and protein levels [58]. Although MGF, the ligand of c-Kit, was aberrantly expressed by several of the melanoma cell lines tested (it is not expressed in normal melanocytes), the growth factor probably did not contribute to autonomous growth, because these cells lacked the receptor [58].

Met, phosphorylated in response to HGF, activates several substrates and intermediates through a cascade of tyrosine phosphorylations. In melanomas, Met is not constitutively activated but, as in normal melanocytes, is stimulated by exogenous ligand, suggesting that melanoma cells do not themselves express the growth factor [142]. Met activation through extrinsic HGF probably promotes melanoma growth in synergy with intrinsic bFGF. Because HGF is known to be not only a growth factor but also a cell-scatter factor and to increase the motility of melanocytes and other cell types, including keratinocytes [138,142], the peptide may contribute to the dissemination of melanoma cells from primary to ectopic, metastatic sites. Preferential metastasis to the liver was shown to be the result of a melanoma growth factor produced by hepatocytes [140]. This growth factor may be HGF.

## REFERENCES


1. J. A. Abraham, A. Mergia, J. L. Whang, A, Tumolo, J. Friedman, K. A. Hjerrild, D. Gospodarowicz, and J. C. Fiddes, *Science 233*, 545 (1986).
2. M. Jaye, J. T. Howk, W. Burgess, G. A. Ricca, I.-M. Chiu, M. W. Ravera, S. J. O'Brien, W. S. Modi, T. Maciag, and W. N. Drohan, *Science 233*, 541 (1986).
3. R. Moore, G. Casey, S. Brookes, M. Dixon, G. Peters, and C. Dickson, *EMBO J. 5*, 919 (1986).
4. C. Dickson and G. Peters, *Nature 326*, 833 (1987).
5. P. Delli Bovi and C. Basilico, *Proc. Natl. Acad. Sci. USA 84*, 5660 (1987).
6. M. Taira, T. Yoshida, K. Miyagawa, H. Sakamoto, M. Terada, and T. Sugimura, *Proc. Natl. Acad. Sci. USA 84*, 2980 (1987).
7. X. Zhan, B. Bates, X. Hu, and M. Goldfarb, *Mol. Cell. Biol. 8*, 3487 (1988).
8. I. Marics, J. Adelaide, F. Raybaud, M. G. Mattei, F. Coulier, J. Planche., O. de Lapeyriere, and D. Birnbaum, *Oncogene 4*, 335 (1989).
9. P. W. Finch, J. S. Rubin, T. Miki, D. Ron, and S. A. Aaronson, *Science 245*, 752 (1989).
10. A. Baird and M. Klagsbrun, *Cancer Cells 3*, 239 (1991).
11. M. Goldfarb, R. Deed, D. MacAllan, W. Walther, C. Dickson, and G. Peters, *Oncogene 6*, 65 (1991).
12. D. Talarico and C. Basilico, *Mol. Cell. Biol. 11*, 1138 (1991).
13. J. Zhang, L. S. Cousens, P. J. Barr, and S. R. Sprang, *Proc. Natl. Acad. Sci. USA 88*, 3446 (1991).
14. A. E. Eriksson, L. S. Cousens, L. H. Weaver, and B. W. Matthews, *Proc. Natl. Acad. Sci. USA 88*, 3441 (1991).
15. X. Zhu, H. Komiya, A. Chirino, S. Faham, G. M. Fox, T. Arakawa, B. T. Hsu, and D. C. Rees, *Science 251*, 90 (1991).
16. J.-C. Jeanny, N. Fayein, M. Moenner, B. Chavallier, D. Barritault, and Y. Courtois, *Exp. Cell. Res. 171*, 63 (1987).
17. I. Vlodavsky, J. Folkman, R. Sullivan, R. Fridman, R. Ishai-Michaeli, J. Sasse, and M. Klagsbrun, *Proc. Natl. Acad. Sci. USA 84*, 2292 (1987).
18. J. DiMario, N. Buffinger, S. Yamada, and R. C. Strohman, *Science 244*, 688 (1989).
19. A.-M. Gonzalez, M. Buscaglia, M. Ong, and A. Baird, *J. Cell Biol. 10*, 753 (1990).
20. W. H. Burgess and T. Maciag, *Annu. Rev. Biochem. 58*, 575 (1989).
21. D. B. Rifkin and D. Moscatelli, *J. Cell. Biol. 109*, 1 (1989).
22. J. Drago, M. Murphy, S. M. Carroll, R. P. Harvey, and P. F. Bartlett, *Proc. Natl. Acad. Sci. USA 88*, 2199 (1991).
23. S. Rogelj, M. Klagsbrun,, R. Atzmon, M. Kurokawa, A. Hamovitz, Z. Fuks, and I. Vlodavsky, *J. Cell Biol. 109*, 823 (1989).

24. D. H. Damon, P. A. D'Amore, and J. A. Wagner, *J. Cell Biol. 110*, 1333 (1990).
25. J. Folkman and M. Klagsbrun, *Science* (Wash.) 235, 442 (1987).
26. R. Tsuboi, Y. Sato, and D. B. Rifkin, *J. Cell Biol. 110*, 511 (1990).
27. Y. Sato and D. B. Rifkin, *J. Cell Biol. 107*, 1199 (1988).
28. J. Jouanneu, J. Gavrilovic, D. Caruelle, M. Jaye, G. Moens, J.-P. Caruelle, and J.-P. Thiery, *Proc. Natl. Acad. Sci. USA 88,* 2893 (1991).
29. D. Kimelman, J. A. Abraham, T. Haaparanta, T. M. Palisi, and M. W. Kirschner, *Science 242*, 1053 (1988).
30. D. Kimelman and M. Kirschner, *Cell 51*, 869 (1987).
31. E. Amaya, T. J. Musci, and M. W. Kirschner, *Cell 66*, 257 (1991).
32. T. G. Parker, K.-L. Chow, R. J. Schwartz, and M. D. Schneider, *Proc. Natl. Acad., Sci. USA 87*, 7066 (1990).
33. M. Gabbianelli, M. Sargiacomo, E. Pelosi, U. Testa, G. Isacchi, C. Peschle, *Science 249*, 1561 (1990).
34. J. A. Thompson, C. C. Haudenschild, K. D. Anderson, J. M. DiPietro, W. F. Anderson, and T. Maciag, *Proc. Natl. Acad. Sci. USA 86*, 7928 (1989).
35. H. Sano, R. Forough, J. A. M. Maier, J. P. Case, A. Jackson, K. Engleka, T. Maciag, and R. L. Wilder, *J. Cell Biol. 110*, 1417 (1990).
36. P. L. McNeil, L. Muthukrishnan, E. Wardern, and P. A. D'Amore, *J. Cell Biol. 109*, 811 (1989).
37. H.-J. Ristow and T. O. Messmer, *J. Cell. Physiol. 137*, 277 (1988).
38. R. Halaban, S. Ghosh, and A. Baird, *In Vitro Cell. Dev. Biol. 23*, 47 (1987).
39. M. T. Story, *In Vitro Cell. Dev. Biol. 25*, 402 (1989).
40. G. D. Shipley, W. W. Keeble, J. E. Hendrickson, R. J. Coffey Jr., and M. R. Pittelkow, *J. Cell. Physiol. 138*, 511 (1989).
41. R. Halaban, B. S. Kwon, S. Ghosh, P. Delli Bovi, and A. Baird, *Oncogene Res. 3*, 177 (1988).
42. P. A. Hebda, C. K. Klingbeil, J. A. Abraham, and J. C. Fiddes, *J. Invest. Dermatol.* 95, 626 (1990).
43. R. Halaban, *Pigment Cell Res. 1*, 18 (1988).
44. R. Halaban, in *Human Melanoma* (S. Ferrone, ed.), New York, 1989, p. 3.
45. R. Halaban, in *Melanoma Research: Genetics, Growth Factors, Metastases, and Antigens* (L. Nathanson, ed.), Kluwer Academic Publishers, Boston, 1991, p. 19.
46. J. S. Rubin, A. M.-L. Chan, D. P. Bottaro, W. H. Burgess, W. G. Taylor, A. C. Cech, W. D. Hirschfield, J. Wong, T. Miki, P. W. Finch, and S. A. Aaronson, *Proc. Natl. Acad. Sci USA 88*, 415 (1991).
47. K. Nakamura, H. Tajima, and T. Nakamura, *Biochem. Biophys. Res. Commun. 176*, 45 (1991).
48. G. Scott, M. Stoler, S. Sarkar, and R. Halaban, *J. Invest. Dermatol. 96*, 318 (1991).
49. K. Schulze-Osthoff, W. Risau, E. Vollmer, and S. Clemens, *Am. J. Pathol. 173*, 85 (1990).
50. A. P. Albino, B. M. Davis, and D. M. Nanus, *Cancer Res. 51*, 4815 (1991).

51. R. Halaban, R. Langdon, N. Birchall, C. Cuono, A. Baird, G. Scott, G. Moellmann, and J. McGuire, *J. Cell. Biol. 107*, 1611 (1988).
52. M. De Luca, F. D'Anna, S. Bondanza, A. T. Franzi, and R. Cancedda, *J. Cell Biol. 107*, 1919 (1988).
53. D. E. Williams, J. Eisenman, A. Baird, C. Rauch, K. Van Ness, C. J. March, L. S. Park, U. Martin, D. Y. Mochizuki, H. S. Boswell, G. M. Burgess, D. Cosman, and S. D. Lyman, *Cell 63*, 167 (1990).
54. J. G. Flanagan and P. Leder, *Cell 63*, 85 (1990).
55. K. M. Zsebo J. Wypych, I. K. McNiece, H. S. Lu, K. A. Smith, S. B. Karkare, R. K. Sadchev, V. N. Yuschenkoff, N. C. Birkett, L. R. Williams, V. N. Satyagal, W. Tung, R. A. Bosselman, E. A. Mendiaz, and K. E. Langley, *Cell 63*, 195 (1990).
56. F. H. Martin, S. V. Sugs, K. E. Langley, H. S. Lu, J. Ting, K. H. Okino, C. F. Morris, I. K. McNiece, F. W. Jacobsen, E. A. Mendiaz, N. C. Birkett, K. A. Smith, M. J. Johnson, V. P. Parker, J. C. Flores, A. C. Patel, E. Fisher, H. O. Erjavec, C. H. Herrera, J. Wypych, R. K. Sachdev, J. A. Pope, I. Leslie, D. Wen, C.-H. Lin, R. L. Cupples, and K. Zsebo, *Cell 63*, 203 (1990).
57. E. Huang, K. Nocka, D. R. Beier, T.-Y. Chu, J. Buck, H.-W. Lahm, D. Wellner, P. Leder, and P. Besmer, *Cell 63*, 225 (1990)
58. Y. Funasaka, T. Boulton, M. Cobb, Y. Yarden, B. Fan, S. D. Lyman, D. E. Williams, D. M. Anderson, R. Zakut, Y. Mishima, and R. Halaban, *Mol. Biol. Cell 3*, 197 (1992).
59. R. M. Lavker and T.-T. Sun, *J. Invest. Dermatol. 81* (Suppl.), 121 (1983).
60. K. S. Stenn, L. A. Fernandez, and S. J. Tirrell, *J. Invest. Dermatol. 90*, 409 (1988).
61. D. L. du Cros, K. Isaacs, and G. P. M. Moore, *Ann. N.Y. Acad. Sci.* in press.
62. I. K. Rosdahl, *Acta Dermatovener* (Stockholm), 58, 217 (1978).
63. K. M. Stocker, L. Sherman, S. Rees, and G. Ciment, *Development 111*, 635 (1991).
64. R. Halaban, S. H. Pomerantz, S. Marshall, D. T. Lambert, and A. B. Lerner, *J. Cell. Biol. 97*, 480 (1983).
65. B. S. Kwon, R. Halaban, G. S. Kim, L. Usack, S. Pomerantz, and A. K. Haq, *Molec. Biol. Med. 4*, 339 (1987).
66. B. S. Kwon, M. Wakulchik, A. K. Haq, R. Halaban, and D. Kestler, *Biochem. Biophys. Res. Commun. 153*, 1301 (1988).
67. P. Dotto, G. Moellmann, S. Ghosh, M. Edwards, and R. Halaban, *J. Cell. Biol. 109*, 3115 (1989).
68. G. Neufeld and D. Gospodarowicz, *J. Biol. Chem. 260*, 13860 (1985).
69. S. S. Huang and J. S. Huang, *J. Biol. Chem. 261*, 9568 (1986).
70. T. Imamura, Y. Tokita, and Y. Mitsui, *Biochem. Biophys. Res. Comm. 155*, 583 (1988).
71. S. R. Coughlin, P. J. Barr, L. S. Cousens, L. J. Fretto, and L. T. Williams, *J. Biol. Chem. 263*, 988 (1988).
72. R. Friesel, W. H. Burgess, and T. Maciag, *Mol. Cell. Biol. 9*, 1857 (1989).
73. P. L. Lee, D. E. Johnson, L. S. Cousens, V. A. Fried, and L. T. Williams, *Science 245*, 57 (1989).

74. M. Ruta, M. Burgess, D. Givol, J. Epstein, N. Neiger, J. Kaplow, G. Crumley, C. Dionne, M. Jaye, and J. Schlessinger, *Proc. Natl. Acad. Sci. USA 86*, 8722 (1989).
75. E. G. Pasquale and S. J. Singer, *Proc. Natl. Acad. Sci. USA 86*, 5449 (1989).
76. D. E. Johnson, P. L. Lee, J. Lu, and L. T. Williams, *Mol. Cell. Biol. 10*, 4728 (1990).
77. D. P. Bottaro, J. S. Rubin, D. Ron, P. W. Finch, C. Florio, and S. A. Aaronson, *J. Biol. Chem. 265*, 12767 (1990).
78. A. Safran, A. Avivi, A. Orr-Urtereger, G. Neufeld, P. Lonai, D. Givol, and Y. Yarden, *Oncogene 5*, 635 (1990).
79. Y. Hattori, O. Odagiri, H. Nakatani, K. Miyagawa, K. Naito, H. Sakamoto, O. Katoh, T. Yoshida, T. Sugimura, and M. Terada, *Proc. Natl. Acad. Sci. USA 87*, 5983 (1990).
80. C. A. Dionne, G. Crumley, F. Bellot, J. M. Kaplow, G. Searfoss, M. Ruta, W. H. Burgess, M. Jaye, and J. Schlessinger, *EMBO J. 9*, 2685 (1990).
81. H. H. Reid, A. F. Wilks, and O. Bernard, *Proc. Natl. Acad. Sci. USA 87*, 1596 (1990).
82. A. Mansukhani, D. Moscatelli, D. Talarico, V. Levytska, and C. Basilico, *Proc. Natl. Acad. Sci. USA 87*, 4378 (1990).
83. J. Partanen, T. P. Mäkelä, R. Alitalo, H. Lehväslaiho, and K. Alitalo, *Proc. Natl. Acad. Sci. USA 87*, 8913 (1990).
84. T. Miki, T. P. Fleming, D. P. Bottaro, J. S. Rubin, D. Ron, and S. A. Aaronson, *Science 251*, 72 (1991).
85. J. Hou, M. Kan, K. McKeehan, G. McBride, P. Adams, and W. L. McKeehan, *Science 251*, 665 (1991).
86. A. Eiseman, J. A. Ahn, G. Graciani, S. R. Tronick, and D. Ron, *Oncogene 6*, 1195 (1991).
87. J. Partanen, T. P. Mäkelä, E. Eerola, J. Korhonen, H. Hirvonen, L. Claesson-Welsh, and K. Alitalo, *EMBO J. 10*, 1347 (1991).
88. A. Avivi, Y. Zimmer, A. Yayon, Y. Yarden, and D. Givol, *Oncogene 6*, 1089 (1991).
89. K. Keegan, D. E. Johnson, L. T. Williams, and M. J. Hayman, *Proc. Natl. Acad. Sci. USA 88*, 1095 (1991).
90. O. Barnard, M. Li, and H. H. Reid, *Proc. Natl. Acad. Sci. USA 88*, 7625 (1991).
91. M. C. Kiefer, J. C. Stephans, K. Crawford, K. Okino, and P. H. Barr, *Proc. Natl. Acad. Sci. USA 87*, 6985 (1990).
92. A. Yayon, M. Klagsbrun, J. D. Esko, P. Leder, and D. M. Ornitz, *Cell 64*, 841 (1991).
93. A. C. Rapraeger, A. Krufka, and B. B. Olwin, *Science 252*, 1705 (1991).
94. K. Sakagushi, M. Yanagishita, Y. Takeuchi, G. D. Auerbach, *J. Biol. Chem. 266*, 7270 (1991).
95. Y. Yarden and A. Ullrich, *Ann. Rev. Biochem. 57*, 443 (1988).
96. W. H. Burgess, C. A. Dionne, J. Kaplow, R. Mudd, R. Friesel, A. Zilberstein, J. Schlessinger, and M. Jaye, *Mol. Cell. Biol. 10*, 4770 (1990).
97. A. Cuadrado and C. J. Molley, *Mol. Cell. Biol. 10*, 6069 (1990).

98. M. J. Berridge and R. F. Irvine, *Nature 312*, 315 (1984).
99. M. Presta, J. A. M. Maier, and G. Ragnotti, *J. Cell Biol. 109*, 1877 (1989).
100. G. L'Allemain, J. Pouyssegur, and M. J. Weber, *Cell Reg. 2*, 675 (1991).
101. L. C. Cantley, K. R. Auger, C. Carpenter, B. Duckworth, A. Graziani, R. Kapeller, and S. Soltoff, *Cell 64*, 281 (1991).
102. V. Baldin, A.-M. Roman, I. Bosc-Bierne, F. Almaric, and G. Bouche, *EMBO J. 9*, 1511 (1990).
103. S. Tessler and G. Neufeld, *J. Cell. Physiol. 145*, 310 (1990).
104. T. Imamura, K. Engleka, X. Zhan, Y. Tokita, R. Forough, D. Roder, A. Jackson, and J. A. M. Mailer, *Science 249*, 1567 (1990).
105. A. Isacchi, M. Statuto, R. Chiesa, L. Bergonzoni, P. S. Rusnati, G. Ragnotti, and M. Presta, *Proc. Natl. Acad. Sci. USA 88*, 2628 (1991).
106. N. Quarto, F. P. Finger, and D. B. Rifkin, *J. Cell. Physiol. 147* (1991).
107. D. Moscatelli, M. Presta, J. Joseph-Silverstein, and D. B. Rifkin, *J. Cell. Physiol. 129*, 273 (1986).
108. R. Lobb, J. Sasse, R. Sullivan, Y. Shing, P. D'Amore, J. Jacobs, and M. Klagsbrun, *J. Biol. Chem. 261*, 1924 (1986).
109. S. Ogata, Y. Furuhashi, and M. Eisinger, *Biochem. Biophys. Res. Commun. 146*, 1204 (1987).
110. D. Becker, C. B. Meier, and M. Herlyn, *EMBO J. 8*, 3685 (1989).
111. M. H. Greene, J. W. Clark Jr., M. A. Tucker, K. H. Kraemer, D. E. Elder, and M. C. Fraser, *Ann. Int. Med. 102*, 458 (1985).
112. C. Theillet, X. Le Roy, O. De Lapeyrière, J. Grosgeorges, J. Adnane, S. D. Raynaud, J. Simony-Lafontaine, M. Goldfarb, C. Escot, D. Birnbaum, and P. Gaudray, *Oncogene 4*, 915 (1989).
113. R. Halaban, Y. Funasaka, P. Lee, J. Rubin, D. Ron, and D. Birnbaum, *Ann. NY Acad. Sci. 638*, 232 (1991).
114. A. Mergia, R. Eddy, J. A. Abraham, J. C. Fiddes, and T. B. Shows, *Biochem. Biophys. Res. Commun. 138*, 644 (1986).
115. M. Lafage-Pochitaloff, F. Galland, J. Simonetti, H. Prats, M.-G. Mattei, and D. Birnbaum, *Oncogene Res. 5*, 241 (1990).
116. G. Balaban, M. Herlyn, D. Guerry IV, R. Bartolo, H. Koprowski, W. H. Clark, and P. C. Nowell, *Cancer Genet. Cytogenet. 11*, 429 (1984).
117. J. M. Cowan, R. Halaban, and U. Francke, *J. Natl. Cancer Inst. 80*, 1159 (1988).
118. J. M. Cowan, and U. Francke, in *Melanoma Research: Genetics, Growth Factors, Metastases, and Antigens* (L. Nathanson, ed.), Kluwer Academic Publishers, Boston, 1991, p. 3.
119. J. M. Trent, F. L. Meyskens, S. E. Salmon, K. Ryschon, S. P. L. Leong, J. R. Davis, and D. L. McGee, *N. Engl. J. Med. 322*, 1508 (1990).
120. J. Adelaide, M.-G. Mattei, I. Marics, R. Raybaud, J. Planche, O. De Lapeyriere, and D. Birnbaum, *Oncogene 2*, 413 (1988).
121. Y. Yarden, W.-J. Kuang, T. Yang-Feng, L. Coussens, S. Munemitsu, T. J. Dull, E. Chen, J. Schlessinger, U. Francke, and A. Ullrich, *EMBO J. 6*, 3341 (1987).

122. F. Qiu, P. Ray, K. Brown, P. E. Barker, S. Jhanwar, F. H. Ruddle, and P. Besmer, *EMBO J. 7*, 1003 (1988).
123. E. N. Geissler, M. A. Ryan, and D. E. Housman, *Cell 55*, 185 (1988).
124. B. Chabot, D. A. Stephenson, V. M. Chapman, P. Besmer, and A. Bernstein, *Nature 335*, 88 (1988).
125. D. P. Bottaro, J. S. Rubin, D. L. Faletto, A. M.-L. Chan, T. E. Kmiecik, G. P. Vande Woude, and S. A. Aaronson, *Science 251*, 802 (1991).
126. L. Naldini, E. Vigna, R. P. Narsimhan, G. Gaudino, R. Zarnegar, G. K. Michaolopoulos, and P. M. Comoglio, *Oncogene 6*, 501 (1991).
127. N. Copeland, D. J. Gilbert, B. C. Cho, P. J. Donovan, N. A. Jenkins, D. Cosman, D. Anderson, S. D. Lyman, and D. E. Williams, *Cell 63*, 175 (1990).
128. K. Zsebo, D. A. Williams, E. N. Geissler, V. C. Broudy, F. H. Martin, H. L. Atkins, R.-Y. Hsu, N. C. Birkett, K. H. Okino, D. C. Murdock, F. W. Jacobsen, K. E. Langley, K. A. Smith, T. Takeishi, B. M. Cattanach, S. J. Galli, and S. Suggs, *Cell 63*, 213 (1990)
129. K. Nocka, S. Majumder, B. Chabot, P. Ray, M. Cervone, A. Bernstein, and P. Besmer, *Genes and Development 3*, 816 (1989).
130. K. Nocka, J. C. Tan, E. Chiu, T. Y. Chu, P. Ray, P. Traktman, and P. Besmer, *EMBO J. 9*, 1805 (1990).
131. A. D. Reith, R. Rottapel, E. Giddens, C. Brady, L. Forrester, and A. Bernstein, *Genes and Development 4*, 390 (1990).
132. J. C. Tan, K. Nocka, P. Ray, P. Traktman, and P. Besmer, *Science 247*, 209 (1990).
133. C. I. Brannan, S. D. Lyman, D. E. Williams, J. Eisenman, D. Anderson, D. Cosman, M. A. Bedell, N. A. Jenkins, and N. G. Copeland, *Proc. Natl. Acad. Sci. USA 88*, 4671 (1991).
134. J. G. Flanagan, D. G. Chan, and P. Leder, *Cell 64*, 1025 (1991).
135. L. B. Giebel and R. A. Spritz, *Proc. Natl. Acad. Sci. USA 88*, 8696 (1991).
136. S. Lev, Y. Yarden, and D. Givol, *Mol. Cell. Biol. 10*, 6064 (1990).
137. C. S. Cooper, M. Park, D. G. Blair, M. A. Tainsky, K. Huebner, C. M. Croce, and G. P. Vande Woude, *Nature 311*, 29 (1984).
138. E. Gherardi and M. Stoker, *Cancer Cells 3*, 227 (1991).
139. N. S. Sargent, M. Oestreicher, H. Haidvogl, H. M. Madnick, and M. M. Burger, *Proc. Natl. Acad. Sci. USA 85*, 7251 (1988).
140. R. Halaban, L. Tyrrell, J. Longley, Y. Yarden, and J. Rubin, *J. Ann. NY Acad. Sci. 680*, 290 (1993).
141. J. Longley, C. S. Morganroth, L. Tyrrell, T. G. Ding, D. M. Anderson, D. E. Williams, and R. Halaban, *N. Engl. J. Med. 328*, 1302 (1993).
142. R. Halaban, J. Rubin, Y. Funasaka, M. Cobb, T. Boulton, D. Faletto, E. Rosen, A. Chan, K. Yoko, W. White, C. Cook, G. Moellmann, *Oncogene 7*, 2195 (1992).

# III
# THE EPIDERMAL CYTOKINE NETWORK

# 13

# The Second Decade of Epidermal Cytokines: An Overview

**Thomas S. Kupper**
*Harvard Medical School and Brigham & Women's Hospital*
*Boston, Massachusetts*

Discovery of a novel and unanticipated biological phenomenon leads to a flurry of scientific activity, as investigators seek to confirm and extend the initial observations. So it was with the first reports of cytokine production by epidermal keratinocytes in the early 1980s. The idea that cells previously regarded as little more than living precursors to stratum corneum could participate actively in host defense was, to say the least, iconoclastic. These early studies disrupted the paradigm that bone marrow derived cells were necessary and sufficient for the induction of inflammation and raised the important possibility that resident epithelial cells might initiate, if not actually orchestrate, cutaneous inflammation.

It is important to reflect on the degree to which these observations have changed our perspectives on skin diseases and mechanisms of inflammation in the skin. First, they provide a logical explanation for the fact that local cutaneous responses to injury or infection do not require global or systemic activation of leukocytes (Kupper et al., 1988a; Kupper, 1990b). That is to say, the discovery that keratinocytes could produce cytokines suggested that the local environment of the injury could potentially modify the behavior and level of activation of resting leukocytes that circulate through it. Second, these observations make it likely that the behavior of resident bone marrow-derived epidermal cells (e.g., Langerhans cells) is influenced directly by cytokines released by contiguous keratinocytes. Finally, the idea that keratinocytes make cytokines relevant to inflammation and immunity has fundamentally changed how we think about the mechanism of action of current therapies for skin diseases, as well as how we design new ones.

The first decade of keratinocyte cytokine biology was understandably dedicated primarily to the description and characterization of all the cytokines that could be produced by cultured keratinocytes. Just as taxonomy is important to biology, the extension of the compendium of keratinocyte cytokines provides us with a dictionary that we can use to help unravel the secrets of cutaneous inflammation. The challenge of the second decade of keratinocyte cytokine biology is to formulate testable hypotheses that incorporate keratinocyte cytokines into cutaneous pathology and to use the "cytokine dictionary" wisely and well. Though I shall discuss some approaches to these challenging issues at the end of this chapter, it is useful to revisit the history of keratinocyte cytokines.

While the idea that keratinocytes could produce factors that influenced T-cell behavior was suggested by individuals studying diseases such as cutaneous T-cell lymphoma, it was not until 1981 that Luger et al. showed that a transformed keratinocyte line called Pam 212 could produce a factor that was biochemically and functionally indistinguishable from interleukin 1 (IL-1). A contemporaneous study by Sauder et al. (1982) extended this observation to human keratinocytes and further showed that normal epidermal cell preparations depleted of Langerhans cells still produced substantial amounts of the IL-1-like factor, then termed epidermal cell–derived thymocyte activating factor or ETAF, in deference to the thymocyte assay then in vogue as an assay of IL-1. The cloning of two different IL-1s permitted molecular analysis of ETAF, and Kupper et al. (1986) showed that keratinocytes did indeed contain mRNA's identical to monocyte IL-1$\alpha$ and IL-1$\beta$ mRNAs. Surprisingly, only biologically active IL-1$\alpha$ could be identified in keratinocyte cultures in this study, an observation confirmed years later by a variety of approaches.

Following the description of IL-1 production by keratinocytes, a logical course of action was to search for other cytokines produced by cultured keratinocytes. It was readily shown that neither IL-2 nor IL-4 could be produced by keratinocytes (Kupper et al., 1989), consistent with the emerging understanding that these cytokines were nearly completely restricted to T cells. IL-3 production by keratinocytes is somewhat more controversial. For example, it is now clear that both Pam 212 keratinocytes and neonatal murine keratinocytes produce authentic IL-3 identical to that derived from T cells (Luger et al., 1985; Peterseim, 1993). Adult murine keratinocytes probably do not make significant amounts of IL-3. In contrast, it has been difficult to find mRNA or protein homologous to human T-cell–derived IL-3 in human keratinocytes, even neonatal cells (Kupper et al., 1988a). Since human keratinocyte IL-3 is based on a growth-promoting activity of keratinocyte supernatants on indicator cell lines, and since cell lines once considered monoresponsive are now known to be rather promiscuous, it is probably best to reconsider the idea that human keratinocytes produce authentic IL-3 in the absence of more direct data.

A family of molecules first characterized by their potential to mediate distinct patterns of differentiation and growth of hematopoietic precursor cells are known as the colony-stimulating factors or CSFs (Metcalf, 1990). Since their molecular cloning, it is now clear that the biological activity of such cells extends to mature counterparts of their respective progenitor target cells. Keratinocytes were found to produce GM-CSF, M-CSF, and G-CSF (Kupper et al., 1988a; Chodakawitz et al., 1990). While the evidence for the first two CSFs is compelling and has been confirmed at the level of mRNA, protein, and biological activity, the evidence for G-CSF production is somewhat more indirect. The production of CSFs by keratinocytes in vivo probably influences the biological behavior of mature cells or Langerhans cells, though potential effects directly on keratinocytes or on circulating hematopoietic progenitor cells cannot be dismissed. IL-3, sometimes called multi-CSF, has been discussed above. It is also likely that a newly described colony-stimulating factor, awkwardly known as steel factor, c-*kit* ligand, and mast cell growth factor, is produced by keratinocytes (J. Longley, personal communication), although formal proof awaits more rigorous study. Again, the known effects of this factor on melanocyte and mast cell function, rather than its effects on hematopoietic progenitor cells, are likely to predominate in cutaneous tissues.

Production of TNF-$\alpha$ has been conclusively demonstrated in keratinocyte cultures and in vivo in cutaneous tissues (Kock, 1990). In contrast to IL-1, TNF-$\alpha$ gene expression in keratinocytes appears to require an inductive stimulus. The probable and potential roles of this cytokine as well as IL-1 are discussed in Section I. In addition, the multifunctional cytokine IL-6 can be produced by keratinocytes (Kupper, 1990a; Kirnbauer, 1989), which has been shown in vivo and in vitro in both human and murine systems. Space does not permit a thorough discussion of the potential roles of IL-6 in skin. IL-7 production by keratinocytes has been suggested by preliminary studies (Heufler et al., 1992), while production of IL-9, IL-11, and IL-12 by keratinocytes has not yet been explored sufficiently to merit comment in this context. Keratinocyte production of IL-10, a molecule that can indirectly inhibit cytokine production by a subset of T-helper cells, has recently been demonstrated (Enk, 1992).

Much recent work on keratinocyte cytokines have focused on their potential to produce IL-8 and other members of the intercrine or chemokine family after appropriate stimulation (Schroder, 1992). Though an exhaustive description of the members of this rapidly growing group of factors is undertaken in Chapter 4, an acceptable generalization is that the chemokine $\alpha$ or C-X-C group (of which IL-8 is the prototype) function to attract and activate cells of the granulocyte series, while members of the chemokine $\beta$ or C-C family (of which monocyte chemotactic and activating factor, or MCAF, is the prototype) tend to act upon monocytes and T cells. The widespread interest in this family of molecules is obvious, since they are likely to play an important role in the microenvironmental activation and chemotaxis of leukocytes from the circulatory system.

I shall restrict my discussion of cytokines to those listed above and will somewhat arbitrarily ignore the transforming growth factor $\alpha$ and $\beta$ families, as well as other factors that function primarily as growth factors for mesenchymal or epithelial cells. Nevertheless, this leaves us to ponder the role of a population of epidermal epithelial cells capable of producing cytokines that can attract and activate every family of leukocyte, induce an acute phase response, induce the growth and differentiation of every hematopoietic lineage, and mediate many of the deleterious features of septic shock. That the outermost 100 $\mu$m of one's body may have such prodigious properties is impressive. There is, upon reflection, a certain logic to the placement of such powerful mediators at the interface between the host and the environment, the site at which most injurious events are likely to occur. Clearly, however, some cytokines must be more relevant than others in different biological settings, and the production of some cytokines must precede that of others in the inflammatory cascade. This has led to a classification of cytokines in skin as either "primary" or "secondary" (Kupper, 1990a), a strategy that is more instructive than absolute.

Primary cytokines were first defined in 1990 based on their capacity to mediate several requisite steps in the induction of inflammation. Both IL-1s and TNFs were designated as primary cytokines. A primary cytokine is both necessary and sufficient for the recruitment of an activated infiltrate of leukocytes to the site of a cutaneous challenge. Primary cytokines must first regulate the adhesion molecule profile of endothelial cells in the dermis, leading to the expression of vascular adhesion molecules such as P- and E-selectin, ICAM-1, and VCAM-1 (Butcher, 1991). While this is necessary for the trapping of leukocytes in the vessels at the site of primary cytokine release, it is not sufficient to induce their egress across the vessel wall. thus, a second property of primary cytokines is that they induce the de novo gene expression of secondary cytokines, which include members of the chemokine family including IL-8 and MCAF, as well as other molecules relevant to inflammation such as IL-6 and the CSFs. Several of these molecules, notably members of the chemokine families, can activate leukocytes that have been captured and slowed to a roll by selectin-expressing dermal endothelium (Oppenheim, et al., 1991). Leukocytes thus activated by secondary cytokines emanating from the abluminal side of the vessel can now bind via $\beta_2$ integrins (LFA-1,

MAC-1) to ICAM-1 and 2, as well as to VCAM, via VLA-4, and to collagen, laminin, and fibronectin via other members of the $\beta_1$ integrin family. Apart from activation of leukocytes which permits their avid binding to primary cytokine-activated endothelium, chemokine release by cutaneous cells (including keratinocytes) forms a concentration gradient along which leukocytes travel via chemotaxis, seeking out the source of the highest level of chemokine release. Since this should be identical to the site of maximal primary cytokine release, such mechanisms provide a process by which primary cytokines can directly and indirectly orchestrate inflammation. Central to this idea is the fact that keratinocytes can produce primary cytokines, meaning that keratinocytes can initiate inflammation.

## I. PRIMARY CYTOKINE PRODUCTION BY THE EPIDERMIS: THE SPECIAL CASE OF INTERLEUKIN 1

The epidermis contains substantial amounts of IL-1, and most if not all biologically active IL-1 in the epidermis is composed of IL-1$\alpha$ (Kupper, 1990a; Cooper et al., 1990), extending to the in vivo setting previous observations that keratinocytes made principally IL-1$\alpha$ mRNA and biological activity in vitro (Kupper et al., 1986). While keratinocytes can produce IL-1$\beta$, they cannot process it efficiently from its 31 kD precursor form to an active 17 kD molecule (Mizutani et al., 1991a). However, keratinocyte IL-1$\beta$ can be cleaved by proteases, including mast cell chymase, to generate an active IL-1$\beta$ species (Mizutani et al., 1991b; Black et al., 1991). A variety of stimuli will enhance IL-1 gene expression by human keratinocytes, including UVB irradiation and protein kinase C agonists (Kupper et al., 1987; Blanton et al., 1989).

Keratinocytes also respond to IL-1 by producing secondary cytokines such as GM-CSF (Kupper et al., 1988b), IL-6 (Kirnbauer et al., 1989), and IL-8 (Larsen et al., 1989). That keratinocytes can produce secondary cytokines in response to an autocrine stimulus (e.g., IL-1) led to the proposal of the "activated keratinocyte" as a cytokine-producing effector cell responsible for inflammatory responses in skin (Kupper et al., 1989; Kupper, 1990a). Whether or not a keratinocyte responds to IL-1 (and thus produces secondary cytokines) was considered to be dependent upon two variables: the level of IL-1 receptor expression on keratinocytes and the amount extracellular active IL-1 species released by the keratinocyte (or by contiguous keratinocytes). Thus, in normal skin, high levels of IL-1 coupled with low levels of receptor expression would not lead to keratinocyte activation. However, stimuli that upregulated IL-1 receptors (e.g., PKC agonists) and/or led to active or passive release of IL-1 from cells might be expected to activate keratinocytes, thus leading to the release of secondary cytokines so important in localizing inflammatory cells to skin.

Recent findings have added additional levels of complexity to this equation. For example, the gene for an additional member of the IL-1 family has been found at a contiguous site on chromosome 2 (Arend, 1991). Unlike IL-1$\alpha$ and IL-1$\beta$, this molecule appears to have pure antagonist activity. This factor, commonly known as the IL-1 receptor antagonist or IL-1ra, binds with high affinity to both IL-1 receptors (IL-1R) and competes with active IL-1 in this regard. Keratinocytes contain a form of the IL-1ra that lacks a leader sequence and signal peptide (Haskill et al., 1991; Bigler et al., 1992) so that this epithelial IL-1ra, like IL-1$\alpha$ and IL-1$\beta$ and basic FGF, is not efficiently secreted from cells. Thus, injury to epidermis will release not only preformed IL-1 but also preformed IL-1ra. Levels of IL-1ra in keratinocyte cultures are often higher than those of active IL-1$\alpha$ (Bigler et al., 1992). This observation places additional importance on the level of receptor expression on keratinocytes. It has been shown for a variety of cells that a certain minimum number of IL-1 receptors need to be occupied for a given response (i.e., activation) to ensue (Curtis et al., 1989). Clearly, for a keratinocyte with few IL-1R, excessive IL-1ra might successfully compete with active IL-1 such that this minimal number of receptors will not be occupied by agonist. However, a keratinocyte with many receptors can respond to active IL-1 even in the face of a vast excess of IL-1ra provided the same number of sites are bound by agonist. In theory, this is true even if 100-fold more receptors are occupied by antagonist rather than agonist.

Yet another element of complexity may occur at the level of type of IL-1 receptor expressed by keratinocytes. Recently, a second IL-1 receptor found predominantly on B cells, monocytes, and other hemapoietic cells was cloned and characterized. Most cells that express this type II IL-1R also express low levels of type I IL-1R. Although these studies are preliminary, it appears that the type II receptor is the biological analog of the IL-1ra; that is, it serves to antagonize IL-1–mediated responses. It appears that this receptor will bind ligand efficiently (both IL-1 and IL-1ra) but will not transduce a signal. Furthermore, PKC agonist treatment of cells leads to release of soluble type II IL-1 receptor release. The type II and type I receptors appear not to cooperate in the binding and internalization of IL-1. Recent evidence suggests that keratinocytes may express both type I and type II receptors (T.S. Kupper et al., unpublished). Their regulation is currently under study.

Taken together, these findings suggest that conditions that will favor generation of an activated keratinocyte include upregulation of IL-1$\alpha$ and (perhaps) IL-1$\beta$ gene expression and upregulation of type I IL-1R expression. Events that oppose this end include upregulation of IL-1ra gene expression and upregulation of type II IL-1R expression or release. In retrospect, it should not be surprising that such elaborate controls on the activity and function of such a powerful pleiotropic mediator exist. This degree of complexity does, however, make it nearly impossible to predict a priori whether a given stimulus will result in an IL-1–mediated response. A corollary to this statement is that the analysis of only one of these variables to the exclusion of others in any setting is unlikely to yield useful information.

## II. NEW CHALLENGES AND OLD PROBLEMS

The complexity of the IL-1 system in skin is daunting and may not be unique. Certainly, the activity of TNF-$\alpha$ (another primary cytokine can be regulated by soluble receptors and by expression of different receptors on different cells. While a TNF-$\alpha$ receptor antagonist has not been described, it is likely that the number of variables that positively and negatively affect TNF-$\alpha$-mediated processes may increase as new molecules are discovered. Are secondary cytokine activities regulated at the level of receptor antagonists and soluble receptors? If so, identification of elevated levels of individual cytokines in lesions of skin disease may not be as informative as one would like.

Given our limitations, can we ever know what individual cytokines really do in skin? While there is no shortage of speculation, most hypotheses are based upon known activities of individual cytokines in vitro extrapolated to the in vivo situation. Experiments wherein cytokines are injected into murine or human skin are useful because they accommodate the complexities of the in vivo system (Granstein, 1986; Groves et al., 1992). Ultimately, these approaches are limited by the fact that they are anatomically and kinetically artificial. Recently, an exciting alternative approach was introduced. Different layers of mammalian epidermis express different keratin pairs; for example, basal keratinocytes express K14 and K5, while suprabasilar cells express K1 and K10 (Fuchs, 1990). Promotors for each keratin have been cloned and characterized. Experiments wherein transgenic mice have been created using known genes linked to keratin promoters have indicated that tissue specificity is maintained under these conditions. For example, the transgene containing TGF-$\alpha$ linked to the K14 promotor is expressed in the basal epidermis of transgenic mice, leading to epithelial hyperproliferation as predicted (Vasser and Fuchs, 1991). However, the histopathology of the skin of these mice differs in some fundamental ways from psoriatic skin, suggesting that overexpression of TGF-$\alpha$ per se is not the fundamental lesion in psoriasis. Thus, overexpression of TGF-$\alpha$ in psoriasis may contribute to but is not responsible for the psoriatic phenotype.

We have employed this approach with cytokines known to have inflammatory properties with interesting results. For example, it has been shown previously that IL-6 (like TGF-$\alpha$) was overexpressed in psoriatic epidermis (Grossman et al., 1989) and that in vitro, IL-6 enhanced keratinocyte proliferation. This led to speculation that IL-6 was central to the pathogenesis of psoriasis. One way of testing this hypothesis was to create a transgenic mouse that overexpressed IL-6 in the epidermis. Would this lead to psoriasis or psoriasiform dermatitis? Surprisingly, the principal cutaneous lesion in the K14/IL-6 transgenic mouse appears to be a thickened stratum corneum, and hyperproliferation of epidermal keratinocytes was absent (Turksen et al., 1992). While these studies do not exclude a role for IL-6 in psoriasis, they imply that other factors must be required.

Each approach has its limitations, and the transgenic one is no exception. The beauty of the transgenic approach is that different lines of transgenic mice can be interbred, creating progeny that may overexpress combinations of cytokines or their receptors that may accumulate and result in disease. Such experiments have the virtue of directly testing previously untestable hypotheses about the role of epidermal cytokines in skin disease. To the extent that this approach is successful in creating animal models of human skin disease, such animals will also provide the best system for testing the efficacy of therapies designed to treat diseased skin.

As we enter the second decade of epidermal cytokine study, the blush of enthusiasm and wonder over the scope and range of keratinocyte cytokines must give way to rigorous analysis of the role of these cytokines in experimental and pathyphysiological systems. Important discoveries may come more slowly, but it is anticipated that the depth of understanding from successful completion of such analyses will change the way we think about skin disease.

## REFERENCES

W. J. Arend, *Clin. Invest. 88*, 445 (1991).

C. F. Bigler, D. Norris, W. L. Weston, and W. P. Arend, *J. Invest. Dermatol. 98*, 38 (1992).

R. Black, S. Kronheim, P. Sleath, T. Greenstreet, G. D. Virca, C. March, and T. S. Kupper, *Agents Actions 35*, 85 (1991).

B. Blanton, T. S. Kupper, J. K. McDougall, and S. Dower, *Proc. Natl. Acad. Sci. 86*, 1273 (1989).

E. Butcher, *Cell 67*, 1033–1036 (1991).

J. A. Chodoakewitz, J. Lacy, S. Edwards, N. Birchall, and D. Coleman, *J. Immunol. 144*, 2190 (1990).

K. D. Cooper, C. Hammerberg, O. Baadsgaard, J. Elder, L. Chan, D. Sauder, J. Vorhees, and G. Fisher, *J. Immunol. 144*, 4593 (1990).

B. Curtis, B. Gallis, R. Overell, C. McMahan, P. DeRoos, R. Ireland, J. Eisenman, S. Dower, and J. Sims, *Proc. Natl. Acad. Sci. 86*, 3045 (1989).

J. T. Elder, G. Fisher, P. Lindquist, G. Bennet, M. R. Pittelkow, R. Coffey, R. D. Granstein, R. Margolis, S. Mizel, and D. N. Sauder, *J. Clin. Invest. 77*, 1020 (1986).

A. Enk and S. Katz, *J. Immunol. 149*, 92–95 (1992).

E. Fuchs, *J. Cell Biol. 111*, 2807–2814 (1991).

R. Granstein, R. Margolis, S. Mizel, and D. Sander, *J. Clin. Invest. 77*, 1220–1227 (1986).

R. M. Grossman, J. Krueger, A. Granelli-Piperno, D. Murphy, L. May, T. S. Kupper, P. B. Sehgal, and A. Gottlieb, *Proc. Natl. Acad. Sci. 86*, 6367 (1989).

R. Groves, E. Ross, J. Ross, J. Barker, R. Campt, and D. MacDonald, *J. Invest. Dermatol. 98*, 384 (1992).

S. Haskill, G. Martin, L. Van Le, J. Morris, A. Peace, C. Bigler, G. Jaffe, C. Hammerberg, S. Sport, and S. Fong, *Proc. Natl. Acad. Sci. 88*, 3681 (1991).

C. Heufler, D. Young, G. Peschel, and G. Schuler, *J. Invest. Dermatol. 94*, 534a (1992).

R. Kirnbauer, A. Kock, T. Schwarz, A. Urbanski, J. Krutman, W. Borth, D. Damm, G. Shipley, J. Ansel, and T. Luger, *J. Immunol. 142*, 1922 (1989).

A. Kock, T. Schwarz, R. T. Kirnbauer, A. Urbanski, P. Perry, J. Ansel, and T. A. Luger, *J. Exp. Med. 172*, 1069 (1990).

T. S. Kupper, D. W. Ballard, A. Chua, J. McGuire, P. Flood, M. Horowitz, R. Langdon, L. Lightfoot, and U. Gubler, *J. Exp. Med. 164*, 2095 (1986).

T. S. Kupper, P. M. Flood, A. Chua, J. McGuire, U. Gubler, *J. Clin. Invest. 80*, 430 (1987).

T. S. Kupper, F. Lee, P. Flood, M. Horowitz, and D. Coleman. *Ann. NY Acad. Sci. 548*, 283 (1988a).

T. S. Kupper, F. Lee, N. Birchall, S. Clark, and S. Dower, *J. Clin. Invest. 82*, 1787 (1988b).

T. S. Kupper, K. Min, P. Sehgal, H. Mizutani, N. Birchall, A. Ray, and L. May, *Ann. NY Acad. Sci. 557*, 454 (1989).

T. S. Kupper, *Arch. Dermatol. 125*, 1406 (1989).

T. S. Kupper, *J. Invest. Dermatol. 94*, 146 (1990a).

T. S. Kupper, *J. Clin. Invest. 86*, 1783 (1990b).

C. Larsen, A. Anderson, J. Oppenheim, and K. Matsushima, *Immunology 68*, 31 (1989).

M. B. Lawrence, and T. A. Springer, *Cell 65*, 859 (1991).

T. Luger, B. Stadler, S. Katz, and J. Oppenheim, *J. Immunol. 127*, 1493 (1981).

T. Luger, A. Uchida, A. Kock, M. Colot, and M. Micksche, *J. Immunol. 143*, 2477 (1985).

T. Luger, A. Kock, R. Kirnbauer, T. Schwartz, and J. Ansel, 548, 253 (1988).

D. Metcalf, *Cancer 65*, 2185 (1990).

H. Mizutani, R. Black, and T. S. Kupper, *J. Clin. Invest. 87*, 1066 (1991a).

H. Mizutani, N. Schechter, R. Black, G. Lazarus, and T. S. Kupper, *J. Exp. Med. 174*, 821 (1991b).

J. J. Oppenheim, C. Zachariae, N. Mukaida, and K. Matsushima, *Annu. Rev. Immunol. 9*, 671 (1991).

U. Peterseim, S. Sarkar, and T. S. Kupper, *Cytokine* (in press), 1993.

D. Sauder, C. Carter, S. Katz, and J. Oppenheim. *J. Invest. Derm. 79*, 34 (1982).

J. M. Schroder, *Exp. Derm. 1*, 12 (1992).

T. A. Springer, *Nature 346*, 425 (1990).

K. Turksen, T. S. Kupper, L. Degenstein, I. Williams, and E. Fuchs, *Proc. Natl. Acad. Sci. 89*, 5068 (1992).

R. Vasser, and E. Fuchs, *Genes and Devel. 5*, 714 (1991).

# 14
# Ultraviolet Light and Epidermal Cell-Derived Cytokines

**Thomas Schwarz, Agatha Urbanski, and Thomas A. Luger**
*Ludwig Boltzmann Institute for Cell Biology and Immunobiology of the Skin*
*University of Münster*
*Münster, Germany*

## I. INTRODUCTION

Ultraviolet (UV) light has a great impact on human life: on the one hand, it is essential for life, on the other it can cause severe damage. The damaging effects of UV light are increasingly evident as a result of modern human behavior.

The UV spectrum is separated into three parts [1]. Wavelengths below 290 nm are referred to as UVC. For humans, UVC is of minor importance because it is completely absorbed by the ozone layer in the stratosphere. UVB is located between 290 and 320 nm. The division between UVB and UVA at 320 nm separates the most erythemogenic wavelengths from the less erythemogenic. UVA (320–400 nm) recently has been divided into UVA1 (340–400 nm) and UVA2 (320–340 nm), because UVA2 is more related to the UVB than to the long wave range [2]. However, one must be aware that all these classifications are arbitrary. In addition, it is important to remember that there is a great variation in the biological effects of different wavelength regions within these subdivisions. This is important when comparing studies using different light sources claiming to emit the same spectra. Thus, the most exact information is given by indicating the emission spectra of the respective light sources instead of using the terms UVA, UVA1, or UVB. Therefore, in this chapter the type of light source used is mentioned as far as this information is provided in the original publication.

## II. BIOLOGICAL EFFECTS OF UV LIGHT

Solar irradiation causes a variety of biological reactions in the skin, which may be both useful and harmful [3]. Exposure to small amounts of UVB is a requirement for photosynthesis of vitamin D in the skin. Larger amounts, depending upon skin type, cause sunburn; this is characterized by erythema, pain, swelling, blistering, and in severe cases epidermal necrosis. Sunburn is a classical cutaneous inflammatory reaction whose pathogenesis is not completely understood. Besides the immigration of inflammatory cells, the release of inflammatory mediators including eicosanoids and cytokines seems to be of relevance [4]. In addition, UVB exposure can compromise the immune system [5]. It is well known that immune reactions are decreased in areas that have been exposed to UV light. Moreover, there are indications that solar exposure can cause systemic immunosuppression [6]. Although the pathomechanisms involved are not quite clear, there is no doubt that the release of cytokines is of primary importance during these events [7].

Chronic UV exposure results in accelerated aging called photoaging [8]. This is characterized by changes in the dermis including solar elastosis. There is no doubt that both UVB and UVA contribute to photoaging. The role of UVA seems plausible because UVA penetrates through the epidermis reaching the dermis, while most of the UVB is absorbed in the upper layers of the epidermis. Recent data indicate that the release of cytokines induced by UV light is of relevance during the process of photoaging [9]. In addition, chronic UV exposure supports the generation of skin cancer [10]. The oncogenic effect of UV light in mammalian skin is primarily due to UVB irradiation. Although the major target in UV-induced carcinogenesis seems to be the DNA itself, it is important to emphasize that there is evidence for suppressive immunological effects of solar radiation in the skin, which could play an important role in the pathogenesis of these neoplasms [10]. In this context, the release of mediators with immunosuppressive properties upon UV exposure seems to be of relevance [7].

## III. THE EPIDERMIS AS A SOURCE FOR CYTOKINES

Within the last decade, it has been demonstrated that the epidermis is much more than just a mechanical barrier to the outside. Meanwhile, it is well established that the epidermis is a site where immune responses and inflammatory reactions can originate independently [11]. The concept of the epidermis as an active immune organ is based on the findings that it appears to contain constituents necessary for the initiation of an immune response. Accordingly, the epidermis harbors dendritic Langerhans cells, which can present antigens [12], cells belonging to the T-cell family (in the murine system) [13], and cells exhibiting the capacity to release a variety of inflammatory and immunological mediators including cytokines, growth factors, hormones, and eicosanoides [14]. Although keratinocytes appear to be the major source of epidermal cytokines, there is evidence that Langerhans cells [15, 16] and melanocytes also can produce immunomodulating factors [17].

The initial observations have been primarily based on biological as well as biochemical data and confirmed by detection of cytokine-specific mRNAs in epidermal cells. Murine keratinocytes are known to express mRNAs specific for interleukin (IL)-1$\alpha$, IL-1$\beta$, IL-3, IL-6, IL-7, IL-10, granulocyte-macrophage colony-stimulating factor (GM-CSF), macrophage colony-stimulating factor (M-CSF), tumor necrosis factor $\alpha$ (TNF-$\alpha$), transforming growth factor $\beta$ (TGF-$\beta$), and nerve growth factor (NGF) [18–29]. Human keratinocytes produce mRNA encoding for IL-1$\alpha$, IL-1$\beta$, IL-3, IL-6, IL-8, GM-CSF, granulocyte colony-stimulating factor (G-CSF), M-CSF, TNF-$\alpha$, basic fibroblast growth factor (bFGF), TGF-$\alpha$, platelet derived growth factor (PDGF), and TGF-$\beta$ [30–40]. There is ample evidence that the constitutive production both in vitro and in vivo is quite low, but dramatically enhanced upon injurious stimuli. UV light has turned out to be one of these inducers [7]. As exposure to UV light leads to local and systemic inflammatory reactions and alterations of the immune response, keratinocyte-derived mediators seem to play an important role in the pathogenesis of UV-induced reactions. This chapter will include epidermal cell-derived cytokines, whose release is known to be induced by UV-light either in vitro or in vivo. Furthermore, the implications of these findings for the pathogenesis of UV-induced dermatoses will be discussed.

## IV. INTERLEUKIN 1

Interleukin 1 (IL-1) is a multifunctional nonspecific cytokine which plays an important role in the mediation of immunological and inflammatory reactions [41, 42]. IL-1 was the first cytokine demonstrated to be secreted by keratinocytes. The epidermal cell product was initially described according to its property to costimulate the proliferative response of thymocytes to mitogens and thus was originally named epidermal cell–derived thymocyte-activating factor (ETAF) [43, 44]. ETAF soon turned out to be biochemically as well as biologically indistinguishable from IL-1. Definite proof that the two molecules are identical was finally provided by the demonstration that both murine and human keratinocytes express the mRNA specific for both IL-1$\alpha$ and IL-1$\beta$ [18, 30].

In contrast to macrophages, which mainly produce IL-1$\beta$, the major active IL-1 species released by keratinocytes seems to be IL-1$\alpha$. This may be due to the fact that biologically inactive 31-kd IL-1$\beta$ has to be cleaved into the active 17-kd form by a specific protease, which is not present in keratinocytes [45]. The release of IL-1 by keratinocytes both in vitro and in vivo seems to be low, however, it can be significantly upregulated by appropriate stimuli, including lipopolysaccharide (LPS), tumor promotors, silica, and other cytokines [46]. In addition, keratinocytes express IL-1 receptors [47]. The amount of IL-1 receptors found on epidermal cells appears to depend on stimulation since they are not detected on normal resting keratinocytes. Therefore, IL-1 receptor expression may be one of the determinants as to whether IL-1 will regulate function and growth of epidermal cells.

As the keratinocyte is the primary target for UV light, one can expect that a variety of UV-induced inflammatory and immunological reactions are mediated by epidermal cell–derived cytokines. This anticipation was first supported by the in vitro demonstration of an increase in both the extracellular and the intracellular ETAF activity of UVB-exposed (Westinghouse FS 20) murine epidermal cells, a murine transformed keratinocyte cell line (PAM 212), and a human keratinocyte cell line (SCC) [48]. The UV-induced ETAF activity was cycloheximide sensitive, suggesting that de novo synthesis of ETAF rather than cell membrane leakage was responsible for the increased activity. These observations were confirmed by another group, demonstrating presence of ETAF/IL-1 in the serum of UV light–exposed (Westinghouse FS 40) but not normal mice [48]. The UV-induced release of IL-1 by PAM 212 cells could be reduced by the addition of hydrocortisone, suggesting that this activity might account for the anti-inflammatory effect of glucocorticosteroids on the skin [50]. The induction of IL-1 by UV light was also confirmed at the transcriptional level showing significantly increased steady-state levels of IL-1$\alpha$ and IL-1$\beta$ mRNA in UVB-exposed (Westinghouse FS 20) human keratinocytes [51]. This was reflected also in the production of increased IL-1 bioactivity by the respective cultures in vitro. The level of actin mRNA, however, was unaffected by UVB light [51]. Another study could show that the outcome appears to depend on the UVB dose used [18]. High-dose UVB (3 $kJ/m^2$) inhibited PAM 212 IL-1$\alpha$ expression at 4, 8, 24, and 48 hours post-UV, whereas a lower dose of UVB (1 $kJ/m^2$) inhibited IL-1 at 4 and 8 hours, but induced IL-1 expression at 24 and 48 hours post-UV. The IL-1–inducing effect of UVB light appears not to be specific for keratinocytes, as similar findings have been reported with murine peritoneal adherent cells and a murine macrophage cell line (P388D1) [52].

Findings based on in vitro studies always raise the question of their in vivo relevance. By using an in vivo skin chamber method, increased release of IL-1–like activity was demonstrated at the site of irradiation with three times the minimal erythema dose of UVB (Philips TL12) [53]. UVB-augmented release peaked one hour after irradiation and levels returned to baseline by 2 hours. There is further evidence that IL-1 is induced in vivo by UV light; IL-1 levels were found enhanced in the sera of UVB-exposed (Westinghouse FS 40) rabbits and mice [49, 54]. Human volunteers given one minimal erythema dose of UVB light (Westinghouse FS 40) developed increased serum IL-1 activity as assessed by the thymocyte co-stimulator assay [55]. This activity peaked 1–4 hours after exposure and returned to baseline by 8 hours after irradiation. Recently IL-1 plasma levels have been found elevated in psoriatics undergoing phototherapy [56]. In order to remove plasma proteins that may inhibit IL-1 bioactivity, each sample was chromatographed and each fraction assayed for IL-1 activity. There was no detectable IL-1 before and one hour after UVB irradiation; IL-1 appeared 4 hours after treatment and was absent after 24 hours. Plasma IL-1 was neutralized by antibodies to recombinant human IL-1$\alpha$ and IL-1$\beta$. Since the predominant keratinocyte-derived subspecies is IL-1$\alpha$, this suggests that UV-induced IL-1 in the circulation may originate from both keratinocyte and nonkeratinocyte sources [56].

The combination of 8-methoxypsoralen (8-MOP) plus UVA light (PUVA, oral photochemotherapy) is a widely used efficient therapy for various skin disorders including psoriasis and cutaneous T-cell lymphoma [57]. From animal studies it is well established that PUVA suppresses inflammatory and immune reactions [58]. In order to obtain more insight into the mode of action of PUVA, the effect of 8-MOP plus UVA on IL-1 production by murine keratinocytes was studied [59]. Freshly isolated murine epidermal cells were exposed to various doses of 8-MOP (5–100 ng/ml) followed by UVA exposure (10 kJ/m$^2$, black light fluorescent bulbs filtered through 4-mm windowglass). Treatment resulted in a clear reduction of IL-1 bioactivity. The suppression was dependent on the dose of 8-MOP and not due to the induction of IL-1 inhibitors as described for UVB treatment [60].

A similar effect of in vitro PUVA was observed by using peripheral blood mononuclear cells (PBMC) as a source for IL-1$\beta$ [61]. Treatment of PBMC with 8-MOP (10–1000 ng/ml) followed by UVA exposure (20 kJ/m$^2$, Philips TL09) resulted in a significant reduction of IL-1$\beta$ protein in the supernatants. The data were confirmed by Northern blot analysis showing reduced IL-1$\beta$–specific transcripts in PUVA-treated PBMC. Neither 8-MOP nor UVA alone had any effect on the cytokine secretion by PBMC.

## V. INTERLEUKIN 6

Interleukin 6 (IL-6) functions as an important mediator of immunity and inflammation [62]. IL-6 is released by a variety of cells, and recently it has been shown that normal human epidermal cells, in particular keratinocytes, melanocytes, epidermoid carcinoma, and melanoma cell lines produce IL-6 [17, 32]. Human epidermal cells in culture spontaneously release only small amounts of IL-6. Addition of stimuli such as IL-1, tumor promotors, bacterial endotoxins, or concanavalin A significantly increases IL-6 production by keratinocytes [32]. As was the case for IL-1, the effect of UV light on the release of IL-6 by epidermal cells was an obvious subject for studies. Supernatants derived from UVB-exposed (Westinghouse FS 20) normal human keratinocytes or keratinocyte cell lines contained significantly increased levels of IL-6 bioactivity [63]. This was also confirmed by Western blot analysis resulting in specific bands at 23 and 27 kd. Northern blot analysis revealed increased IL-6 mRNA expression after UVB exposure. Addition of different corticosteroid preparations was able to reverse the UVB-induced induction of IL-6 suggesting that the therapeutic effect of corticosteroids may be partly due to their downregulating capacity of IL-6 production [63]. In the same study the effect of UVA1 light (UVASUN Mutzhas) in a dose range from 100 to 1500 $kJ/m^2$ did not have a significant effect on the IL-6 release by keratinocytes. However, it seems too premature to claim that UVA does not influence IL-6 production by keratinocytes at all, because there are preliminary observations that doses in the lower range do have an effect (Schwarz, unpublished observation).

There are indications that the induction of IL-6 by UV light takes place also in vivo. Because severe sunburn reaction is associated with fever, chills, and induction of an acute phase response—events that principally could be mediated via IL-6 [62]—the effect of a single UVB dose eliciting severe sunburn reaction was studied. Human volunteers underwent total body UVB exposure (Dr. Hönle blue light without filters) causing severe sunburn reaction [64]. In contrast to plasma samples obtained before UV exposure, post-UV specimens contained significant levels of IL-6 peaking at 12 hours after UV irradiation. Plasma IL-6 activity correlated remarkably with fever course followed by an increase of acute phase proteins such as C-reactive protein. These data indicate that IL-6, which is released by keratinocytes following UV exposure, may gain access to the circulation and via its pyrogenic as well as acute phase–inducing effects could function as an important mediator of systemic sunburn reaction.

In recent years the particular mechanisms involved in photoaging have been studied intensively. It is known that UVA reaches the reticular dermis making fibroblasts an accessible target. In addition, it has been shown that UVA induces the release of collagenase by fibroblasts [65]. Since IL-6 has been reported to stimulate collagenase production by fibroblasts [9, 66], it was studied whether the UV-induced collagenase increase is mediated via IL-6. Confluent fibroblast layers exposed to UVA1 light (50–350 $kJ/m^2$; UVASUN Mutzhas) released significantly enhanced levels of IL-6 as detected in an IL-6–specific bioassay [9]. These data were also confirmed by Northern blot analysis showing enhanced IL-6 transcripts in UVA1-exposed fibroblasts.

Incubation of irradiated cells with IL-6 antisense oligonucleotides resulted in a significant but not complete downregulation of collagenase. The failure of complete blocking may be due to the fact that UVA-induced release of other mediators such as IL-1 by fibroblasts may be of importance in the induction of collagenase as well [66].

As was the case for IL-1, the effect of PUVA on the release of IL-6 was studied [67]. Treatment of PBMC with 8-MOP (10–1000 ng/ml) followed by UVA exposure (20 kJ/m$^2$, Philips TL09) resulted in a significant reduction of IL-6 protein in the supernatants. The data were confirmed by Northern blot analysis showing reduced IL-6–specific transcripts in PUVA-treated PBMC.

## VI. TUMOR NECROSIS FACTOR ALPHA

Tumor necrosis and cachexia were found to be mediated by a macrophage-derived cytokine that was named cachectin/tumor necrosis factor $\alpha$ (TNF-$\alpha$) [68]. Another cytotoxic mediator released by lymphocytes was initially named lymphotoxin and now is called TNF-$\beta$. TNF-$\alpha$ and TNF-$\beta$ are antigenically distinct proteins, but they have similar biological activities and bind to a common receptor [69].

Like many other cytokines, TNF-$\alpha$ is produced by a variety of cells including keratinocytes [36]. Unstimulated epidermal cells express low levels of TNF-$\alpha$ mRNA and release minimal amounts of biologically active TNF-$\alpha$. Synthesis and release of TNF-$\alpha$ is significantly upregulated by tumor promotors and LPS. The production of TNF-$\alpha$ by human keratinocytes is also under control by UV light. Supernatants of UVB-exposed (Westinghouse FS 20) normal human keratinocytes and epidermoid carcinoma cell lines were found to contain significant amounts of TNF-$\alpha$, while in supernatants of untreated epidermal cells, no or minimal TNF-$\alpha$ activity was detected [36]. The biological data were also confirmed by Western and Northern blot analysis. These findings are in accordance with immunohistological observations using polyclonal TNF-$\alpha$ antibodies [70]. TNF-$\alpha$ was located on the epidermal cell membranes of the stratum granulosum and stratum spinosum in unexposed skin. After UVB exposure (Philips TL 12), the staining intensity for TNF-$\alpha$ was markedly increased, and the epidermal staining included the basal cell layer. Further evidence for the in vivo release of TNF-$\alpha$ after UV exposure results from the detection of increased TNF-$\alpha$ levels in the serum obtained from humans 12 and 24 hours after a single total body UVB exposure (Dr. Hönle blue light without filters) [36]. These findings suggest that keratinocytes upon stimulation are able to synthesize and release TNF-$\alpha$, which may gain access to the circulation.

Because IL-1 and IL-6 have been demonstrated to be downregulated by treatment of the combination of 8-MOP plus UVA, the effect of PUVA on the release of TNF-$\alpha$ has been studied [61]. Treatment of PBMC with 8-MOP (10–1000 ng/ml) followed by UVA exposure (20 kJ/m$^2$, Philips TL09) resulted in a significant reduction of TNF-$\alpha$ protein in the supernatants. The data were confirmed by Northern blot analysis showing reduced TNF-$\alpha$–specific transcripts in PUVA-treated PBMC.

## VII. COLONY-STIMULATING FACTORS

Colony-stimulating factors (CSFs), which induce stem-cell colony formation in soft agar cultures, include IL-3, GM-CSF, G-CSF, and M-CSF [71]. IL-3, also called multi-CSF, and GM-CSF stimulate the proliferation of multilineage colonies, whereas G-CSF induces mainly colonies of neutrophils and M-CSF causes primarily monocyte colony formation [72, 73].

A variety of cells throughout the body are capable of producing mainly the non–lineage-specific CSF, IL-3, and GM-CSF. Normal cells constitutively do not produce significant amounts of CSF; however, upon stimulation with endotoxins, interferons, or tumor promotors, monocytes, endothelial cells, and fibroblasts express high levels of G-CSF and M-CSF. Moreover, human and murine keratinocytes upon stimulation with tumor promotors synthesize and release GM-CSF, G-CSF, and M-CSF [25, 26, 34, 35]. Although murine keratinocytes have been shown to produce IL-3 [20], for a long period of time there was a debate as to whether human keratinocytes are also able to make IL-3. Finally, IL-3 protein and IL-3–specific transcripts have been recently detected in human keratinocyte cell lines [31].

Currently, it was shown that UVB exposure (Westinghouse FS-40) to PAM 212 cells results in increase of IL-3 and GM-CSF–specific mRNA [74]. By using slot blot analysis, enhanced levels of mRNA were found within one hour after UV treatment. However, only GM-CSF–specific bioactivity, as determined by antibody neutralization studies, was shown increased above baseline in cell supernatants. These effects were only observed when cells were cultured to subconfluency. Under confluent conditions a decrease in bioactivity was detected after UV exposure for both growth factors, and no change in mRNA levels was found. In addition to cell density, calcium and sodium levels during irradiation altered the release of IL-3 and GM-CSF. These data demonstrate that UV light influences the release of CSFs and suggests that the state of cell growth and conditions of membrane ion transport influence the mechanisms regulating the secretion of those factors. Moreover, it was shown that UVB-induced (Westinghouse FS 20) GM-CSF secretion by PAM 212 cells is mediated by enhanced release of IL-1$\alpha$ [75]. The increase of IL-1$\alpha$ preceded the rise of GM-CSF mRNA, addition of recombinant IL-1$\alpha$ to the medium increased GM-CSF mRNA expression, and IL-1$\alpha$ antibodies could completely inhibit UV-induced GM-CSF mRNA expression.

There is also evidence that CSF induction by UV light takes place in vivo. Albino hairless mice (SKH-1) were treated i.p. with a single dose of 5-fluorouracil sufficient to cause complete transient bone marrow suppression [76]. Daily UVB exposure resulted in the following observations: soluble extracts of UVB-irradiated skin stimulated proliferation of normal murine bone marrow cells, CSF activity present in normal murine skin was enhanced, and recovery of neutropenia was accelerated. Thus one may conclude that UVB irradiation leads to the cutaneous release of CSFs in amounts sufficient to reverse acute myelosuppression.

## VIII. OTHER CYTOKINES

When investigating the effect of UV light on the release of cytokines by epidermal cells, most of the research groups focused on the nonspecific inflammatory mediators like IL-1, IL-6, and TNF-$\alpha$. Consequently, a reasonable number of studies have broadened our knowledge about the mechanisms involved in UV-induced inflammation. However, there are also indications that other, more specific mediators are affected by UV light as well, although the data available so far are not as detailed.

Interleukin 8 (IL-8) is a potent chemotactic mediator that mainly attracts neutrophils and mediates their function [77]. Based on its biological functions, IL-8 seems to play an important role during inflammatory reactions. The main source of IL-8 are macrophages and fibroblasts, however, it has recently been shown that IL-8 can be produced by keratinocytes as well [33]. In addition, other IL-8–related peptides like melanoma growth-stimulating activity (MGSA), also called GRO, are found in the epidermis [78, 79]. Because UV light is supposed to be a contributing factor in the generation of malignant melanoma, the question of whether UV light affects the release of these peptides by keratinocytes appears obvious. Currently, GRO-specific transcripts were found to be increased in human keratinocytes within 0.5 hour after UVB exposure (70 $J/m^2$) [80]. GRO levels remained elevated for up to 6 hours after UV treatment. In addition, IL-8 seems to be an important mediator in the pathogenesis of psoriasis. Thus the effect of in vitro PUVA on the IL-8 release by PBMC was studied, demonstrating reduced expression of IL-8 both at the protein and at the mRNA levels after treatment of PBMC with 8-MOP (10–1000 ng/ml) followed by UVA exposure (20 kJ/cm$^2$, Philips TL09) [61].

IL-10 was originally described according to its capacity to inhibit lymphokine production by $T_H2$ cells and thus was initially called cytokine synthesis inhibitory factor [81]. Based on this capacity IL-10 is supposed to play an important role in the downregulation of inflammatory responses. In addition to being made by macrophages and T cells, IL-10 is made by keratinocytes as recently demonstrated [23, 24]. IL-10 production is enhanced upon application of contact allergens, while tolerogens or irritants have no effect [24]. UV light is known to inhibit inflammatory and immune reactions, and the selective nature of the UV-induced suppression is similar to the biological activity of IL-10. Accordingly, it could be demonstrated that UVB light upregulates IL-10 production by murine keratinocytes [23]. This was demonstrated both on the protein and the mRNA level. Moreover, there is evidence that keratinocyte derived IL-10 is involved in the systemic suppression of delayed type hypersensitivity caused by UV-light [23].

## IX. GROWTH FACTORS

Growth factors are a heterogeneous group of cytokines that comprises several mediators originally regarded as exclusive regulators of cell growth [82–84]. The family includes epidermal growth factor, TGF-$\alpha$, FGF, NGF, and platelet-derived growth factor (PDGF). In addition to controlling the growth of normal and malignant cells as well as matrix protein formation, some members of the family are important mediators of cell surface marker expression and immunoregulation [85]. Certain growth factors are also produced by keratinocytes [29, 37, 38], however, the mechanisms involved in the regulation of the release are not well characterized as are cytokines. At present there is evidence that UV light can induced the release of bFGF, TGF-$\alpha$, and NGF by keratinocytes [29, 37, 86]. Consequently, TGF-$\alpha$ has been suggested to be involved in the generation of UVB-induced epidermal hyperplasia [86]. In addition, TGF-$\alpha$ release by melanocytes and melanoma cell lines was found to be increased upon UV irradiation [87]. Although a possible autocrine mechanism for the epidermal melanocytic response as well as for UV-induced tumor promotion has been suggested, the in vivo relevance of those findings is questionable due to the use of a light source exhibiting its emission peak at 254 nm, which is not relevant in the solar spectrum reaching the earth because of absorption by the ozone layer in the stratosphere. Thus the in vivo implications of the growth factor–inducing effect of UV light remain to determined.

# X. UV-INDUCED RELEASE OF UNCHARACTERIZED FACTORS

## A. UV-Induced Immunosuppressive Factors

One of the most important biological effects of UV light is the induction of immunosuppression [5]. This immunomodulation may contribute at least partially to UV-induced carcinogenesis [10]. Immunological alterations that follow UV exposure can be divided into local and systemic immunosuppression. Local alterations result from a direct interaction between UV light and immunocompetent cells, e.g., Langerhans cells, in the irradiated area [88].

Higher doses of UV light influence immune responses, e.g., induction of contact hypersensitivity (CHS), at sites not exposed directly to UV light ("systemic" immunosuppression) [6]. How the events occurring at the irradiated site lead to an abnormal response to an antigen applied at a distant non–UV-exposed skin area remains unanswered so far. The most attractive hypothesis for this immunosuppression involves soluble mediators. Accordingly, the keratinocyte representing the main target for UVB light must be considered as the primary source of such putative inhibitors. In fact, it has been shown that intravenous injection of supernatants obtained from UV-exposed (Osram Ultravitalux) PAM 212 cells into naive mice 5 days before sensitization with dinitrofluorobenzene, a potent contact allergen, results in suppression of induction of CHS [89]. Since this suppressive activity was not observed in conditioned medium of unirradiated cells, one may suggest that UV irradiation induces the release of soluble suppressive mediator(s) by keratinocytes. Upon HPLC gel filtration this factor exhibited a molecular weight between 25 and 50 kd. For the first time, this study could at least partially explain the phenomenon of UV-induced systemic immunosuppression by showing that exposure of epidermal cells to UV light in vitro causes the release of immunoregulatory factors that mimic some of the immunosuppressive effects of in vivo UV irradiation.

Meanwhile the concept that UV-exposed keratinocytes secrete immunosuppressive factors has also been supported by other investigators. Accordingly, injection of supernatants from UVB-exposed (Westinghouse FS 40) PAM 212 cells suppressed the induction of delayed-type hypersensitivity (DTH) to alloantigen and trinitrophenyl-modified self antigens in syngeneic and allogeneic mice [90]. However, in this study application of supernatants from UVB-irradiated PAM 212 cells had no effect on the induction of CHS to trinitrochlorobenzene. On the other hand, treatment of keratinocytes with extremely low doses of UVA (Dermalight 2001 with H-1 filters) resulted in the release of a mediator that blocked CHS [90]. These findings indicate that more than one suppressor factor is released upon UV exposure by keratinocytes and that which factor is released depends on the UV spectrum. The DTH inhibitor was further characterized and appeared to be cycloheximide and trypsin sensitive and to bind to concanavalin A, suggesting it to be a glycoprotein of approximately 68 kd [91].

In addition, supernatants obtained from PAM 212 or fresh murine keratinocytes were found to suppress the proliferative response of KLH-specific $T_H1$ clones in the presence of KLH-coupled Langerhans cells [92]. Preincubation of Langerhans cells, but not of $T_H1$ cells, with the supernatants from irradiated keratinocytes suppressed $T_H1$ proliferation, suggesting that Langerhans cells and not $T_H1$ cells are the initial target of the suppressive activity.

Since all these suppressor factors have not yet been purified, it cannot be answered whether they are new mediators or well-known cytokines with a so-far-undescribed activity. In spite of that, there is evidence that TNF-$\alpha$ is involved in the suppression of CHS in mice as well. Recent studies with inbred strains of mice have revealed that impairment of CHS by UVB is a polymorphic trait polygenically dictated by susceptibility alleles at the LPS and TNF-$\alpha$ loci [93]. In particular, it was shown that strains of mice homozygenous both for the TNF-$\alpha^b$ and for the $LPS^n$ allele fall into the UVB-susceptible category. Accordingly, it could be demonstrated that injection of TNF-$\alpha$ prevents the induction of CHS and that administration of a TNF-$\alpha$ antibody prevents UVB-induced suppression of CHS [94]. These findings are supplemented by the observation that the release of TNF-$\alpha$ by keratinocytes can be induced by UVB light [36]. Taken together, the studies addressing the pathomechanisms involved in the UVB-induced immunosuppression indicate that more than one factor appear to be involved.

Recently, treatment of keratinocytes with 8-MOP plus UVA (Sylvania F15T8) was shown to release a mediator that depresses the DTH reaction to alloantigen [95]. The suppressive factor was secreted regardless of whether the psoralen formed monofunctional or bifunctional adducts with DNA and regardless of its phototoxicity. In addition, keratinocytes treated with 8-MOP (400 ng/ml) and lower doses of UVA (50–100 $J/m^2$) released a factor that inhibited CHS, but not DTH. Interestingly, the CHS inhibitor was induced by low UVA doses (100–500 $J/m^2$) alone as well [95]. This suggests that more than one immunosuppressive factor are released following treatment of keratinocytes with appropriate doses of psoralen and UVA light. Moreover, evidence is provided that immunosuppressive factors released by keratinocytes may play a role in the induction of systemic immune suppression following PUVA treatment [58].

The question of whether the release of these yet uncharacterized suppressor factors also happens in vivo is supported by other observations. Injection of plasma obtained from UVB-exposed (Westinghouse FS 40) mice into normal animals suppresses the ability of the recipient mice to respond adequately to contact allergens [96]. In addition, it has been shown that this results in the generation of antigen-specific T-suppressor cells. Whether the suppressor factor found in the serum of UV-treated mice is related to one of the keratinocyte-derived inhibitors [89, 90] is not yet clear because all these factors have not been purified to homogeneity. A UVB-inducible (Sylvania fluorescent bulbs F75/85W/UV21) serum factor that suppresses allergic contact dermatitis has also been found in guinea pigs [97].

In addition, in supernatants of UV-irradiated (Osram Ultravitalux) PAM 212 and freshly isolated murine epidermal cells, an inhibitory activity was found which blocked particular functions of IL-1 [60]. This observation was both interesting and surprising, since it was well established that supernatants derived from UV-exposed epidermal cells contain high levels of IL-1 [48, 51]. Consequently, this inhibitor (EC-contra-IL-1) was only found after chromatographic removal of the high amounts of IL-1 present in the supernatants. As in all previous studies, only crude supernatants were tested, and this inhibitor was always overlooked. Partially purified EC-contra-IL-1 blocked both natural and recombinant IL-1 in a dose-dependent manner and exhibited a molecular weight of approximately 40 kd and an isoelectric point of 8.8. In subsequent studies, an IL-1 inhibitor with similar biochemical characteristics was found in the sera of total body UVB-exposed (Philips TL12) mice, suggesting that the production of EC-contra-IL-1 is obviously not only an in vitro phenomenon [98]. This circulating factor could not be detected in unirradiated animals; maximum levels appeared between 12 and 24 hours after UV exposure. These observations support the view that epidermal cells upon UV exposure release contra-IL-1, which may gain access to the circulation and probably cause systemic immunosuppression. The biological in vivo functions of such inhibitors are not yet clear; however, they may be part of a physiological feedback mechanism downregulating IL-1 activity after excessive release of IL-1.

## B. Other Uncharacterized UV-Induced Factors

Exposure to sunlight has been implicated as a contributing factor in the etiology of melanoma [99]. Therefore it was studied whether the exposure of mouse epidermal cells to UVB light (Westinghouse FS 40) induces the release of factors that can stimulate the in vitro and in vivo growth of syngeneic melanoma cells [100]. Supernatants obtained from epidermal sheets exposed to UVB light, but not control supernatants, stimulated the in vitro and in vivo growth of murine melanomas, but not of other malignant tumors (fibrosarcoma, hepatocellular carcinoma, squamous cell carcinoma). The nature of the melanoma cell growth-stimulatory activity is not yet clear; possible candidates, however, include bFGF, melanoma growth-stimulatory activity (MGSA/GRO), and IL-8, factors that have been detected in the epidermis and shown to induce melanoma cell growth [37, 79, 80, 101].

## XI. BIOLOGICAL IMPLICATIONS OF THE CYTOKINE-MODULATING EFFECT BY ULTRAVIOLET LIGHT

The effect of UV light on the release of epidermal cytokines has been extensively investigated, and quite a number of studies address that issue. The majority of these papers used in vitro techniques, mostly exposing normal keratinocytes or keratinocyte cell lines to UV light and then measuring bioactivity or protein levels of the respective factor in the supernatants. In addition, most of these data have been confirmed by Northern blot analysis demonstrating increased mRNA levels after UV exposure. However, no detailed studies have been performed addressing whether this increase in mRNA is due to real enhanced transcription or to a change in mRNA stability. Moreover, it is not quite clear whether there are unique UV-responsive elements on the respective genes encoding for cytokines in epidermal cells.

In vitro studies raise the question of the in vivo relevance. This has been addressed by the use of immunohistochemistry demonstrating that the staining pattern, e.g., with TNF-$\alpha$ in UV-exposed skin, is more pronounced than in unirradiated controls [70]. Such studies, however, do not answer whether the cells stained with the antibodies are the source of the respective cytokine. Alternatively, cytokines released from other cells, e.g., inflammatory ones, may be bound to the receptors present on the epidermal cells. Accordingly, it has been reported that keratinocytes express receptors for IL-1, IL-4, IL-2, and the 55 kd TNF-$\alpha$ type I receptor [47, 102]. Another approach to prove in vivo induction is measuring cytokine levels in suction blister fluid raised in UV-exposed skin or using the skin chamber method [53]. Stronger evidence for in situ production of various cytokines by keratinocytes upon UV exposure may be generated from in situ hybridization studies, but to the best of our knowledge, no definite data have been published so far. There are only preliminary reports, for example, that TNF-$\alpha$ transcripts are greater expressed by keratinocytes in PUVA-treated skin (Petzelbauer, personal communication). Transgenic mice bearing a chloramphenicol acetyltransferase (CAT) construct that reports the synthesis of TNF in a tissue-specific manner express CAT as well as TNF in several extrathymopoietic tissues when injected with LPS [103]. In the same model, it was shown that in vivo UV exposure results in CAT expression within the skin.

Moreover, there is recent evidence that TNF-$\alpha$ is involved in the formation of sunburn cells, which are commonly found in UV-exposed epidermis.

The formation of sunburn cells could be significantly reduced by injection of a TNF-$\alpha$ antiserum immediately after UV exposure into irradiated murine skin [104]. Sunburn cells supposedly undergo apoptosis due to DNA fragmentation [105]. Accordingly, in DNA extracted from UV-exposed murine skin treated with the TNF-$\alpha$ antiserum, fragmentation was found to be less pronounced than in DNA from skin treated with UV light only [104].

Further evidence for the in vivo induction of cytokines by UV light is provided by detecting increased levels in the circulation after in vivo UV exposure. The first respective studies were performed in animals [49, 54]. Subsequently enhanced IL-1, IL-6, and TNF-$\alpha$ serum levels have been found in human volunteers after total body UVB exposure [36, 55, 56, 64]. The release of these mediators may be relevant in the pathogenesis of systemic sunburn reaction, which is characterized by fever, leukocytosis, and induction of an acute phase response. IL-1, IL-6, and TNF-$\alpha$ are nonspecific inflammatory cytokines exhibiting activities that could mediate these effects. Definite proof that these mediators are in fact involved in sunburn reaction can be achieved only by blocking experiments with antibodies; these studies of course have not been performed for ethical reasons. A likely alternative to address that issue in the future will be the application of physiological cytokine antagonists, such as the recently cloned IL-1 receptor antagonist [106], or drugs that inhibit the secretion of cytokines, as was recently shown to be true for pentoxifylline blocking the release of TNF-$\alpha$ by leukocytes [107, 108].

The cellular source of the cytokines detected to be enhanced in the circulation upon UV exposure is not yet completely clear. Since keratinocytes are the main target for UVB light and exhibit the capacity to release these mediators, it is easy to speculate that the circulating factors are keratinocyte derived, however, definite proof is lacking. This is also complicated by the fact that there is strong evidence for an in vivo network of interacting cytokines [109, 110]. This is based on several findings: cytokines usually have multiple overlapping activities, and they may induce each other, interfere with the expression of their receptors and those of other mediators, and thus can affect cell function in a synergistic, additive, or antagonistic way. For example, IL-1 can induce IL-6, thus it is possible that the enhanced IL-6 levels found in the circulation are not a direct effect of UV light, but at least partially indirect via the release of IL-1.

Adhesion molecules are newly recognized cell-surface receptors that play an important role in various immunological and inflammatory reactions by mediating lymphocyte–target cell and lymphocyte–accessory cell communication [111]. In the human epidermis keratinocytes were found to express intercellular adhesion molecule I (ICAM-1) [112]. ICAM-1/LFA-1 binding appears to be the major pathway by which lymphocytes and/or monocytes are able to attach to keratinocytes [113]. Thus the regulation of the expression of ICAM-1 on keratinocytes appears to be of relevance for immunological and inflammatory reactions within the skin. UV light has been demonstrated to influence ICAM-1 expression on keratinocytes significantly [114, 115]. UVB exposure of keratinocytes pretreated with interferon gamma, TNF-$\alpha$, or TNF-$\beta$ results in a significant reduction of ICAM-1 expression within 24 hours. After 48 hours, however, UV light alone is found to remarkably upregulate constitutive ICAM-1 expression on keratinocytes. This induction can be significantly blocked by addition of antibodies directed against TNF-$\alpha$ or IL-1 [116, 117]. These data suggest that UV light influences ICAM-1 expression on keratinocytes in a biphasic manner and also that the induction of ICAM-1 in the late phase is not a direct effect of UV light but indirect via the autocrine release of TNF-$\alpha$ and IL-1 by keratinocytes upon UV exposure [116, 117]. Similar observations have been made during studies of melanocytes and melanoma cells [118]. The in vivo relevance of this late-phase induction of keratinocyte ICAM-1 expression is supported by the observation that repeated exposure of humans to irradiation from a solar simulator (Sol-3 solar simulator) over 3 days results in significant ICAM-1 expression on keratinocytes [119]. Moreover, these data demonstrate that some of the immunomodulatory effects of UV light may not be direct, but indirect via the UV-induced release of epidermal cell–derived cytokines.

UVB light is known to induce the release of eicosanoids like prostaglandin $E_2$ by keratinocytes [120]. The secretion of these substances plays an important role in the mediation of UVB-induced erythema, which can be efficiently suppressed by the application of cyclooxygenase inhibitors [121]. There are also recent indications that prostaglandin release is not direct due to UV light, but may be mediated by UV-modulated cytokine secretion. TNF-$\alpha$ and IL-1 are known to stimulate prostaglandin release [122, 123]. Recently it has been shown that culture of UVB-irradiated (Westinghouse FS 40) keratinocytes in the presence of a TNF-$\alpha$ antibody results in a 50% reduction of prostaglandin $E_2$ production, indicating that endogenous TNF-$\alpha$ substantially contributes to increased prostaglandin synthesis by UV-treated keratinocytes [124]. Failure of complete suppression of prostaglandin secretion by TNF-$\alpha$ antibodies may be due to the fact that other UV-induced cytokines like IL-1 are involved as well [125].

The great majority of the studies addressing the implications of UV light on epidermal cytokine release has focused on the effects of UVB light. This may be due to the fact that UVB is the most relevant part of the solar spectrum in terms of biological activity. UVB exhibits potent proinflammatory properties, induces immunosuppression, and contributes to carcinogenesis [5, 10]. The fact that most of the studies focus on UVB, however, must not result in the conclusion that UVA has no effects, as frequently claimed. There is growing evidence that UVA may be involved in carcinogenesis too and that UVA may play an important role in premature skin aging [126–128]. Therefore, like several other aspects, the effects of UVA light on the release of cytokines need to be studied in the future. However, one has to be aware that the UVA range is much broader than the UVB part and that within the UVA spectrum distinct wavelengths exhibit different biological activities. There is no doubt that the lower wavelengths between 320 and 340 nm differ from the longer waves (340–400 nm). Awareness of this fact is extremely important when comparing studies using different UVA sources. Therefore definition of the spectrum of the light source should be as exact as possible.

There are some indications that, in contrast to previous expectations, UVA has an effect on the release of cytokines. Fibroblasts seem to respond quite well to UVA1 with enhanced production of IL-1 and IL-6 [66]. Keratinocytes obviously release mediators with immunosuppressive properties upon very low doses of UVA light [95]. However, much more needs to be done to elucidate the relationship between UVA light and cytokine secretion within the skin.

## XII. CONCLUDING REMARKS

Based on the present studies, there is no doubt that many of the biological activities of UV light are due to the induced release of cytokines by different cells. However, one has to be aware that there is strong evidence for a complicated network of interacting cytokines [109], thus it would be too simple to attribute one activity of UV light to a particular mediator. Additional studies of the cytokine cascade, in particular its regulatory mechanisms, will contribute to the further understanding of physiological and pathological reactions within the skin. This will also increase the knowledge of the mechanisms of the biological actions of UV light.

## NOTE ADDED IN PROOF

1. H. Christoph, A. Budnik, F. Parlow, R. Block, M. Grewe, and J. Krutmann, UVA1- and UVB-radiation affect human keratinocyte expression of intercellular adhesion molecule-1 by different mechanisms. *J. Invest. Dermatol. 100*, 443, 1993.

   In this abstract it is reported that in addition to UVB, UVA1 also affects ICAM-1 expression which ultimately may be mediated by cytokine release. In addition, there is evidence that UVB and UVA1 may act via different mechanisms.
2. A. Takashima, K. Ariizumi, L. Ellinger, P. R. Bergstresser, Mechanisms for UVB-induced depletion of dendritic epidermal T-cells. *J. Invest. Dermatol. 100*, 521, 1993.

   In this abstract it is reported that UVB depletes dendritic epidermal T-cells by induction of apoptosis. This effect can be reversed by IL-7. Moreover, it is shown that UVB downregulates the release of IL-7 by keratinocytes. This is the first observation that UVB is also able to suppress the release of particular cytokines like IL-7.

3. J. M. Rivas and S. E. Ullrich, Essential role of keratinocyte-derived interleukin 10 in the UV-induced suppression of delayed type hypersensitivity but not contact hypersensitivity. *J. Invest. Dermatol. 100*, 522, 1993.

   This abstract yields evidence that IL-10 primarily mediates UV-induced suppression of the induction of delayed type hypersensitivity, whereas TNF primarily mediates UV-induced suppression of contact hypersensitivity.
4. M. Simon, Y. Aragane, A. Schwarz, T. A. Luger, and T. Schwarz, UVB light induces NF-kappa-B activation by cytosolic NFkB-IkB complex dissociation in cell free protein extracts of human epidermal cells. *J. Invest. Dermatol. 100*, 526, 1993.

   This abstract shows that UVB-light causes activation of the transcription factor NFkB by inducing the dissociation of the NFkB-IkB complex. This event can be observed in DNA free protein cell extracts, suggesting a direct DNA damage independent mechanism of NFkB-IkB complex dissociation by UVB-light.

## REFERENCES

1. I. E. Kochevar, M. A. Pathak, and J. A. Parrish, in *Dermatology in General Medicine* (T. B. Fitzpatrick, A. Z. Eisen, K. Wolff, I. M. Freedberg, K. F. Austen, ed.), McGraw-Hill Book Company, New York, 1987, p. 1441.
2. M. Pathak, in *Biological Effects of UVA-Light* (F. Urbach, ed.), Valdenmar Publishing Co., Overland Park, KS, 1992, p. 1.
3. R. W. Gange, in *Dermatology in General Medicine* (T. B. Fitzpatrick, A. Z. Eisen, K. Wolff, I. M. Freedberg, K. F. Austen, ed.), McGraw-Hill Book Company, New York, 1987, p. 1451.
4. L. C. Harber, and D. R. Bickers, in *Photosensitivity Diseases* (L. C. Harber, D. R. Bickers, ed.), B.C. Decker Inc., Toronto, 1989, p. 112.
5. M. L. Kripke, *Photochem. Photobiol. 52*, 919 (1990).
6. M. Jessup, N. Hanna, E. Plaszynski, and M. L. Kripke, *Cell. Immunol. 38*, 105 (1978).
7. T. Schwarz and T. A. Luger, *J. Photochem. Photobiol. B4*, 1 (1989).
8. B. A. Gilchrest, *J. Am. Acad. Dermatol. 21*, 610 (1989).
9. K. Scharffetter, F. Wilmroth, M. Wlaschek, K. Bolsen, P. Lehmann, T. Krieg, G. Goerz, G. Plewig, and P. C. Heinrich, *Arch. Dermatol. Res. 283*, 58A (1991).
10. M. L. Kripke, *J. Am. Acad. Dermatol. 14*, 149 (1986).
11. J. Bos and M. L. Kapsenberg, *Immunol. Today 7*, 235 (1986).
12. G. Stingl, K. Tamaki, and S. I. Katz, *Immunol. Rev. 53*, 149 (1980).
13. G. Stingl, K. C. Gunter, E. Tschachler, H. Yamada, R. J. Lechler, W. M. Yokoyama, G. Steiner, R. N. Germain, and E. M. Shevach, *Proc. Natl. Acad. Sci. USA 84*, 2430 (1987).
14. T. Schwarz and T. A. Luger, in *Pharmacology of the Skin* (H. Mukhtar, ed.), CRC Press, Boca Raton, FL, 1992, p. 283.
15. S. Schreiber, O. Kilgus, E. Payer, R. Kutil, A. Elbe, C. Mueller, and G. Stingl, *J. Immunol. 149*, 3525 (1992).
16. A. H. Enk and S. I. Katz, *Proc. Natl. Acad. Sci. USA 98*, 1398 (1992).
17. A. Köck, T. Schwarz, M. Micksche, and T. A. Luger, in *Melanoma Research: Genetics, Growth Factors, Metastases and Antigens* (L. Nathanson, ed.), Kluwer Academic Publishers, Boston, 1991, p. 41.

18. J. C. Ansel, T. A. Luger, D. Lowry, P. Perry, D. Roop, and J. D. Mountz, *J. Immunol. 140*, 2274 (1988).
19. T. A. Luger and T. Schwarz, in *Epidermal Langerhans Cells* (G. Schuler, ed.), CRC Press, Boca Raton, FL, 1991, p. 217.
20. T. A. Luger, A. Köck, R. Kirnbauer, T. Schwarz, and J. C. Ansel, *Ann. NY Acad. Sci. 548*, 253 (1988).
21. T. S. Kupper, M. Horowitz, F. Lee, D. Coleman, and P. Flood, *J. Invest. Dermatol. 88*, 501A (1987).
22. C. Heufler, D. Young, G. Peschel, and G. Schuler, *J. Invest. Dermatol. 94*, 534A (1990).
23. J. M. Rivas and S. E. Ullrich, *J. Immunol. 149*, 3865 (1992).
24. A. H. Enk and S. I. Katz, *J. Immunol. 149*, 92 (1992).
25. T. S. Kupper, F. Lee, D. Coleman, J. Chodakewitz, P. Flood, and M. Horowitz, *J. Invest. Dermatol. 91*, 185 (1988).
26. J. A. Chodakewitz and D. L. Coleman, *Fed. Proc. A1472* (1988).
27. J. C. Ansel, M. Heinrich, S. Hefeneider, and P. Perry, *Clin. Res. 36*, 630A (1988).
28. R. J. Akhurst, F. Lee, and A. Balmain, *Nature 331*, 363 (1988).
29. V. A. Tron, M. D. Coughlin, D. E. Jang, J. Stanisz, and D. N. Sauder, *J. Clin. Invest. 85*, 1085 (1990).
30. T. S. Kupper, D. Ballard, A. O. Chua, J. S. McGuire, P. Flood, M. C. Horowitz, R. Langdon, L. Lightfood, and U. Gubler, *J. Exp. Med. 164*, 2095 (1986).
31. A. H. Dalloul, M. Arock, C. Fourcade, J. Y. Beranger, P. Jaffray, P. Debre, and M. D. Mossalayi, *J. Clin. Invest. 90*, 1242 (1992).
32. R. Kirnbauer, A. Köck, T. Schwarz, A. Urbanski, J. Krutmann, W. Borth, D. Damm, G. Shipley, J. C. Ansel, and T. A. Luger, *J. Immunol. 142*, 1922 (1989).
33. C. G. Larsen, A. O. Anderson, J. J. Oppenheim, and K. Matsushima, *Immunology 68*, 31 (1989).
34. T. S. Kupper, F. Lee, N. Birchall, S. Clark, and S. Dower, *J. Clin. Invest. 82*, 1787 (1988).
35. N. Birchall, L. Park, and T. S. Kupper, *Clin. Res. 36*, 374A (1988).
36. A. Köck, T. Schwarz, R. Kirnbauer, A. Urbanski, P. Perry, J. C. Ansel, and T. A. Luger, *J. Exp. Med. 172*, 1609 (1990).
37. R. Halaban, R. Langdon, N. Birchall, C. Cuono, A. Baird, G. Scott, G. Moellmann, and J. McGuire, *Proc. NY Acad. Sci. 548*, 180 (1988).
38. G. Fisher, J. Elder, J. Voorhees, J. Kawalki, C. Petersen, R. Derynck, and L. Ellingsworth, *Clin. Res. 36*, 645A (1988).
39. D. C. Damm, G. D. Shipley, C. E. Hart, and J. C. Ansel, in *Molecular and Cellular Biology of Cytokines* (J. J. Oppenheim, M. C. Powanda, M. J. Kluger, and C. A. Dinarello, eds.), Wiley Liss, New York, 1990, p. 111.
40. R. J. Coffey, R. Derynck, J. N. Wilcox, T. S. Bringman, A. S. Goustin, H. L. Moses, and M. R. Pittelkow, *Nature 328*, 817 (1987).
41. J. J. Oppenheim, E. J. Kovacs, K. Matsushima, and S. K. Durum, *Immunol. Today 7*, 45 (1986).
42. C. A. Dinarello, *FASEB J. 2*, 108 (1988).
43. T. A. Luger, B. M. Stadler, S. I. Katz, and J. J. Oppenheim, *J. Immunol. 127*, 1493 (1981).

44. D. N. Sauder, C. Carter, S. I. Katz, and J. J. Oppenheim, *J. Invest. Dermatol. 79*, 34 (1982).
45. H. Mizutani, R. Black, and T. S. Kupper, *J. Clin. Invest. 87*, 1066 (1989).
46. T. A. Luger, M. B. Sztein, J. A. Schmidt, P. Murphy, G. Grabner, and J. J. Oppenheim, *Fed. Proc. 42*, 2772 (1983).
47. R. A. Blanton, T. S. Kupper, J. K. McDougall, and S. Dower, *Proc. Natl. Acad. Sci. USA 86*, 1273 (1989).
48. J. C. Ansel, T. A. Luger, and I. Green, *J. Invest. Dermatol. 81*, 519 (1983).
49. L. Gahring, M. Baltz, M. B. Pepys, and R. Daynes, *Proc. Natl. Acad. Sci. USA 81*, 1198 (1984).
50. T. S. Kupper and J. McGuire, *J. Invest. Dermatol. 87*, 570 (1986).
51. T. S. Kupper, A. O. Chua, P. Flood, J. McGuire, and U. Gubler, *J. Clin. Invest. 80*, 430 (1987).
52. J. Ansel, T. A. Luger, A. Köck, D. Hochstein, and I. Green, *J. Immunol. 133*, 1350 (1984).
53. G. M. Murphy, P. M. Dowd, B. N. Hudspith, J. Brostoff, and M. W. Greaves, *Photodermatology 6*, 268 (1989).
54. J. C. Ansel, T. A. Luger, and I. Green, *J. Invest. Dermatol. 89*, 32 (1987).
55. R. D. Granstein and D. N. Sauder, *Lymphokine Res. 6*, 187 (1987).
56. N. Konnikov, S. H. Pincus, and C. A. Dinarello, *J. Invest. Dermatol. 91*, 235 (1989).
57. A. K. Gupta and T. F. Anderson, *J. Am. Acad. Dermatol. 17*, 703 (1987).
58. M. L. Kripke, W. Morison, and J. A. Parrish, *J. Invest. Dermatol. 81*, 87 (1983).
59. Y. Tokura, J. Yagi, R. L. Edelson, and F. P. Gasparro, *Photochem. Photobiol. 53*, 517 (1991).
60. T. Schwarz, A. Urbanska, F. Gschnait, and T. A. Luger, *J. Immunol. 138*, 1457 (1978).
61. P. Neuner, B. Charvat, R. Knobler, A. Urbanski, T. A. Luger, and T. Schwarz, *J. Invest. Dermatol. 98*, 654A (1992).
62. G. G. Wong and S. C. Clark, *Immunol. Today 9*, 137 (1988).
63. R. Kirnbauer, A. Köck, P. Neuner, E. Förster, J. Krutmann, A. Urbanski, E. Schauer, J. C. Ansel, T. Schwarz, and T. A. Luger, *J. Invest. Dermatol. 96*, 484 (1991).
64. A. Urbanski, T. Schwarz, P. Neuner, J. Krutmann, R. Kirnbauer, A. Köck, and T. A. Luger, *J. Invest. Dermatol. 94*, 808 (1990).
65. K. Scharffetter, M. Wlaschek, A. Hogg, K. Bolsen, A. Schothorst, G. Goerz, T. Krieg, and G. Plewig, *Arch. Dermatol. Res. 283*, 506 (1991).
66. M. Wlaschek, G. Herrmann, K. Bolsen, A. Urbanski, T. Krieg, G. Goerz, G. Plewig, and K. Scharffetter-Kochanek, *Arch. Dermatol. Res. 284*, 63 (1992).
67. P. Neuner, A. Möller, R. Knobler, Ch. Grünwald, A. Urbanski, R. Kirnbauer, T. A. Luger, and T. Schwarz, *J. Invest. Dermatol. 96*, 584A (1991).
68. E. A. Carswell, L. J. Old, R. L. Kassel, S. Green, N. Fiore, and B. Williamson, *Proc. Natl. Acad. Sci. USA 72*, 3666 (1975).
69. B. Beutler and A. Cerami, in *Immunophysiology; The Role of Cells and Cytokines in Immunity and Inflammation* (J. J. Oppenheim and E. M. Shevach, eds.), Oxford University Press, New York, 1990, p. 226.
70. A. Oxholm, P. Oxholm, B. Staberg, and K. Bendtzen, *Br. J. Dermatol. 118*,

369 (1988).
71. S. C. Clark and R. Kamen, *Science 236*, 1229 (1987).
72. C. Sieff, *J. Clin. Invest. 79*, 1549 (1987).
73. D. Metcalf, *Cancer 65*, 2185 (1990).
74. R. L. Gallo, R. Stazewski, D. N. Sauder, T. L. Knisely, and R. D. Granstein, *J. Invest. Dermatol. 97*, 203 (1991).
75. S. Nozaki, J. S. Abrams, M. K. Pearce, and D. N. Sauder, *J. Invest. Dermatol. 97*, 10 (1991).
76. N. Birchall, C. Gamba, and T. S. Kupper, *Clin. Res. 36*, (1988).
77. M. Baggioloini, A. Walz, and S. L. Kunkel, *J. Clin. Invest. 84*, 1045 (1989).
78. A. Richmond, E. Balentein, H. G. Thomas, G. Flaggs, D. E. Barton, J. Spiess, R. Bordoni, U. Francke, and R. Derynck, *EMBO J. 7*, 2025 (1988a).
79. J. M. Schröder, H. Gregory, J. Young, and E. Christophers, *J. Invest. Dermatol. 98*, 241 (1992).
80. R. C. McKenzie, C. Feliciani, T. J. Venner, and D. N. Sauder, *J. Invest. Dermatol. 98*, 565A (1992).
81. D. R. Fiorentino, M. W. Bond, and T. R. Mosmann, *J. Exp. Med. 170*, 2081 (1989).
82. M. D. Waterfield, *Lancet 1*, 1243 (1989).
83. K. A. Thomas, *FASEB J. 1*, 4334 (1987).
84. R. Ross, *Lancet 2*, 1179 (1986).
85. M. B. Sporn and A. B. Roberts, *J. Clin. Invest. 78*, 329 (1986).
86. G. M. Murphy, D. G. Quinn, R. D. R. Camp, J. I. M. Hawk, and M. W. Greaves, *Br. J. Dermatol. 125*, 566 (1991).
87. K. A. O. Ellem, M. Cullinan, K. C. Baumann, and A. Dunstan, *Carcinogenesis 9*, 797 (1988).
88. O. Baadsgaard, *Arch. Dermatol. 127*, 99 (1991).
89. T. Schwarz, A. Urbanska, F. Gschnait, and T. A. Luger, *J. Invest. Dermatol. 87*, 289 (1986).
90. T. Y. Kim, M. L. Kripke, and S. E. Ullrich, *J. Invest. Dermatol. 94*, 26 (1990).
91. S. E. Ullrich, B. W. McIntyre, and J. M. Rivas, *J. Immunol. 145*, 489 (1990).
92. K. J. Eerkes, A. Takashima, P. R. Bergstresser, and P. D. Cruz, *J. Invest. Dermatol. 98*, 557A (1992).
93. J. W. Streilein and P. R. Bergstresser, *Immunogenetics 27*, 252 (1988).
94. T. Yoshikawa and J. W. Streilein, *Immunogenetics 32*, 398 (1990).
95. F. Aubin, M. L. Kripke, and S. E. Ullrich, *J. Invest. Dermatol. 97*, 995 (1991).
96. R. P. Swartz, *J. Invest. Dermatol. 83*, 305 (1984).
97. O. B. Christensen, M. B. Christensen, and L. M. Wall, *Contact Dermatitis 16*, 208 (1987).
98. T. Schwarz, A. Urbanski, R. Kirnbauer, A. Köck, F. Gschnait, and T. A. Luger, *J. Invest. Dermatol. 91*, 536 (1988).
99. H. K. Koh, B. E. Kligler, and R. A. Lew, *Photochem. Photobiol. 51*, 765 (1990).
100. C. Q. Wang, M. L. Kripke, and I. J. Fidler, *Photodermatol. Photoimmunol. Photomed. 7*, 128 (1990).
101. E. Förster, R. Kirnbauer, A. Urbanski, A. Köck, T. A. Luger, and T. Schwarz, *J. Invest. Dermatol. 96*, 608A (1991).

102. U. Trefzer, M. Brockhaus, H. Loetscher, F. Parlow, A. Kapp, E. Schöpf, and J. Krutmann, *J. Invest. Dermatol. 97*, 911 (1991).
103. B. Beutler, *Eur. Cytokine Netw. 3*, 120 (1992).
104. T. Schwarz, A. Urbanski, F. Trautinger, P. Neuner, and T. A. Luger, in *Basic Mechanisms of Physiological and Aberrant Lymphoproliferation in the Skin* (W. A. Van Vloten, W. C. Lambert, eds.), Plenum Publ. Corp., New York, in press.
105. K. Danno and T. Horio, *Photochem. Photobiol. 45*, 683 (1987).
106. S. P. Eisenberg, R. J. Evans, W. P. Arend, E. Verderber, M. T. Brewer, C. H. Hannum, and R. C. Thompson, *Nature 343*, 341 (1990).
107. R. M. Stieter, D. G. Remick, and P. A. Ward, *Biochem. Biophys. Res. Comm. 155*, 1230 (1988).
108. A. Schwarz, C. Krone, F. Trautinger, Y. Aragane, P. Neuner, T. A. Luger, and T. Schwarz, *J. Invest. Dermatol.*, in press.
109. F. R. Balkwill and F. Burke, *Immunol. Today 10*, 299 (1989).
110. T. A. Luger and T. Schwarz, *J. Invest. Dermatol. 95*, 100S (1990).
111. T. A. Springer, *Nature 346*, 425 (1990).
112. K. H. Singer, D. T. Tuck, H. A. Sampson, and R. P. Hall, *J. Invest. Dermatol. 92*, 746 (1989).
113. M. L. Dustin, K. H. Singer, D. T. Tuck, and T. A. Springer, *J. Exp. Med. 167*, 1323 (1988).
114. J. Krutmann, A. Köck, E. Schauer, F. Parlow, A. Möller, A. Kapp, E. Förster, E. Schöpf, and T. A. Luger, *J. Invest. Dermatol. 95*, 127 (1990).
115. D. A. Norris, B. Lyons, M. H. Middleton, J. J. Yohn, and M. Kashihara-Sawami, *J. Invest. Dermatol. 95*, 132 (1990).
116. J. Krutmann, W. Czech, F. Parlow, U. Trefzer, A. Kapp, E. Schöpf, and T. A. Luger, *J. Invest. Dermatol. 98*, 923 (1992).
117. J. Krutman, U. Trefzer, A. Kapp, E. Schöpf, and T. A. Luger, *J. Invest. Dermatol. 98*, 578A (1992).
118. R. Kirnbauer, B. Charvat, E. Schauer, A. Köck, A. Urbanski, E. Förster, P. Neuner, I. Assmann, T. A. Luger, and T. Schwarz, *J. Invest. Dermatol. 98*, 320 (1990).
119. D. A. Norris, S. D. Bennion, and M. H. Middleton, *J. Invest. Dermatol. 94*, 560 (1990).
120. M. W. Greaves, *Curr. Probl. Derm. 15*, 18 (1986).
121. D. S. Snyder and W. M. Eaglestein, *Br. J. Dermatol. 90*, 91 (1974).
122. S. M. Krane, J. M. Dayer, L. S. Simon, and S. Byrne, *Collagen Relat. Res. 5*, 99 (1985).
123. C. A. Dinarello, J. G. Cannon, S. M. Wolff, H. A. Bernehiem, B. Beutler, A. Cerami, I. S. Figari, and M. A. Palladino, *J. Exp. Med. 163*, 1433 (1988).
124. M. Grewe, U. Trefzer, M. Brockhaus, A. Kapp, E. Schöpf, and J. Krutmann, *Arch. Dermatol. Res. 284*, 40 (1992).
125. A. Pentland and M. G. Mahoney, *J. Invest. Dermatol. 94*, 43 (1990).
126. P. T. Strickland, *J. Invest. Dermatol. 87*, 272 (1986).
127. H. J. C. M. Sterenborg and J. C. van der Leun, *Photochem. Photobiol. 51*, 325 (1990).
128. L. H. Kligman, *J. Am. Acad. Dermatol. 21*, 623 (1989).

# 15
# Cytokines and Wound Healing

**Cornelia Mauch, Takashi Oono, Beate Eckes, and Thomas Krieg**
*University of Cologne*
*Cologne, Germany*

## I. INTRODUCTION

The normal wound-healing process has been divided into five overlapping phases: inflammation, granulation tissue formation, epithelialization, matrix production, and remodeling [1, 2] (Table 1). During injury blood vessels are disrupted, resulting in extravasation of blood constituents and concomitant platelet aggregation. In addition, blood coagulation generates biologically active substances, which promote cell migration and growth into the site of injury.

Neutrophils are the first leukocytes that infiltrate the area of inflammation, followed by monocytes, seen shortly thereafter. The major function of neutrophils during the early inflammation phase is to eliminate contaminating bacteria. The influx of monocytes and their activation to macrophages, in contrast, has an important impact on the initiation of tissue repair. Although macrophages like neutrophils consume pathogenic microorganisms and remove tissue debris, they release a large number of biologically active cytokines (e.g., IL-1, TGF-$\beta$, TGF-$\alpha$, PDGF, bFGF, TNF), which are important for the formation of granulation tissue in the next phase of wound repair [2–8].

Granulation tissue formation includes accumulation of macrophages, ingrowth of fibroblasts, deposition of a loose connective tissue composed of collagen, fibronectin, and hyaluronic acid, and angiogenesis. Wound fibroblasts derive from cells in the close vicinity of the wound. Stimulated

**Table 1** Phases During Wound Healing

| |
|---|
| Inflammation |
| Granulation tissue formation |
| Epithelialization |
| Matrix deposition |
| Remodeling |

by a variety of growth and chemotactic factors, they become mobile and migrate into the area of injury [4, 8]. They proliferate and deposit a loose extracellular matrix (ECM). In addition, these cells align along the radial axes of the wound, exert mechanical forces, and generate a concerted tension that results in wound contraction. The directed growth of microvascular endothelial cells occurs simultaneously with the migration of fibroblasts, stimulated by active factors released from platelets and macrophages [10]. The increased angiogenesis results in a rich microvascularization of the granulation tissue and gives a deep red color. It also provides the new tissue with oxygen and nutrients needed for growth of the tissue.

Reepithelialization of a wound begins within hours after injury. Epithelial cells surrounding the defect become mobile and move into the defect. At the wound edge epithelial cells begin to proliferate and the new cells migrate either on an intact basement membrane, or, if the basement membrane is destroyed by injury or subsequent enzymatic degradation, cells migrate across a provisional matrix of fibrin and fibronectin which is then replaced with basement membrane. The stimuli for epithelial proliferation are unknown, however, local release of growth factors, e.g., EGF, is likely to induce epidermal proliferation and was found to increase movement of epithelial cells and reepithelialization when added exogenously [11]. Once reepithelialization is complete, epithelial cells reform hemidesmosomes, revert to their normal phenotype, and attach to the new basement membrane, thus reforming a barrier to further contamination.

Wound healing therefore appears to be a highly complex process that involves several regulatory mechanisms. Characteristic for wound healing is the interaction of a variety of different cell types, which communicate by direct cell-cell interaction (Fig. 1) or by the secretion of cytokines. Although most of the initial events following tissue injury seem to involve endothelial cells and fibroblasts, keratinocytes have also been found to release a large number of cytokines, which could potentially be active in all phases of wound healing (Table 2).

The fifth phase of wound repair involves matrix formation and remodeling. This phase requires months for completion, during which time the loose

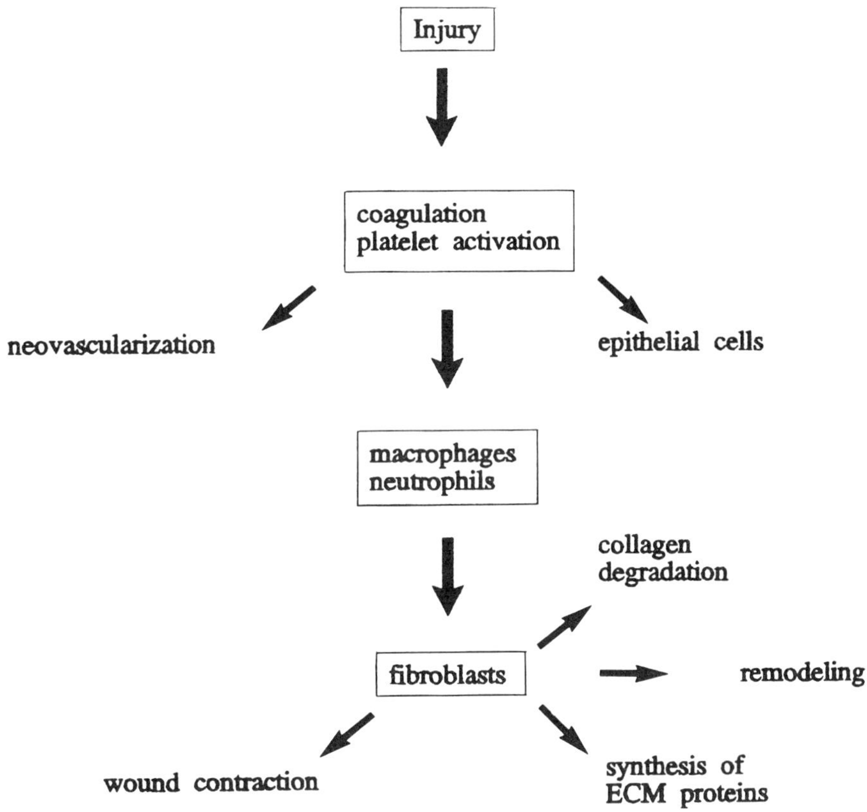


**Fig. 1** Interaction of different cell types during wound healing.

**Table 2** Cytokines Produced by Keratinocytes with Activity on Wound Healing Process

| Cytokine | Activity |
|---|---|
| PDGF | granulation tissue formation |
| bFGF | granulation tissue formation |
| TGF-$\alpha$ | epithelialization |
| TGF-$\beta$ | matrix deposition |
| IL-1 | matrix deposition, tissue remodeling |
| IL-6 | inflammation |
| TNF | tissue remodeling |
| IL-8 | inflammation |
| CSF | inflammation |

extracellular matrix consisting of fibronectin and large amounts of highly hydrated hyaluronic acid in granulation tissue that is easily penetrated by ingrowing cells is removed and replaced by collagen fibrils, which then provide the residual scar with increasing tensile strength. As the matrix becomes mature over several weeks, fibronectin and hyaluronic acid disappear and proteoglycans as well as fibrils of collagen types I, III, and V are deposited and grow in size. Recent studies have shown that de novo synthesis of collagen I during wound repair is time-dependently controlled. Using in situ hybridization techniques, collagen gene expression was localized on a cellular level and activation of collagen synthesis was first found within fibroblastic cells around the deep layers of the granulation tissue as early as 16 hours after wounding. After 6 days most of the cells in the granulation tissue synthesized collagen, and they decreased to basal activity after 26 days [9].

## II. CONTROL OF CONNECTIVE TISSUE METABOLISM BY CYTOKINES

The extracellular matrix (ECM) in skin has a complex composition and contains many components (Table 3). The remodeling of connective tissue during wound healing involves both the degradation of the extracellular matrix and the coordinated synthesis of new matrix components. Both pathways normally are maintained under tight control and balanced but are altered in repair processes such as wound healing. Over the last years studies from a number of different investigators have demonstrated that products of inflammatory cells play a role in the regulation of extracellular matrix proteins and their degradation. Although in vivo these processes are controlled by the complex interaction of different cytokines with synergistic and antagonistic effects, the availability of pure cytokines through recombinant DNA technologies allowed the selective study on a molecular level of the

**Table 3** Composition of the ECM in Skin

| Basement membrane components | Interstitial connective components |
|---|---|
| Laminin | Collagen I, III |
| Collagen IV | Collagen V |
| Nidogen/Entactin | Collagen VI |
| BM 40 | Fibrillin |
| Collagen VII | Elastin |
| Heparansulfate proteoglycan | Proteoglycans |
| Bullous pemphigoid antigen | |

influence of defined molecules on migration, proliferation, and biosynthesis in different cell types in vitro.

## A. Regulation of Collagen Synthesis by Various Cytokines

The collagens constitute a large group of triple helical matrix proteins which give connective tissues their strength. Several proteins are synthesized in the skin by fibroblasts or fibroblastlike connective tissue cells (Table 4). However, other cell types (e.g., keratinocytes, endothelial cells) contribute to the synthesis of collagenous proteins. Type I collagen is the major structural component of the skin, which is found to be associated with type III and type V collagens. Normal dermis contains about 80% type I and 20% type III collagen [13]. The amount of type III collagen in healing wounds and in granulation tissue is higher than in normal skin [14]. During maturation of the scar, type III collagen is gradually replaced by type I collagen and the normal ratio of these collagen types is reestablished.

Biosynthesis of collagen I is a highly complex process involving transcription of the pro $\alpha_1$ (I) and pro $\alpha_2$ (I) genes, processing of the pre-mRNAs to mature mRNAs, and translation of these mRNAs into pre–pro $\alpha$-chains. These precursor molecules are modified posttranslationally by hydroxylation of some proline and lysine residues and subsequent glycosylation of hydroxylysine. Triple helices form, which are secreted into the extracellular space where the procollagen molecules are processed by cleavage of the N- and C-terminal propeptides, and the resulting mature collagen molecules containing two $\alpha_1$ (I) and one $\alpha_2$ (I) chain can aggregate to fibrils [15]. Various cytokines stimulate or inhibit some of these processes and thereby regulate the level of type I collagen in the tissue. The most important factors that directly influence collagen synthesis include PDGF, TGF-$\beta$, IL-1, TNF-$\alpha$, EGF, and different interferons.

**Table 4** Collagens Synthesized by Fibroblasts

| Collagen type | Chain composition |
|---|---|
| Collagen I | $\alpha$1(I) $\alpha$2(I) |
| Collagen III | $\alpha$1(III) |
| Collagen V | $\alpha$1(V) $\alpha$2(V) |
| Collagen VI | $\alpha$1(VI) $\alpha$2(VI) $\alpha$3(VI) |
| Collagen VII | $\alpha$1(VII) |
| Collagen XII | |
| Collagen XIV | |

*Platelet-Derived Growth Factor*

Platelet-derived growth factor (PDGF) has been suggested to play an important role in wound healing. It is a mitogen and acts as chemoattractant for several cell types [8]. Although a direct activity on connective tissue synthesis is not very pronounced, recent reports [10, 12] demonstrate that skin injury can induce the expression of the PDGF receptor b and the c-*sis*/PDGF-2 in epithelial cells and the c-*sis* in fibroblasts. The expression levels correlated well with the stage of tissue repair. The studies provide further evidence that PDGF plays an important part in controlling connective tissue cell activation and, therefore, in an indirect fashion matrix deposition in wound healing.

*Transforming Growth Factor*

Transforming growth factor (TGF-$\beta$) is one of the most powerful mediators released during wound-healing processes. It was found to display pleiotropic effects on proliferation, cell migration, and biosynthesis of a variety of target cell types. In vivo studies of wound healing have shown that TGF-$\beta$ has an important role as an endogenous mediator of wound repair [16–18]. When injected subcutaneously in newborn mice, TGF-$\beta$ results in the formation of granulation tissue with angiogenesis and collagen deposition [16, 26] at the site of injection. In another study TGF-$\beta$ was topically applied to linear incisions made through the skin of rats. A dose-dependent, direct stimulatory effect on the breaking strength of the healing wounds was demonstrated [17]. The increase in wound strength was found to be accompanied by an increased influx of mononuclear cells and fibroblasts and by a marked increase in collagen deposition at the site of application of TGF-$\beta$ [16–18, 26]. These studies implicate that TGF-$\beta$ is a potent agent that can accelerate wound healing.

The family of TGF-$\beta$ peptides consists currently of four TGF-$\beta$, which display a strong homology within different species. Among them TGF-$\beta$1 is the best characterized. TGF-$\beta$1 is released in large quantities by platelets during degranulation, however, a wide variety of other cell types were found to synthesize and secrete this mediator as well [19, 21]. TGF-$\beta$ is synthesized as a large precursor of about 390 amino acids, which is processed by cleavage of the C-terminal domain. The mature TGF-$\beta$ is a homodimeric peptide of 25 kd, which remains associated in a latent complex with a binding protein. This latent complex is incapable of binding to the TGF-$\beta$ receptor and must be activated by dissociation from the protein for full activity. Although in vitro this activation can be achieved by acidification or plasmin treatment [21, 22], the physiological process of activation in vivo is unknown. Coculture experiments of smooth muscle cells and endothelial cells indicate that cell-cell interactions may play an important role in this activation. Whereas both cell types alone produced latent TGF-$\beta$, activation was only found in co-cultures [22]. Activated TGF-$\beta$ has divergent effects on different cell types depending on the amount of TGF-$\beta$ present. At femtomolar concentrations, TGF-$\beta$1 is a potent chemoattractant for macrophages and fibroblasts [23, 24] and causes their activation. Higher concentrations also induce the secretion of other factors such as IL-1, FGFs, TNF-$\alpha$, PDGF, and TGF-$\alpha$, which in turn control connective tissue metabolism [24]. Macrophages that have been activated by TGF-$\beta$ increase their expression of TGF-$\beta$1 mRNA [25] and therefore potentiate the effect of this cytokine.

The effect of TGF-$\beta$ on wound repair and granulation tissue formation has been reproduced in cell culture systems with isolated fibroblasts. Here, TGF-$\beta$1 was shown to stimulate collagen and fibronectin production in a variety of fibroblastic cell lines [26–28]. The increase in protein synthesis was accompanied by elevated mRNA levels, suggesting that transcriptional regulation of synthesis of both proteins is involved. In addition, this stimulation was found to proceed rapidly, since increased mRNA levels could already be detected 2 hours after addition of TGF-$\beta$, reaching a maximum after about 10 hours, which remained constant for at least 24 hours following a single addition of TGF-$\beta$1 to the cultures.

Transcriptional stimulation involves complicated interactions between *cis*-acting DNA sequences and *trans*-acting protein factors. Several regulatory proteins have been identified within the promotor and in the first intron of the collagen type I genes [29]. In particular, a TGF-$\beta$ activation region has been located in the mouse $\alpha_2$ (I) gene to about 300 base pairs before the transcription start site [30]. Using DNA transfection, it has been shown that promoter activity was stimulated 5- to 10-fold by TGF-$\beta$; a 3 bp substitution mutation that abolished binding of the DNA-binding protein NF1 resulted in the loss of induction by the cytokine [30]. Recent studies on the $\alpha_1$ (I) gene located a *cis*-acting element within sequences 1.600 bases upstream of the transcription start site, which is similar to the previously characterized $\alpha_2$ (I) element but is located in a different region [31]. In addition, de novo transcription of the gene after TGF-$\beta$ treatment was not dependent on synthesis of new proteins, since inhibitors, e.g., cycloheximide, did not influence de novo transcription, suggesting the presence of preexisting DNA-binding proteins [31]. Other investigators have shown that TGF-$\beta$ is not only capable of controlling de novo transcription of collagen genes, but can also increase selectively the stability of synthesized collagen mRNA leading to up to 20-fold higher de novo synthesis of collagen proteins [32, 33].

### *Interleukin 1 and Tumor Necrosis Factor*

Among the large number of factors released by monocytes, interleukin 1 (IL-1) and tumor necrosis factor alpha (TNF-$\alpha$) have been well characterized and appear to play a role in regulation of collagen synthesis during wound healing [34–36]. Although IL-1 and TNF-$\alpha$ share a variety of properties, they are distinct polypeptides and bind to different specific receptors [37]. IL-1 exists in two different forms, IL-1$\alpha$ and IL-1$\beta$, which display only low homology but bind to the same cell surface receptor. They share the same biological properties, however, they were found to differ in their quantitative effect on the response by various cell types [34, 38]. Both IL-1 and TNF-$\alpha$ are released by macrophages and monocytes during inflammation, however, they are also expressed by other cells including endothelial cells and fibroblasts. Several studies have reported that IL-1 and TNF-$\alpha$ can increase as well as inhibit collagen production of fibroblasts depending on the experimental conditions used. A two- to fourfold stimulation of collagen synthesis could only be observed in serum-free conditions, whereas in presence of serum no effect or even inhibition was demonstrated [39–41]. In all circumstances the observed changes in collagen synthesis were paralleled by alterations in mRNA levels, suggesting control mechanisms on a transcriptional level. In addition, IL-1 and TNF-$\alpha$ were found to display different effects when tested individually or in combination. Whereas collagen synthesis was stimulated in serum-free conditions, no induction could be observed when both cytokines were applied in combination, suggesting a complex interaction in the cytokine network in vivo [39].

### *Interferons*

An inverse inhibitory effect on collagen synthesis has been demonstrated for interferon gamma (IFN-$\gamma$), a cytokine produced by activated lymphocytes. IFN-$\gamma$ belongs to a multigene family whose protein products have been divided into three main types: IFN-$\alpha$, -$\beta$, and -$\gamma$. These polypeptides exhibit antiproliferative and antitumor effects and also have immunoregulatory functions [42]. All interferons were found to inhibit collagen synthesis; among then IFN-$\gamma$ had the most powerful effect [43]. Interestingly, IFN-$\gamma$ was found to reduce type III collagen synthesis to a larger extent than type I, resulting in an increased ratio of type I and type III collagen, whereas fibronectin production was induced by the cytokine. In vitro transcription experiments further elucidated that IFN-$\gamma$ can display regulatory effects on different levels [45–47]. Whereas the amount of collagen protein was decreased, de novo synthesis of collagen mRNA was unaltered, indicating regulation on a posttranscriptional level. In contrast, increased synthesis of fibronectin was paralleled by induced transcription of the corresponding gene [47]. IFN-$\gamma$ also can reverse the stimulatory effect of TGF-$\beta$ on collagen production, which results in a net inhibition of collagen synthesis [46]. Simultaneously, the increase of fibronectin production induced by TGF-$\beta$ was augmented further by IFN-$\gamma$. This additive increase in the synthesis of fibronectin was accompanied by parallel alterations in the corresponding mRNA levels. These findings suggest that IFN-γ modulates expression of the collagen gene by a combination of transcriptional and posttranscriptional events, whereas fibronectin gene expression is controlled by transcriptional mechanisms. IFN-γ also displays synergistic effects on collagen synthesis when applied in combination with TNF-α. Whereas TNF-α reduces collagen synthesis about twofold in presence of serum, combined exposure results in an almost complete downregulation of collagen production, which was found to be more than an additive effect [36]. The importance of these observations is not clear, however, recent evidence indicates that IFN-γ induces specific receptors for TNF-α in a variety of cell types, which might be the basis, at least in part, for the synergism of both cytokines [48].

## B. Regulation of Metalloproteinase Activity by Cytokines

The remodeling of connective tissue during inflammation and wound healing involves degradation of the extracellular matrix (ECM). Macrophages participate in modulation of matrix turnover both directly by secretion of proteinases and proteinase inhibitors and indirectly by the release of cytokines such as IL-1, TNF-α, and TGF-β that induce or repress gene expression of metalloproteinases and their inhibitors in fibroblasts, endothelial cells, and epidermal cells.

Two families of proteases and inhibitors are involved in degradation of connective tissue proteins. The plasminogen activator system includes two different plasminogen activators, urokinase-type (u-PA) and tissue-type (t-PA), which activate plasminogen, leading to the formation of plasmin, which is capable of degrading a number of proteins present in the ECM such as fibronectin, laminin, and fibrin. In addition, plasmin activates procollagenases and prostromelysins. The activity of the plasminogen activator is controlled by the amount of enzymes produced and the presence of their inhibitors [49]. The second family of proteinases represents the family of matrix metalloproteinases [50, 51] (Table 5). These include a large number of proteinases, which share similarities. They all have a zinc ion at the active center, which is necessary for their activity. All proteinases are secreted as inactive precursors, and the zymogens can be activated by proteases, e.g., plasmin, or by organomercurials, and this activation is accompanied by the loss of about 10 kd molecular mass. The members of this family specifically cleave one or more components of the ECM and are inhibited by tissue inhibitors of metalloproteinases (TIMPs). In addition, all members share amino acid similarities and a domain structure [50, 51].

Thus far, the matrix metalloproteinases (MMPs) have been divided into three subclasses with respect to their substrate specificity (Table 5): (a) col-

**Table 5** Family of Matrix Metalloproteinases

| Groups | Enzyme names | Matrix substrates |
|---|---|---|
| I | Interstitial collagenase | collagen types I, II, III, VII, X |
| | Neutrophil collagenase | collagen types I, II, III |
| II | 72 kd gelatinase | gelatin type I<br>collagens IV, V, VII, X<br>fibronectin, elastin |
| | 92 kd gelatinase | gelatin type I, V<br>collagens, IV, V |
| III | Stromelysin<br>(transin) | proteoglycans, fibronectin<br>laminin<br>gelatins I, III, IV, V |
| | Stromelysin-2<br>(transin-2) | gelatins I, III, IV, V<br>fibronectin |
| | Pump-1<br>(uterine metalloproteinase) | gelatins I, III, IV, V<br>proteoglycans, fibronectin |

lagenases that can cleave native triple helical collagens into characteristic 3/4 (TCA) and 1/4 (TCB) fragments that denature and can be further degraded by unspecific proteases as well as metalloproteinases, (b) 72 and 92 kd IV collagenases (gelatinases), which degrade basement membrane collagens as well as denatured collagens and gelatins, and (c) the stromelysins. Stromelysin-1 and -2 are very similar in size and amino sequence, while Pump-1 (putative metalloproteinase) is a smaller truncated version of the stromelysins. Recently, a new member of this class has been described in stromal cells of breast carcinomas, which, with respect to the strong homology to stromelysin-1 and -2, was named stromelysin-3 [52]. The class of stromelysins has a wider substrate specificity and is active on gelatins, fibronectin, proteoglycans, and laminin. The cellular control of the metalloproteinases is exerted at several levels including their synthesis and secretion, activation of the zymogens, and inhibition by the complexing of the specific matrix metalloproteinase inhibitors, TIMPs, to the enzymes (Fig. 2). Activation of the proenzymes occurs by proteolytic enzymes, e.g., trypsin, kallikrein, and plasmin, which cleave the propeptide of the proteins. Caused by a conformational change, the zinc atom at the active center, which is complexed by a cysteine in the proenzyme domain, becomes exposed and the enzymes activated. In a second step, these active forms can be autolytically cleaved by the activated metalloproteinases to remove the propeptide and provide permanent activity [53].

In recent years it has become increasingly clear that the control of proteolysis of the extracellular matrix is regulated by the amount of metallo-

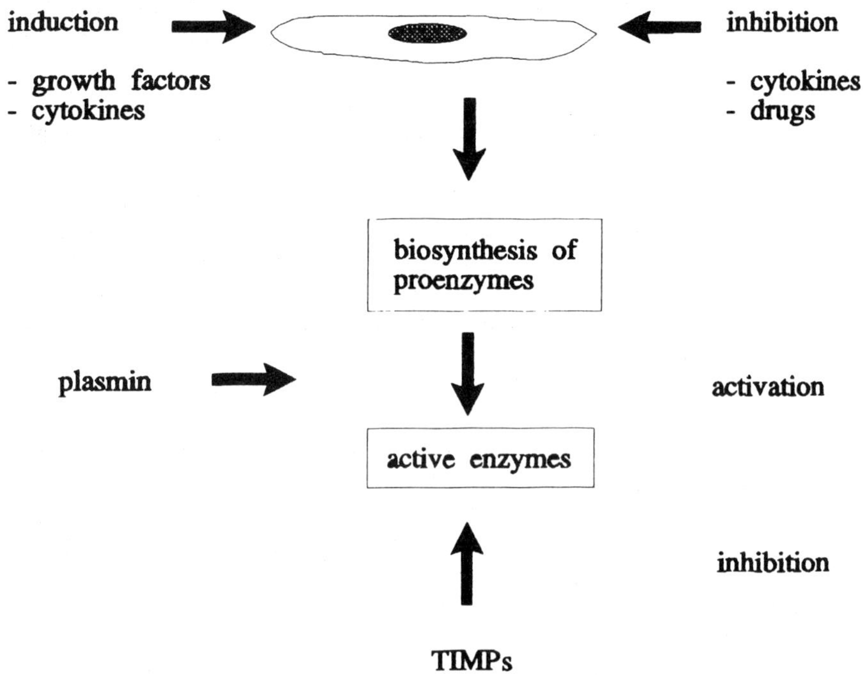


**Fig. 2** Regulation of metalloproteinase activity.

proteinases and their inhibitors present in the tissue. The balance of these proteins finally determines the degradation process in the tissue. Like the metalloproteinases, the inhibitors also appear to be a multigene family that includes at least four members. TIMP-1 and TIMP-2 are the best characterized. They both bind noncovalently to active metalloproteinases in a 1:1 ratio and specifically inhibit their enzyme activity [50, 51]. TIMP-1 also forms a complex with the inactive 92 kd type IV collagenase/gelatinase [54]. A larger TIMP-like inhibitor (LIMP) of 76 kd has recently been purified from fibroblast culture medium [55]. It binds to type I collagenase and stromelysin-1 as well as to the 72 kd gelatinase and is not recognized by TIMP antibodies.

The metalloproteinases are not stored in most skin cell types, except macrophages and neutrophils, but synthesized as soon as a clear signal arrives. These regulatory signals work almost exclusively at the level of transcription. Synthesis of mRNA for the metalloproteinases can be induced by a variety of agents such as growth factors, cytokines, oncogenes, and tumor promoters [56]. Type I collagenase and stromelysin are often coordinately regulated, and their genes are located close together on chromosome 11, whereas others (e.g., the gene for 92 kd collagenase) were located on chromosome 16. However, a coordinate regulation is not always the rule [57, 58]. IL-1$\alpha$ and IL-1$\beta$ and TNF were found to induce both type I collagenase and stromelysin gene expression, where IL-1 was more potent than TNF in the induction of stromelysin. In addition, these cytokines in combination synergistically enhanced stromelysin mRNA expression resulting in stromelysin mRNA levels three to fourfold higher than would be expected from a simple additive effect of both cytokines. IL-1 and TNF, in contrast, had only additive effect on collagenase gene expression. Under the same conditions expression of TIMP-1 was not affected using IL-1 and TNF separately or in combination, which results in a net increase of metalloproteinases versus inhibitors [57]. A stronger indication for a dissociable control of metalloproteinase expression has been demonstrated for IFN-$\gamma$, which was found to decrease the collagenolytic activity induced by IL-1$\beta$ in human fibroblasts. Whereas IL-1$\beta$ induction of collagenase gene expression was not altered by IFN-$\gamma$, stromelysin synthesis was found to be significantly inhibited by the addition of this cytokine. Since stromelysin is able to act as an activator of procollagenase, its expression can serve as a control mechanism to regulate collagen degradation. The decrease in collagenolytic activity, in addition, was not mediated by alterations of the levels of inhibitors, which were found to be unaltered by IL-1$\beta$ and IFN-$\gamma$ [58].

Several studies have been done to elucidate the molecular mechanisms involved in transcription processes. Many growth factors and cytokines are known to induce the expression of the proto-oncogene products c-Fos and c-Jun. These proteins have recently been shown to be transcription factors which recognize a specific DNA sequence called TPA-responsible element (TRE) or an activator protein-1 (AP-1)–binding site [59].

These sequences are present in the promotors of the type I collagenase and stromelysin genes, whereas the 72 kd gelatinase does not show a phorbol ester–responsive element. The response to IL-1 and TNF-$\alpha$ is mediated by this regulatory sequence, and cycloheximide blocks the induction of metalloproteinase gene expression, which suggests that the response is dependent on the synthesis of c-Fos and c-Jun protein [60, 61]. Induction of metalloproteinase expression can also be negatively regulated. Glucocorticoids and TGF-$\beta$ have been reported to block the induction of metalloproteinase expression. This inhibition is mediated by a 10 bp element at -709/-700, which was found to be highly conserved in several TGF-$\beta$–inhibited genes including collagenase, stromelysin, and urokinase and was called TGF-$\beta$ inhibitory element (TIE). This sequence has been shown to be bound by a complex that contains the c-Fos protein [62, 63]. In addition, TGF-$\beta$ stimulates synthesis of enzyme inhibitors. Expression of the metalloproteinase inhibitor TIMP was increased two- to threefold, whereas synthesis of the plasminogen activator inhibitor PAI-1 in fibroblasts was found to be elevated more than 10-fold under the same experimental conditions [63]. TGF-$\beta$ stimulation of cells during wound healing could therefore markedly inhibit degradation of the extracellular matrix by its dual effects on inhibiting metalloproteinase transcription as well as stimulating expression of inhibitors.

## III. ROLE OF THE EXTRACELLULAR MATRIX IN REGULATION OF WOUND HEALING

The extracellular matrix has a complex structure composed of a variety of different molecules (Table 3), which not only acts as a structural scaffold of the tissue but can also control several cellular functions. This includes migration, chemotaxis, cell morphology, and proliferation, as well as the regulation of connective tissue synthesis and differentiation of the cells. Cell-matrix interaction has turned out also to play a critical role in wound healing by controlling connective tissue production by fibroblasts. Several years ago an in vitro model was established that is considered to be an equivalent of the process of wound contraction [64]. Skin fibroblasts that are seeded into a reconstituted three-dimensional type I collagen gel adhere to the collagen fibers and contract the gel to a dense connective tissue matrix. Although the mechanism of contraction is not really understood, forces generated by the cells during spreading and consecutive aligning of collagen fibers in the direction of the cells and migration of fibroblasts seems to be important. The functional integrity of the cytoskeleton and protein synthesis are a requirement for gel contraction [64–66]. The cytokines TGF-$\beta$ and PDGF are both reported to enhance the contraction process [67, 68]. Interestingly, fibroblasts from granulation tissue of different stages were found to vary in their ability to contract a collagen gel. Cells from 21- to 28-day-old granulation tissue showed an increased contraction of the tissue equivalent to cells from 7- to 14-day-old granulation tissue or normal skin fibroblasts [69].

The interaction of fibroblasts with collagen in a three-dimensional matrix leads to major changes in cell morphology and a strict organization of cytoskeletal proteins, which enables them to interact with each other and to generate forces within the cells [73]. On the other hand, collagen can interact with the cytoskeleton via specific cell membrane receptors and thus allow migration of fibroblasts within and contraction of the collagen gels. The reorganization of the collagen matrix results in the modulation of different fibroblast functions. These include reduced proliferation and reprogramming of protein and collagen metabolism when compared to monolayer cultures.

Synthesis of types I and III collagen is particularly decreased as retraction of the gels progresses and reaches values of about 10% of those in monolayer cultures, which is similar to the biosynthetic activity of fibroblasts in normal skin [65, 70]. The decreased collagen synthesis is partly due to a reduced de novo transcription of the collagen genes, however, changes of the half-life of the mRNA seem also to be involved in the regulation process [87]. Whereas synthesis of interstitial collagens is downregulated, production of type VI collagen and fibronectin that function as adhesion proteins is not altered, indicating the specificity of this process [65, 72].

Contact of fibroblasts with collagen also results in a rapid increase of collagenolytic activity, and the removal of serum inhibitors leads to a complete breakdown of the collagenous scaffold within several days, liberating the cells [71]. In contrast to monolayer cultures with low levels of collagenase and most of the enzyme being present in an inactive, latent precursor form, in collagen gels the enzyme was found to be already activated. Recent data have shown that synthesis of other members of the metalloproteinase family, e.g., stromelysin and 72 kd type IV collagenase/gelatinase, is also induced, however, it is unclear which mechanisms lead to the activation of these enzymes (C. Mauch, unpublished).

Elevated collagenase protein was paralleled by a strong induction of de novo synthesis of collagenase mRNA, which was found to increase after 9 hours of culture and reached a maximum of 30-fold induction after 3 days, when compared to monolayer cultures. A divergent regulation of collagen and collagenase synthesis has already been reported for cytokines, e.g., TNF-$\alpha$ and IL-1 [36, 41]. Although it is unclear whether similar mechanisms are active in vivo, they could play a role in wound-healing processes, where in injured tissue a fast degradation of the debris and replacement by new collagen occurs.

The mechanisms underlying signal transmission from the surrounding extracellular matrix to the fibroblasts in three-dimensional collagen gels are not clearly understood. Recent investigations, however, indicate that adhesion receptors of the integrin family are involved. The integrins are heterodimeric complexes consisting of one $\alpha$ and one $\beta$ subunit, which are non-covalently linked. Both subunits have a transmembrane segment, a large N-terminal extracellular domain, and a small C-terminal cytoplasmic domain connected to the cytoskeleton [74]. It was found that synthesis and transcription of the $\alpha 2\ \beta 1$ (VLA-2) integrin is selectively upregulated when fibroblasts are seeded into collagen gels. The high synthetic levels of $\alpha 2\ \beta 1$ paralleled the gel-contraction process and returned to baseline production after the contraction was completed. In addition, gel contraction could be inhibited by using monoclonal antibodies against both $\alpha$ and $\beta$ chains [75]. Other studies have demonstrated that transfection of $\alpha$2-cDNA into cell lines, which express minimal levels of this integrin and fail to contract collagen gels, obtain de novo capacity to contract collagen matrices [76].

So far, it is not clear how integrins may transduce signals from the extracellular matrix to the cell interior. A recent report provides evidence that protein phosphorylation on tyrosine residues might be involved in integrin signaling [77].

The importance of integrin receptors in processes such as wound contraction was further substantiated by the observation that expression and de novo synthesis of integrins can be modulated by cytokines such as TGF-$\beta$. In vitro studies have shown that addition of TGF-$\beta$ to fibroblasts results in an elevated expression of $\alpha 1$, $\alpha 2$, $\alpha 3$, and $\beta 1$ subunits and an increased exposure on the cell surface [78], which coincides with an increased ability of fibroblasts to contract collagen gels.

Beside the interstitial collagens, other components of the ECM seem to have specific effects on wound healing. One example is collagen VI, which has several biological activities. Recently, in vitro experiments have shown that intact collagen VI mediates attachment and spreading of several cell types [79]. Furthermore, the globular domains of collagen VI contain motifs similar to type A domains of von Willebrand's factor, which has been shown to bind to extracellular matrix such as type I collagen, implying a possible bridging role of type VI collagen with other matrix proteins in connective tissue [79–82]. Collagen VI was also increased in active fibrotic diseases [83, 84]. All these findings indicate that collagen VI can play an important role in the organization of a coordinate matrix deposition in wound healing. This is further supported by the influence of IFN-$\gamma$ on collagen VI gene expression [85] and the increase of collagen VI mRNA levels observed in early phases of wound healing (T. Oono, unpublished).

On the other hand, degradation products of collagen and fibronectin have been found to activate collagen synthesis as well as migration of fibroblasts. Tissue destruction generates those biologically active fragments by the activation of metalloproteinases as discussed before and can initiate connective tissue formation.

In addition, several growth factors have been found to have a high affinity to components of the extracellular matrix and bind to distinct sequences of these large multifunctional proteins [86, 87]. The extracellular matrix therefore provides a storage pool of cytokines, which can be released and become biologically active after proteolytic cleavage of the connective tissue molecules. This can occur during early phases of wound healing but also later during remodeling. Here keratinocytes and other cells in the dermis could activate TNF-$\alpha$ synthesis or stimulate directly metalloproteinase production. Figure 3 summarizes the complex interaction between cytokines and the extracellular matrix, which play together in a concert of information provided between

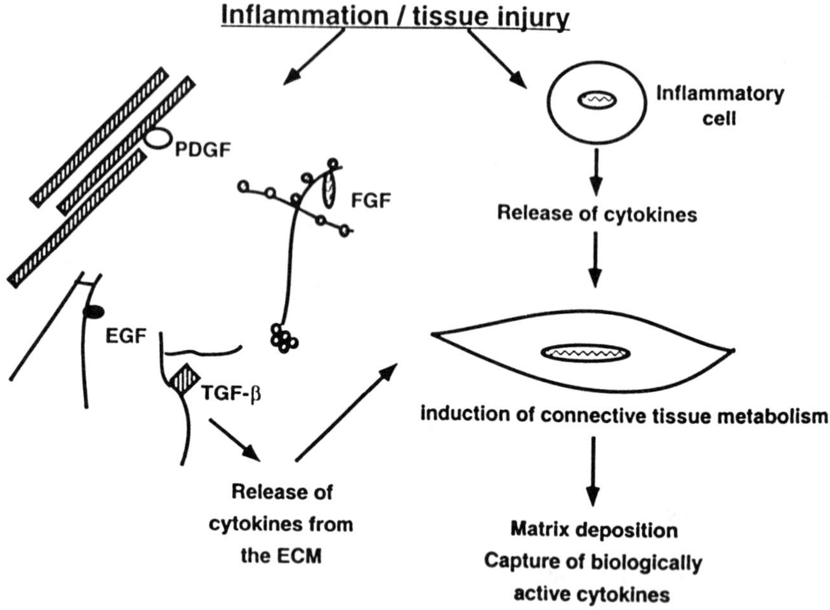


**Fig. 3** The role of the extracellular matrix and cytokines in wound repair.

the various cells. All these steps are strictly controlled in order to guarantee physiological tissue repair and to avoid formation of hypertrophic scars and keloids.

## REFERENCES


1. R. A. F. Clark and P. M. Henson, *The Molecular and Cellular Biology of Wound Repair*, Plenum Press, New York (1988).
2. R. W. Jennings and T. K. Hunt, in *Fetal Wound Healing* (N. S. Adzick and M. T. Longacker, eds.), Elsevier, p. 25 (1992).
3. R. K. Assoian, A. Komoriya, C. A. Meyers, D. M. Miller, and M. B. Sporn, *J. Biol. Chem. 258*, 7155 (1983).
4. S.M. Wahl, H. Wong, and N. McCartney-Francis, *J. Cell Biochem. 40*, 193 (1989).
5. H. R. Ford, R. A. Hoffmann, E. J. Wing, D. M. Magree, L. McIntyre, and R. L. Simmons, *Arch. Surg. 124*, 1422 (1989).
6. G. G. Nemeth, M. E. Bolander, and G. R. Martin, *Growth Factors and Other Aspects of Wound Healing: Biological and Clinical Implications*, Alan R Liss, Inc., New York, p. 19 (1987).

7. R. Snyderman and E. J. Goetzel, *Science 213*, 830 (1981).
8. H. E. J. Seppa, G. R. Grotendorst, and S. I. Seppa, *J. Cell. Biol. 92*, 584 (1982).
9. K. Scharffetter, M. Kulozik, W. Stolz, B. Lankat-Buttgereit, A. Hatamochi, R. Söhnchen, and T. Krieg, *J. Invest. Dermatol. 93*, 405 (1989).
10. H. N. Antoniades, T. Galanopoulos, J. Neville-Golden, C. P. Kiritsy, and S. E. Lynch, *Proc. Natl. Acad. Sci. USA 88*, 565 (1991).
11. S. E. Lynch, R. B. Colvin, and H. N. Antoniades, *J. Clin. Invest. 84*, 640 (1989).
12. S. E. Lynch, J. C. Nixon, R. B. Colvin, and H. N. Antoniades, *Proc. Natl. Acad. Sci. USA 84*, 7696 (1987).
13. L. Weber, E. Kirsch, P. K. Müller, and T. Krieg, *J. Invest. Dermatol. 82*, 156 (1984).
14. J. N. Clare, I. K. Cohen, and R. F. Diegelman, *Proc. Soc. Exp. Biol. Med. 161*, 337 (1979).
15. K. Kühn, in *Structure and Function of Collagen Types* (R. Mayne, R. E. Burgeson, eds.), Academic Press, New York, p. 1 (1987).
16. D. Quaglino Jr., L. B. Nanney, J. A. Ditesheim, and J. M. Davidson, *J. Invest. Dermatol. 97*, 34 (1991).
17. T. A. Mustoe, G. F. Pierce, A. Thomason, P. Gramates, M. B. Sporn, and T. F. Deuel, *Science 237*, 1333 (1987).
18. E. F. Bernstein, L. Harisiadis, G. Salomon, J. Norton, S. Sollberg, J. Uitto, E. Glatstein, J. Glass, T. Talbot, A. Russo, and J. B. Mitchell, *J. Invest. Dermatol. 97*, 430 (1991).
19. R. K. Assoian, A. Komoriya, C. A. Meyers, D. M. Miller, and M. B. Sporn, *J. Biol. Chem. 258*, 7155 (1983).
20. G. F. Pierce, T. A. Mustoe, J. Lingelbach, V. R. Masakowski, G. L. Griffin, R. M. Senior, and T. F. Deuel, *J. Cell Biol. 109*, 429 (1989).
21. L. M. Wakefield, D. M. Smith, K. C. Flanders, and M. B. Sporn, *J. Biol. Chem. 263*, 7646 (1988).
22. Y. Sato, R. Tsuboi, R. Lyans, H. Moses, and D. B. Rifkin, *J. Cell Biol. 111*, 757 (1990).
23. A. E. Postlethwaithe, J. Keski-Oja, H. Moses, and A. Kang, *J. Exp. Med. 165*, 251 (1987).
24. S. M. Wahl, D. A. Hunt, L. M. Wakefield, N. McCartney, L. M. Wahl, A. B. Roberts, and M. B. Sporn, *Proc. Natl. Acad. Sci. USA 84*, 5788 (1987).
25. E. V. Obberghen-Schilling, N. S. Roche, K. L. Flanders, M. B. Sporn, and A. B. Roberts, *J. Biol. Chem. 263*, 7741 (1988).
26. A. B. Roberts, M. B. Sporn, R. K. Assoian, J. M. Smith, N. S. Roche, L. M. Wakefield, U. I. Heine, L. A. Liotta, V. Falanga, J. H. Kehrl, and A. S. Fauci, *Proc. Natl. Acad. Sci. USA 83*, 4167 (1986).
27. R. A. Ignotz, T. Endo, and J. Massagué, *J. Biol. Chem. 262*, 6443 (1987).
28. R. A. Ignotz and J. Massagué, *J. Biol. Chem. 261*, 4337 (1986).
29. B. de Crombrugghe, J. Karsenty, S. Maity, T. Vuorio, P. Rossi, E. C. Rutes-houser, S. H. McKinney, and G. Lozano, *Ann. NY Acad. Sci. 580*, 88 (1990).
30. P. Rossi, G. Karsenty, A. B. Roberts, N. S. Roche, M. B. Sporn, and B. de Crombrugghe, *Cell 52*, 405 (1988).

31. J. D. Ritzenthaler, R. H. Goldstein, A. Fine, A. Lichtler, D. W. Rowe, and B. D. Smith, *Biochem. J. 280*, 157 (1991).
32. R. Raghow, A. E. Postlethwaite, J. Keski-Oja, H. L. Moses, and A. H. Kang, *J. Clin. Invest. 79*, 1285 (1987).
33. R. P. Penttinen, S. Kobayashi, and P. Bornstein, *Proc. Natl. Acad. Sci. USA 85*, 1105 (1988).
34. A. Mauviel, J. Heino, V.-M. Kähäri, D.-J. Hartmann, G. Loyau, J.-P. Pujol, and E. Vuorio, *J. Invest. Dermatol. 96*, 243 (1991).
35. M. B. Goldring and S. M. Krane, *J. Biol. Chem. 262*, 16724 (1987).
36. K. Scharffetter, M. Heckmann, A. Hatamochi, C. Mauch, B. Stein, G. Riethmüller, H.-W. L. Ziegler-Heitbrock, and T. Krieg, *Exp. Cell Res. 181*, 409 (1989).
37. C. J. March, B. Mosley, A. Larsen, D. P. Ceretti, G. Braedt, V. Price, S. Gillis, C. S. Henney, S. R. Kronhein, K. Grabstein, P. J. Conlon, T. P. Hopp, and D. Cosman, *Nature 315*, 641 (1985).
38. J. Le and J. Vilcek, *Lab. Invest. 56*, 234 (1987).
39. J. A. Elias, B. Freundlich, S. Adams, and J. Rosenbloom, *Ann. NY Acad. Sci. 580*, 233 (1990).
40. A. E. Postlethwaite, R. Raghow, G. P. Stricklin, H. Poppleton, J. M. Seyer, and A. H. Kang, *J. Cell. Biol. 106*, 311 (1988).
41. M. R. Duncan and B. Berman, *J. Invest. Dermatol. 92*, 699 (1989).
42. G. Gastl and C. Huber, *Blut 56*, 193 (1988).
43. M. R. Duncan and B. Berman, *Arch. Dermatol. Res. 281*, 11 (1989).
44. M. L. Stephenson, S. M. Krane, E. P. Amento, P. A. McCroskery, and M. Byrne, *FEBS Lett. 180*, 43 (1985).
45. J. Rosenbloom, G. Feldman, B. Freundlich, and S. A. Jimenez, *Biochem. Biophys. Res. Commun. 123*, 365 (1984).
46. J. Varga, A. Olsen, J. Herhal, G. Constantine, J. Rosenbloom, and S. A. Jimenez, *Eur. J. Clin. Invest. 20*, 487 (1990).
47. M. J. Czaja, F. R. Weiner, M. Eghbali, M.-A. Giambrone, M. Eghbali, and M. A. Zern, *J. Biol. Chem. 262*, 13348 (1987).
48. B. B. Aggerwal and T. E. Eessalu, *J. Biol. Chem. 262*, 10000 (1987).
49. O. Saksela and D. B. Rifkin, *Ann. Rev. Cell Biol. 4*, 93 (1988).
50. L. M. Matrisian, *TIG 6*, 121 (1990).
51. J. F. Woessner Jr., *FASEB J. 5*, 2145 (1991).
52. P. Basset, J. P. Bellocq, C. Wolf, I. Stoll, P. Hutin, J. M. Limacher, M. P. Podhajcer, M. C. Rio, and P. Chambon, *Nature 348*, 699 (1990).
53. E. B. Springman, E. L. Angleton, H. Birkedal-Hansen, and H. E. van Wart, *Proc. Natl. Acad. Sci. USA 87*, 364 (1990).
54. W. G. Stetler-Stevenson, H. C. Krutzsch, and L. A. Liotta, *J. Biol. Chem. 264*, 17374 (1989).
55. T. E. Cawston, V. A. Curry, I. M. Clark, and B. L. Hazelman, *Biochem. J. 269*, 183 (1990).
56. S. M. Frisch and Z. Werb, in *Collagen, Molecular Biology* (B. R. Olsen and M. E. Nimni, eds.), Vol. IV, CRC Press, Boca Raton, FL, p. 85 (1989).

57. K. L. Mac Naul, N. Chartrain, M. Lark, M. J. Tocci, and N. I. Hutchinson, *J. Biol. Chem. 265*, 17238 (1990).
58. E. N. Unemori, M. J. Bair, E. A. Bauer, and E. P. Amento, *J. Biol. Chem. 266*, 23477 (1991).
59. P. Angel, M. Imagawa, R. Chin, B. Stein, R. J. Imbra, H. J. Rahmsdorf, C. Jonat, P. Herrlich, and M. Karin, *Cell 49*, 729 (1987).
60. D. A. Brenner, M. O'Hara, P. Angel, M. Chojkier, and M. Karin, *Nature 337*, 661 (1989).
61. A. Schönthal, P. Herrlich, H. J. Rahmsdorf, and H. Ponta, *Cell 54*, 325 (1988).
62. L. D. Kerr, D. B. Miller, and L. M. Matrisian, *Cell 61*, 267 (1990).
63. C. M. Overall, J. L. Wrana, and J. Sodek, *J. Biol. Chem. 264*, 1860 (1989).
64. E. Bell, B. Ivarsson, and C. Merrill, *Proc. Natl. Acad. Sci. USA 76*, 1274 (1979).
65. C. Mauch, A. Hatamochi, K. Scharffetter, and T. Krieg, *Exp. Cell Res. 178*, 493 (1988).
66. C. Guidry and F. Grinell, *J. Cell Sci. 79*, 67 (1985).
67. R. Montesano and L. Orci, *Proc. Natl. Acad. Sci. USA 85*, 4894 (1988).
68. R. A. F. Clark, J. M. Folkvard, C. E. Hart, M. J. Murray, and J. M. McPherson, *J. Clin. Invest. 84*, 1036 (1989).
69. T. H. Finesmith, K. N. Broadley, and J. M. Davidson, *J. Cell Phys. 144*, 99 (1990).
70. B. Nusgens, C. Merrill, C. Lapiere, and E. Bell, *Collagen Rel. Res. 4*, 351 (1984).
71. C. Mauch, B. C. Adelmann-Grill, A. Hatamochi, and T. Krieg, *FEBS Lett. 250*, 301 (1989).
72. A. Hatamochi, M. Aumailley, C. Mauch, M.-L. Chu, R. Timpl, and T. Krieg, *J. Biol. Chem. 264*, 3494 (1989).
73. J. J. Tomasek, E. D. Hay, and K. Fujiwara, *Dev. Biol. 92*, 107 (1982).
74. E. Ruoslathi, in *Cell Biology of Extracellular Matrix* (E. Hay, ed.), Plenum Press, New York, 1991.
75. C. E. Klein, D. Dressel, T. Steinmayer, C. Mauch, B. Eckes, T. Krieg, R. B. Bankert, and L. Weber, *J. Cell Biol. 115*, 1427 (1991).
76. J. A. Schiro, B. M. Chan, W. T. Roswit, P. D. Kassner, A. P. Pentland, M. E. Hemler, A. Z. Eisen, and T. S. Kupper, *Cell 67*, 403 (1991).
77. L. J. Kornberg, H. S. Earp, C. E. Turner, C. Prockop, and R. L. Juliano, *Proc. Natl. Acad. Sci. USA 88*, 8392 (1991).
78. J. Heino, R. A. Ignatz, M. E. Hemler, C. Crouse, and J. Massagué, *J. Biol. Chem. 264*, 380 (1989).
79. M. Aumailley, K. Mann, H. von der Mark, and R. Timpl, *Exp. Cell Res. 182*, 463 (1989).
80. P. Bonaldo, V. Russo, F. Bucciotti, R. Dolicina, and A. Colombatti, *Biochemistry 29*, 1245 (1990).
81. E. Keller, A. W. Kaspar, and B. Trueb, *EMBO J. 8*, 1073 (1989).
82. M. L. Chu, R. Z. Zhang, T. C. Pam, D. Stokes, D. Conway, H. J. Kuo, R. Glanville, U. Mayer, K. Mann, R. Deutzmann, and R. Timpl, *EMBO J. 9*, 385 (1990).
83. J. Peltonen, J. Varga, S. Sollberg, J. Uitto, and S. A. Jimenez, *J. Invest. Dermatol. 50*, 20 (1991).

84. J. Peltonen, L. Kähäri, J. Uitto, and S. A. Jimenez, *Arth. Rheum. 33*, 1829 (1990).
85. M. Heckmann, M. Aumailley, A. Hatamochi, M. L. Chu, R. Timpl, and T. Krieg, *Eur. J. Biochem. 182*, 719 (1989).
86. K. Elenius, S. Vainio, M. Laato, M. Salmivirta, I. Thesleff, and M. Jalkanen, *J. Cell Biol. 114*, 585 (1991).
87. E. Ruoslathi and Y. Yamaguchi, *Cell 64*, 867 (1991).
88. B. Eckes, C. Mauch, G. Hüppe, and T. Krieg, *FEBS Lett. 318*, 129 (1993).

# 16
# Cytokines and Langerhans Cells

**Nikolaus Romani, Christine Heufler, Franz Koch, Gerda Topar, Eckhart Kämpgen,* and Gerold Schuler**
*University of Innsbruck*
*Innsbruck, Austria*

## I. LANGERHANS CELLS AS A PART OF THE DENDRITIC CELL SYSTEM

### A. The Dendritic Cell System

Dendritic cells constitute a widely distributed system of antigen-presenting cells specialized to initiate primary immune responses ("nature's adjuvant") [1]. They occur as trace populations (<1–2%) in lymphoid organs, in the circulation (blood, afferent lymph), and in nonlymphoid tissues. Detailed studies of epidermal Langerhans cells revealed how the different populations of dendritic cells are interconnected and how they cooperate to initiate immune responses [1–3]. Two main conclusions were derived from these investigations: dendritic cells in the nonlymphoid tissues ("tissue dendritic cells") including epidermal Langerhans cells as the first and best-studied example are (a) immature precursors of dendritic cells in the lymphoid organs ("lymphoid dendritic cells") and (b) highly specialized to process antigen. "Lymphoid dendritic cells" (i.e., mature dendritic cells) are particularly specialized to sensitize T lymphocytes.

### B. The Position of Langerhans Cells Within the Dendritic Cell System

Langerhans cells are leukocytes that reside in the epidermis [4] and are considered to be part of the dendritic cell system [1, 2]. Some hallmarks clearly

**Current affiliation*: University of Würzburg, Würzburg, Germany.

distinguish cells of the dendritic cell system from cells of the monocyte/macrophage system.

1. Dendritic cells display a characteristic morphology. While resident in the tissues, for example as Langerhans cells in the epidermis, they possess dendritic cell processes which have a round cross section and contain cell organelles; after some time in cell culture they develop highly characteristic sheetlike cytoplasmic processes ("veils"), which are typically devoid of organelles. They are constantly being extended and retracted. No other leukocyte exhibits such a behavior.
2. Dendritic cells constitutively express large amounts of MHC class II molecules on their cell surfaces. This is true for both freshly isolated Langerhans cells and even more so for cultured Langerhans cells.
3. Dendritic cells lack or express comparably low levels of typical macrophage markers.
4. Their phagocytic potential is relatively limited when compared to professional phagocytes. This has been shown for both fresh and cultured Langerhans cells.
5. Most importantly, dendritic cells were found to serve as specialized accessory cells for the initiation of primary T-cell–mediated immunity. Depending on their state of maturation, they are excellent in processing native protein antigens (immature dendritic cells) or they show strong stimulatory capacity for resting T lymphocytes (mature dendritic cells).

Langerhans cells share all of these characteristics with dendritic cells; in fact, some of these features have been detected and first described with epidermal Langerhans cells as a model [5–7]. In addition to these general markers for cells of the dendritic cell system, resident and freshly isolated Langerhans cells possess highly characteristic rod- and tennis-racket–shaped cytoplasmic organelles, the so-called Birbeck granules or Langerhans cell granules [4]. In summary, dendritic cells represent a cell lineage distinct from monocytes/macrophages but possibly with a common precursor. For a comprehensive review on dendritic cells, the reader is referred to a recent article by R. M. Steinman [1]. More detailed aspects of dendritic cell and Langerhans cell biology can be found in volume 140 of *Research in Immunology*, volume 6 of *International Reviews in Immunology*, and the book *Epidermal Langerhans Cells* (CRC Press, 1991).

## C. Immunological Functions of Langerhans Cells

Stingl and colleagues were the first to show that Langerhans cells are efficient epidermal antigen-presenting cells for proliferative and cytotoxic T-cell responses (see Ref. 8). Later, the experiments of Schuler and Steinman established the dendritic cell nature of Langerhans cells: they showed that when epidermal Langerhans cells are cultured for 2–3 days, they undergo a number of changes which make them fully resemble blood dendritic cells or lymphoid dendritic cells in morphology, phenotype, and function [5, 6]. The cytokine granulocyte/macrophage colony-stimulating factor (GM-CSF) turned out to be the key mediator for this maturation process in culture [9, 10].

Freshly isolated Langerhans cells, which are considered in vitro equivalents of resident Langerhans cells, are poor stimulators of resting T lymphocytes in the allogeneic mixed leukocyte reaction or in polyclonal T-cell responses. After short-term culture they upregulate their T-cell stimulatory capacity for resting T lymphocytes 30- to 100-fold [5, 6]. They become identical to splenic dendritic cells in that regard. Preactivated T cells (blasts), however, are stimulated similarly well by both fresh and cultured Langerhans cells. As could be demonstrated for lymphoid dendritic cells [11], cultured but not fresh Langerhans cells are also able to bind ("cluster") resting T cells in an antigen-*in*dependent fashion [6, 12]. This, rather than the increase in MHC class II expression that also occurs during culture, may explain the special ability of cultured Langerhans cells and dendritic cells to activate resting T cells [1]. Stingl et al. first reported that Langerhans cells serve as effective antigen-presenting cells for protein antigens such as ovalbumin in an MHC class II–restricted way [8]. The presentation of protein antigens to T cells typically requires intracellular processing, i.e., the enzymatic digestion of the proteins into small peptides and their binding to the "groove" of the MHC molecule [13]. Using peptide-specific T-cell lines as well as in vivo primed T cells, it could be shown that freshly prepared Langerhans cells are very potent in presenting exogenous protein antigens to peptide-specific T cells [7, 14]. After 3 days of culture, Langerhans cells downregulate their processing capacity for native protein antigens and thus become like spleen dendritic cells. Defined peptides, however, which do not need intracellular processing, are readily presented both by cultured Langerhans cells and spleen dendritic cells [7, 14]. Thus, the studies on epidermal Langerhans cells reveal that two crucial properties needed to stimulate resting T cells are expressed at distinct stages of cell differentiation and are regulated differentially. The *function of generating the ligand* (i.e., the MHC class II/peptide complex) for the antigen-specific T-cell receptor and the *function of sensitizing T cells* (i.e., antigen-unspecific T-cell binding and delivery of necessary signals) are reciprocally expressed in fresh and cultured Langerhans cells: fresh Langerhans cells are outstanding in antigen processing but weak in stimulating resting T cells, whereas cultured Langerhans cells show the inverted pattern [1, 2].

The mediator responsible for the development of Langerhans cells in culture was shown to be GM-CSF [9, 10]: when freshly isolated Langerhans cells are enriched to a high degree of purity, exogenous GM-CSF has to be added to the cultures to prevent Langerhans cells from dying and to enhance immunostimulatory function [9, 10]; when epidermal cell suspensions containing 1–3% Langerhans cells are cultured for 2–3 days, the necessary GM-CSF is supplied by the keratinocytes in the culture [15, 16].

## D. The Concept of Dendritic Cell Maturation

The in vitro data from the experiments with fresh and cultured Langerhans cells demonstrate a maturation process that goes on in culture and that turns Langerhans cells, as they typically occur in the epidermis, into dendritic cells as they are typically found in the lymphoid organs [2]. This process is mediated by the cytokine GM-CSF. Therefore, Langerhans cells as they appear in situ in the epidermis (i.e., "tissue dendritic cells") may be regarded as immature precursors to the mature dendritic cells in the lymphoid tissues (i.e., "lymphoid dendritic cells"). Resident Langerhans cells may form a reservoir of dendritic cells, which, presumably upon antigenic stimulus, migrate to the draining lymphoid organs, where they arrive as mature dendritic cells ideally suited to initiate a primary immune response.

Based on the in vitro findings, the mechanisms that lead to immunity in vivo can be considered in terms of three broad functions, which develop in sequence as a primary immune response evolves [1]:

1. Dendritic cells in peripheral tissues such as the epidermis act as *sentinels*, which efficiently capture and process antigen.
2. Since the chances to find antigen-specific T cells for a primary immune response in the skin are low, Langerhans cells move to the lymph nodes. This *migratory function* serves to find antigen-specific T cells. The evidence for migration stems from a number of investigations using contact hypersensitivity to haptens as a model (reviewed in Refs. 1, 4, 17): upon application of contact sensitizers Langerhans cells leave the epidermis, increased numbers of "veiled cells" can be observed in the afferent lymph, and hapten-carrying dendritic cells containing Birbeck granules can be found in the draining lymph nodes. The capacity of Langerhans cells to emigrate from the epidermis was also demonstrated in an organ culture model [18].
3. The *adjuvant function* enables Langerhans cells to bind and activate resting T cells, that is, to provide the necessary signals needed by the resting T cells to start proliferation and cytokine synthesis [19].

It is obvious that all three functions are regulated by the action of cytokines.

After briefly reviewing what we know about cytokine production/mRNA expression of epidermal cells, including Langerhans cells, we want to discuss the—unfortunately still sparse—data on the regulation of each of the three dendritic cell/Langerhans cell functions and on Langerhans cell viability.

## II. CELLULAR SOURCES FOR CYTOKINES IN THE EPIDERMIS

Here, we shall emphasize Langerhans cells and keratinocytes as cellular sources for cytokines. It must not be forgotten, however, that other epidermal cells such as melanocytes (see Chapter 21) or epidermal T cells can contribute to the epidermal cytokine pool. It is also conceivable that cytokines produced by cells in the dermis may diffuse into the overlying epidermis and act there in a manner analogous to experimentally injected cytokines [20].

### A. Keratinocytes

Langerhans cells are embedded in an epithelium composed primarily of keratinocytes. Therefore, soluble mediators synthesized and secreted by these cells should be of crucial importance for the regulation of Langerhans cell behavior. (Cytokine production patterns of keratinocytes are dealt with in several chapters of this book. In addition, the reader is referred to an excellent recent review covering this topic in depth [16]. We would like to emphasize some points of general significance.)

When considering the cytokine production of cells such as keratinocytes, it seems very important to clearly distinguish whether the cells have the potential to make a cytokine as can be shown in culture (with or without certain—sometimes unphysiological—stimuli), or whether the cells actually make the cytokine in situ. Freshly isolated keratinocyte suspensions are often considered as an equivalent or an approximation to keratinocytes in situ. Caution is warranted in that regard, because it recently became evident that certain cytokine mRNAs may be upregulated during the experimental preparation of cell suspensions [21].

It must also be stressed that it is essential to distinguish between expression of mRNA, synthesis of cytokine proteins, and secretion of bioactive cytokine proteins. These terms must not automatically be equated with each other. For example, mRNA may be expressed, but the corresponding cytokine may not be secreted. Alternatively, cytokines may be detectable by antibodies but prove biologically inactive [22].

Few data are available regarding cytokine expression of keratinocytes in situ. Polymerase chain reaction (PCR) data from our [23, G. Topar et al., manuscript in preparation] and other laboratories [21, 24, 25] indicate that murine keratinocytes synthesize clearly fewer cytokines in situ or freshly isolated than they do in culture. In preparations of heat-separated murine epidermal sheets we could detect no cytokine mRNAs at all [3, G. Topar et al., manuscript in preparation]. Immunoreactive IL-1$\alpha$ and IL-1$\beta$ [22, 26], IL-8 [27, 28], and TNF-$\alpha$ [29] were found in normal human skin in situ. However, only IL-1$\alpha$ [22, 30] could so far be extracted from normal human epidermis in a bioactive form.

Changes in the in vivo cytokine expression patterns under the influence of physicochemical treatments such as contact allergens [24, 31, 32] or UV irradiation [G. Topar et al., manuscript in preparation] or in disease states [33, 34] are being investigated.

## B. Langerhans Cells

The availability of techniques that allow the analysis of mRNA from very small cell numbers such as the PCR [35, 36] or in situ hybridization [37] has meant a "great leap forward." The four main groups currently trying to unravel the cytokine production patterns of Langerhans cells have chosen different approaches. The Dallas group [25] and the NIH group [24] use cell depletion methods: epidermal cells are analyzed prior to or after selective depletion of Langerhans cells. This strategy allows positive identification of cytokines expressed by Langerhans cells but not by keratinocytes; cytokines that are produced by both cell types cannot be evaluated with regard to Langerhans cells. In other words, if a given PCR signal does not change (provided that quantitative or semi-quantitative PCR is applied) following removal of Langerhans cells from the epidermal cell suspension, it may be concluded that keratinocytes are the principal source for this cytokine. Unless Langerhans cells express huge amounts of mRNA for the cytokine in question, a possible contribution of Langerhans cells would not be detected by depleting these cells. Alternatively, the Austrian groups [23, 38] and the Dallas group (for part of their experiments) apply additional positive selection methods. Epidermal cells are prepared and Langerhans cells are enriched to high purity by density gradient, sorting, or panning methods. The strategy of screening by PCR and selective analysis by Northern blotting or in situ hybridization makes possible an answer to the question whether cytokines that are expressed by keratinocytes are also expressed by Langerhans cells.

Very recent data from the above-mentioned research groups suggest the following cytokine expression pattern for murine Langerhans cells. We and others detected mRNA for only four cytokines in Langerhans cells (Table 1): Freshly isolated Langerhans cells and Langerhans cells in situ express MIP-1$\alpha$ [23, 25], MIP-2 [23, 24], little IL-1$\beta$, and no IL-1$\alpha$ [23–25] mRNA. Upon short-term culture (2–3 days) IL-1$\beta$ expression is strongly upregulated [23], thus clearly representing the most abundant cytokine mRNA found in Langerhans cells. IL-1$\alpha$ is not induced during culture [23, 38]. Moreover, IL-6 mRNA [23, 38] as well as bioactivity [38] was discovered in cultured Lan-

**Table 1** Regulation of Cytokine mRNA Expression of Langerhans Cells and Keratinocytes During In Vitro Culture and Specifically Upon Application of Contact Sensitizers

| Cytokine | LC in culture | LC upon sensitizer | Keratinocytes upon sensitizer |
|---|---|---|---|
| IL-1α | 0 | 0 | Up |
| IL-1β | Up | Up | unchanged |
| IL-6 | Up | — | — |
| IP-10 | — | 0 | Up |
| IL-10 | — | 0 | Up |
| MIP-1α | Down | — | — |
| MIP-2 | Down | — | Up |

Langerhans cells (LC) were cultured for 2–4 days. From Ref. 24, only those cytokines were selected that were selectively influenced by contact sensitizers; cytokines showing a general response to any kind of irritation (TNF-α, GM-CSF) are not included here. —, not done; 0, mRNA expression not detectable; IP-10, interferon-induced protein-10 [79].
*Source*: Refs. 23–25, 38, 80.

gerhans cells. The expression of mRNAs for the cytokines MIP-1α and MIP-2 was downregulated in the course of the three-day culture period [23]. Mature dendritic cells from other sources have yet to be examined with the same technology. The same applies for human Langerhans cells and dendritic cells, where even less data are available.

The new findings are complemented by the sparse earlier data on Langerhans cell cytokines. IL-1β [39] and TNF-α [40] mRNAs were found in Langerhans cells upon LPS and PMA stimulation. These data indicate that under certain conditions Langerhans cells may have the potential to express TNF-α mRNA. Clearly, however, the LPS/PMA stimulation does not correspond to the physiological model of Langerhans cell maturation in culture. In the first report on Langerhans cell cytokines, namely, the description of IL-1 bioactivity in supernatants of cultured human Langerhans cells by Sauder et al. [41], it could not be absolutely excluded that the IL-1 was derived from contaminating keratinocytes. More recently the capacity of human Langerhans cells to make bioactive IL-8 was reported [42].

## III. CYTOKINE RECEPTORS EXPRESSED ON LANGERHANS CELLS

### A. Methodical Considerations

The classical method of receptor quantification is to measure the binding of radioactively labeled ligand to the cells in the presence or absence of an excess of unlabeled ligand. The use of this approach for receptor determination on Langerhans cells or dendritic cells is limited for several reasons. The number of cytokine receptors expressed on the surfaces of cells is generally very low; often only a few hundred or thousand receptor molecules are present per cell. In order to compensate for the low receptor number, large numbers of cells have to be used for the binding assays ($1 \times 10^6$ or more cells per point). It is hard, time consuming, and expensive to obtain sufficient numbers of enriched Langerhans cells or dendritic cells for extensive use in such binding assays. Alternative approaches are becoming available [37]. The number of antibodies, cDNA probes, and PCR primers is rapidly increasing. Binding assays employing fluorescent cytokines rather than radioactive ligands are being developed. Therefore, data on cytokine receptors on Langerhans cells are still very sparse; the most important are reviewed here.

## B. IL-1 Receptors

Prompted by the observation that IL-1 contributes to the amplification of the accessory functions of Langerhans cells [9], we searched for IL-1 receptor expression on Langerhans cells in comparison with dendritic cells from the spleen. Using classical radioligand binding assays as well as immunolabeling, we could detect high affinity (type I) receptors for IL-1$\alpha/\beta$ on both freshly isolated Langerhans cells and cultured Langerhans cells [43]. The number of cell surface–expressed receptors appeared to be downregulated during culture from around 2000 or more receptors per fresh Langerhans cells to approximately 500 receptors per cultured Langerhans cells [43]. Spleen dendritic cells had even fewer receptors than cultured Langerhans cells. These data indicate that the enhancing effect of IL-1 on the maturation of Langerhans cells in culture is a direct effect. Moreover, the data underscore that the role of IL-1 may be most important in the early phases of Langerhans cell maturation.

## C. GM-CSF Receptors

The maturation of Langerhans cells is mediated by GM-CSF. On cultured murine Langerhans cells and on mature spleen dendritic cells we found comparably large numbers of GM-CSF receptors by radioligand binding assays [44, 45]. One would expect that freshly isolated Langerhans cells express even more of these receptors since Langerhans cells must be highly responsive to GM-CSF at that time. Data on fresh Langerhans cells are not available, however, because GM-CSF receptors are digested by the trypsin treatment necessary to obtain an epidermal cell suspension.

## D. M-CSF Receptors

There is a single report that resident human Langerhans cells express mRNA for c-*fms*, which is homologous to the receptor for M-CSF [46]. By immunocytochemistry as well as radioligand binding assays, we failed to detect M-CSF receptors on cultured Langerhans cells and spleen dendritic cells (E. Kämpgen et al., unpublished).

## E. IL-2 Receptors

Cultured Langerhans cells and dendritic cells both in mouse and in human express the low-affinity $\alpha$ chain of IL-2 receptor ("Tac-antigen," CD25) (reviewed in Refs. 45, 47). Radioligand binding data indicated a low-affinity interaction of the receptor with IL-2 [48]. Moreover, the 75 kd $\beta$ chain of the IL-2 receptor could not be detected on human Langerhans cells [49]. The function of these receptors is still unclear; they do not induce proliferative responses in Langerhans cells but may be involved in Langerhans cell migration [49].

# IV. REGULATION OF LANGERHANS CELL FUNCTIONS INVOLVED IN THE GENERATION OF SPECIFIC IMMUNE RESPONSES BY CYTOKINES

## A. Regulation of the Sentinel Function of Langerhans Cells by Cytokines

In vitro data have shown that Langerhans cells, when freshly isolated from the epidermis, are very efficient in taking up and processing native protein antigens, thereby generating immunogenic peptide/MHC ligands for the T-cell receptor. Thus, in vivo resident Langerhans cells appear ideally suited to act in the epidermis as sentinels that capture antigen and transform it into immunogen.

Little is known about the influence of cytokines on the steps that lead to antigen processing (antigen uptake) and on antigen processing itself. A prerequisite for efficient processing is the availability of newly synthesized MHC class II and invariant chain molecules for association with the peptides generated in the acidic organelles of the Langerhans cells [13, 50, 51]. One might therefore expect that cytokines that can influence the biosynthesis of MHC molecules such as interferon-$\gamma$, TNF-$\alpha$, or IL-4 exert effects on antigen processing. Unfortunately, however, neither the cytokine dependence of MHC class II upregulation during Langerhans cell culture [45] nor the influence of the above-mentioned cytokines on processing have been systematically studied as yet.

A number of observations, however, suggest a downregulatory role for TNF-α on antigen presentation at another level. Our own findings indicate that TNF-α might influence the capacity of Langerhans cells to retain immunogenic peptide/MHC complexes on their surface rather than directly interfering with the processing events [52]. When freshly isolated, highly purified Langerhans cells are pulsed with native protein antigen (e.g., myoglobin), they process the protein into immunogenic peptide/MHC class II complexes, and they are able to retain these complexes on their surface during a 2- to 3-day culture period in the presence of keratinocyte-conditioned medium or GM-CSF. This is demonstrated by their ability to stimulate an appropriate peptide-specific T-cell hybridoma 3 days after the antigen pulse [14, 52]. If, however, the very same antigen-pulsed Langerhans cells are cultured in the presence of TNF-α, they cannot retain the immunogenic peptides—the T-cell hybridoma is not stimulated [52]. In contrast, the response of a peptide-specific T-cell hybridoma to fresh Langerhans cells and native myoglobin protein is not affected by the simultaneous presence of TNF-α implying that this cytokine does not interfere with the processing of antigens but obviously causes a loss of already processed immunogenic peptides from the peptide-binding "groove" of MHC class II molecules [52].

Simon and colleagues have shown a similar phenomenon [53]. Epidermal cell suspensions containing about 10% Langerhans cells were pulsed with protein antigen, washed, and subsequently cocultured with antigen-specific T-cell clones in the presence or absence of TNF-α. A marked reduction of T-cell clone proliferation was noted in the presence of TNF-α [53]. This might be explained in the same way, namely, TNF-α may have led to a loss of processed peptides from the MHC molecules.

Epidermal Langerhans cells can be pulsed with tumor cells and injected into syngeneic recipient mice, which become successfully immunized to a subsequent in vivo challenge with these tumor cells [54]. It was recently shown that TNF-α, induced by IL-1α, could drastically inhibit the development of protective immunity [55].

It has been known for a long time that UVB irradiation impairs the development of contact hypersensitivity (reviewed in Ref. 56). In in vivo experiments in order to define more precisely the mechanism of action of the UV light, Vermeer and Streilein observed that intradermal injection of TNF-α could inhibit subsequent contact sensitization just like UVB irradiation [57].

These examples show that the sentinel function of Langerhans cells is critically regulated by cytokines. Yet, caution is warranted when transferring in vitro data to an in vivo situation. In vivo, Langerhans cells are probably exposed to a mixture of different cytokines, which might synergize or antagonize with each other. In vitro, however, the effect of one isolated cytokine is studied. Nevertheless, in vitro studies on the regulation of antigen processing by cytokines are valuable, and epidermal Langerhans cells represent a convenient model for such experiments. Data from in vitro experiments will have to be combined and compared with data derived from in situ analyses of cytokine production within the epidermal environment under different conditions.

## B. Regulation of the Migratory Function of Langerhans Cells by Cytokines

There is evidence that after the generation of immunogenic ligands (i.e., antigen processing) antigen-laden Langerhans cells leave the epidermis and migrate to the draining lymphoid organs to find the appropriate T-cell clones specific for the antigens they processed while still in the epidermis [1, 2].

It is not yet known which cytokine or which combination of cytokines trigger the emigration of Langerhans cells out of the epidermis. Recent experiments [58] present evidence that TNF-$\alpha$ might be one of the possible stimuli for emigration of Langerhans cells out of the epidermis. Injection of TNF-$\alpha$—but not GM-CSF-into the dermis led to a dose-dependent increase in the number of dendritic cells in draining lymph nodes. Data from two groups [57, 58] strongly suggest a role for TNF-$\alpha$ as a cytokine that may get Langerhans cells to move: intradermal injection of TNF-$\alpha$ resulted in a decrease in Langerhans cell density as determined by immunolabeling of epidermal sheets. The authors concede, however, that the mere loss of surface markers rather than the physical disappearance of Langerhans cells might be an alternative explanation for the phenomenon. A clue might come from combining earlier studies describing the partial disappearance of Langerhans cells from the epidermis after application of contact sensitizers but not after nonsensitizers or tolerogens [59, 60] and recent studies investigating the cytokine production profiles of epidermal cells under similar conditions. Whereas TNF-$\alpha$ and GM-CSF were upregulated by epidermal cells in response to irritants as well as sensitizers, mRNAs for IL-1$\alpha$, interferon-induced protein 10 (IP10), macrophage inflammatory protein-2 (MIP-2) and IL-10 were specifically enhanced by contact allergens [24, 80]. It is therefore tempting to test experimentally whether these cytokines—by themselves or in concert with other cytokines—really have the potential to make Langerhans cells emigrate from the epidermis in appropriate model systems such as organ culture [18, 61].

Adhesion molecules play crucial roles when Langerhans cells, on their way from the epidermis through the afferent lymph to the lymphoid organs, have to migrate across endothelial barriers and eventually have to home to the T-cell areas of the lymph nodes. The expression of adhesion molecules is regulated by cytokines on various cell types [62]. It is known that in delayed type hypersensitivity reactions adhesion molecules such as ELAM-1,

ICAM-1 (CD54), and VCAM-1 are induced or upregulated on keratinocytes and/or endothelial cells [63–65]. It is also known from in vitro studies that the surface expression of several of the known adhesion molecules on Langerhans cells is induced (ICAM-1/CD54, LFA-3/CD58 [66, 67]) during culture. How this is regulated by cytokines is still unknown, however.

## C. Regulation of the Adjuvant Function of Langerhans Cells by Cytokines

When antigen-laden Langerhans cells arrive in the draining lymph nodes it is thought that they have undergone a maturation process that is analogous to the events during short-term culture of Langerhans cells. We do not know exactly where the maturation takes place. The experiments of Larsen and coworkers [18] using murine skin transplantation and organ culture systems indicated that an initial maturation of Langerhans cells occurs still in the epidermis. On epidermal sheets it became evident that only a few hours after the start of the organ culture Langerhans cells displayed increased levels of MHC class II expression and were enlarged in size. McPherson et al. studied veiled cells from the afferent lymphatics of the rat. They found that phenotypical features (IL-2 receptor expression) and immunostimulatory capacity of these cells could still be enhanced during culture [68, 69]. This would suggest that veiled cells are not yet fully mature. Hence it appears that Langerhans cells may mature gradually, commencing still in the epidermis, continuing in the afferent lymph, and ending possibly upon arrival in the lymph node.

Few data are available about the regulation of the Langerhans cells maturation process. Clearly, the cytokine GM-CSF mediates the development of fresh Langerhans cells into immunostimulatory potent dendritic cells during culture [9, 10]. Although both TNF-$\alpha$ and GM-CSF sustain the viability of Langerhans cells (see below), only GM-CSF enhances the immunostimulatory capacity of Langerhans cells during culture: highly purified Langerhans cells cultured for 3 days in the presence of GM-CSF show a 30- to 100-fold increase of stimulatory capacity for resting T cells in in vitro assays such as the allogeneic MLR or the oxidative mitogenesis [9, 10, 70]; Langerhans cells cultured in the presence of TNF-$\alpha$, however, remain poor stimulators of resting T cells [52, 70]. The precise maturation-promoting effects of GM-CSF on Langerhans cells are not clear. The cytokine is not responsible for the increase in MHC class II expression during culture [70, 71]. Presumably, the capacity of dendritic cells to bind resting T cells in an antigen-independent fashion is enhanced by the cytokine, as could be shown for thymic dendritic cells [45, 72].

A T-cell stimulation-enhancing effect on Langerhans cells was also described for IL-1$\alpha$ in concert with GM-CSF: the addition of IL-1 to Langerhans cells cultures containing GM-CSF led to another twofold increase in T-cell–sensitizing function [9]. The mechanisms underlying these observations have been studied in dendritic cells from other sources (reviewed in Ref. 71). When IL-1$\alpha$ was added to an allogeneic mixed leukocyte reaction (MLR) with dendritic cells as stimulators, the T-cell response was clearly increased; the same happened when IL-1 was preincubated with stimulator dendritic cells, rather than continuously added to the assay [73, 74]. Clustering experiments proved that IL-1$\alpha$ directly increased the capacity of dendritic cells to bind resting T cells [73], possibly by upregulating the expression of an unknown dendritic cell surface molecule ("clustering molecule"). MHC class II expression was not upregulated by IL-1 [73].

Although the known adhesion molecules do not mediate the initial antigen-unspecific binding of T cells to dendritic cells [75], they do contribute to the later T cell–dendritic cell interactions. During the activation (sensitization) of T cells by dendritic cells, the adhesion of the two cell types to each other is reinforced and signals are delivered by the following pairs of molecules on dendritic cells and T cells, respectively: MHC—T cell receptor; MHC class I—CD8; MHC class II—CD4; CD54/ICAM-1—CD11a/LFA-1; CD58/LFA-3—CD2; B7/BB1—CD28 [19, 76]. It was observed that Langerhans cells [47, 66, 67, 81, 82] and blood dendritic cells [76, 81] upregulate these molecules upon culture. A detailed study of how the upregulation is influenced by the various cytokines has not been undertaken.

In search for an explanation for the exclusive capacity of mature dendritic cells, including cultured Langerhans cells, to efficiently stimulate resting T cells, soluble factors elaborated by dendritic cells were also considered. Double chamber experiments ruled out the possibility that Langerhans cells made large amounts of T-cell stimulatory cytokines [12]. However, these experiments did not exclude the additional possibility that Langerhans cells produced small amounts of highly potent short-range factors, which might be operative in the Langerhans cell/T cell clusters. In situ hybridization experiments on preparations of dendritic cell/T cell aggregates ("clusters") may help to answer this question.

The in vitro experiments described here deal with facets of the whole picture, i.e., the effects of single cytokines were investigated rather than the synergistic or antagonistic interactions of cocktails of cytokines, which would be closer to the in vivo situation. The main conclusion that can be drawn from these data is that the specialized function of mature dendritic cells to sensitize resting T cells ("adjuvant function") is highly influenced and regulated by cytokines, GM-CSF being the key mediator. In vivo, a delicate balance of up- and downregulating cytokines may be crucial to the kind of response following antigenic challenge: immunity or nonresponsiveness/tolerance.

## V. CYTOKINES AND LANGERHANS CELL VIABILITY

Resident Langerhans cells in the epidermis are relatively long-lived (reviewed in Ref. 77). In contrast, when freshly isolated and highly enriched (i.e., keratinocyte-depleted) Langerhans cells are cultured in plain culture medium, they die within the first day of culture. If, however, they are cultured together with keratinocytes or in keratinocyte-conditioned medium, most Langerhans cells survive as determined on day 3 of culture. This indicated that cultured keratinocytes were able to provide the necessary factors for survival. In vitro experiments have shown that out of a wide spectrum of cytokines only two mediators can sustain the viability: GM-CSF [9, 10] and TNF-$\alpha$ [70]. If either GM-CSF or TNF-$\alpha$ is added to the plain medium, 40–80% of all highly enriched Langerhans cells survive the 3-day culture. Neutralizing antibodies against the cytokines block this effect. Among many other cytokines tested, IL-1 also proved ineffective in that regard. The viability-enhancing effect of GM-CSF has also been shown for other types of dendritic cells [68] (reviewed in Ref. 45).

There is evidence that mRNAs for both GM-CSF [21, 25] and TNF-$\alpha$ [21, 25, 70] are expressed by freshly prepared, unstimulated epidermal cells either in suspension [25, 70] or in dispase sheets [21]. Whether this corresponds perfectly to the in situ situation remains to be established (see above) [3]. In murine epidermis the detection of GM-CSF and TNF-$\alpha$ in epidermal extracts by immunohistochemistry and/or bioassay has not been attempted yet; TNF-$\alpha$ was found by antibody staining in human epidermis [29]. If we assume that the epidermal environment in situ does provide the necessary GM-CSF and/or TNF-$\alpha$ for Langerhans cell survival, it is still not clear how exactly the two cytokines cooperate to fulfill this task. Two sets of data have to be taken into account:

1. GM-CSF is a maturation-enhancing cytokine (see above), but there is no evidence that the bulk of Langerhans cells mature while still resident in the epidermis.
2. TNF-$\alpha$ appears to distort the antigen-presenting function of Langerhans cells (see above), but the epidermis would be the very locale where this ability is needed.

So, it may be that a certain ratio of GM-CSF to TNF-$\alpha$ concentrations—possibly influenced by other cytokines—ensures the viability of Langerhans cells in the epidermis. Clearly, this point needs to be studied in more detail.

## VI. CYTOKINES AND OTHER FUNCTIONS OF LANGERHANS CELLS NOT RELATED TO SPECIFIC IMMUNE RESPONSES

A longstanding concept of *epidermal homeostasis* maintains that the growth and proliferation of keratinocytes in epidermal tissue may be regulated by Langerhans cells. This was based on microscopic observations that keratinocytes appeared to be regularly arranged around and above Langerhans cells (reviewed in Refs. 4 and 77). The detection of MIP-1-alpha mRNA in freshly prepared LC might revive speculations along these lines: MIP-1$\alpha$ inhibits the proliferation of bone marrow stem cells [78] as well as of murine and human keratinocytes (E. K. Parkinson et al., unpublished). Thus, resident epidermal Langerhans cells might in fact actively regulate keratinocyte proliferation. Implications for diseases caused by a dysregulation of keratinocyte growth (e.g., psoriasis) are obvious and are beginning to be explored.

Apart from their prime function in the initiation of specific immune responses, Langerhans cells most likely also participate in *inflammatory reactions*. They seem to be well suited for this task since they express mRNA for the inflammatory cytokines IL-1$\beta$, IL-6, and MIP-1$\alpha$.

## VII. CONCLUSIONS

As can be seen from the relatively large number of abstracts cited here, the field is very active at the moment. Methods are still being adapted to the specific needs of Langerhans cell researchers. Hard data are still sparse. It remains to be seen which of the many interesting and fascinating observations will pass all the necessary experimental controls. Yet, some trends are emerging.

1. Epidermal cells as well as Langerhans cells in situ synthesize surprisingly few cytokines under normal circumstances.
2. Epidermal cells, i.e., keratinocytes, react to various physicochemical stimuli by expression of a rather broad spectrum of cytokines, but in response to certain contact allergens switch on a more selected pattern. This indicates that certain cytokines are relevant for delivering immunizing signals.
3. Langerhans cells can also mount specific cytokine responses to antigenic stimuli, such as application of contact sensitizers.
4. The specialized functions of Langerhans cells in the course of the initiation of a primary immune response are critically regulated by cytokines; GM-CSF and IL-1 are positive regulators, TNF-$\alpha$ is predominantly a downregulating mediator.

Important questions for the future remain. We are sure that a few years from now it will be easier to write a conclusive review about Langerhans cells and cytokines. We are looking forward to that day.

## ACKNOWLEDGEMENTS

Our own work on Langerhans cells and dendritic cells was supported by grants of the Austrian Science Foundation (FWF grant P8549MED) and of the Austrian National Bank (Jubiläumsfonds No. 3872) to GS. The support of Prof. Dr. P. Fritsch, Department of Dermatology, Innsbruck, is greatly appreciated. We thank Prof. Dr. W. Platzer and the Senate of the University of Innsbruck for generous financial help with experimental animals.

## REFERENCES

1. R. M. Steinman, *Annu. Rev. Immunol. 9*, 271 (1991).
2. N. Romani, M. Witmer-Pack, M. Crowley, S. Koide, G. Schuler, K. Inaba, and R. M. Steinman, in *Epidermal Langerhans Cells* (G. Schuler, ed.), CRC Press, Inc., Boca Raton, FL, 1991, p. 191.
3. G. Schuler and N. Romani, in *Hematopoietic Growth Factors and Mononuclear Phagocytes* (R. VanFurth, ed.), Adelphi Communication, Macclesfield, UK, 1992, p. 63.
4. G. Schuler, N. Romani, H. Stössel, and K. Wolff, in *Epidermal Langerhans Cells* (G. Schuler, ed.), CRC Press Inc., Boca Raton, FL, 1991, p. 87.
5. G. Schuler and R. M. Steinman, *J. Exp. Med. 161*, 526 (1985).
6. K. Inaba, G. Schuler, M. D. Witmer, J. Valinski, B. Atassi, and R. M. Steinman, *J. Exp. Med. 164*, 605 (1986).
7. N. Romani, S. Koide, M. Crowley, M. Witmer-Pack, A. M. Livingstone, C. G. Fathman, K. Inaba, and R. M. Steinman, *J. Exp. Med. 169*, 1169 (1989).
8. G. Stingl and E. M. Shevach, in *Epidermal Langerhans Cells* (G. Schuler, ed.), CRC Press Inc., Boca Raton, FL, 1991, p. 159.
9. C. Heufler, F. Koch, and G. Schuler, *J. Exp. Med. 167*, 700 (1988).
10. M. D. Witmer-Pack, W. Olivier, J. Valinsky, G. Schuler, and R. M. Steinman, *J. Exp. Med. 166*, 1484 (1987).
11. K. Inaba and R. M. Steinman, *J. Exp. Med. 163*, 247 (1986).
12. K. Inaba, N. Romani, and R. M. Steinman, *J. Exp. Med. 170*, 527 (1989).
13. J. J. Neefjes and F. Momburg, *Curr. Op. Immunol. 5*, 27 (1993).
14. E. Puré, K. Inaba, M. T. Crowley, L. Tardelli, M. D. Witmer-Pack, G. Ruberti, G. Fathman, and R. M. Steinman, *J. Exp. Med. 172*, 1459 (1990).
15. T. S. Kupper, F. Lee, D. Coleman, J. Chodakewitz, P. Flood, and M. Horowitz, *J. Invest. Dermatol. 91*, 185 (1988).
16. T. A. Luger and T. Schwarz, in *Epidermal Langerhans Cells* (G. Schuler, ed.), CRC Press, Boca Raton, FL, 1991, p. 217.
17. N. Romani and G. Schuler, in *Springer's Seminars in Immunopathology 13*, 265 (1992).

18. C. P. Larsen, R. M. Steinman, M. Witmer-Pack, D. F. Hankins, P. J. Morris, and J. M. Austyn, *J. Exp. Med. 172*, 1483 (1990).
19. R. M. Steinman and J. W. Young, *Curr. Op. Immunol. 3*, 361 (1991).
20. G. Kaplan, A. Nusrat, M. D. Witmer, I. Nath, and Z. A. Cohn, *J. Exp. Med. 165*, 763 (1987).
21. O. Kilgus, E. Payer, S. Schreiber, A. Elbe, R. Strohal, and G. Stingl, *J. Invest. Dermatol. 100*, 674 (1993).
22. A. J. H. Gearing, N. J. Fincham, C. R. Bird, M. Wadhwa, A. Meager, J. A. Cartwright, and R. D. R. Camp, *Cytokine 2*, 68 (1990).
23. C. Heufler, C. Topar, F. Koch, B. Trockenbacher, E. Kämpgen, N. Romani, and G. Schuler, *J. Exp. Med. 176*, 1221 (1992).
24. A. H. Enk and S. I. Katz, *Proc. Natl. Acad. Sci. USA 89*, 1398 (1992).
25. H. Matsue, P. D. Cruz, P. R. Bergstresser, and A. Takashima, *J. Invest. Dermatol. 99*, 537 (1992).
26. H. S. I. Anttila, S. Reitamo, P. Erkko, A. Miettinen, L. Didierjean, and J.-H. Saurat, *J. Invest. Dermatol. 95*, 31 (1990).
27. H. S. I. Anttila, S. Reitamo, P. Erkko, M. Ceska, B. Moser, and M. Baggiolini, *J. Invest. Dermatol. 98*, 96 (1992).
28. M. Sticherling, E. Bornscheuer, J.-M. Schröder, and E. Christophers, *J. Invest. Dermatol. 96*, 26 (1991).
29. A. Oxholm, P. Oxholm, B. Staberg, and K. Bendtzen, *Br. J. Dermatol. 118*, 369 (1988).
30. C. Hauser, J.-H. Saurat, A. Schmitt, F. Jannin, and J. M. Dayer, *J. Immunol. 136*, 3317 (1986).
31. A. B. Kay, S. Ying, V. Varney, M. Gaga, S. R. Durham, R. Moqbel, A. J. Wardlaw, and Q. Hamid, *J. Exp. Med. 173*, 775 (1991).
32. U. Malorny, J. Knop, G. Burmeister, and C. Sorg, *Clin. Exp. Immunol. 71*, 164 (1988).
33. R. M. Grossman, J. Krueger, D. Yourish, A. Granelli-Piperno, D. P. Murphy, L. T. May, T. S. Kupper, P. B. Sehgal, and A. B. Gottlieb, *Proc. Natl. Acad. Sci. USA 86*, 6367 (1989).
34. B. J. Nickoloff, G. D. Karabin, J. N. W. N. Barker, C. E. M. Griffiths, V. Sarma, R. S. Mitra, J. T. Elder, S. L. Kunkel, and V. M. Dixit, *Am. J. Pathol. 138*, 129 (1991).
35. A. M. Lew, *Curr. Op. Immunol. 3*, 242 (1991).
36. D. A. Rappolee, A. Wang, D. Mark, and Z. Werb, *J. Cell. Biochem. 39*, 1 (1989).
37. P. M. Beckmann and P. J. Morissey, *Curr. Op. Immunol. 3*, 247 (1991).
38. S. Schreiber, O. Kilgus, E. Payer, R. Kutil, A. Elbe, C. Mueller, and G. Stingl, *J. Immunol. 149*, 3525 (1992).
39. V. B. Morhenn, S. Lee, E. M. Euqui, and A. C. Allison, *J. Invest. Dermatol. 84*, 285 (1989) (abstract).
40. J. W. Larrick, V. Morhenn, Y. L. Chiang, and T. Shi, *J. Leukocyte Biol. 45*, 429 (1989).
41. D. N. Sauder, C. A. Dinarello, and V. B. Morhenn, *J. Invest. Dermatol. 82*, 605 (1984).

42. T. Bieber, M. Sticherling, R. Rupec, and J.-M. Schröder, *J. Invest. Dermatol. 96*, 1013 (1991) (abstract).
43. E. Kämpgen, A. Lenz, F. Koch, C. Mikolajewski, A. Hartmann, N. Romani, and G. Schuler, *Arch. Dermatol. Res. 284*, 17 (1992) (abstract).
44. E. Kämpgen, C. Heufler, F. Koch, and G. Schuler, *Arch. Dermatol. Res. 281*, 546 (1990) (abstract).
45. N. Romani, E. Kämpgen, F. Koch, C. Heufler, and G. Schuler, *Int. Rev. Immunol. 6*, 151 (1990).
46. R. Wolff, A. T. Healy, R. M. Crawford, and M. S. Meltzer, *Fed. Proc. 46*, 1223 (1987) (abstract).
47. N. Romani, P. Fritsch, and G. Schuler, in *Epidermal Langerhans Cells* (G. Schuler, ed.), CRC Press, Boca Raton, FL, 1991, p. 49.
48. G. Steiner, E. Tschachler, M. Tani, T. R. Malek, E. M. Shevach, W. Holter, W. Knapp, K. Wolff, and G. Stingl, *J. Immunol. 137*, 155 (1986).
49. I. Strobel, R. Rupec, E. Sander, A. Wollenberg, and T. Bieber, *J. Invest. Dermatol. 100*, 462 (1993) (abstract).
50. E. Kämpgen, N. Koch, F. Koch, P. Stöger, C. Heufler, G. Schuler, and N. Romani, *Proc. Natl. Acad. Sci. USA 88*, 3014 (1991).
51. H. Stössel, F. Koch, E. Kämpgen, P. Stöger, A. Lenz, C. Heufler, N. Romani, and G. Schuler, *J. Exp. Med. 172*, 1471 (1990).
52. F. Koch, E. Kämpgen, B. Trockenbacher, C. Heufler, P. Stöger, N. Romani, and G. Schuler, *J. Invest. Dermatol. 98*, 510 (1992) (abstract).
53. J. C. Simon, D. Edelbaum, P. D. Cruz, A. Kapp, J. Krutman, E. Schöpf, and P. R. Bergstresser, *Arch. Dermatol. Res. 284*, 69 (1992) (abstract).
54. S. Grabbe, S. Bruvers, R. L. Gallo, T. L. Knisely, R. Nazareno, and R. D. Granstein, *J. Immunol. 146*, 3656 (1991).
55. S. Grabbe, S. Bruvers, A. M. Lindgren, J. Hosoi, K. C. Tan, and R. D. Granstein, *J. Leukocyte Biol. 52*, 209 (1992).
56. P. D. Cruz and P. R. Bergstresser, in *Epidermal Langerhans Cells* (G. Schuler, ed.), CRC Press, Inc., Boca Raton, FL, 1991, p. 253.
57. M. Vermeer and J. W. Streilein, *Photodermatol. Photoimmunol. Photomed. 7*, 258 (1990).
58. M. Cumberbatch and I. Kimber, *Immunology 75*, 257 (1992), and *J. Invest. Dermatol. 100*, 561 (1993) (abstract).
59. G. Weinlich, N. Sepp, F. Koch, G. Schuler, and N. Romani, *Arch. Dermatol. Res. 281*, 556 (1990) (abstract).
60. P. A. Botham, N. J. Rattray, S. T. Walsh, and E. J. Riley, *Br. J. Dermatol. 117*, 1 (1987).
61. R. Rupec, C.-G. Schirren, and T. Bieber, *J. Invest. Dermatol. 96*, 1022 (1991) (abstract).
62. Y. Shimizu, W. Newman, Y. Tanaka, and S. Shaw, *Immunol. Today 13*, 106 (1992).
63. W. Sterry, N. Künne, K. Weber-Matthiesen, J. Brasch, and V. Mielke, *J. Invest. Dermatol. 96*, 459 (1991).
64. P. Norris, R. N. Poston, D. S. Thomas, M. Thornhill, J. Hawk, and D. O. Haskard, *J. Invest. Dermatol. 96*, 763 (1991).

65. M. Goebeler, J. Gutwald, J. Roth, G. Meinardus-Hager, and C. Sorg, *Int. Arch. Allergy Appl. Immunol. 93*, 294 (1990).
66. N. Romani, A. Lenz, H. Glassel, H. Stössel, U. Stanzl, O. Majdic, P. Fritsch, and G. Schuler, *J. Invest. Dermatol. 93*, 600 (1989).
67. M. B. M. Teunissen, J. Wormmeester, S. R. Krieg, P. J. Peters, I. M. C. Vogels, M. L. Kapsenberg, and J. D. Bos, *J. Invest. Dermatol. 94*, 166 (1990).
68. G. G. MacPherson, *Immunology 68*, 102 (1989).
69. G. G. MacPherson, S. Fossum, and B. Harrison, *Immunology 68*, 108 (1989).
70. F. Koch, C. Heufler, E. Kämpgen, D. Schneeweiss, G. Böck, and G. Schuler, *J. Exp. Med. 171*, 159 (1990).
71. R. M. Steinman, *Immunol. Lett. 17*, 197 (1988).
72. K. Naito, K. Inaba, Y. Hirayama, M. Inaba-Miyama, T. Sudo, and S. Muramatsu, *J. Immunol. 142*, 1834 (1989).
73. S. L. Koide, K. Inaba, and R. M. Steinman, *J. Exp. Med. 165*, 515 (1987).
74. K. Inaba, M. D. Witmer-Pack, M. Inaba, S. Muramatsu, and R. M. Steinman, *J. Exp. Med. 167*, 149 (1988).
75. J. P. Metlay, M. D. Witmer-Pack, R. Agger, M. T. Crowley, D. Lawless, and R. M. Steinman, *J. Exp. Med. 171*, 1753 (1990).
76. J. W. Young, L. Koulova, S. A. Soergel, E. A. Clark, R. M. Steinman, and B. Dupont, *J. Clin. Invest. 90*, 229 (1992).
77. S. M. Breathnach, in *Epidermal Langerhans Cells* (G. Schuler, ed.), CRC Press Inc., Boca Raton, FL, 1991, p. 23.
78. G. J. Graham, E. G. Wright, R. Hewick, S. D. Wolpe, N. M. Wilkie, D. Donaldson, S. Lorimore, and I. B. Pragnell, *Nature 344*, 442 (1990).
79. A. D. Luster and J. V. Ravetch, *J. Exp. Med. 166*, 1084 (1987).
80. A. H. Enk and S. I. Katz, *J. Immunol. 149*, 92 (1992).
81. C. P. Larsen, S. C. Ritchie, T. C. Pearson, P. S. Linsley, and R. P. Lowry, *J. Exp. Med. 176*, 1215 (1992).
82. F. W. Symington, W. Brady, and P. S. Linsley, *J. Immunol. 150*, 1286 (1993).

# 17

# Epidermal Cell–Derived Cytokines and Delayed-Type Hypersensitivity

**Detlef Becker and Jürgen Knop**
*University of Mainz*
*Mainz, Germany*

## I. INTRODUCTION

Delayed type hypersensitivity (DTH) is defined as T-cell–mediated immune response that takes more than 12 hours to develop. DTH, originally described by Gell and Coombs, can be divided into four different types with respect to the dynamic of development and differences in the cells involved. The Jones-Mote reaction, contact hypersensitivity (CH), and tuberculin-type hypersensitivity occur during the first 72 hours after antigen challenge, whereas the granulomatous reaction is not seen for 2 weeks.

CH is a model widely used to study basic mechanisms of DTH. This reaction is well defined in animals like mice or guinea pigs and of important clinical relevance in humans. At the present time only rare data are available on the role of cytokines for development and regulation of other types of DTH. For this reason we will focus on the role of cytokines in CH. Although it is not clear whether the details of our present knowledge on the role of epidermal cell cytokines in CH are representative for other types of DTH, the principal mechanisms are probably comparable.

CH has two phases—sensitization and elicitation—both involving mechanisms of cellular activation and migration as well as antigen presentation and cytotoxicity, all of which are known to be induced or regulated by cytokines. Of course cytokines involved in CH are not solely produced by epidermal cells, they are also released by infiltrating leukocytes in epidermal tissue.

This chapter will review presently available data and present a critical discussion of the models used to determine how epidermal cell cytokines may influence CH. First a short overview of immunological events during CH will be given. Then we focus on the role of cytokines in sensitization to contact allergens, which involves the activation and emigration of antigen-presenting dendritic cells from the skin into regional lymphatic structures after encountering contact sensitizers. The role of epidermal cell cytokines during elicitation of CH, which is superimposed by release of cytokines from T cells undergoing intraepidermal secondary activation, will be discussed. Finally, comments on experimental systemic or local application of epidermal cell cytokines may provide insight into the relevance of cytokine production and release for development and regulation of CH.

## II. IMMUNOLOGICAL MECHANISMS OF CONTACT HYPERSENSITIVITY

CH is normally induced by penetration of contact allergens into epidermal and dermal structures and coupling to extracellular or cell membrane–associated molecules. The structural features of reactive haptens and chemical mechanisms of coupling to their carrier proteins will not be discussed in this chapter (a general overview is given in Ref. 1).

As a result of this haptenization, cellular activation of epidermal cells like keratinocytes, melanocytes, dendritic T cells, and, more important, Ia-antigen bearing dendritic cells like epidermal Langerhans cells and dermal dendritic cells is seen. Langerhans cells are believed to be the most important cell type for induction of primary T-cell response to contact allergens [2, 3], but it should be noted that this capability has also been described for dermal dendritic cells [4].

Successful T-cell activation requires establishment of an immunogenic antigen–MHC class II molecule complex on the cell surface of antigen-presenting cells. For the majority of protein antigens, effective intracellular antigen processing has been found to be a prerequisite for this process [5, 6]. Presently it is unknown whether this is also necessary for contact allergens, but it should be noted that mechanisms like formation of endocytotic organelles have been seen after in vivo application of contact allergen on murine skin [7]. In the murine system there is direct evidence for profound in vivo activation of Langerhans cells by several contact allergens [8], which results in significant upregulation of Ia-antigen expression by Langerhans cells as well as their functional capabilities. Most authors favor the hypothesis that primary antigen presentation of contact allergens to naive T cells occurs in regional lymphatic structures. This is supported by data on emigration of dendritic cells from the skin into regional lymphatic vessels and lymph nodes, where they resemble veiled cells and interdigitating cells [9].

Beside an immunogenic antigen–MHC class II molecule complex costimulatory signals given by antigen-presenting dendritic cells like Langerhans cells are required for a complete and successful activation of naive T cells [10]. These signals are composed of adhesion molecules and probably also of cytokines. According to present knowledge the T-helper cell type 1 ($T_H1$) is the most important cell type mediating CH in mice [11]. Its regulatory influence on T-helper cells type 2 ($T_H2$) and the conditions for primary induction of the latter cell type as well as the development of suppressive mechanisms needs to be further elucidated and cannot be discussed in this paper.

However, it is well documented that antigen-specific T cells undergo clonal expansion and infiltrate dermal and epidermal structures, especially under the influence of contact allergens [12]. Restimulation of these T cells with the corresponding antigen in the context of MHC class II molecules results in cytokine secretion followed by increased vascular permeability and immigration of a mononuclear cellular infiltrate [13–15]. This infiltrate is the main cause for the inflammation leading to the clinical diagnosis of manifest contact dermatitis.

## III. CYTOKINES IN SENSITIZATION

### A. Langerhans Cells Activation

The earliest events after contact of epidermal structures with sensitizing compounds (Fig. 1) may involve the processing of hapten–carrier complexes by Langerhans cells and formation of a MHC–contact allergen complex. Nothing is known about the role of cytokines for these mechanisms. During the first 24 hours after contact allergen application, Langerhans cells upregulate their expression of MHC class II molecules [8] either by stimulatory influence of haptens or by external signals derived from surrounding cells like keratinocytes or epidermal dendritic T cells. Evidence for cytokine-independent upregulation of MHC class II molecule expression came from in vitro experiments with highly enriched murine Langerhans cell preparations [16, 17]. The authors were able to show that Langerhans cells upregulate their Ia-antigen expression independently from the presence of GM-CSF or TNF-$\alpha$, which are critical for survival of highly enriched Langerhans cells during short-term culture. On the other hand, in vitro culture of murine epidermal tissue with various cytokines (GM-CSF, IL-1, IL-2, IL-3, IL-4, IL-6, TNF-$\alpha$, and IFN-$\tau$) results in upregulation of MHC class II molecule expression by Langerhans cells [18]. Among these cytokines GM-CSF, IL-1, IL-3, IL-6, and TNF-$\alpha$ are produced by epidermal cells, as discussed in other chapters. However, it needs to be shown whether these in vitro data reflect the cellu-

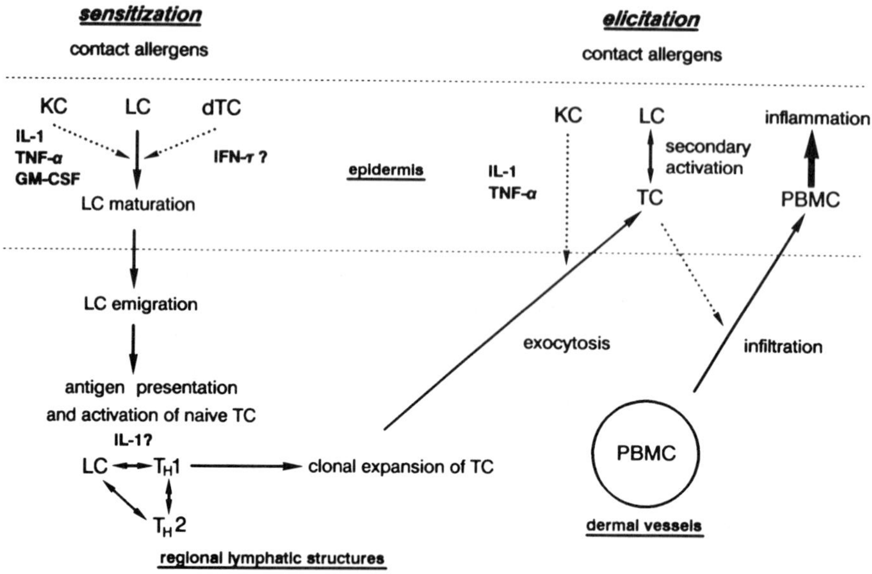


**Figure 1** Immunological events during sensitization and elicitation of CH and the probable involvement of epidermal cell cytokines. KC, keratinocytes; LC, Langerhans cells; dTC, dendritic epidermal T cells; TC,T cells; $T_H1$,T helper cells type 1; $T_H2$,T helper cells type 2; PBMC, peripheral blood mononuclear cells. Regulatory influence of cytokines is indicated by dotted arrows. Bidirectional arrows represent mechanisms of antigen presentation or cellular interaction. Epidermal cell-cytokines are indicated near the probably modulated immunological mechanism.

lar mechanisms of Ia-antigen upregulation by Langerhans cells under the influence of contact allergens.

The latest results presented by different groups suggest increased mRNA levels for TNF-$\alpha$, IL-1$\alpha$, IL-1$\beta$, IFN-$\tau$ as well as IFN-induced protein 10 (IP-10) and macrophage inflammatory protein 2 (MIP-2) in epidermal cells a few hours after application of contact sensitizers and in part also under the influence of tolerogenic and irritant compounds [19–21] (Table 1). For IL-1$\alpha$ and TNF-$\alpha$, these data could be confirmed by detection of augmented cytokine release in vitro after cell isolation [21]. In addition, immunohistochemical methods revealed evidence for augmented production of TNF-$\alpha$ by keratinocytes in allergic patch test reactions before infiltration by lymphoid cells [22].

As discussed later, secretion of these cytokines might have consequences for various immunological mechanisms during CH. Whether they are the

**Table 1** Upregulation of mRNA Levels for Several Cytokines in Epidermal Cell Populations After In Vivo Application of Contact Sensitizers, Tolerogens, and Irritants on Murine Skin

| | KC | LC | TC |
|---|---|---|---|
| TNF-α | all/cs | - | - |
| IFN-τ | - | - | all |
| IL-1α | cs | - | - |
| IL-1β | - | cs | - |
| IP-10 | cs | - | - |
| MIP-2 | cs | - | - |

KC, keratinocytes; LC, Langerhans cells; TC, intraepidermal T cells; all, under influence of contact sensitizers, tolerogens or irritants; cs, only after application of contact sensitizers.
*Source*: Refs. 19–21.

cause for upregulated expression of Ia-antigen expression by Langerhans cells during sensitization remains to be elucidated.

## B. Langerhans Cell Maturation and Emigration

Another prerequisite for effective primary T-cell activation by dendritic cells is the expression of co-stimulatory signals. It is believed that resident Langerhans cells are immature with respect to this capacity and undergo maturation after in situ activation in the epidermal environment. This maturation can be studied in vitro during short-term culture of isolated epidermal cells [16, 17, 23, 24]. From these experiments the crucial role of GM-CSF for this process became apparent, whereas TNF-α and IL-1 only supported the stimulatory influence of GM-CSF. The constitutive expression of mRNA for GM-CSF in keratinocytes during sensitization [20, 21] may reflect a role of this cytokine during Langerhans cell maturation in vivo. Its release may be regulated directly by stimulatory influence of contact allergens or by IL-1, which mediates augmented translation of GM-CSF in human keratinocytes in vitro [25]. Further work is required to understand the complex interactions in the epidermal cytokine network under these conditions.

As a result of maturation, somehow some of these cells leave the epidermis and enter regional lymphatic structures [9]. The role of epidermal cell cytokines in this migration remains to be defined.

## C. Resident and Early Infiltrating T Cells

Another unknown factor for induction of CH is the role of resident epidermal T cells. These cells and, more likely, early infiltrating T cells [26] may be an intraepidermal source of IFN-$\tau$ (see Ref. 21) with implications for the regulation of CH. Early infiltrating T cells may be guided to epidermal structures during sensitization by chemoattractant properties of epidermal cell cytokines like IL-1 and IL-8 [27], TNF-$\alpha$ [28], and IFN-$\tau$ [29,30]. Their exact role is presently unknown.

### D. Primary T-Cell Activation by Langerhans Cells

After reaching lymphatic structures Langerhans Cells induce T-cell–mediated immune reactions by stimulating naive T-helper cells. As reported for macrophages, IL-1 may serve as a-costimulating factor for this mechanism. Upregulated levels of IL-1$\beta$ mRNA in Langerhans cells were found recently after in vivo stimulation with contact sensitizers [21]. On the other hand, it is not known whether these data are representative for emigrated Langerhans cells after their maturation to dendritic cells. It cannot be excluded that co-stimulating effect on T cells may also be caused by keratinocyte-derived IL-1 due to the vast reservoir of this cytokine in the epidermis. Augmented production and release under the influence of contact sensitizers may result in relevant concentrations in draining lymphatic structures. Evidence for an important functional role of IL-1 in induction of CH came from experiments with $\alpha$-melanocyte-stimulating hormone ($\alpha$-MSH), a potent IL-1 antagonist [31]. Application of $\alpha$-MSH together with sensitizing compounds abolished sensitization, suggesting an important role of IL-1 for this process [32].

## IV. EPIDERMAL CELL CYTOKINES IN ELICITATION

The complex mechanism of CH regulation with regard to the role of different T-cell subsets cannot be discussed in this review due to the pivotal role of T-cell derived cytokines for this mechanism. Possible involvement of epidermal cell cytokines in this process will be discussed in the last section. However, after successful sensitization, a polyclonal population of hapten-specific effector T cells is found, which can be activated by rechallenge with the corresponding contact allergen. Again this involves the formation of an antigen–MHC complex on the cell surface of an antigen-presenting cell like epidermal Langerhans cells. A prerequisite for this activation of T cells is their exocytosis in the epidermis, which may be regulated by adhesion molecules on dermal vascular endothelial cells probably under the influence of epidermal cell-cytokines. This exocytosis may be enhanced by secretion of chemoattractant allergen-induced epidermal cell-cytokines like TNF-$\alpha$ and IFN-$\tau$ [22, 28–30]. Infiltrating lymphocytes are probably retained in the epidermis by augmented expression of adhesion molecules like ICAM-1 on keratinocytes [33] under the stimulatory influence of TNF-$\alpha$ and IFN-$\tau$ [34].

Manifest contact dermatitis is the result of cytokine release by different subsets of T-cells [35, 36] after their intraepidermal antigen-specific activation. These cytokines recruit an inflammatory cellular infiltrate [13–15]. Cellular recruitment may be further supported by contact allergen-induced release of proinflammatory EC-derived proteins MIP-2 and IP-10 [21]. Discussion of the complex interactions between these infiltrating leucocytes and epidermal cells can not be the purpose of this review.

## V. EPIDERMAL CELL CYTOKINES AND REGULATION OF CONTACT HYPERSENSITIVITY

The following sections summarize data obtained by application or functional inhibition of epidermal cytokines during sensitization and elicitation (Table 2). Much of these findings support the ideas about pathophysiological mechanisms of CH discussed in this chapter.

### A. TNF-$\alpha$

The central role of TNF-$\alpha$ is stressed by Piguet et al. [19], who showed that injection of TNF-$\alpha$–specific antibody abrogated elicitation of CH to trinitrochlorobenzene as well as inflammatory response in irritant dermatitis. Antibodies to IFN-$\tau$, GM-CSF, and IL-3 were only in part able to inhibit CH, whereas IL-2–specific antibodies had no effect at all. These findings

**Table 2** Regulatory Effect of Epidermal Cell Cytokine or the Corresponding Neutralizing Antibody on CH

| | Sensitization | Elicitation | Ref. |
|---|---|---|---|
| TNF-$\alpha$ | ↑ | ↑ | 19 |
| | ↑ | | 37 |
| | | ↓ | 38 |
| IL-6 | ↑ | | 37 |
| IL-1 | | ↓ | 38–40 |
| $\alpha$-MSH | ↓ | ↓ | 32 |
| IFN-$\tau$ | ↑ | | 43 |
| | | ↓ | 44 |
| | | ↓ | 45 |

The up- or downregulatory role of the cytokines indicated upon application or injection in rodents during sensitization or elicitation is demonstrated by arrows.

may underline the role of TNF-$\alpha$ as chemoattractant as well as its influence on ICAM-1 expression by epidermal cells. The authors also suggest a stimulating influence on infiltrating lymphocytes and direct cytotoxic effect on epidermal cells. Other authors studied the induction of CH by haptenated murine spleen cells after preincubation with several cytokines and found an augmenting effect of TNF-$\alpha$ and IL-6 [37].

In contrast, Robertson et al. [38] showed depressive influence of IL-1 and TNF-$\alpha$ on the effector phase of CH responses in animals given an adoptive transfer of primed lymphocytes from hapten-sensitized donors. These different findings suggest that route and point of time of TNF-$\alpha$ application determine the expected effect on CH response.

## B. IL-1

Similar data to those obtained with TNF-$\alpha$ were found for IL-1. Systemic application of IL-1 before elicitation resulted in depressed CH [38–40]. The authors suggest an upregulated level of prostaglandins mediated by IL-1 to be responsible for this effect, and reduced capacity of effector cells to infiltrate epidermal structures was seen. Whether elevated levels of IL-1 found during elicitation of CH [41] really play a downregulatory role needs to be elucidated.

Indirect evidence for an essential role of IL-1 during sensitization as well as elicitation was obtained by local application of $\alpha$-MSH [32]. This neuropeptide is a potent functional inhibitor of IL-1–mediated effects [39, 40]. In a preliminary report it was shown that IL-1 upregulates $\alpha$-MSH production by keratinocytes [42]. One may speculate that these data reflect self-limitation of IL-1 effects by augmented release of $\alpha$-MSH. Further work is needed to prove this hypothesis.

## C. IFN-$\tau$

There is some evidence for elevated intraepidermal levels of IFN-$\tau$ early after application of contact sensitizers on murine [21] as well as human skin (unpublished observations from our laboratory). Whether IFN-$\tau$ is produced by T cells or Langerhans cells under these conditions and whether the secreted quantities are able to modify immunological mechanisms during sensitization is still a matter of debate.

However, several authors described profound modulation of CH after application of IFN-$\tau$ as well as IFN-$\alpha/\beta$, suggesting an important role for this cytokine. Local injection at the side of sensitization resulted in enhanced aquisition of CH in mice [43]. Application of IFN-$\tau$ before contact allergen challenge of sensitized rats resulted in a reduced local response [44], whereas an IFN-$\tau$–specific antibody augmented CH in this experimental system [45].

Interferons seem to have profound influences on regulation of CH by inhibition of suppressive mechanisms. This has been shown for IFN-$\alpha/\beta$ [46–48] as well as IFN-$\tau$ [49]. Whether these regulatory effects result from IFN release by extraepidermal cells and especially activated $T_H1$ cells or may be somehow in part mediated by intraepidermal IFN-$\tau$ release during sensitization is presently unknown.

### D. Suppressor Factors

The possible role of $\alpha$-MSH has been outlined in the context of its relationship to IL-1. Another factor found to inhibit induction of CH is UVB radiation of keratinocytes [50]. There is evidence that this inhibitor is related to epidermal cell contra-IL-1 [51] and may play an important role in the prevention of CH development under the influence of UV light by blocking the biological activity of IL-1.

## VI. CONCLUSIONS

The most important cytokines during sensitization and elicitation of CH seem to be TNF-$\alpha$ and IL-1. Both are important proinflammatory mediators and exhibit complex interactions with different cell types and regulation of other cytokines. The role of IFNs as regulatory cytokines in the epidermal environment needs further elucidation. They may be necessary for enhancing the mechanisms resulting in the induction of a hapten-specific T-cell response, nevertheless there is no doubt about their involvement in regulation of suppressive mechanisms.

Research on epidermal cell cytokines during DTH is hampered by the complexity of this immunological reaction. In situ detection of cytokine production under the various conditions may be helpful, and more sensitive methods like polymerase chain reaction are available. In vitro experiments with isolated cells are often poorly representative for the in vivo situation, but they may give valuable hints to pathophysiological mechanisms involved in CH.

For experiments with in vivo application of cytokines or cytokine-specific antibodies during sensitization and elicitation, one must carefully consider parameters like cytokine dosage and location, as well as time of application. Interesting new findings may be expected from further work on recently described epidermal cell-derived mediators like IP-10, MIP-2, and $\alpha$-MSH as well as presently poorly defined suppressive factors.

## NOTE ADDED IN PROOF

Data presented by Bromberg et al. confirmed the important role of TNF-$\alpha$ for sensitization to contact allergens [52]; evidence for the crucial role of

IL-1β during development of CS is coming from a report by Enk et al. [53]. This group was also able to demonstrate upregulated synthesis of IL-10-specific mRNA by keratinocytes under these conditions [54]. Another report by Schwarz et al. suggests a suppressive effect of this cytokine on the effector phase of CS [55]. Downregulation of this inflammatory response was also noticed after application of IL-4 [56], TGF-β [57] as well as after psoralen plus UVA radiation, which was attributed to the release of soluble suppressive factors [58].

## REFERENCES


1. G. Dupuis and C. Benezra, in *Allergic contact dermatitis to simple chemicals. A molecular approach*, Marcel Dekker, New York, 1982, p. 47.
2. G. B. Toews, P. R. Bergstresser and J. W. Streilein, *J. Immunol. 124*, 445 (1980).
3. S. Sullivan, P. R. Bergstresser, R. E. Tigelaar, and J. W. Streilein, *J. Immunol. 137*, 2460 (1986).
4. Y. Tse and K. D. Cooper, *J. Invest. Dermatol. 94*, 267 (1990).
5. P. M. Allen, *Immunol. Today 8*, 270 (1987).
6. T. J. Braciale and V. L. Braciale, *Immunol. Today*, *12*, 124 (1991).
7. G. Kolde and J. Knop, *J. Invest. Dermatol. 89*, 19 (1987).
8. S. Aiba and S. I. Katz, *J. Immunol. 145*, 2791 (1990).
9. M. L. Kripke, C. G. Munn, A. Jeevan, J-M. Tang, and C. Bucana, *J. Immunol. 145*, 2833 (1990).
10. P. D. King and D. R. Katz, *Immunol. Today 11*, 206 (1990).
11. D. J. Cher and T. R. Mosman, *J. Immunol. 138*, 3688 (1987).
12. R. J. Scheper, A. C. H. M. van Dinther-Janssen, and L. Polak, *J. Immunol. 134*, 1333 (1985).
13. E. M. McMillian, L. Stoneking, S. Burdick, I. Cowan, and S. L. Husian-Hamzavi, *J. Invest. Dermatol. 84*, 229 (1985).
14. G. S. Wood, A. S. Volterra, E. A. Abel, B. J. Nickoloff, and R. M. Adams, *J. Invest. Dermatol. 87*, 688 (1986).
15. C. Avnstorp, E. Ralfkiaer, J. Jorgensen, and G. L. Wantzin, *Contact Dermatitis 16*, 239 (1987).
16. M. D. Witmer-Pack, W. Olivier, J. Valinsky, G. Schuler, and R. M. Steinmann, *J. Exp. Med. 166*, 1484 (1987).
17. F. Koch, C. Heufler, E. Kämpgen, D. Schneeweiss, G. Böck, and G. Schuler, *J. Exp. Med. 171*, 159 (1990).
18. D. V. Belsito, S. P. Epstein, J. M. Schultz, R. L. Baer, and G. J. Thorbecke, *J. Immunol. 143*, 1530 (1989).
19. P. F. Piguet, G. E. Grau, C. Hauser, and P. Vassalli, *J. Exp. Med. 173*, 673 (1991).
20. J. Haas, T. Lipkow, M. Mohamadzadeh, G. Kolde, and J. Knop, *Exp. Dermatol. 1*, 76 (1992).
21. A. H. Enk and S. I. Katz, *Proc. Natl. Acad. Sci. USA 89*, 1398 (1992).

22. C. E. M. Griffiths, J. N. W. N. Barker, S. Kunkel, and B. J. Nickoloff, *Br. J. Dermatol. 124*, 519 (1991).
23. N. Romani, A. Lenz, H. Glassel, H. Stössel, U. Stanzl, O. Majdic, P. Fritch, and G. Schuler, *J. Invest. Dermatol. 93*, 600 (1989).
24. S. Kolenik, T. G. Ding, and J. Longley, *J. Invest. Dermatol. 95*, 359 (1990).
25. T. S. Kupper, N. Birchall, J. S. McGuire, and F. Lee, *Clin. Res. 35*, 581 (1987).
26. G. Kolde and J. Knop, *J. Invest. Dermatol. 92*, 463 (1989) (abstract).
27. R. D. R. Camp, N. J. Fincham, J. S. Ross, K. B. Bacon, and A. J. H. Gearing, *J. Invest. Dermatol. 95*, 108S (1990).
28. A. N. Kalaaji, K. McCullough, and J. B. Hay, *Immunol. Lett. 23*, 143 (1989).
29. T. B. Issekutz, J. M. Stoltz, and D. M. Webster, *Cell. Immunol. 99*, 322 (1986).
30. T. B. Issekutz, J. M. Stoltz, and P. V-d-Meide, *J. Immunol. 140*, 2989 (1988).
31. R. A. Daynes, B. A. Robertson, B. H. Cho, D. K. Burnham, and R. Newton, *J. Immunol. 139*, 103 (1987).
32. L. A. Rheins, A. L. Cotleur, R. S. Kleier, W. B. Hoppenjans, D. N. Saunder, and J. J. Nordlund, *J. Invest. Dermatol. 93*, 511 (1989).
33. C. E. Griffiths and B. J. Nickoloff, *Am. J. Pathol. 135*, 1045 (1989).
34. D. A. Norris, *J. Invest. Dermatol. 95*, 111S (1990).
35. W. R. Herzog, I. Millet, N. R. Ferreri, R. Ramabhadran, J. Schreurs, and P. W. Askenase, *J. Immunol. 144*, 3667 (1990).
36. W. Sterry, S. Bruhn, N. Künne, B. Lichtenberg, K. Weber-Matthiesen, J. Brasch, and V. Mielke, *Br. J. Dermatol. 123*, 59 (1990).
37. S. Jayaraman, C. A. Martin, and M. E. Dorf, *J. Immunol. 144*, 942 (1990).
38. B. Robertson, K. Dostal, and R. A. Daynes, *J. Immunol. 140*, 4300 (1988).
39. B. Robertson, L. Gahring, R. Newton, and R. Daynes, *J. Invest. Dermatol. 88*, 380 (1987).
40. R. A. Daynes, B. A. Robertson, B. H. Cho, D. K. Burnham, and R. Newton, *J. Immunol. 139*, 103 (1987).
41. C. G. Larsen, T. Ternowitz, F. G. Larsen, and K. Thestrup-Pedersen, *J. Invest. Dermatol. 90*, 230 (1988).
42. A. Köck, E. Schauer, T. Schwarz, and T. A. Luger, *J. Invest. Dermatol. 95*, 476 (1990) (abstract).
43. H. C. Maguire Jr, M. Guidotti, and W. P. Weidanz, *Int. Arch. Allergy. Appl. Immunol. 88*, 345 (1989).
44. C. Skoglund and A. Scheynius, *Arch. Dermatol. Res. 282*, 318 (1990).
45. C. Skoglund, A. Scheynius, R. Holmdahl, and P. H. Van-der-Meide, *Clin. Exp. Immunol. 71*, 428 (1988).
46. J. Knop, R. Stremmer, Ch. Neumann, E. De Maeyer, and E. Macher, *Nature 296*, 757 (1982).
47. J. Knop, R. Stremmer, U. Taborski, W. Freitag, J. de-Maeyer-Guignard, and E. Macher, *J. Immunol. 133*, 2412 (1984).
48. J. Knop, B. Taborski, and J. DeMaeyer-Guignard, *J. Immunol. 138*, 3684 (1987).
49. U. Taborski, W. Freitag, H. Heremans, and J. Knop, *Immunobiology 171*, 329 (1986).

50. T. Schwarz, A. Urbanska, F. Gschnait, and T. A. Luger, *J. Invest. Dermatol. 87*, 289 (1986).
51. T. Schwarz, A. Urbanska, F. Gschnait, and T. A. Luger, *J. Immunol. 138*, 1457 (1987).
52. J. S. Bromberg, K. D. Chavin, and S. L. Kunkel, *J. Immunol. 148*, 3412 (1992).
53. A. H. Enk, V. L. Angeloni, M. C. Udey, and S. I. Katz, *J. Invest. Dermatol. 100*, 447 (1992) (abstract).
54. A. H. Enk and S. I. Katz, *J. Immunol. 149*, 92 (1992).
55. A. Schwarz, S. Grabbe, M. Simon, Y. Aragane, T. A. Luger, A. Zlotnik, and T. Schwarz, *J. Invest. Dermatol. 100*, 521 (1993) (abstract).
56. S. C. Gautam, N. F. Chikkala, and T. A. Hamilton, *J. Immunol. 148*, 1411 (1992).
57. S. P. Epstein, R. L. Baer, G. J. Thorbecke, and D. V. Belsito, *J. Invest. Dermatol. 96*, 832 (1991).
58. F. Aubin, M. L. Kripke, and S. E. Ullrich, *J. Invest. Dermatol. 97*, 995 (1991).

# 18
# Epidermal Cytokines and Mast Cells

**Annelie Möller and Beate M. Czarnetzki**
*Rudolf Virchow Clinics, Free University*
*Berlin, Germany*

## I. INTRODUCTION

### A. Posing the Problem

The epidermis consists of nonvascularized tissue that depends on the underlying dermis for support and communication with the body's interior. This means that physiological signals as well as mediators of inflammatory and immunological defense must be transferred from the dermis to the epidermis and vice versa. One of the few candidate cells for such function in the dermis are mast cells. Until now, these cells have not been specifically examined regarding their communicative tasks with the epidermis. In this chapter, experimental data suggesting such activity will be examined. First, an up-to-date review will be provided of the basic properties and functions of mast cells. Then, the potential influence of mast cell–derived factors on epidermal cells will be discussed as well as possible pathways by which epidermal cytokines might affect mast cells. Finally, the significance of the epidermal cell–mast cell interactions will be reviewed regarding the pathological events in cutaneous disease processes.

### B. Defining Mast Cells

Mast cells are resident cells of connective tissue in all organs of the body and are particularly abundant in the gastrointestinal and respiratory tracts and in the skin. The cells were originally differentiated from macrophages by their metachromatically staining cytoplasmic granules and have been viewed ever since primarily as effector cells of immediate-type hypersensitivity reactions [1]. Other distinguishing characteristics of the cells are:

1. Their special morphology, particularly regarding their electron dense cytoplasmic granules.
2. Their contents of unique and potent mediators of inflammation like histamine, of glycosaminoglycans, and of special enzymes like tryptase and chymase.
3. Their expression of the high-affinity IgE receptor (FcεRI) on their surface membranes (Table 1).

## C. Mast Cell Heterogeneity

Almost none of these features are unique for mast cells. Thus, the dogma that mast cells and basophils are the only cells that bear the FcεRI has recently been shattered, since both cell types share this receptor with epidermal and dermal Langerhans cells [2, 3]. Peripheral blood basophils also have features of mast cells but move into the tissue only in rare pathological situations (cutaneous basophil hypersensitivity or Jones-Mote reaction). They derive from a different lineage than tissue mast cells and resemble the so-called mucosal mast cells (MMC) (see Table 2) because of their smaller size, their lower quantity of intracellular histamine, and the presence of less sulfated glycosaminoglycans rather than heparin in their cytoplasmic granules.

Tissue mast cells also differ from each other depending on the microenvironment they reside in. This was first noted in the murine system when mast cells from the gastrointestinal mucosa were studied and compared to those from lung and skin (Tables 2 and 3). One distinguishes MMC from the so-called connective tissue mast cells (CTMC) in the skin and the peritoneal cavity according to the quantitative and qualitative expression of mediators and enzymes, the responsiveness to stimulating and modulating chemicals, and the ability of T-cell–derived factors to modulate the differentiation and maturation of the cells (reviewed in Refs. 4, 5). Whether MMC can also be found in the skin has not yet been resolved.

**Table 1** Characteristic Features of Mast Cells

| | |
|---|---|
| Morphology: | histology—metachromatic granules |
| | electronmicroscopy—electrondense granular crystal structure or whorls |
| Mediators: | histamine, heparin, and other glycosaminoglycans |
| Enzymes: | chymase, tryptase |
| Receptor: | high-affinity IgE (FcεRI) |

**Table 2** Distinguishing Characteristics of Connective Tissue and Mucosal Mast Cells

| | CTMC | MMC |
|---|---|---|
| Localization | skin, peritoneal cavity | lung, intestinal mucosa |
| Heparin | + + + | − |
| Chondroitin sulfate E | + | + + + |
| Histamine | + + + | + |
| RMCPI (chymase) | + + + | − |
| RMCPII (tryptase) | +/− | + + + |
| Responsive to | | |
| compound 48/80 | + | − |
| substance P | + | − |
| Inhibition by DSCG | + | − |
| T-cell growth dependence | − | + |

DSCG = disodiumcromoglycate.

In humans, there is no exact equivalent to CTMC and MMC, although human mast cells can also be distinguished by their ultrastructure, their granule contents, their pharmacological modulation, and their T-cell dependence during maturation (Table 3) [4, 6–11].

## D. Mast Cell Ontogeny

Mast cells derive from myeloid precursors in the bone marrow, with the precursors residing in many organs, the peripheral blood monocyte fraction,

**Table 3** Heterogeneity of Human Mast Cells

| | TC | T |
|---|---|---|
| Localization | skin, conjunctiva intestinal submucosa | lung intestinal mucosa |
| Carboxypeptidase | 0.5–16 pg/cell | − |
| Tryptase | 35 pg/cell | 11 pg/cell |
| Chymase | 4.5 pg/cell | − |
| Cathepsin G-like protein | + + + | − |
| Responsive to | | |
| compound 48/80 | + + + | − |
| substance P | + + + | − |
| Inhibition by DSCG | − | + |
| T-cell growth dependence | − | + + + |

DSCG = disodiumcromoglycate.

and the peritoneal cavity [12–14]. During in vitro culture, these precursors can be induced to develop into cells with features of CTMC under the influence of fibroblast but not lymphocyte products [12, 13]. Repeated injections of crude supernatants from both cell types into rat skin induced an increase in dermal and fatty tissue mast cells, with the fibroblast supernatants being more effective [15]. In the murine system, interleukin 3 (IL-3)–dependent MMC can be switched to CTMC under the influence of fibroblast feeder layers [16], and precursors develop into different phenotypes depending on the different body organs of mice into which they are injected [17]. These processes of mast cell differentiation and maturation are controlled by a variety of cytokines and growth factors [18], as discussed below.

## E. Mast Cells in the Skin

Within the skin, mast cells reside in greater abundance in the loose subepidermal, perivascular, and periappendageal connective tissue. At times, they can also be found close to or even invading into muscle and nerve bundles. On very rare occasions, one can detect mast cells in epidermal locations (Fig. 1). Mast cells are identified routinely in the skin by the metachromatic stain-

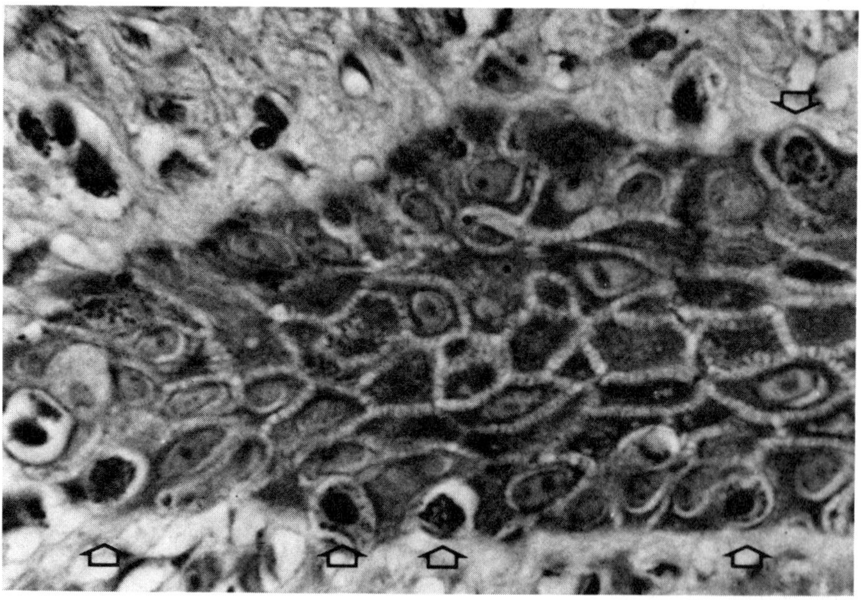

**Fig. 1** Localization of mast cells (arrows) between epidermal cells in stasis eczema, a very rare finding. (Toluidine blue stain, magnification 400×.)

**Table 4** Mediators of Inflammation and Growth Factors Present in Mast Cells in a Preformed State or Newly Generated on Mast Cell Stimulation

| Preformed mediators | Newly generated mediators |
|---|---|
| Histamine | Peptides: IL-1, IL-3, IL-4, IL-5, IL-6, IL-8, |
| Enzymes | TNF-α, TGF-β, GM-CSF, |
| TNF-α | IFN-τ, MIP, I-309 |
| Clq | Lipids: LTs, HETEs, PGs |
| PF4 | TXs, PAF |
| Glycosaminoglycans | |

ing of their granules with toluidine blue, Giemsa stain, and by specific enzymatic reactions (chloroacetate esterase, tryptase, chymase). By immunochemical methods, a monoclonal antibody (AAI) against the mast cell tryptase is the most reliable mast cell marker in our hands. With rare exceptions [19], the other so-called mast cell-specific monoclonal antibodies also react with epidermal, endothelial, smooth muscle, and sweat gland cells in the skin [20].

## II. MAST CELLS INFLUENCING EPIDERMAL CELLS

### A. Mast Cell Mediators

Mast cells are a storehouse of preformed and newly generated mediators (Table 4). These agents are released after cross-linking of antigens with antigen-specific, cell-bound IgE, but also after stimulation with a wide array of other stimuli, including hormones, neuropeptides, and the so-called histamine-releasing factors (HRF) (Fig. 2) [21–25]. The most exciting recent ob-

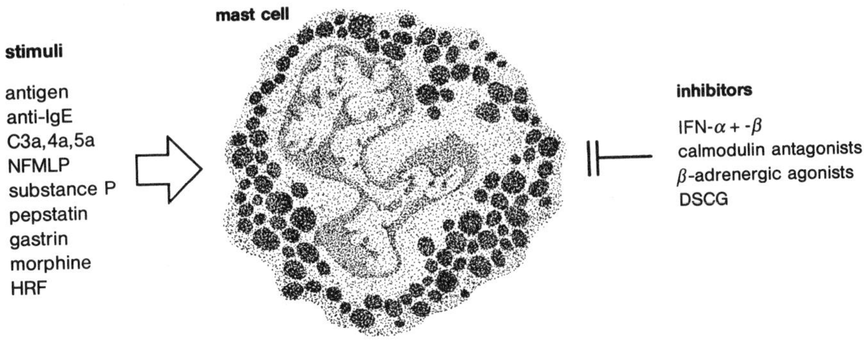


**Fig. 2** The most common agents known to induce or inhibit mast cell mediator release.

servation regarding mast cells relates to the identification of a number of cytokines produced by the cells together with many other well-known mediators (Table 4).

## B. Functional Significance of Mast Cell Mediators

### *IgE Production*

The pattern of mast cell–derived cytokines includes that of type 2 T-helper lymphocytes [26–31] which favor IgE-dependent immunological processes such as IL-4 production by B cells, with additional boosting via IL-5, IL-6, and IL-10 (Fig. 3). Binding of antigens to specific IgE which is bound to the FcεRI on mast cells and Langerhans cells, sets the stage for epidermal and dermal IgE-dependent allergic reactions. Furthermore, IgE production can be sustained in this process via additional IL-4 production from mast cells. Thus, mast cell stimulation results in a circuit of complex, potentially self-sustaining immediate-type immunological and inflammatory reactions.

### *Diverse Effects on the Epidermis*

Mediators other than cytokines are released during mast cell stimulation. These include vasoactive agents like histamine, leukotrienes (LT) $C_4/D_4$, prostaglandins, and platelet activating factor (PAF) which induce dermal and epidermal edema (Fig. 3) [25]. Several of the arachidonate metabolites ($PGE_2$, $PGI_2$) have recently been shown to modulate tumor necrosis factor

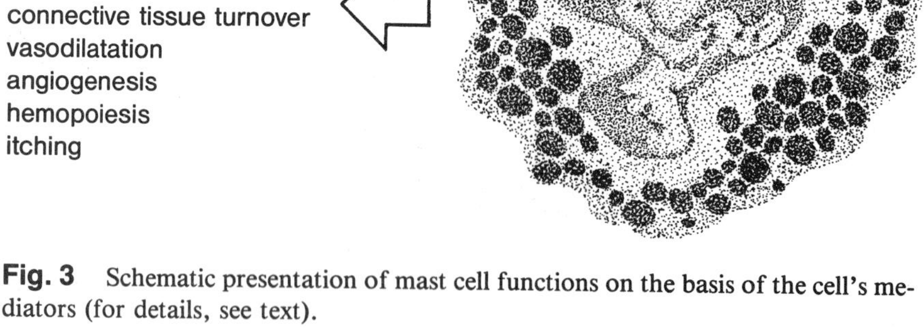


**Fig. 3** Schematic presentation of mast cell functions on the basis of the cell's mediators (for details, see text).

alpha (TNF-$\alpha$), IL-1, IL-4, and IL-6 expression and secretion [32]. The rapidly generated, immediately released mast cell mediators can thus influence mast cell and epidermal cell cytokine production which is necessary to induce and sustain immunological and inflammatory reactions. Several lipid mediators as well as histamine have been shown to stimulate keratinocyte proliferation in vitro [33]. Histamine, LTs, heparin, and most likely also the c-kit ligand, stem cell growth factor, induce epidermal pigmentation, and heparin, IL-1, IL-6, and mast cell enzymes can affect connective tissue turnover which in turn is necessary to sustain epidermal cell function. Heparin, histamine, and TNF-$\alpha$ are well-known angiogenesis factors (Fig. 3).

### *TNF-$\alpha$ and the Dermal Vasculature*

Among all of the proinflammatory mediators from mast cells mentioned so far, TNF-$\alpha$ deserves special mention. The mast cell is the only cell in the skin that stores this mediator in a preformed state, with the kinetics of release therefore differing from those of other cytokines [34]. Upon stimulation of mast cells, TNF-$\alpha$ is quickly released into the cell environment to induce the expression of endothelial leukocyte adhesion molecule I [34, 35], thus setting the stage for the action of leukocyte emigration in response to the various mast cell chemotactic factors (Fig. 3). TNF-$\alpha$, together with IL-1 and IL-8, also activates endothelial and epithelial $\beta_2$ integrins and selectins [36]. Via TNF-$\alpha$, interleukins, and the classical vasoactive mediators, mast cells function as gatekeepers of dermal vessels, in whose close vicinity they are preferentially located.

Interestingly, mast cells also exhibit mechanisms by which they can downregulate the proinflammatory events on vessels. Thus, mast cell–derived histamine antagonizes the production of TNF-$\alpha$ from monocytes via its $H_2$-receptor [37], and calcitonin gene–related peptide, a potent vasodilator, is hydrolyzed by mast cells [38].

### *Mast Cell–Induced Chemotaxis*

The process of leukocyte emigration into tissues is complex and requires the expression of adhesion molecules on the endothelium and the connective tissue to allow leukocyte attachment as well as the directional stimulation via an increasing gradient of specific chemotactic factors for translocation of the migrating cells towards the source of the factors. During the last several decades, a number of investigators have demonstrated eosinophil chemotactic factor (ECF) in mast cell and basophil supernatants and in the serum and the tissue fluid of patients with mast cell–dependent diseases [39–41]. These factors represent most likely $LTB_4$, TAF [40], GM-CSF, and IL-5 [27] (Table 5). IL-5 is unique among the eosinophil chemotactic factors in that it is specific for eosinophils and has eosinopoietic and eosinophil-activating properties.

**Table 5** Chemotactic Factors from Mast Cells and Their Potential Target Cells

| Chemotactic factors from mast cells | Target cells |
|---|---|
| IL-5, $LTB_4$, PAF (ECF) | eosinophils |
| IL-8, $LTB_4$, PAF (NCF) | neutrophils |
| IL-8, MIP$\alpha$, MIP$\beta$ | lymphocytes |
| $LTB_4$, PAF, MIP$\alpha$, MIP$\beta$ | monocytes |

Besides ECFs, neutrophil chemotactic factors (NCF) have been identified in mast cell supernatants which may in part represent $LTB_4$ and PAF since these small lipids are potent chemotactic factors for neutrophils, eosinophils, and, under certain conditions, monocytes [39, 42–44] (Table 5). Higher molecular weight NCFs which have also been identified in body fluids of mast cell–dependent diseases [43], could represent mast cell–derived IL-8. We have recently demonstrated for the first time that human and rodent mast cell lines can be induced to express and secrete this potent chemotactic factor [30]. These observations could be confirmed in human skin mast cells by immunoelectronmicroscopy.* Other potential sources of IL-8 in the skin are monocytes, endothelial cells, melanocytes, and keratinocytes. IL-8 also has T-lymphocyte chemotactic properties, which it shares with two recently described mast cell–derived cytokines, MIP-1$\alpha$ and MIP-1$\beta$ [45]. Thus, mast cells which are located in close proximity to vessels, can not only regulate transudation of plasma into the tissue, but can also initiate and sustain the emigration of formed elements from the blood into the dermis by promptly producing a wide range of rapidly as well as more slowly acting chemotactic factors with specificities for a wide range of cell types. Additional cells in epidermis and dermis can potentiate this effect by further secretion of chemotactic factors, thus allowing the directed locomotion of cells from the vessels through the dermal connective tissue to the epidermis.

### *Mast Cell Growth Factors*

In addition to the proinflammatory and proallergic cytokines discussed so far, mast cells can also generate and release hematopoietic growth factors like IL-3 and GM-CSF [29]. The significance of these findings is currently not clear. Hemopoiesis occurs in the skin only in the newborn period or during leukemic processes. IL-3 has been shown to cause basophil histamine release, and IL-1 can potentiate this process [46, 47]. Since CTMC have no IL-3 receptor [48], the IL-3–mediated effects can only have significance for

*A. Möller, U. Lippert, D. Lessmann, G. Kolde, K. Hamann, P. Welker, D. Schadendorf, J. Grabbe, T. Rosenbach, T. Luger, B. M. Czarnetzki. *J. Immunol.*, in press.

MMC and for basophils. The enhancement of mast cell growth by GM-CSF might, on the other hand, represent another autocrine regulatory loop of mast cell growth (see below).

*Downmodulation of Inflammation*

Finally, mast cells can function not only as initiators and enhancers, but also as downmodulators of allergic and inflammatory processes. They accomplish this in part by taking up into and storing in their cytoplasmic granules a great variety of substances that may act as antigens as well as mediators of inflammation [49]. Heparin and other glycosaminoglycans within the granules apparently bind these mediators effectively, a process that also occurs outside the mast cell when heparin is released into the cell environment. Extracellular heparin and mast cell granules can in turn be taken up and phagocytosed by fibroblasts [50, 51]. What happens thereafter to the mediators is uncertain. Although the phagocytosed or pinocytosed material might be degraded by mast cell enzymes, it can also be released again from the cells in an active form, as is known for serotonin and for eosinophil-derived peroxidase, with the latter enhancing mast cell cytotoxicity [52].

Some mast cell mediators can apparently also inhibit mediator release from other cells. IL-10, for example, inhibits IL-2 and IFN-$\gamma$ release from murine $T_H2$ lymphocytes [52], and rat mast cell proteases can inactivate the calcitonin gene–related peptide and neurotensin [38, 54].

## III. EPIDERMAL CYTOKINES INFLUENCING MAST CELL FUNCTION

### A. Source of Epidermal Cytokines

As reviewed in other chapters of this volume, several different epidermal cell types can potentially generate almost all of the presently known cytokines and growth factors. These in turn can modulate dermal cells, including mast cells, by affecting their growth and differentiation, their metabolic activities, and their secretory activities (Fig. 4).

### B. Mast Cell Growth Factors

In recent years, IL-3, IL-4, IL-6, IL-9, IL-10, nerve growth factor, and GM-CSF have been shown to support rodent mast cell growth in an autocrine and paracrine manner [18, 55–59] (Table 6). In humans, none of these factors are effective, except for IL-3 on basophils [60]. Instead, the well-known fibroblast dependence of human mast cells [13, 16] can be at least partially explained by the c-kit product from fibroblasts [61, 62]. IL-3 downmodulates c-kit mRNA expression, thus favoring the production of the MMC [63]. In serial biopsies of IFN-$\alpha$ injection sites, we have noted marked increases

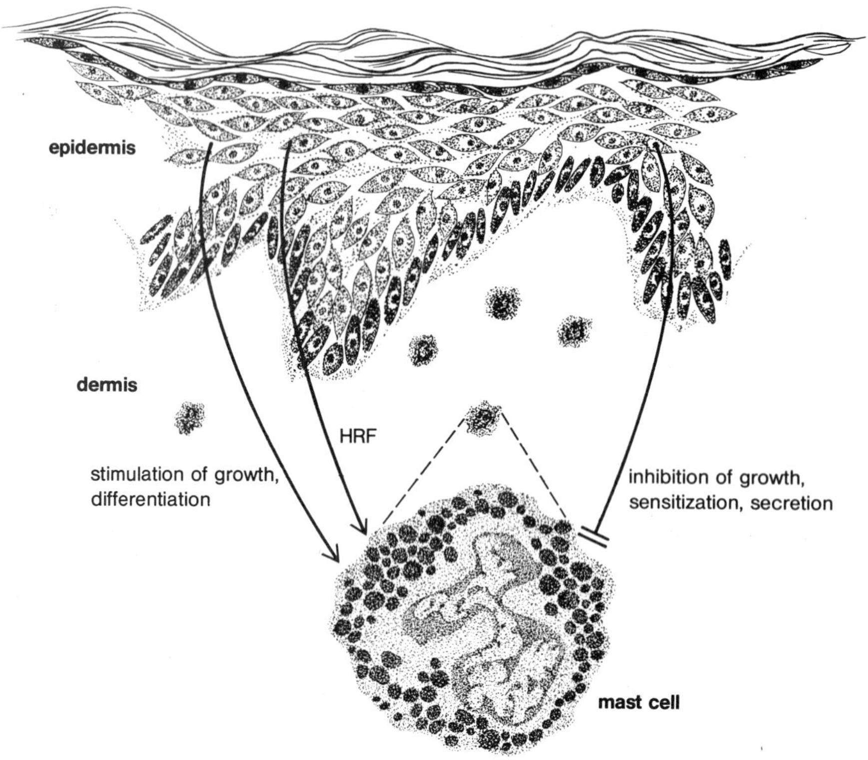


**Fig. 4** Potential influence of epidermal cells on dermal mast cells.

**Table 6** Factors Causing Growth and Maturation of Mast Cells (or Basophils) and Inhibitors of This Process

| | |
|---|---|
| Stimulation | |
| rodent: | IL-3, IL-4, IL-6, IL-9, IL-10 |
| | NGF, GM-CSF |
| | c-kit ligand |
| human: | IL-3 (basophil) |
| | fibroblast products |
| | c-kit ligand |
| Inhibition | |
| IFN-$\gamma$, TGF-$\beta$, corticosteroids | |

of dermal mast cells.* Whether these effects are mediated directly or only indirectly by IFN-$\alpha$ needs to be further examined. Similarly, it is unknown whether epidermal cells are also capable of producing mast cell growth factors like c-kit ligand. Since murine mast cells differentiate and also migrate in response to IL-3 [64], epidermis-derived IL-3 could explain dermal mast cell increase in this species.

Viewed as a whole, it is apparent that differentiation and maturation of mast cells in the tissue are orchestrated by a complex interplay of different factors from different cell types in the microenvironment of the cells and that human mast cells are regulated by very different factors than murine cells.

## C. Histamine-Releasing Factors

The stimulatory and modulatory role of cytokines on mast cell secretion is currently under intense study, with some controversy regarding findings from different laboratories. Most of the data available so far apply to basophils only. The so-called histamine-releasing factor (HRF) or release-enhancing factors include IL-1, IL-3, IL-5, IL-8, SCF, and GM-CSF, as well as several monocyte- and platelet-derived factors with homologies to connective tissue-activating peptide (CTAPIII) and neutrophil-activating peptide (NAP)2. In addition, several not well-characterized HRFs from mononuclear cells, neutrophils, T and B cells have been described, with those whose action depends on IgE being generally less potent [65–68]. These factors represent an alternative pathway to immunoglobulin-dependent mast cell activation, so that mast cell function is not restricted to IgE-dependent allergic processes.

## D. Interferons

Although interferons can enhance cytotoxicity of natural killer cells and monocytes, they have the opposite effect on mast cells, causing downregulation of cytotoxicity in these cells by suppressing TNF-$\alpha$ production [69, 70]. Moreover, IFN-$\alpha$ and IFN-$\beta$ suppress histamine release from mast cells [71], while IFN-$\gamma$ inhibits sensitization of mast cells either via IgE-binding or via Fc$\epsilon$RI regulation. IFNs derived from epidermal cells are thus generally downmodulators of mast cell function. The same holds for corticosteroids and transforming growth factor beta (TGF-$\beta$) which affect primarily mast cell proliferation (Table 6). Topically applied corticosteroids also decrease mast cell numbers in the skin [72, 73].

*F. Nowak, N. Haas, J. Grabbe, D. Schadendorf, A. Möller, B. M. Czarnetzki. *Hautarzt*, in press.

# IV. MAST CELLS IN CUTANEOUS DISEASE

## A. Effects on Disease Processes

Mast cells have been found to be increased in a great variety of chronic inflammatory and proliferative processes. In a few of them, there is also evidence for active participation of mast cells in the pathological events [5] (Table 7). Cutaneous whealing reactions are the prototype of mast cell–dependent processes which can be explained by classical, rapidly released and highly active mediators like histamine and arachidonate metabolites. Epidermal cells are hardly affected during these events, except for edema and, in small children, a rare subcutaneous blistering reaction. In vasculitic reactions, mast cell histamine is thought to enhance the deposition of immune complexes in the vessel walls.

Mast cell enzymes have also been implicated in blister formation in bullous pemphigoid. Hypogranulated mast cells are increased in the upper papillary dermis in this condition, and endothelial cell damage, a perivenular infiltrate of predominantly eosinophils, but also of lymphocytes, and a few basophils are seen on histology, together with elevated serum IgE levels [40, 74, 75]. These features fit well with the functions of mast cell mediators such as IL-3, IL-4, IL-5, IL-6, and TNF-$\alpha$.

The effect of chronic mast cell stimulation on the epidermis is perhaps best seen in urticaria pigmentosa, a benign mast cell–proliferative disease. The epidermis above the mast cell accumulation is normal except for a moderate increase of pigmentation which might be due to mast cell–derived mediators (Fig. 3) or to mediators from other cells that cause both mast cell proliferation and increased melanogenesis, such as the c-kit ligand from fibroblasts [62]. Postinflammatory pigmentation may be produced by the same mechanisms.

The possible role of mast cells in delayed-type hypersensitivity eczematous reactions and atopic eczema is controversial. The cells have been implicated

**Table 7** Cutaneous Disease Processes in Which Mast Cells are Thought to Actively Participate

| |
|---|
| Urticaria |
| Bullous pemphigoid |
| Vasculitis |
| Eczema |
| Wound healing |
| Fibrosis |

in T-lymphocyte activation during immunological sensitization [76], and the itching, edema, and leukocyte infiltration in these processes might in part be caused by mast cell mediators like histamine, LTs, and ILs [77, 78] (Fig. 3).

## B. Increase in Mast Cell Numbers

Mast cell numbers have been found to be increased in a wide spectrum of cutaneous diseases (Table 8). They include psoriasis [79], neurofibromatosis [80], and many other solid tumours, particularly lymphomas [81]. Their numbers have been reported to fluctuate during various phases of graft-versus-host disease [82]. The association of mast cells with healing wounds, keloids, and scleroderma [83–85] has recently led to much speculation about the role of the cells in fibrosis.

## C. Significance of Mast Cells in Cutaneous Disease

After having gone through this literature, the implication of mast cell participation in such a great variety of very different pathological processes leaves one puzzled and confused. A first reaction might be that, due to the multiple possible ways of mast cell activation, the cell is an innocent bystander, releasing some of its mediators in all kinds of processes without being specifically involved in the central pathogenetic process. Alternately, one could view the mast cell as a central effector cell of a great variety of pathological events, a role it is particularly well equipped for because of its great spectrum of potent, rapidly acting and more slowly released mediators. Depending on the local tissue environment, the mast cell might not only change its morphology, but also its basic function, causing an upregulation as well as a downregulation of the ongoing events. Clearly, this cell will have to be studied much more thoroughly regarding both its basic capabilities and its function in disease in order to clarify the large quantity of apparently meaningless data amassed in the literature.

**Table 8** Pathological Conditions of the Skin in Which Mast Cells Have Been Shown to Be Increased in Number

| | |
|---|---|
| Chronic urticaria | Epidermal tumors |
| Eczema | Fibromas |
| Psoriasis | Mastocytosis |
| Bullous pemphigoid | Keloids |
| Vasculitis | Scleroderma |
| Behçet's syndrome | Prurigo nodularis |
| Lichen planus | Lichen sclerosus et atrophicus |
| Graft-versus-host disease | |

## V. CONCLUSIONS

Mast cells are dermal cells of myeloid origin which are preferentially located in the vicinity of vessels. This fact, together with their great store of preformed mediators and the wide range of newly generated immediate and delayed-acting mediators, makes them particularly suitable to function as conveyors of chemical and formed elements from the blood to the epidermis (Fig. 5). Mast cells are in turn receptive to signals released from the epidermis, which can regulate their growth and function. Specifically, epidermal cytokines can induce the release of rapidly acting preformed and newly generated mediators of inflammation from mast cells and also a number of cytokines. Additional mediators from the epidermis can boost or downmodulate inflammatory processes that have thus been initiated. In chronic inflammation and in cutaneous proliferative diseases, mast cell numbers are often increased, a process that can be influenced by well-known cytokines from the epidermis as well as from the dermal cell compartment.

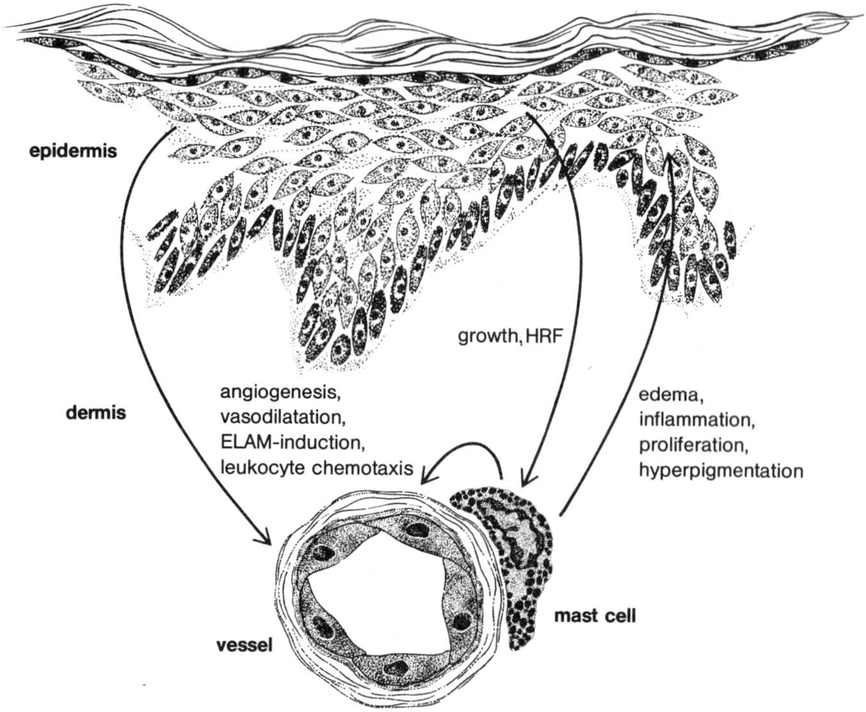


**Fig. 5** Presentation of the most important potential interactions of mast cells and epidermal cells, including effects on the vasculature.

Most of the fascinating and potentially important interactions between epidermal cells and dermal mast cells and their cytokines, as discussed here, are still deductive and speculative since they are based on a number of artificial in vitro systems and on complex in vivo observations. Their true significance in specific disease processes requires further clarification.

## REFERENCES


1. P. Ehrlich, Thesis, Leipzig, 1878, in *The Collected Papers of Paul Ehrlich* (R. Himmelweit, M. Marquardt, and H. Dale, eds.), Pergamon Press, London, 1956, vol. 1, p. 29.
2. B. Wang, A. Rieger, O. Kilgus, K. Ochiai, D. Fodinger, J.-P. Kinet, and G. Stingl, *J. Exp. Med. 175*, 1353 (1992).
3. N. Haas, K. Mamann, J. Grabbe, B. Cremer, and B. M. Czarnetzki, *Acta Dermatovener. 72*, 271 (1992).
4. S. J. Galli, *Lab. Invest. 62*, 5 (1990).
5. A.-M. Irani and L. B. Schwartz, *Clin. Exp. Allergy 19*, 143 (1989).
6. S. S. Craig, N. M. Schechter, and L. B. Schwartz, *Lab. Invest. 58*, 682 (1988).
7. M. K. Church, R. C. Benyon, P. H. Rees, M. A. Lowman, A. M. Campbell, C. Robinson, and S. T. Holgate, in *Mast Cell and Basophil Differentiation and Function in Health and Disease* (S. J. Galli and K. F. Austen, eds.), Raven Press, New York, 1989, p. 161.
8. N. Weidner and K. F. Austen, *J. Invest. Dermatol. 96*, 26S (1991).
9. A. A. Irani, S. M. Goldstein, B. U. Wintroub, T. Bradford, and L. B. Schwartz, *J. Immunol. 147*, 247 (1991).
10. F. L. Pearce, P. B. Boulos, H. Y. A. Lau, W. L. Liu, and K. R. Tainsh, *Int. Arch. Allergy Appl. Immunol. 94*, 239 (1991).
11. E. S. Schulman, A. Kagey-Sobotka, D. W. MacGlashan, N. F. Adkinson, St. P. Peters, R. P. Schleimer, and L. M. Lichtenstein, *J. Immunol. 131*, 1936 (1983).
12. B. M. Czarnetzki, C. G. Figdor, G. Kolde, T. Vroom, R. Aalberse, and J. E. de Vries, *Immunology 51*, 549 (1984).
13. B. M. Czarnetzki, W. Sterry, H. Bazin, and K. J. Kalveram, *Int. Archs. Allergy Appl. Immunol. 67*, 44 (1982).
14. J. W. Schrader, R. Scollay, and F. Battye, *J. Immunol. 130*, 558 (1983).
15. B. M. Czarnetzki and G. Mecklenburg, *J. Dermatol. Sci. 2*, 1 (1991).
16. F. Levi-Schaffer, K. F. Austen, P. M. Gravallese, et al., *Proc. Natl. Acad. Sci. USA 83*, 6485 (1986).
17. T. Kobayashi, T. Nakano, N. Tatsutoshi, et al., *J. Immunol. 136*, 1378 (1986).
18. A. Möller, J. Grabbe, and B. M. Czarnetzki, *Skin Pharmacol. 4* (Suppl. 1), 56 (1991).
19. P. Valent, L. K. Ashman, W. Hinterberger, F. Eckersberger, O. Majdic, K. Lechner, and P. Bettelheim, *Blood 73*, 1778 (1989).
20. K. Hamann, N. Haas, J. Grabbe, A. Möller, E. Bauer, and B. M. Czarnetzki, *Arch. Derm. Res. 284*, 16 (1992).
21. G. Marone, N. Casolaro, C. Raffaele, C. Stellato, and A. Genovese, *Clin. Immunol. Immunopathol. 50*, 524 (1989).

22. M. A. Lettbrown, R. Lalm, and J. A. Grant, *Yearbook Immunol. 5*, 195 (1989).
23. B. M. Czarnetzki, *Scand. J. Immunol. 15*, 581 (1982).
24. P. H. Rees, K. Hillier, and M. K. Church, *Immunology 65*, 437 (1988).
25. C. C. Fox, A. Kagey-Sobotka, R. P. Schleimer, S. P. Peters, D. W. MacGlashan, and L. M. Lichtenstein, *Int. Arch. Allergy Appl. Immunol. 77*, 130 (1985).
26. P. R. Burd, H. W. Rogers, J. R. Gordon, C. A. Martin, S. Jayaraman, S. D. Wilson, A. M. Dvorak, S. J. Galli, and M. E. Dorf, *J. Exp. Med. 170*, 245 (1989).
27. R. A. Seder, W. E. Paul, S. Z. Ben-Sasson, G. S. LeGros, A. Kagey-Sobotka, F. D. Finkelman, J. H. Pierce, and M. Plaut, *Int. Arch. Allergy Appl. Immunol. 94*, 137 (1991).
28. A. Wodnar-Filipowicz, C. H. Heusser, and C. Moroni, *Nature 339*, 150 (1989).
29. A. Wodnar-Filipowicz and C. Moroni, *Proc. Natl. Acad. Sci. USA 87*, 777 (1990).
30. A. Möller, D. Schadendorf, U. Lippert, E. Förster, T. A. Luger, and B. M. Czarnetzki, *Am. J. Allergy Clin. Immunol. 87*, 277 (1991).
31. J. R. Gordon, P. R. Burd, and S. J. Galli, *Immunol. Today 11*, 458 (1990).
32. J. Marcinkiewicz, *Cytokine 3*, 327 (1991).
33. T. Rosenbach and B. M. Czarnetzki, in *Eicosanoids and the Skin* (T. Ruzicka, ed.), CRC Press, Boca Raton, FL, 1989, p. 127.
34. L. J. Walsh, G. Trinchieri, H. A. Waldorf, D. Whitaker, and G. F. Murphy, *Proc. Natl. Acad. Sci. USA 88*, 4220 (1991).
35. C. Nathan and M. Sporn, *J. Cell Biol. 113*, 984 (1991).
36. L. M. Klein, R. M. Lavker, W. L. Matis, and G. F. Murphy, *Proc. Natl. Acad. Sci. USA 86*, 8972 (1989).
37. E. Vannier, L. C. Miller, and C. A. Dinarello, *J. Exp. Med. 174*, 281 (1991).
38. S. D. Brain and T. J. Williams, *Nature* (London) *335*, 73 (1988).
39. B. M. Kzarnetzki, K. König, and L. M. Lichtenstein, *Inflammation 1*, 201 (1975).
40. B. M. Czarnetzki, K. J. Kalveram, and U. Dierksmeier, *J. Invest. Dermatol. 72*, 163 (1979).
41. R. N. Boswell, K. F. Austen, and E. J. Goetzl, *J. Immunol. 126*, 15 (1978).
42. B. M. Czarnetzki, *Int. Arch. Allergy Appl. Immunol. 67*, 181 (1982).
43. P. C. Atkins, M. Norman, H. Weiner, and B. Zweiman, *Ann. Int. Med. 86*, 415 (1977).
44. B. M. Czarnetzki, *Clin. Exp. Immunol. 54*, 486 (1983).
45. P. R. Burd, H. W. Rogers, J. R. Gordon, C. A. Martin, S. Jayaraman, S. D. Wilson, A. M. Dvorak, S. J. Galli, and M. E. Dorf, *J. Exp. Med. 170*, 245 (1989).
46. S. M. MacDonald, R. P. Schleimer, A. Kagey-Sobotka, S. Gillis, and L. M. Lichtenstein, *J. Immunol. 142*, 3527 (1989).
47. W. A. Massey, T. C. Randall, A. Kagey-Sobotka, J. A. Warner, S. M. MacDonald, S. Gillis, A. C. Allison, and L. M. Lichtenstein, *J. Immunol. 143*, 1875 (1989).
48. P. Valent, J. Besemer, C. Sillaber, J. H. Butterfield, R. Eher, O. Majdic, K. Kishi, W. Klepetko, F. Eckersberger, K. Lechner, and P. Bettelheim, *J. Immunol. 145*, 3432 (1990).

49. J. Padawer, in *Hypersensitivity* (M. D. Bach, ed.), Marcel Dekker, New York, 1979, p. 301.
50. F. M. Atkins and D. D. Metcalfe, *J. Immunol. 131*, 1420 (1983).
51. A. M. Dvorak, T. Ishizaka, and S. J. Galli, *Lab. Invest. 53*, 57 (1985).
52. W. R. Henderson, E. Y. Chi, E. C. Jong, and S. J. Klebanoff, *J. Immunol. 137*, 2695 (1986).
53. T. R. Mosmann, *Int. Arch. Allergy Appl. Immunol. 94*, 110 (1991).
54. H. Le Trong, H. Neurath, and R. G. Woodbury, *Proc. Natl. Acad. Sci. USA 84*, 364 (1987).
55. Y. Hamaguchi, Y. Kanakura, J. Fujita, S. I. Takeda, T. Nakano, S. Tarui, T. Honjo, and Y. Kitamura, *J. Exp. Med. 165*, 237 (1987).
56. K. Ikebuchi, G. G. Wong, S. C. Clark, J. N. Ihle, Y. Hirai, and M. Ogawa, *Proc. Natl. Acad. Sci. USA 84*, 9035 (1987).
57. L. Thompson-Snipes, V. Dhar, K. Moore, M. Band, and D. Rennick, *Exp. Hematol. 18*, 612 (1990).
58. L. Hultner, C. Druez, J. Moeller, C. Uyttenhove, E. Schmitt, E. Rude, and P. Dormer, *Eur. J. Immunol. 20*, 1413 (1990).
59. L. Thompson-Snipes, V. Dhar, M. W. Bond, T. R. Mosmann, K. W. Moore, and D. M. Rennik, *J. Exp. Med. 173*, 507 (1991).
60. T. Ishizaka, T. Furitsu, and N. Inagaki, *Int. Arch. Allergy Appl. Immunol. 94*, 116 (1991).
61. K. M. Zsebo, P. H. Martin, S. V. Suggs, J. Wypych, H. S. Lu, I. McNiece, E. Medlock, F. Morris, R. Sachdev, W. Tung, N. Birkett, K. Smith, V. Yuschenkoff, E. M. Mendiaz, F. W. Jacobsen, and K. E. Langley, *Exp. Hematol. 18*, 703 (1990).
62. M. Tsai, S. Takeishi, H. Thompson, K. E. Langley, K. M. Zsebo, D. D. Metcalfe, E. N. Geissler, and S. J. Galli, *Proc. Natl. Acad. Sci. USA 88*, 6382 (1991).
63. M. J. Welham and J. W. Schrader, *Mol. Cell. Biol. 11*, 2901 (1991).
64. N. Matsuura and B. R. Zetter, *J. Exp. Med.*, 1421 (1989).
65. M. V. White, H. Baer, Y. Kubota, and M. Kaliner, *J. Allergy Clin. Immunol. 84*, 773 (1989).
66. A. P. Kaplan, M. Baeza, S. Reddigari, and P. Kuna, *Int. Arch. Allergy Appl. Immunol. 94*, 148 (1991).
67. K. Hirai, M. Yamagouchi, Y. Misaki, T. Takaishi, K. Ohta, K. Ito, and T. Miyamoto, *J. Exp. Med. 172*, 1525 (1990).
68. J. A. Grant, R. Alam, and M. A. Lett-Brown, *Int. Arch. Allergy. Appl. Immunol. 94*, 141 (1991).
69. E. Y. Bissonnette and A. D. Befus, *J. Immunol. 145*, 3385 (1990).
70. J. W. Coleman and A. G. Morris, *Int. Arch. Allergy Appl. Immunol. 94*, 179 (1991).
71. M. Swieter, W. A. Ghali, C. Rimmer, and A. D. Befus, *Immunology 66*, 606 (1989).
72. R. M. Lavker and N. M. Schlechter, *J. Immunol. 135*, 2368 (1985).
73. D. H. Broide, S. I. Wasserman, J. Alvaro-Gracia, N. J. Zvaifler, and G. S. Firestein, *J. Immunol. 143*, 1591 (1989).

74. B. U. Wintroub, M. C. Mihm, E. J. Goetzl, et al., *N. Engl. J. Med. 298*, 417 (1978).
75. A. M. Dvorak, B. U. Wintroub, M. C. Mihm, et al., *J. Invest. Dermatol. 78*, 91 (1982).
76. H. Van Loveren, W. D. Otter, R. Meade, P. M. Terheggen, and P. W. Askenase, *J. Immunol. 134*, 1292 (1985).
77. M. C. Mihm, N. A. Soter, and H. F. Dvorak, *J. Invest. Dermatol. 67*, 305 (1976).
78. F. A. Kerdel, D. V. Belsito, R. Scotto-Chinnici, and N. A. Soter, *J. Invest. Dermatol. 8*, 686 (1987).
79. S. Toyry, J. Fraki, and R. Tammi, *Arch. Dermatol. Res. 280*, 282 (1988).
80. V. M. Riccardi, *Birth Defects 17*(2), 129 (1981).
81. W. R. Roche, *Am. J. Pathol. 119*, 57 (1985).
82. H. N. Claman, *J. Invest. Dermatol. 84*, 246 (1985).
83. M. H. Amler, M. S. Jacobson, and R. W. Amler, *Ann. Dent. 46*, 16 (1987).
84. C. W. Kischer, H. Bunce, and M. R. Shetlar, *J. Invest. Dermatol. 70*, 355 (1978).
85. H. N. Claman, *JAMA 262*, 1206 (1989).

# 19
# Epidermal Cell Cytokines and Endothelial Cells

**Sergij Goerdt, Hans-Hermann Hagemeier, and Clemens Sorg**
*University of Münster*
*Münster, Germany*

## I. INTRODUCTION

Vascular organization in skin comprises both blood and lymphatic vascular systems (reviewed in Refs. 8, 105). The blood vessels are organized in two plexus in the dermis: an upper horizontal plexus from which the capillary loops of the dermal papillae arise and a lower horizontal plexus at the dermal-subcutaneous interface. Both plexus have a separate system of arterioles, terminal arterioles, precapillary sphincters, arterial and venous capillaries, postcapillary venules, and larger venules, but are connected to each other through arterioles and venules. The capillary loop is composed of an ascending limb, a papillary loop with a hairpin turn, and a descending limb. The ascending limb and the intrapapillary portion display characteristics of an arterial capillary with a smaller tube diameter and a homogeneous basement membrane. The descending limb abruptly turns into a venous capillary with a larger tube diameter and a multilayered basement membrane. Throughout the skin blood vasculature, the endothelium is of the continuous type, but contains more pinocytotic vessels and fewer Weibel-Palade bodies than is typical of other organs. In healthy skin, endothelial cells are not fenestrated, though at the tip of the capillary loop the endothelium may become extremely attenuated. Mural cells around skin vessels consist of smooth muscle cells on the arterial side and predominantly pericytes on the capillary and venous segments. Both smooth muscle cells and pericytes are an integral part of the vascular wall embedded in the mural basement membrane and form occasional tight junctions with endothelial cells. Intradermal cells of bone marrow origin, including subpopulations of macrophages, mast cells, and T cells, can be found in close vicinity to the dermal microvascular wall. Among these, the veil cells, which are thought to be of macrophage/dendritic cell lineage and constitute a considerable proportion of the factor XIIIa-positive "dermal dendrocytes," appear unique to the skin microvasculature.

The lymphatics in the skin consist of a subpapillary plexus of initial lymphatics, displaying interendothelial openings and endothelial bridges. They are connected to the epifascial and subfascial collectors by precollectors at the dermal-subcutaneous interface.

In addition to these morphological characteristics, blood vascular endothelial cells express antigens normally found in continuous microvascular endothelia, such as von Willebrand's factor (vWF) [7], CD31 [78, 86], CD34 [30, 108], and CD36 [2, 58, 82]. In contrast, NCAM seems to be expressed in cultured skin microvascular endothelial cells, but not in cultured human umbilical vein endothelial cells. Lymphatic endothelial cells may express only low amounts of vWF, but lack CD31, CD34, and CD36.

In many skin diseases, morphological and functional changes of blood vascular endothelial cells constitute part of the pathobiological process. In psoriasis, papillary capillaries become hyperplastic and tortuous and endothelial cells acquire fenestrations. In allergic contact dermatitis, venular endothelial cells become swollen and begin to replicate. In granuloma pyogenicum, an inflammatory, tumorlike vascular proliferation is the main feature of the lesion, while in Kaposi's sarcoma the tumor cells themselves seem to be derived from some endothelial source. In all these lesions, endothelial changes do not appear to occur as effects of primary or autonomous endothelial disease processes, but rather seem to be induced by previous alterations of other cellular components in skin. These primary disease targets, such as keratinocytes, melanocytes, Langerhans cells, mast cells, dermal dendrocytes and other tissue macrophages, and skin-seeking T cells, are first activated to secrete large amounts and a vast array of different cytokines. These cytokines in turn reach the dermal endothelial cells in the vicinity of their producers and are thought to cause the endothelial reactions observed. Cytokine-induced redifferentiation processes are not restricted to endothelial cells in skin and have largely been investigated in vitro. In general, endothelial cells exposed to cytokines may undergo one of three processes: (a) endothelial activation (reviewed in Ref. 97), i.e., the reversible expression of newly synthesized proteins important in inflammatory reactions, (b) angiogenesis [31], i.e., the formation of new vessels from preexisting ones, and (c) tumor induction [28, 29, 77, 83]. Each of these processes may be induced largely separately or combined depending on the cytokines produced, which can act additively, synergistically [54], or mutually inhibitory [21]. Some cytokines, such as TNF-$\alpha$, exhibit both activating and angiogenic properties. In addition, cytokines can induce endothelial cells to secrete cytokines, themselves acting in autocrine and paracrine fashion, to complete the local and systemic cytokine network. On the other hand, cytokine actions are imposed on endothelial cells that already exhibit a special differentiative state depending on (a) their positions along the vascular trees of the blood vascular and lymphatic systems and (b) the local organ microenvironment in which they are embedded. The most prominent differences in differentiation have been noticed morphologically and antigenically between continuous and noncontinuous, sinusoidal endothelial cells [36]. The preexisting differentiative state modulates the endothelial response to infectious and inflammatory agents. For example, the same agent induces bacillary angiomatosis in organs with continuous blood vessels, such as skin, and peliosis in organs with noncontinuous, sinusoidal blood vessels, such as liver and spleen [26, 92, 101, 113]. Another example for the interaction of differentiation and activation are the phenotypes ;and functions of high endothelial venular endothelial cells in various secondary lymphatic tissues [11, 44, 134]. High endothelial venular endothelial cells express different adhesion molecules for recirculating lymphocytes, collectively called vascular addressins, due to differentiative processes (reviewed in Ref. 11) while they maintain their morphology and other aspects of their functional status through continuous activation by interferon gamma (IFN-$\gamma$) [24] and/or other as yet undefined cytokines. In conclusion, the source of cytokines (e.g., T cell, keratinocyte, mast cell) seems to be less important than the actual pattern of the cytokines secreted and the differentiative state of the resting endothelial cell at a local tissue site. In this chapter, we will describe general mechanisms of endothelial activation, show how they apply to endothelial activation in skin, and discuss what is known about skin-specific homing of lymphocytes. Since skin-specific and, even less so, epidermal cell–specific mechanisms of angiogenesis and tumor induction have as yet not been elucidated, we will not discuss these events here in further detail.

## II. INFLAMMATION AND GENERAL MECHANISMS OF ENDOTHELIAL ACTIVATION

Blood vascular endothelial cells play a number of important roles in inflammatory reactions. Four important functions performed by endothelium that contribute to inflammation are (a) relaxation of smooth muscle tone allowing increased blood flow, (b) opening of intercellular spaces, causing increased permeability with extravascular leakage of plasma proteins, (c) adhesion of circulating leukocytes on postcapillary venules, a prelude to leukocyte extravasation, and (d) activation of the adherent leukocytes, converting immotile circulating forms into motile forms which can migrate into inflammatory sites. To a certain extent, these functions can be performed by differentiated endothelia in their normal resting state when elicited by mediators such as histamine or leukotriene $C_4$ ($LTC_4$). Such elicited responses, which we call *endothelial stimulation*, are rapid (minutes) and occur independently of new protein synthesis. Inflammatory cytokines, such as interleukin 1 (IL-1) and TNF, can induce endothelial cells to increase their capacity to perform inflammatory functions. Most altered capacities result from a process we call *endothelial activation*, which is dependent on new or altered protein synthesis occurring as a result of altered levels of gene transcription. We will describe both stimulation and activation in more detail.

## A. Rapid Responses: Stimulation of Resting Endothelium

As noted above, endothelial stimulation consists of a group of rapid and often transient responses elicited by agents such as histamine. The best studied examples of stimulation are synthesis of prostacyclin ($PGI_2$) [131], synthesis of platelet-activating factor (PAF) [132], synthesis of nitric oxide (NO) [32, 90], release of stored von Willebrand's factor (vWF) [17], surface expression of granule-membrane protein 140 (GMP-140), also known as platelet activation-dependent granule-external membrane protein (PADGEM) or CD62 [41], and endothelial cell contraction [69]. Certain other responses, such as secretion of Protein S [119] or expression and shedding of prothrombinase [40], may also be examples of stimulation, but these processes are less well understood and will not be further discussed. The agents that cause stimulation vary somewhat among species and with the vascular bed. Such agonists include histamine, $LTC_4$ and its breakdown products, $LTD_4$ and $LTE_4$, bradykinin, C5a, $\alpha$-thrombin, platelet-activating factor, and, most recently, vascular permeability factor (VPF), also known as vascular endothelial growth factor (VEGF).

All features of the stimulation response can be mimicked by calcium ionophores, and all known agents that trigger endothelial stimulation cause alterations of the concentration of cytoplasmic calcium ion ($[Ca^{2+}]_i$). Thus $[Ca^{2+}]_i$ is thought to be a key second messenger in the stimulation pathway. Different patterns of elevation in $[Ca^{2+}]_i$ (oscillations, long-lasting transients, plateaus [49] and formation of $[Ca^{2+}]_i$/calmodulin complexes [9]) may trigger different aspects of the stimulation responses. Oscillations in $[Ca^{2+}]_i$ may be sufficient to cause $PGI_2$ and PAF synthesis, while NO formation [9], vWF release, GMP-140 translocation [41, 135], and endothelial contraction [133] seem to require $[Ca^{2+}]_i$/calmodulin complexes.

Endothelial stimulation may contribute to inflammation in several ways. $PGI_2$, NO, and PAF can cause smooth muscle cells of precapillary sphincters to dilate, increasing blood flow and delivery of leukocytes to tissues [100]. Endothelial contraction occurs mostly in postcapillary venules whose endothelial cells are enriched for expression of histamine 1 (H1) receptors [43], which mediate this response. Endothelial contraction leads to extravasation of fluid and plasma proteins and to leukostasis and enhanced leukocyte adhesion to the endothelial surface due to reduced shear forces. GMP-140 cell surface expression could serve to bind neutrophils [33]. GMP-140 contains an amino-terminal mammalian C-type lectin domain [55] and has been shown to bind asialyl Lewis X glycan moieties (CD15) attached to macromolecules on the surface of neutrophils and monocytes [63]. It has been proposed that these events also take place at postcapillary venules in vivo, but it should be pointed out that Weibel-Palade bodies, the storage location of intracellular GMP-140 and vWF, are more numerous in arteriolar endothelium. In contrast to GMP-140 translocation, secretion of vWF has not been directly linked to inflammation. Instead, endothelial-derived vWF acts as a molecular bridge to stabilize platelet attachment to subendothelium exposed at sites of vascular injury [118, 128]. This stabilization of platelet adhesion is most critical under arterial sheer stress, and arteries are the location of the highest concentration of Weibel-Palade bodies. Thus, vWF release is thought to be an important determinant of arterial hemostasis rather than of inflammation. PAF, however, may actually be involved in inflammation by triggering increased neutrophil adhesion and extravasation, since it acts on neutrophils to augment the expression and avidity of CD11/CD18 adhesion molecules, especially Mac-1 (CD11b/CD18) and lymphocyte function-associated antigen 1 (LFA-1, also called CD11a/CD18) [127]. LFA-1 [25] and Mac-1 [20] bind to intercellular adhesion molecule-1 (ICAM-1, CD54) on endothelium. LFA-1 also binds to intercellular adhesion molecule 2 (ICAM-2) [117]. Both LFA-1 and Mac-1 may have as yet unidentified additional endothelial ligands.

## B. Activation of Endothelium by Cytokines

As noted above, resting endothelial cells, upon stimulation, perform functions that can contribute to the development of inflammation. However, these actions may not be sufficient. For example, histamine causes endothelial cells to make vasodilators, to contract, to express GMP-140, and to synthesize PAF, yet it cannot cause inflammation as defined by the accumulation of leukocytes. In response to cytokines such as IL-1 and TNF, endothelial cells undergo a series of changes that serve to increase their capacity to promote the inflammatory process. Some of these changes augment or complement those produced by stimulation. For example, IL-1 and TNF increase transcription of genes encoding the enzymes responsible for $PGI_2$ synthesis [68]. As a result, cytokine-treated cells synthesize much greater amounts of $PGI_2$ in response to the same concentrations of histamine [135]. In addition, cytokines cause long-lived changes in the organization of endothelial cytoskeletal proteins, which contribute to more sustained vascular leakage than that elicited by endothelial contraction [10, 120]. Furthermore, cytokines cause synthesis of new endothelial leukocyte adhesion molecules (other than GMP-140) and new leukocyte activating proteins, such as granulocyte-monocyte colony-stimulating factor (GM-CSF), interleukin 8 (IL-8), and monocyte chemotactic protein-1 (MCP-1) (reviewed in Ref. 97). These latter cytokine actions appear to be crucial for inflammation and will be discussed in more detail.

*Endothelial/Leukocyte Adhesion Molecules*

In humans, IL-1 and TNF have been found to increase synthesis and expression of three endothelial leukocyte adhesion molecules: endothelial leukocyte adhesion molecule 1 (ELAM-1), vascular cell adhesion molecule 1 (VCAM-1), and intercellular adhesion molecule 1 (ICAM-1). These molecules differ in their specificity for leukocytes and in the timing of their expression. IL-1 or TNF cause endothelium to begin de novo transcription, translation, and surface expression of ELAM-1 [4], a 110 kd cell surface glycoprotein that binds neutrophils, certain subsets of lymphocytes [66, 94, 110] and perhaps monocytes. In vivo, ELAM-1 is readily expressed by cytokine-activated venular and sometimes capillary endothelial cells of most vascular beds but generally not by arteriolar or arterial endothelial cells [15, 76]. Synthesis and expression of ELAM-1 are optimal after about 2–4 hours of cytokine treatment and then slowly decline over the next 24–48 hours. Interestingly, ELAM-1 is structurally related to GMP-140; like GMP-140, ELAM-1 contains an amino-terminal mammalian C-type lectin domain [5], and recent evidence indicates that ELAM-1 acts as a lectin to bind leukocytes. However, ELAM-1 recognizes sialylated Lewis X determinants as opposed to asialylated Lewis X determinants recognized by GMP-140. Transfection of a specific $\alpha$-(1,3)fucosyltransferase cDNA into nonmyeloid cell lines causing expression of $\alpha$-(2,3)sialylated, $\alpha$-(1,3)fucosylated lactosaminoglycans (the sialylated Lewis C carbohydrate determinant) can confer ELAM-1–dependent endothelial adhesion [65, 93, 130]. The identities of the protein or lipid molecules that display the involved oligosaccharides on the leukocyte surface are as yet unknown. Furthermore, the core structure of the carbohydrate-bearing molecules may additionally participate in the adhesive interactions and contribute to their specificity.

VCAM-1 is the second endothelial leukocyte adhesion molecule to be induced by IL-1 and TNF [89, 102]. In contrast to ELAM-1, VCAM-1 may be expressed at low levels on unactivated endothelial cells. VCAM-1 expression rises by 4 hours, and peak expression probably occurs by 24 hours. Structurally, VCAM-1 is a 110 kd glycoprotein (it was originally called inducible cell adhesion molecule 110, or INCAM-110) and is a member of the immunoglobulin (Ig) gene superfamily [89], containing six or seven (depending on mRNA splicing) tandem extracellular Ig-like domains. The leukocyte receptor for VCAM-1 is the $\beta_1$-integrin protein, VLA-4 (CD29/CD49d) [27, 109].

The third of the well-studied endothelial leukocyte adhesion molecules is ICAM-1. Like VCAM-1, ICAM-1 is basally expressed on endothelial cells, and its IL-1- or TNF-induced expression rises by 4 hours and reaches plateau levels at 24 hours or later [80, 98]. Also like VCAM-1, ICAM-1 is a member of the Ig gene superfamily. ICAM-1 contains five extracellular tandem Ig-like domains. The amino-terminal Ig-like domains of ICAM-1 are highly homologous to ICAM-2, a protein expressed constitutively on endothelium with only two Ig-like domains. ICAM-2 levels on unactivated endothelium appear higher than those of ICAM-1, but ICAM-2 is not increased by cytokine treatment. As noted earlier, both ICAM-1 and ICAM-2 interact with the leukocyte $\beta_2$-integrin protein, LFA-1 (CD11a/CD18); ICAM-1, but not ICAM-2, also interacts with Mac-1 (CD11b/CD18) [20], a $\beta_2$-integrin expressed on polymorphonuclear leukocytes and blood monocytes.

Studies of tissues by immunohistochemistry [80; D. Briscoe and J. S. Pober, unpublished] suggest that the onset of ELAM-1 expression is correlated with neutrophil accumulation in tissues, whereas increasing VCAM-1 and ICAM-1 expression is better correlated with mononuclear cell infiltration. These observations are consistent with the fact that ligands for ELAM-1 are predominantly expressed on neutrophils, whereas ligands for VCAM-1 are predominantly expressed on monocytes and lymphocytes. In vitro, ICAM-1 is an important ligand for neutrophil adhesion as well as lymphocyte adhesion; ICAM-1 is also involved in transmigration through cultured endothelial cell monolayers by both neutrophils and lymphocytes [88, 114, 129].

### *Endothelial-Derived Leukocyte-Activating Cytokines*

Expression of ELAM-1, VCAM-1, and ICAM-1 is neither sufficient nor entirely necessary for the accumulation of leukocytic infiltrates. For example, ELAM-1 expression may be found on arteries in septic shock, but neutrophil adhesion and migration are still confined to microvessels, especially postcapillary venules. On the other hand, intradermal injection of neutrophil (and T-cell) activating substances, such as IL-8 and chemoattractants like $LTB_4$, can cause neutrophil (and T-cell) accumulation at the injection site [57, 62] without causing ELAM-1 or enhanced VCAM-1/ICAM-1 expression by the endothelium [81]. Furthermore, recently activated T-cell clones may be able to penetrate through endothelial barriers, even in the brain [103], in the absence of endothelial activation. Neutrophil activation is accompanied by a decrease in adhesivity for ELAM-1. In part, this is explained by the observation that activated neutrophils shed several membrane proteins [57], some of which bear sialylated Lewis X glycans. (Surprisingly, the net level of sialylated Lewis X on the surface of activated neutrophils does not significantly decrease, probably because of concomitant translocation of granule membrane proteins bearing sialylated Lewis X to the cell surface; however, these new proteins appear less interactive with ELAM-1.) Interestingly, among the molecules that are shed (and may bear sialylated Lewis X) is the neutrophil version of the peripheral lymph node homing receptor [57]. This molecule, first identified in mouse by monoclonal antibody (mAb) Mel-14, and in human by mAbs TQ1 and Leu8 [12], has also been called leukocyte adhesion molecule 1 (LAM-1) or LECAM-1 (*l*ectin domain–*E*GF domain–*c*omplement domains—*a*dhesion *m*olecule). This last acronym emphasizes the structural features shared by LECAM-1 with ELAM-1 and GMP-140. These three molecules have been collectively called either LECCAMs (lectin-cell adhesion molecules) or selectins to emphasize their lectinlike functions in cell adhesion. These data raise the possibility that LECAM-1 is a ligand for ELAM-1; LECAM-1 has been found to participate in homing of neutrophils to peripheral sites of inflammation in the mouse [56]. If this is true, the specificity must reside in differences between LECAM-1 expressed on neutrophils vs. T cells, because T cells high in LECAM-1 expression (naive T cells) do not recognize ELAM-1 and home to lymph node rather than inflammatory sites. Although activated neutrophils are less adhesive for ELAM-1, they become more adhesive for resting endothelial cells through a CD18-dependent mechanism [18]. Specifically, both LFA-1 and Mac-1 appear to increase their avidity for endothelial ligands such as ICAM-1. The loss of ELAM-1–dependent binding that accompanies neutrophil activation may thus result in a net decrease in avidity for endothelium, but may actually favor transmigration through the endothelial layer, a process dependent upon CD18 molecules on the leukocyte and ICAM-1 on the endothelial cell [88, 114, 129].

T-lymphocyte adhesion to and transmigration through endothelial monolayers share a number of features with neutrophil recruitment. Homing to inflammatory sites in vitro is a property of memory T cells [14, 67], characterized by the expression of the low molecular weight isoform of CD45 (CD45RO) and also by low or absent levels of LECAM-1 and elevated levels of LFA-1 and VLA-4, as well as other adhesion molecules [96, 106]. Like neutrophils, memory T cells adhere to cytokine-activated endothelial cells in vitro [16], and cytokine-activated endothelial cell cultures can be used to selectively absorb out memory T cells capable of homing to inflammatory sites [48]. Memory T cells bind to cytokine-activated endothelial cells by utilizing a combination of LFA-1 to recognize ICAM-1 (and perhaps ICAM-2) and VLA-4 to recognize VCAM-1. ELAM-1 recognition may also contribute to binding of some T cells, although it is not known if these cells bear sialylated Lewis X determinants or another ligand. Upon activation by antigen or by other signals, T cells may further increase their avidity of LFA-1 and VLA-4 for their ligands (although in the case of VLA-4, it has not been established that this increase is directed towards VCAM-1) [34, 129]. Like neutrophils, activated lymphocytes are better at transmigrating through endothelial cell monolayers, and migration is further augmented if the endothelial monolayer has been activated by cytokines [88].

In conclusion, these studies indicate that the accumulation of leukocytic infiltrates in vivo may be composed of two sequential steps: (a) adherence of resting leukocytes to cytokine-activated endothelial cells through ELAM-1 or VCAM-1, and (b) in loco activation of bound leukocytes to allow them to migrate across the endothelial monolayer. How are leukocytes activated in situ? Presumably, the activation signals are provided by the cytokine-activated endothelium to which the leukocytes adhere. They may be contact dependent, either through the leukocyte adhesion molecules or through other structures (e.g., endothelial LFA-3 (CD59) interacting with T cell CD2 [46], or endothelial cell membrane-associated IL-1 [61] interacting with leukocyte IL-1 receptors). Alternatively, endothelial cells may provide soluble leukocyte-activating signals in the form of cytokines. To date, cytokine-activated endothelial cells have been shown to secrete several cytokines with specific activities directed toward various leukocyte populations. For example, IL-1- or TNF-treated endothelium will secrete GM-CSF, an activator of chemokinesis in neutrophils and monocytes [3, 79]; IL-8, an activator of chemokinesis in neutrophils and T cells [123]; MCP-1 [104, 111, 124], an activator of chemokinesis in monocytes [75]; and IL-6, a general activator of T cells and B cells [53, 112]. Both GM-CSF and IL-8 convert neutrophils from their nonmotile bloodborne form to their motile phenotype, and IL-8 may have similar actions on T cells. MCP-1 appears to be the most important endothelial-derived activator of monocytes [104a]. As already mentioned, extravascular injection of IL-8, like that of $LTB_4$, can cause neutrophils and perhaps T-cell accumulations in local tissues [57, 62]. Moreover, neutrophils treated with IL-8 become less adhesive with ELAM-1–expressing endothelium but increase CD18-dependent adhesion for resting endothelium [18]. IL-8 can actually cause neutrophil detachment from cytokine-activated endothelial monolayers in vitro [34], and intravenously administered IL-8 may inhibit the ability of circulating neutrophils to home to inflammatory sites in vivo [42].

*Supplement: Endothelial Actions of IFN-γ and IL-4*

With regard to synthesis of IL-1 and TNF by epidermal keratinocytes, we have so far emphasized the functions of IL-1- and TNF-activated endothelial cells as participants in inflammation. Two additional cytokines have activating properties on endothelium which may modify inflammatory reactions: IFN-γ and IL-4. IFN-γ can induce increased expression of ICAM-1 [114], albeit to a lesser extent than TNF, and although IFN-γ does not directly affect expression of ELAM-1 or VCAM-1, it displays striking synergy with TNF in upregulation of these molecules. IFN-γ is a direct inducer of MCP-1 [104] and may augment GM-CSF or IL-6 induction by TNF [64]. Although IFN-γ does not influence IL-8, it causes synthesis and secretion of a structurally related molecule, γ-IP10 (104a]; it is not known whether γ-IP10 has IL-8–like activity. IFN-γ also causes endothelial cells to express a 16 kd cell surface antigen, Leu13, which has been proposed as a T-cell interaction molecule [50, 99]. IL-4 directly causes increases in VCAM-1 expression [73] and may synergize with IL-1. IL-4 does not induce ELAM-1 or ICAM-1 and has been reported to partly inhibit their expression [126]. IL-4 causes endothelial cells to secrete MCP-1, but does not induce IL-8 or γ-IP10 [104a]. Cumulatively, the effects of IFN-γ and IL-4 appear to intensify endothelial cell inflammatory functions, especially those involved in mononuclear cell recruitment. Indeed, IFN-γ and IL-4 treatment can selectively increase T-cell adhesion to cultured endothelium without inducing neutrophil adhesion [126].

In addition to its role in stimulating leukocyte adhesion and transmigration, IFN-γ can regulate endothelial expression of class I and class II MHC antigens, molecules involved in antigen-specific activation of T cells. Class I molecules, involved in antigen presentation to CD8+ T cells, can also be upregulated by IFN-α or IFN-β and by TNF or lymphotoxin (LT). TNF and LT act synergistically with IFN-γ to increase class I expression (reviewed in Ref. 47).

Regulation of class II molecules on endothelium, which are involved in antigen presentation to CD4+ T cells, is more complex. In humans and certain other species (e.g., baboons and dogs) [84, 85], there is basal expression of class II MHC antigens on venular endothelial cells in situ. Experiments in dogs suggest that such endothelial expression is not constitutive but rather depends on basal levels of IFN-γ production. This conclusion is based on the observations that cyclosporin A treatment of dogs in vivo diminishes basal expression of class II molecules on endothelium [39] and that cyclosporin A in vitro acts to inhibit IFN-γ secretion by T cells but not the response of cultured endothelial cells to exogenous IFN-$\gamma$ [38]. Neutralizing antibodies to IFN-$\gamma$ can block T cell–mediated induction of endothelial class II molecules in vitro, and no other well-defined cytokine has been shown to cause class II expression on these cells. However, IFN-$\gamma$ may not be the only mediator with the capability to induce class II expression in endothelial cells. CD16+ natural killer cells when binding to endothelial cells in culture are efficient in triggering the expression of class II antigens. Antibodies to IFN-$\gamma$, however, do not inhibit class II antigen induction mediated by CD16+ cells, suggesting that T cells and natural killer cells may use different mechanisms to induce class II antigens on endothelial cells [91]. In vivo, basal levels of class II antigen expression may be increased during inflammatory responses to antigen [80]. In species other than humans and dogs, e.g., mice and guinea pigs, venular endothelial cell class II expression may be induced as a very early event in antigen responses [19, 115]. Rats are an exception, in that class II antigen expression by rat endothelial cells is not readily inducible in vivo [74], although cultured rat endothelial cells do respond to exogenous IFN-$\gamma$ [70]. These species differences suggest that endothelial class II antigen expression and concomitant endothelial cell-dependent antigen presentation to CD4+ T cells may not be essential for primary host defense. They may, however, modify the nature of the immune response, perhaps accounting for the difficulties in eliciting classical lymphocyte-rich delayed-type hypersensitivity reactions in the rat.

## III. CUTANEOUS DELAYED-TYPE HYPERSENSITIVITY AND ENDOTHELIAL ACTIVATION

Because of its easy accessibility by biopsy, more is perhaps known about endothelial activation in skin than in any other organ. Endothelial activation patterns in skin have largely been explored by immunohistological methods using the standard model of experimentally induced cutaneous delayed-type hypersensitivity reactions. Delayed-type hypersensitivity reactions can be divided into three phases. In the first or cognitive phase, antigen-specific CD4+ T cells recognize foreign protein antigens complexed to a self-allelic form of a class II major histocompatibility complex (MHC) molecule on the surface of an antigen-presenting cell. In the second or activation phase, the T cell integrates signals received through the T-cell receptor CD3 complex with additional signals received through other cell surface molecules or through soluble cytokines. If the sum of the signals is sufficient, the T cell will become activated, synthesizing IL-2 and other cytokines. Cytokines secreted by the activated T cell will lead to the third or effector phase of the immune response, involving recruitment and activation of lymphocytes, monocytes, and other leukocytes, producing an inflammatory reaction, which serves to eliminate and destroy the source of foreign antigen. Recruitment of the infiltrate is thought to depend upon cytokine-mediated activation of vascular endothelial cells. Nonimmune inflammatory reactions may resemble the effector phase of a delayed type hypersensitivity reaction, because various inflammatory cytokines (e.g., TNF or IL-1) can be secreted by skin cell types other than infiltrating activated T cells, e.g., by keratinocytes [1, 59, 60, 87], Langerhans cells, melanocytes, resident macrophages/dendritic cells [87], and mast cells [125]. Endothelial cells may participate in the first and second phases of delayed-type hypersensitivity as immune accessory cells (reviewed in Ref. 48). Most data in support of this have been derived from culture experiments or studies of organs other than skin. Here we will concentrate on studies that indicate how skin endothelial cells contribute to the third or inflammatory phase.

## A. Rapid Responses: Migration Inhibitory Factor

Endothelial stimulation responses are indispensible in the effector phase of delayed-type hypersensitivity reactions and have collectively been called the immediate hypersensitivity–like early component of delayed-type hypersensitivity [45]. This immediate hypersensitivity–like early component of delayed-type hypersensitivity peaks about 2 hours after antigen challenge and is caused by local release of vasoactive agents from mast cells that are reported to carry antigen-specific, IgE-analogous T-cell factors on their surface. If the immediate hypersensitivity–like early component of delayed-type hypersensitivity is abrogated, the late component of delayed-type hypersensitivity cannot occur. Furthermore, endothelial and perivascular expression of migration inhibitory factor (MIF), a mediator of macrophage differentiation [116], precedes leukocytic infiltration in delayed-type hypersensitivity and can occur as early as 20 minutes after antigen challenge as assessed by immunohistology using rat anti-mouse MIF monoclonal antibody 7D10 [72]. The severity of the delayed-type hypersensitivity reaction in various strains of mice correlates with endothelial expression of MIF [71]. Since endothelial MIF expression is similar in delayed-type hypersensitivity reactions and in irritant contact dermatitis in a given strain of mice [35, 71], a T-cell–independent mechanism seems to regulate endothelial MIF expression. Early endothelial MIF expression may influence early leukocyte adhesion to endothelium and early endothelium-dependent leukocyte activation and transmigration. This may be especially important with regard to the local emigration of the late-acting, antigen-specific and major histocompatibility antigen–restricted T cell that causes the leukocytic infiltrate during the late component of delayed-type hypersensitivity.

## B. Activation of Skin Endothelium

The leukocytic infiltrate of the late component of delayed-type hypersensitivity predominantly localizes in a perivenular distribution. Neutrophil-rich infiltrates appear early (at 6 hours) and are replaced at 18 hours with mononuclear cell infiltrates. Peak mononuclear infiltration occurs only 24–48 hours after antigenic challenge, and hence the reaction is termed delayed. The major approach used to assess participation of endothelial activation in the recruitment of leukocytes during the inflammatory phase of delayed-type hypersensitivity in the skin is immunocytochemical evaluation of the intensity and the kinetics of the expression of known endothelial leukocyte adhesion molecules. The expression of endothelial adhesion molecules is then compared to the accumulation of leukocytes. ELAM-1 expression in delayed-type hypersensitivity reactions is found on endothelial cells of numerous small vessels in the hypodermis and dermis by 16–24 hours [15, 37]. ELAM-1 expression is most prominent in the deeper venules, which exhibit a dense perivascular infiltrate. At 4 days after elicitation there is still residual ELAM-1 expression in endothelium, though by 6 days most of the endothelial cells have become ELAM-1 negative. VCAM-1 (D. Briscoe and J. S. Pober, unpublished), ICAM-1, and class II MHC molecules are expressed basally in normal skin endothelium, but increase considerably during delayed-type hypersensitivity reactions by 24 hours. Interestingly, the onset and peak of the expression of these adhesion molecules precede or occur concomitantly with, rather than follow, leukocyte infiltration.

It should be noted that, compared with direct cytokine injection into the skin, both endothelial activation and leukocyte accumulation in antigen-elicited reactions appear delayed, possibly due to the necessity of a preceding T-cell–activation step. For example, TNF injected intracutaneously into normal skin can induce expression of ELAM-1 at 2 hours, which is associated with polymorphonuclear cell accumulation at the injection site. Increased expression of ICAM-1 is induced by TNF by 9 hours and is associated with the onset of progressive mononuclear cell accumulation. IFN-$\gamma$ injection induces increased expression of class II molecules, but not of ICAM-1, and minimal accumulation of mononuclear cells by 24 hours. The combination of TNF and IFN-$\gamma$ induces a set of changes that qualitatively resemble those of the antigen-induced delayed-type hypersensitivity reaction [80]. These findings suggest that cytokine-inducible changes in endothelial cell capacities, especially those induced by IFN-$\gamma$ and TNF, could play an important role in delayed-type hypersensitivity. It should be noted that there are species-specific differences in the relevant cytokines; for example, in rat skin IFN-$\gamma$ is more potent than TNF in recruiting T-cell infiltrates [48].

## IV. SKIN ENDOTHELIUM AND SKIN-SPECIFIC HOMING OF LYMPHOCYTES

Many inflammatory skin diseases exhibit striking skin specificity. Some of these disease processes may primarily involve skin-specific cell types such as keratinocytes, Langerhans cells, or melanocytes. Yet other processes just appear to specifically attract different leukocytic infiltrates to localize in skin. Hence, the cells in the extravascular microenvironment of skin, especially during disease processes, could provide characteristic profiles of cytokines produced and thus elicit a characteristic kind of infiltrate by induction of specific sets of leukocyte subset–specific endothelial adhesion molecules or endothelial-derived chemoattractants. Alternatively, skin-specific endothelial differentiation could provide skin-specific endothelial activation programs, including skin-specific vascular addressins, which upon appropriate stimulation would recruit special leukocytic infiltrates. Here we will review this current controversy.

It has been proposed that the skin constitutes a special regional immune system called skin-associated lymphoid tissue (SALT) [122]. Lymphocyte homing to secondary lymphoid organs (e.g., lymph node vs. Peyer's patches) involves specific high endothelial cell adhesion molecules, the vascular addressins, and their lymphocyte counterparts, the lymphocyte homing receptors (reviewed in Refs. 11, 121). By analogy, SALT would constitute a distinctive leukocyte recirculation unit composed of lymphocytes differentiated to home to the skin under certain circumstances and endothelial cells which express, constitutively and/or upon activation, skin-specific sets of vascular addressins. Indeed, it has been shown using binding assays that psoriatic endothelium may express a tissue-specific vascular addressin [13, 14]. Recent interest has focused upon a molecule identified by mAb HECA-452. The HECA-452 epitope was first described as a marker of human high endothelial venules and on activated endothelium in sites of inflammation [23]. In contrast to most organs, however, mAb HECA-452 does not stain high endotheliallike postcapillary venular endothelial cells in skin [23, 52]. The absence of HECA-452 on skin endothelium may imply that skin endothelium is somehow unique and that the putative skin addressin, if any, remains to be identified. Interestingly, skin-associated lymphocytes appear to express the HECA-452 epitope, which is lacking on lymphocytes in other peripheral sites [95]. Therefore, the HECA-452 epitope has been renamed cutaneous lymphocyte-associated antigen (CLA) [94]. Although HECA-452–bearing lymphocytes seem to be chronically activated cells, HECA-452 does not appear to be an easily inducible lymphocyte activation antigen. This has raised the possibility that HECA-452 could mark a lymphocyte subset predestined to home to the skin.

The alternative view of skin-specific homing is simply that the dermal microenvironment produces a unique spectrum of cytokines which favor recruitment of certain lymphocyte subsets. In this model, skin endothelium is not itself unique. In support of this view, it has been shown that the same subpopulations of inflammatory T cells may be attracted to several organs by the same mediators. For example, phytohemagglutinin injection—whether intradermally, into the gut wall, joints, or peripheral lymph nodes—elicits a predominantly CD8+ T-cell infiltrate [6], while the cytokine RANTES [107] seems to selectively attract CD4+ memory T cells (and monocytes). In rats, small peritoneal exudate lymphocytes, but not lymph node lymphocytes, readily migrate into skin inflammatory sites, further suggesting a lack of tissue specificity [48]. These same peritoneal exudate lymphocytes strongly adhere to cytokine-activated cultured endothelial cells and are likely to be memory T cells [16]. T lymphocytes migrating into inflammatory sites are memory T cells [14, 67] and are more adhesive than naive T cells for cytokine-activated endothelial cells in vitro [16]. Compared to naive T cells, memory T cells have diminished expression of LECAM-1, the homing receptor for lymph node, but increased expression of CD44 [96, 106]. CD44, one of the adhesion molecules increased in expression by memory T cells, may be involved in homing of lymphocytes to both inflamed skin [52] and Peyer's patches [51]. Surprisingly, the putative endothelial ligand for these memory T cells has been identified as ELAM-1 [66, 94, 110], the adhesion molecule formerly described as the endothelial adhesion molecule for neutrophils. These observations raise the question how selectivity for neutrophil versus memory T-cell recruitment is achieved. Of the memory T cells, only the HECA-452/CLA$^+$ subpopulation adheres strongly to ELAM-1. In inflamed tissue specimens, endothelial expression of ELAM-1 seems to occur at cutaneous sites in preference to noncutaneous sites [94]. This may be due to characteristic cytokine profiles in inflamed skin. For example, combined treatment of human umbilical vein endothelial cells in vitro with TNF and IFN-$\gamma$, but not with IL-1 and IFN-$\gamma$, both accelerates and prolongs ELAM-1 expression [22]. Whether TNF and IFN-$\gamma$ are the cytokines actually used in inflamed skin to enhance ELAM-1 expression or whether yet other combinations are most important has not yet been established. The observed failure of dermal endothelial cells to express the HECA-452 epitope in settings of inflammation adds to this unsolved puzzle, since IFN-$\gamma$ induces cytoplasmic, though not cell surface, expression of the HECA-452 epitope on endothelial cells in vitro [52]. Thus inflamed skin should either contain little IFN-$\gamma$ or produce inhibitors of endothelial HECA-452 expression. In light of these observations, we believe that more work needs to be done to elucidate the actual cytokine profiles in inflamed skin, to study their influence on dermal endothelial cell activation, and to define how dermal endothelial differentiation interferes with dermal endothelial activation. This may lead us to better understand the mechanisms of lymphocyte and, as yet neglected, monocyte homing to inflamed skin.

## REFERENCES


1. J. Ansel, P. Perry, J. Brown, D. Damm, T. Phan, C. Hart, T. Luger, and S. Hefeneider, *J. Invest. Dermatol. 94*, 101s (1990).
2. A. S. Asch, J. Barnwell, R. L. Silverstein, and R. L. Nachman, *J. Clin. Invest. 79*, 1054 (1987).
3. G. C. Bagby, C. A. Dinarello, P. Wallace, C. Wagner, S. Hefeneider, and F. McCall, *J. Clin. Invest. 78*, 1316 (1986).
4. M. P. Bevilacqua, J. S. Pober, D. L. Mendrick, R. S. Cotran, and M. A. Gimbrone, Jr. *Proc. Natl. Acad. Sci. USA 84*, 9238 (1987).
5. M. P. Bevilacqua, S. Stengelin, M. A. Gimbrone, Jr., and B. Seed, *Science 243*, 1467 (1989).
6. R. M. Binns, S. T. Licence, and F. B. P. Wooding, *Eur. J. Immunol. 20*, 1067 (1990).
7. A. A. Bloom, J. C. Giddings, and C. J. Wilks, *Nature 241*, 217 (1973).
8. I. M. Braverman, *J. Invest. Dermatol. 93*, 2S (1989).
9. D. S. Bredt and S. H. Snyder, *Proc. Natl. Acad. Sci. USA 87*, 682 (1990).
10. J. Brett, H. Gerhach, P. Nawroth, S. Steinberg, G. Goodman, and D. Stern, *J. Exp. Med. 169*, 1977 (1989).
11. E. C. Butcher, *Am. J. Pathol. 136*, 3 (1990).
12. D. Camerini, S. P. James, I. Stamenkovic, and B. Seed, *Nature 342*, 78 (1989).
13. Y. H. Chin, V. Falanga, J. W. Streilein, and R. Sackstein, *J. Invest. Dermatol. 93*, 82S (1989).
14. Y. H. Chin, V. Falanga, R. Taylor, J.-P. Cai, and J. Bax, *J. Invest. Dermatol. 94*, 413 (1990).
15. R. S. Cotran, M. A. Gimbrone, Jr., M. P. Bevilacqua, D. L. Mendrick, and J. S. Pober, *J. Exp. Med. 164*, 661 (1986).
16. N. K. Damle and L. V. Doyle, *J. Immunol. 144*, 1233 (1990).
17. P. G. de Groot, M. D. Gonsalves, C. Loesberg, M. F. van Buul-Wortelboer, W. G. van Aken, and J. A. van Mourik, *J. Biol. Chem. 259*, 13329 (1984).
18. P. A. Detmers, K. Los, E. Olsen-Egbert, A. Walz, M. Baggiolini, and Z. A. Cohn, *J. Exp. Med. 171*, 1155 (1990).
19. R. M. Dewaal, M. J. J. Bogman, C. I. N. Maass, L. M. H. Cornelissen, W. J. M. Tax, and R. A. P. Koene, *Nature 303*, 426 (1983).
20. M. S. Diamond, D. E. Staunton, A. R. de Fougerolles, S. A. Stacker, J. Garcia-Aguilar, M. Hibbs, and T. A. Springer, *J. Cell Biol. 111*, 3129 (1990).
21. J. T. Doukas and J. S. Pober, *J. Immunol. 145*, 1088 (1990).
22. J. T. Doukas and J. S. Pober, *J. Immunol. 145*, 1727 (1990).
23. A. M. Duijvestijn, E. Horst, S. T. Pals, B. N. Rouse, A. C. Steere, L. J. Picker, C. J. L. M. Meijer, and E. C. Butcher, *Am. J. Pathol. 130*, 147 (1988).
24. A. M. Duijvestijn, A. S. Schreiber, and E. C. Butcher, *Proc. Natl. Acad. Sci. USA 83*, 9114 (1986).

25. M. L. Dustin, R. Rothlein, A. K. Bhan, C. A. Dinarello, and T. A. Springer, *J. Immunol. 137*, 245 (1986).
26. B. I. Eisenstein, *N. Engl. J. Med. 323*, 1625 (1990).
27. M. J. Elices, L. Osborn, Y. Takada, C. Crouse, S. Luhowskyj, M. E. Hemler, and R. R. Lobb, *Cell 60*, 577 (1990).
28. B. Ensoli, G. Barillari, S. Z. Salahuddin, R. C. Gallo, and F. Wong-Staal, *Nature 345*, 84 (1990).
29. B. Ensoli, S. Nakamura, S. Z. Salahuddin, P. Biberfeld, L. Larsson, B. Beaver, F. Wong-Staal, and R. C. Gallo, *Science 243*, 223 (1989).
30. L. Fina, H. V. Molgaard, D. Robertson, N. J. Bradley, P. Monaghan, D. Delia, D. R. Sutherland, M. A. Baker, and M. F. Greaves, *Blood 75*, 2417 (1990).
31. J. Folkman and M. Klagsbrun, *Science 235*, 442 (1987).
32. R. F. Furchgott and J. V. Zawadzki, *Nature 288*, 373 (1980).
33. J. G. Geng, M. P. Bevilacqua, and K. L. Moore, *Nature 343*, 757 (1990).
34. M. A. Gimbrone, Jr., M. S. Obin, and A. F. Brock, *Science 246*, 1601 (1989).
35. M. Goebeler, J. Gutwald, J. Roth, and C. Sorg, *Arch. Dermatol. Res. 283*, 246 (1991).
36. S. Goerdt, L. J. Walsh, G. F. Murphy, and J. S. Pober, *J. Cell Biol. 113*, 1425 (1991).
37. S. Goerdt, G. Zwadlo, R. Schlegel, H.-H. Hagemeier, and C. Sorg, *Exp. Cell Biol. 55*, 117 (1987).
38. G. Groenewegen, W. A. Buurman, G. M. M. A. Jeunhomme, and C. J. van der Linden, *Transplantation Baltimore 40*, 21 (1985).
39. G. Groenewegen, W. A. Buurman, and C. J. van der Linden, *Nature 316*, 361 (1985).
40. K. K. Hamilton, R. Hattori, C. T. Esmon, and P. J. Sims, *J. Biol. Chem. 265*, 3809 (1990).
41. R. Hattori, K. K. Hamilton, R. D. Fugate, R. D. McEver, and P. J. Sims, *J. Biol. Chem. 264*, 7768 (1989).
42. D. H. Hechtman, M. I. Cybulsky, J. B. Baker, and M. A. Gimbrone, Jr., *FASEB J. 4*, A890 (1990).
43. C. Heltianu, M. Simionescu, and N. Simionescu, *J. Cell Biol. 93*, 357 (1982).
44. H. R. Hendriks, I. L. Eestermans, and E. C. M. Hoefsmit, *Cell Tissue Res. 211*, 375 (1980).
45. W.-R. Herzog, N. R. Ferreri, W. Ptak, and P. W. Askenase, *J. Immunol. 143*, 3125 (1990).
46. C. C. W. Hughes, C. O. S. Savage, and J. S. Pober, *J. Exp. Med. 171*, 1453 (1990).
47. C. C. W. Hughes, C. O. S. Savage, and J. S. Pober, *Immunol. Rev. 117*, 85 (1990).
48. T. B. Issekutz, *J. Immunol. 144*, 2140 (1990).
49. R. Jacob, J. E. Merritt, T. J. Hallam, and T. J. Rink, *Nature 335*, 40 (1988).
50. E. A. Jaffe, D. Armellino, G. Lam, C. Cordon-Cardo, H. W. Murray, and R. L. Evans, *J. Immunol. 143*, 3961 (1989).
51. S. Jalkanen, R. F. Bargatze, J. de los Toyos, and E. C. Butcher, *J. Cell Biol. 105*, 983 (1987).

52. S. Jalkanen, S. Saari, H. Kalimo, K. Lammintausta, E. Vainio, R. Leino, A. M. Duijvestijn, and K. Kalimo, *J. Invest. Dermatol. 94*, 786 (1990).
53. F. R. Jirik, T. J. Podor, T. Hirano, T. Kishimoto, D. J. Loskutoff, D. A. Carson, and M. Lotz, *J. Immunol. 142*, 144 (1989).
54. D. R. Johnson and J. S. Pober, *Proc. Natl. Acad. Sci. USA 87*, 5183 (1990).
55. G. I. Johnston, R. G. Cook, and R. P. McEver, *Cell 56*, 1033 (1989).
56. M. A. Jutila, L. Rott, E. L. Berg, and E. C. Butcher, *J. Immunol. 143*, 3318 (1989).
57. T. K. Kishimoto, M. A. Jutila, and E. C. Butcher, *Proc. Natl. Acad. Sci. USA 87*, 2244 (1990).
58. D. M. Knowles II, B. Tolidjian, C. Marboe, V. D'Agati, M. Grimes, and L. Chess, *J. Immunol. 132*, 2170 (1984).
59. T. S. Kupper, *Am. J. Dermatopathol. 11*, 69 (1989).
60. T. S. Kupper, *J. Invest. Dermatol. 94*, 146S (1990).
61. E. A. Kurt-Jones, W. Fiers, and J. S. Pober, *J. Immunol. 139*, 2317 (1987).
62. C. G. Larsen, A. O. Anderson, E. Appella, J. J. Oppenheim, and K. Matsushima, *Science 243*, 1464 (1989).
63. E. Larsen, T. Palabrica, S. Sajer, G. E. Gilbert, D. D. Wagner, B. C. Furie, and B. Furie, *Cell 63*, 467 (1990).
64. J. F. T. Leeuwenberg, E. J. U. von Asmuth, T. M. A. A. Jeunhomme, and W. A. Buurman, *J. Immunol. 145*, 2110 (1990).
65. J. B. Lowe, L. M. Stoolman, R. P. L. M. Nair, R. D. Larsen, T. L. Berhend, and R. M. Marks, *Cell 63*, 475 (1990).
66. C. R. Mackay, *Nature 349*, 737 (1991).
67. C. R. Mackay, W. L. Marston, and L. Dudler, *J. Exp. Med. 171*, 801 (1990).
68. J. A. M. Maier, T. Hla, and T. Maciag, *J. Biol. Chem. 265*, 10805 (1990).
69. G. Majno, S. M. Shea, and M. Leventhal, *J. Cell Biol. 42*, 647 (1969).
70. D. K. Male, G. Pryce, and C. C. W. Hughes, *Immunology 60*, 453 (1987).
71. U. Malorny, M. Goebeler, J. Gutwald, J. Roth, and C. Sorg, *Int. Arch. Allergy Appl. Immunol. 92*, 356 (1990).
72. U. Malorny, J. Knop, G. Burmeister, and C. Sorg, *Clin. Exp. Immunol. 71*, 164 (1988).
73. B. Masinovsky, D. Urdal, and M. Gallatin, *J. Immunol. 145*, 2886 (1990).
74. D. W. Mason and A. N. Barclay, *Immunobiology 168*, 167 (1984).
75. K. Matsushima and J. J. Oppenheim, *Cytokine 1*, 2 (1989).
76. D. V. Messadi, J. S. Pober, W. Fiers, M. A. Gimbrone, Jr., and G. F. Murphy, *J. Immunol. 139*, 1557 (1987).
77. S. A. Miles, A. R. Rezai, J. F. Salazar-Gonzalez, M. van der Meyden, R. H. Stevens, D. M. Logan, R. T. Mitsuyasu, T. Taga, T. Hirano, T. Kishimoto, and O. Martinez-Maza, *Proc. Natl. Acad. Sci. USA 87*, 4068 (1990).
78. W. A. Muller, C. M. Ratti, S. L. McDonnell, and Z. A. Cohn, *J. Exp. Med. 170*, 399 (1989).
79. G. Munker, J. Gasson, M. Ogawa, and H. P. Koeffler, *Nature 323*, 79 (1986).
80. J. M. Munro, J. S. Pober, and R. S. Cotran, *Am. J. Pathol. 135*, 121 (1989).
81. J. M. Munro, J. S. Pober, and R. S. Cotran, *Lab. Invest. 64*, 295 (1991).

82. H. Nagura, T. Koshikawa, Y. Fukuda, and J. Asai, *Virchows Arch. (Pathol. Anat.) 409*, 407 (1986).
83. S. Nakamura, S. Z. Salahuddin, P. Biberfeld, B. Ensoli, P. D. Markham, F. Wong-Staal, and R. C. Gallo, *Science 242*, 426 (1988).
84. P. G. Natali, C. Demartino, V. Quaranta, M. R. Nicotra, F. Frezza, M. A. Pellegrino, and S. Ferrone, *Transplantation Baltimore 31*, 75 (1981).
85. P. G. Natali, V. Quaranta, M. R. Nicotra, C. Appoloni, M. A. Pellegrino, and S. Ferrone, *Transplant. Proc. 13*, 1026 (1981).
86. P. J. Newman, M. C. Berndt, J. Gorski, G. C. White, S. Lyman, C. Paddock, and W. A. Muller, *Science 247*, 1219 (1990).
87. B. J. Nickoloff, C. E. M. Griffiths, and J. N. W. N. Barker, *J. Invest. Dermatol. 94*, 151S (1990).
88. N. Oppenheimer-Marks, L. S. Davis, and P. E. Lipsky, *J. Immunol. 145*, 140 (1990).
89. L. Osborn, R. Hession, and R. Tizard, *Cell 59*, 1203 (1989).
90. R. M. J. Palmer, D. S. Ashton, and S. Moncada, *Nature 333*, 664 (1988).
91. R. Pardi, J. R. Bender, and E. G. Engleman, *J. Immunol. 139*, 2585 (1987).
92. L. A. Perkocha, S. M. Geaghan, T. S. B. Yen, S. L. Nishimura, S. P. Chan, R. Garcia-Kennedy, G. Honda, A. C. Stoloff, H. Z. Klein, R. L. Goldman, S. Van Meter, L. D. Ferrel, and P. E. Le Boit, *N. Engl. J. Med. 323*, 1581 (1990).
93. M. L. Phillips, E. Nudelman, F. C. A. Gaeta, M. Perez, A. K. Singhal, S.-I. Hakomori, and J. C. Paulson, *Science 250*, 1130 (1990).
94. L. J. Picker, T. K. Kishimoto, W. C. Smith, R. A. Warnock, and E. C. Butcher, *Nature 349*, 796 (1991).
95. L. J. Picker, S. A. Michie, L. S. Rott, and E. C. Butcher, *Am. J. Pathol. 136*, 1053 (1990).
96. L. J. Picker, L. W. M. M. Terstappen, L. S. Rott, P. R. Streeter, H. Stein, and E. C. Butcher, *J. Immunol. 145*, 3247 (1990).
97. J. S. Pober and R. S. Cotran, *Phys. Rev. 70*, 427 (1990).
98. J. S. Pober, M. A. Gimbrone, Jr., and L. A. Lapierre, *J. Immunol. 137*, 1893 (1986).
99. T. Pumarola-Sune, F. Graus, Y.-X. Chen, C. Cordon-Cardo, and R. L. Evans, *J. Immunol. 137*, 826 (1986).
100. M. Rampart and T. J. Williams, *Am. J. Pathol. 124*, 66 (1986).
101. D. A. Relman, J. S. Loutit, T. M. Schmidt, S. Falkow, and L. S. Tompkins, *N. Engl. J. Med. 323*, 1573 (1990).
102. G. E. Rice and M. P. Bevilacqua, *Science 246*, 1303 (1989).
103. W. Risau, B. Engelhardt, and H. Wekerle, *J. Cell Biol. 110*, 1757 (1990).
104a. B. J. Rollins, T. Yoshimura, E. J. Leonard, and J. S. Pober, *Am. J. Pathol. 136*, 1229 (1990).
104b. B. J. Rollins and J. S. Pober, *Am. J. Pathol. 138*, 1315 (1991).
105. T. J. Ryan, *J. Invest. Dermatol. 93*, 18S (1989).
106. M. E. Sanders, M. W. Makgoba, and S. Shaw, *Immunol. Today 9*, 195 (1988).
107. T. J. Schall, K. Bacon, K. J. Toy, and D. V. Goeddel, *Nature 347*, 669 (1990).

108. R. O. Schlingemann, F. J. R. Rietveld, R. M. W. de Waal, N. J. Bradley, A. I. Skene, A. J. S. Davies, M. F. Greaves, J. Denekamp, and D. J. Ruiter, *Lab. Invest. 62*, 690 (1990).
109. B. R. Schwartz, E. A. Wayner, T. M. Carlos, H. D. Ochs, and J. M. Harlan, *J. Clin. Invest. 85*, 2019 (1990).
110. Y. Shimizu, S. Shaw, N. Graber, T. V. Gopal, K. J. Horgan, G. A. Van Seventer, and W. Newman, *Nature 349*, 799 (1991).
111. A. Sica, J. M. Wang, and F. Colotta, *J. Immunol. 144*, 3034 (1989).
112. M. Sironi, F. Breviario, P. Proserpio, A. Biondi, A. Vecchi, J. van Damme, E. Dejana, and A. Mantovani, *J. Immunol. 142*, 549 (1989).
113. L. N. Slater, D. F. Welch, D. Hensel, and D. W. Coody, *N. Engl. J. Med. 323*, 1587 (1990).
114. C. W. Smith, R. Rothlein, and B. J. Hughes, *J. Clin. Invest. 82*, 1746 (1988).
115. R. A. Sobel, B. W. Blanchette, A. K. Bhan, and R. B. Colvin, *J. Immunol. 132*, 2402 (1984).
116. C. Sorg, E. Michels, U. Malorny, and C. Neumann, *Springer Semin. Immunopathol. 7*, 311 (1984).
117. D. E. Staunton, M. L. Dustin, and T. A. Springer, *Nature 339*, 61 (1989).
118. H. V. Stel, K. S. Sakariassen, P. G. de Groot, J. A. van Mourik, and J. J. Sixma, *Blood 65*, 85 (1985).
119. D. M. Stern, J. Brett, K. Harris, and P. Nawroth, *J. Cell Biol. 102*, 1971 (1986).
120. A. H. Stolpen, E. C. Guinan, W. Fiers, and J. S. Pober, *Am. J. Pathol. 169*, 1977 (1986).
121. L. M. Stoolman, *Cell 56*, 907 (1989).
122. J. W. Streilein, *J. Invest. Dermatol. 80*, 12S (1983).
123. R. M. Streiter, S. L. Kunkel, and H. J. Showell, *Science 243*, 1467 (1989).
124. R. M. Streiter, R. Wiggins, and S. H. Phan, *Biochem. Biophys. Res. Commun. 162*, 694 (1989).
125. M. D. Tharp, *J. Invest. Dermatol. 93*, 107S (1989).
126. M. H. Thornhill, U. Kyan-Aung, and D. O. Haskard, *J. Immunol. 144*, 3060 (1990).
127. M. G. Tonnesen, D. C. Anderson, T. A. Springer, A. Knedler, N. Avdo, and P. M. Henson, *J. Clin. Invest. 83*, 637 (1989).
128. V. T. Turrito, H. J. Weiss, G. A. Zimmerman, and I. I. Sussman, *Blood 65*, 823 (1985).
129. D. E. van Epps, J. Potter, M. Vachula, C. W. Smith, and D. C. Anderson, *J. Immunol. 143*, 3207 (1989).
130. G. Walz, A. Aruffo, W. Kolanus, M. P. Bevilacqua, and B. Seed, *Science 250*, 1132 (1990).
131. B. B. Weksler, C. W. Ley, and E. A. Jaffe, *J. Clin. Invest. 62*, 923 (1978).
132. R. E. Whatley, G. A. Zimmerman, T. M. McIntyre, and S. M. Prescott, *Arteriosclerosis 8*, 321 (1988).
133. R. B. Wysolmerski and D. Lagunoff, *Proc. Natl. Acad. Sci. USA 87*, 16 (1990).
134. T. A. Yednock and S. D. Rosen, *Adv. Immunol. 44*, 313 (1989).
135. G. B. Zavoico, B. M. Ewenstein, A. I. Schafer, and J. S. Pober, *J. Immunol. 142*, 3993 (1989).

# 20

# Regulatory Interactions Between Epidermal Cell Adhesion Molecules and Cytokines

**Jean Krutmann**
*University of Freiburg*
*Freiburg, Germany*

## I. INTRODUCTION

A prominent feature of a variety of inflammatory/immunological skin diseases is the intraepidermal presence of leukocytes [1, 2]. Recently, substantial progress has been made in elucidating the mechanisms responsible for the migration of leukocytes from the circulation into the skin as well as for the consecutive physical interaction of these cells with epidermal cells. Research in this area has mainly been stimulated by the identification of functionally active adhesion molecules on the surface of endothelial cells and, in particular, of epidermal cells including keratinocytes, melanocytes, and Langerhans cells [3, 4].

Adhesion molecules represent a recently identified, still growing, and heterogeneous group of molecules belonging to three families: the integrins, the immunoglobulins, and the selectins [3]. Leukocyte/endothelial cell binding appears to be mediated via at least three different adhesion pathways. Specifically, these pathways are mediated by binding of endothelial cell adhesion molecule-1 (ELAM-1) to cutaneous lymphocyte-associated antigen-1 (CLA) on skin homing memory T cells [5, 6] or sialyl Lewis x molecules on neutrophils/monocytes [7–11], or by binding of endothelial vascular cell adhesion molecule-1 (VCAM-1) to leukocyte very late activation antigen-4 (VLA-4) [12–14], or by binding of endothelial cell intercellular adhesion molecule-1 (ICAM-1) to lymphocyte function-associated antigen-1 (LFA-1) on the surface of leukocytes [14, 15], respectively.

The existence of multiple adhesion pathways for leukocyte/endothelial cell interactions is in marked contrast to intraepidermal adhesion processes, which appear to be primarily mediated via binding of the integrin LFA-1 on the leukocyte surface to the immunoglobulin ICAM-1 on the surface of epidermal cells. As a consequence, great interest has been focused on identifying mechanisms, by which LFA-1/ICAM-1–mediated adhesion processes may be regulated [4]. A common feature of these studies is the interest in regulation of epidermal cell ICAM-1, which, in contrast to its constitutively expressed counterreceptor LFA-1, was found to be highly inducible. From these studies it appears that cytokines as well as modulators of cytokine production and bioactivity such as ultraviolet (UV) radiation represent important regulators of epidermal cell ICAM-1 surface expression [4, 16]. In addition, cytokines may also play a pivotal role in inducing the shedding of soluble ICAM-1 molecules from the surface of epidermal cells [17–19]. This chapter will therefore focus on recent research into the regulatory interactions of cytokines and epidermal cell–associated ICAM-1 molecules.

In addition to ICAM-1, epidermal cells are known to express a variety of other adhesion molecules [20]. Moreover, some of these adhesion molecules were found to function as regulatory structures affecting cytokine production and secretion [21–23]. However, since the functional relevance of epidermal cell adhesion molecules others than ICAM-1 is currently unknown, these studies will only be briefly summarized.

## II. STRUCTURE AND FUNCTION OF EPIDERMAL CELL ADHESION MOLECULES

### A. Intercellular Adhesion Molecules

ICAM-1 is a heavily glycosylated single-chain transmembrane molecule with a molecular weight of 85–105 kd [24, 25]. The extracellular domain of the ICAM-1 molecule consists of 453 residues containing five immunoglobulin-like domains. ICAM-1 is encoded by an inducible 3.3 kb mRNA, and the gene for human ICAM-1 has been mapped to chromosome 19 [26]. ICAM-1 is functionally defined by its capacity to serve as a counterreceptor for the LFA-1 molecule. Accordingly, the ICAM-1 molecule could be identified by generating monoclonal antibodies to lymphocytes from LFA-1–negative patients [27]. One of these antibodies was found to effectively block LFA-1–dependent homotypic adhesion by binding to a novel cell surface molecule, which was subsequently designated as ICAM-1.

There is strong in vitro and in vivo evidence that the interaction of ICAM-1 with its ligand LFA-1 is critical for a variety of adhesion processes among leukocytes and between leukocytes and other cell types [3]. Accordingly, ICAM-1/LFA-1–mediated adhesion appears to contribute to several immunological and inflammatory reactions in the skin by mediating adhesion of leukocytes to epidermal keratinocytes, melanocytes, and/or Langerhans cells, as will be discussed in detail in the following sections. The functional relevance of ICAM-1/LFA-1–mediated adhesion has mainly been derived from in vitro studies in which antibodies directed against LFA-1 and/or ICAM-1 have been used to block cell-cell interactions. It should therefore be noticed that ICAM-1 is an important, but not the only, ligand for LFA-1. Accordingly, two ligands for LFA-1 distinct from ICAM-1 recently have been identified and designated as ICAM-2 and ICAM-3, respectively. As compared with ICAM-1, ICAM-2 is a much smaller molecule with two rather than five immunoglobulinlike domains [28]. Most remarkably, the two immunoglobulinlike domains show 34% identity in their amino acid sequences with the two most N-terminal immunoglobulinlike domains of ICAM-1, indicating that ICAM-1 and ICAM-2 represent a subfamily of immunoglobulinlike ligands binding to the same integrin molecule. In addition to ICAM-1 and ICAM-2, several studies strongly indicate the existence of a third LFA-1–binding molecule, and cloning and characterization of the ICAM-3 molecule recently has been achieved [29, 30, D. Staunton, personal communication]. The relevance of ICAM-2 and ICAM-3 for adhesion processes within the epidermis is currently unknown.

Moreover, it should also be emphasized that ICAM-1, besides binding to LFA-1, is also capable of binding to leukocyte Mac-1 [31], although with a lower affinity, as well as to leukocyte sialophorin (CD43) molecules [32]. The functional relevance of ICAM-1/Mac-1 and/or ICAM-1/CD43 binding for intraepidermal adhesion processes remains to be established. Finally, in addition to functioning as a ligand for adhesion molecules, ICAM-1 was found to serve as a receptor for certain viruses [33–36] and as a sequestration antigen for plasmodium falciparum [37–39]. Again, the pathophysiological relevance of these findings for skin diseases is currently unknown.

Recently, a circulating form of the usually membrane-bound ICAM-1 was identified and characterized in normal human serum [17]. Circulating ICAM-1 contains most, if not all, of the five extracellular domains of membrane ICAM-1 (mICAM-1) and is capable of binding to LFA-1 molecules in a specific fashion. Circulating ICAM-1 molecules are probably derived from mononuclear cells, since supernatants of lymphoid cell lines or peripheral blood mononuclear cells contain significant levels of soluble ICAM-1 molecules (sICAM-1). With regards to epidermal cells, melanocytes as well as keratinocytes recently were identified as a source for sICAM-1 [18, 19]. Although the exact function of sICAM-1 molecules is currently unknown, it is tempting to speculate that they may be able to modulate LFA-1–mediated adhesion events by promoting deadhesion.

## B. Other Adhesion Molecules

In addition to ICAM-1, several other adhesion molecules are found to be expressed by epidermal cells [20]. The function of these molecules for adhesion processes within the epidermis is currently unknown. Very recent studies indicate that keratinocytes express the adhesion molecule B7, which serves as a counterreceptor for the lymphocyte CD28 molecule, and which may facilitate keratinocyte/T-lymphocyte adhesion [40–42]. Moreover, keratinocyte B7 expression is significantly enhanced after PMA stimulation. However, the likely role of cytokines in the regulation of keratinocyte B7 expression remains to be established.

Moreover, LFA-3 as well as CD44 molecules, which were found to be constitutively expressed by the majority of epidermal cells, are fundamental to a variety of immunological reactions including the interaction of T lymphocytes with antigen-presenting cells. Although it is therefore very likely that these molecules contribute to adhesion processes within the epidermis as well, the functional relevance of epidermal cell LFA-3 and CD44 expression remains to be established (for detailed review on the structure and function of these molecules see Refs. 1 and 43).

# III. CYTOKINE REGULATION OF KERATINOCYTE ADHESION MOLECULES

## A. Cytokine Regulation of Keratinocyte ICAM-1 Surface Expression

### *Function of Keratinocyte ICAM-1 Molecules*

Several in vitro studies indicate that LFA-1/ICAM-1–mediated adhesion represents the major, if not the only, adhesion pathway by which lymphocytes bind to epidermal keratinocytes. Accordingly, anti-ICAM-1 antibodies were found to completely block binding of T lymphoblasts to ICAM-1–positive keratinocytes [44]. Similarly, keratinocyte ICAM-1 expression was shown to be a prerequisite for the efficient lysis of human keratinocytes by allogeneic HLA class I–specific cytotoxic T cells or lymphokine-activated killer cells [45, 46]. In addition, binding of keratinocyte ICAM-1 molecules to lymphocyte LFA-1 molecules may deliver a stimulatory signal, which, among other signals, may be crucial for the capacity of PMA-treated, "activated" keratinocytes to induce T-cell proliferation [43, 47].

Several immunohistochemical studies indicate that these in vitro data may have in vivo relevance as well. Accordingly, no or only weak keratinocyte ICAM-1 surface expression could be detected in normal human skin, whereas in skin diseases characterized by an intraepidermal infiltrate (e.g., psoriasis, atopic dermatitis, lichen planus, or allergic contact dermatitis), keratinocytes were found to strongly express ICAM-1 molecules on their surface [48–50]. Most remarkably, keratinocyte ICAM-1 expression in inflammatory skin diseases was focal rather than homogeneous, and typically a close colocalization between intraepidermal lymphocytes and ICAM-1–expressing keratinocytes could be observed, strongly indicating that ICAM-1 expression on human keratinocytes is important for the generation as well as maintenance of an intraepidermal lymphocytic infiltrate. Moreover, ICAM-1 molecules on the keratinocyte surface may also be important for intraepidermal trapping of circulating T lymphocytes in cutaneous lymphomas. This hypothesis is mainly based on the immunohistochemical demonstration of strongly ICAM-1–positive keratinocytes in patch- or plaque-stage cutaneous T-cell lymphoma and, even more important, the absence of ICAM-1–expressing keratinocytes in patients with Sézary syndrome, which represents the leukemic rather than epidermotrophic form of a cutaneous T-cell lymphoma [48–51]. Finally, the in vivo relevance of ICAM-1 molecules contributing to keratinocyte cytotoxicity is suggested by the immunohistochemical demonstration of ICAM-1–expressing keratinocytes in lesional skin from patients with skin diseases, which, as a common denominator, exhibit selective destruction of epidermal keratinocytes. These include subacute cutaneous lupus erythematosus, erythema multiforme, pemphigus vulgaris, and vitiligo [52]. Taken together, these studies indicate that keratinocyte ICAM-1 expression is crucial for a variety of immunological reactions within the epidermis.

*Keratinocyte ICAM-1–Inducing Cytokines*

The notion that keratinocytes in normal human skin are ICAM-1 negative, whereas in inflammatory skin reactions, strong keratinocyte ICAM-1 expression may be observed, has prompted the interest of dermatologists in defining the mechanisms by which keratinocyte ICAM-1 expression may be regulated. From these studies it appears that selected cytokines are capable of inducing human keratinocyte ICAM-1 expression. Accordingly, long-term cultured normal human keratinocytes constitutively did not express ICAM-1 molecules but could be induced to do so upon stimulation with recombinant human (rh) interferon gamma (IFN-$\gamma$), tumor necrosis factor alpha (TNF-$\alpha$), or tumor necrosis factor beta (TNF-$\beta$) [44, 53–55]. Similarly, the same cytokines significantly enhanced low constitutive ICAM-1 expression, which could be observed on transformed human keratinocytes [54, 55].

Moreover, the combination of IFN-$\gamma$ plus TNF-$\alpha$ or IFN-$\gamma$ plus TNF-$\beta$ was found to induce ICAM-1 expression in untransformed as well as transformed human keratinocytes in a synergistic fashion [44, 54, 56]. The exact mechanisms responsible for the synergistic upregulation of keratinocyte ICAM-1 expression by these two cytokines are currently unknown. However, recent studies indicate that the observed synergism may not be attributed to IFN-$\gamma$–induced upregulation of human keratinocyte TNF receptor (TNFR) expression, as suggested previously [57, 58].

Cytokine-induced ICAM-1 expression is highly specific, since IL-2, IL-3, IL-4, IL-5, IL-6, IL-7, IL-8, GM-CSF, and IFN-$\alpha$ did not significantly affect human keratinocyte ICAM-1 expression either alone or in combination. The role of IL-1$\alpha$/IL-1$\beta$ in regulation of human keratinocyte ICAM-1 expression is somewhat controversial and may depend on the activation stage of the keratinocyte. Accordingly, several authors report on the failure of rhIL-1$\alpha$ and IL-1$\beta$ to significantly induce ICAM-1 surface expression in resting human keratinocytes [44, 53, 54]. In this regard it is of great interest that the capacity of a given cell to respond to IL-1 is mainly determined by the density of IL-1 receptors present on the cell surface [59]. Moreover, IL-1 receptor expression on resting human keratinocytes may be markedly upregulated by IFN-$\gamma$ stimulation, which greatly increases the capacity of these cells to respond to stimulation with exogenous IL-1 [60, 61]. Accordingly, Dustin et al. observed that IFN-$\gamma$–induced ICAM-1 expression in human keratinocytes may be superinduced by IL-1, although IL-1 alone did not significantly affect keratinocyte ICAM-1 expression. Moreover, IL-1 was shown to be capable to induce ICAM-1 expression in UV-irradiated keratinocytes, but not in unirradiated cells, and this was associated with a markedly increased capacity of irradiated cells to bind rhIL-1$\alpha$ [62].

The in vitro observation that selected cytokines are capable of upregulating keratinocyte ICAM-1 expression most likely extrapolates to the in vivo situation. Accordingly, intradermal injection of IFN-$\gamma$ was found to markedly increase human keratinocyte ICAM-1 expression, as demonstrated by immunohistochemistry [63]. Moreover, the synergistically acting cytokines IFN-$\gamma$ and TNF-$\beta$ represent T-lymphocyte–derived cytokines, strongly indicating that intraepidermal T cells may be able to generate a dense matrix of ICAM-1 molecules within the epidermis, which in turn allows binding of T-cell LFA-1 to keratinocyte ICAM-1 and thereby facilitates the generation and maintenance of an intraepidermal T-cell infiltrate [54]. In contrast to IFN-$\gamma$ and TNF-$\beta$, TNF-$\alpha$ is mainly produced by monocyte/macrophages and, even more important, by keratinocytes themselves [64].

Due to the great pathogenetic and therapeutic relevance of cytokine-induced upregulation of keratinocyte ICAM-1 expression, extensive studies have been conducted to define the underlying mechanisms more closely. Increased ICAM-1 surface expression may be observed in cytokine-stimulated keratinocytes after 4 hours, reaching a maximum after 16–24 hours [54]. There is strong evidence that cytokine-regulated ICAM-1 expression is, at least in part, controlled at the level of transcription. Accordingly, increased ICAM-1 surface expression in untransformed as well as transformed human keratinocytes is accompanied by a time-dependent increase in steady-state levels of ICAM-1-specific mRNA expression in cytokine-stimulated keratinocytes [54–56]. Recently, cloning of the 5′ region of the human ICAM-1 gene containing a functional promotor has been achieved [65–68]. Analysis of the promoter region revealed the presence of numerous *cis*-acting enhancer elements including interferon-responsive elements as well as binding sites for NFϰB and AP-1. TNF-α–induced ICAM-1 expression in human keratinocytes recently was shown to be mediated via the 55 kd TNFR, and anti-55 kd TNFR antibodies were found to activate the transcription factor NFϰb in a human epithelial cell line [69]. It is therefore tempting to speculate that NFϰb activation may contribute to TNF-α–mediated ICAM-1 induction. In addition, there is circumstantial evidence that TNF-α–induced ICAM-1 expression may be additionally controlled by posttranscriptional mechanisms [68].

### *Role of Cytokines in UV-Induced Modulation of Keratinocyte ICAM-1 Expression*

In addition to cytokines, UV radiation recently was found to be a potent modulator of human keratinocyte ICAM-1 expression [16, 53, 54]. Specifically, in vitro exposure of long-term cultured, normal as well as transformed human keratinocytes to sublethal doses of UV radiation markedly inhibited cytokine (IFN-γ, TNF-α, TNF-β)–induced ICAM-1 expression if the irradiated cells were cytokine-stimulated immediately after exposure to UV light. This novel immunosuppressive property of UV light is thought to represent a thus far undescribed mechanism, by which the therapeutic effectiveness of UV phototherapy in inflammatory skin diseases such as psoriasis or atopic dermatitis (characterized by ICAM-1–expressing keratinocytes) may at least partially be explained [54]. UV light inhibited cytokine-induced ICAM-1 surface expression in a dose-dependent manner, and this inhibition was associated with a UV dose–dependent decrease of ICAM-1 mRNA expression [69, 77]. Specifically, 100 $J/m^2$ UVB were sufficient to reduce IFN-γ–induced upregulation of steady-state levels of ICAM-1 mRNA to background levels. Most remarkably, UV-induced inhibition of cytokine-mediated upregulation of keratinocyte ICAM-1 expression was found to be transient [70]. Accordingly, restoration of responsiveness to IFN-γ was measured by Northern blot analysis and could be observed in UV-irradiated keratinocytes as early as 12 hours postexposure. Restoration of cytokine responsiveness was not specific for IFN-γ, but could also be observed for TNF-α–induced ICAM-1 expression. Most interestingly, cytokine responsiveness of UV-irradiated keratinocytes was found to be differentially restored for IFN-γ versus TNF-α, since restoration of TNF-α responsiveness required at least a 24-hour recovery phase [70]. Human keratinocytes express the 55 kd TNFR, which was shown to mediate TNF-α–induced ICAM-1 upregulation [57]. Moreover, UV exposure of human keratinocytes lead to binding of UV-induced, endogenous TNF-$\alpha$ to 55 kd TNFR on the keratinocyte surface, which in turn caused downregulation followed by reexpression (after 24 hours) of keratinocyte TNFR [71]. Differential restoration of IFN-$\gamma$ versus TNF-$\alpha$ responsiveness is therefore most likely due to an autocrine modulatory effect of UVB radiation on human keratinocyte TNF receptor expression.

In addition to suppressing cytokine-induced ICAM-1 expression, identical doses of UV radiation were found to be capable of enhancing constitutive ICAM-1 expression in normal as well as transformed human keratinocytes after a 48-hour incubation period, strongly indicating that a single exposure to UV light may exert both anti- and proinflammatory effects on keratinocyte ICAM-1 expression [16, 53, 54, 70, 74]. Similarly, UV radiation was found to produce up- and downregulation of contact hypersensitivity reactions in the skin, which may at least partially be due to the UV-induced biphasic modulation of keratinocyte ICAM-1 expression [53, 72, 73]. In addition, subacute cutaneous lupus erythematosus is a photosensitive skin disease, which is characterized by both ICAM-1–expressing keratinocytes and cytotoxic damage to keratinocytes. It has therefore been proposed that UV-induced keratinocyte ICAM-1 expression may promote binding of effector cells to epidermal keratinocytes and thus facilitate keratinocyte cytotoxicity [52]. The in vivo relevance of UV-induced keratinocyte ICAM-1 expression is strongly suggested by studies of Norris et al. [74]. Accordingly, sequential exposure of normal human volunteers to 0.5–200 J/m$^2$ UVB on 3 consecutive days induced keratinocyte ICAM-1 surface expression in a dose-dependent manner, as was assessed by immunohistochemistry. However, in order to achieve induction of keratinocyte ICAM-1 expression in vivo, it appears to be crucial that several consecutive UV exposures are applied to overcome UV-induced inhibition of cytokine unresponsiveness [75].

Further characterization of UV-induced keratinocyte ICAM-1 expression indicates an important role for keratinocyte-derived cytokines in this process. Accordingly, UV-induced expression of ICAM-1 surface and mRNA in transformed human keratinocytes could be superinduced by stimulation of irradiated cells with rhIFN-$\gamma$, but not rhTNF-$\alpha$, indicating that UV-light induced human keratinocyte ICAM-1 expression via a TNF-$\alpha$–like pathway [70]. In this regard it is of interest that UV radiation was shown to induce human keratinocyte TNF-$\alpha$ production and secretion [64]. Moreover, functional TNF receptors could be identified on the surface of human keratinocytes [57], and UV-induced, endogenous TNF-$\alpha$ was shown to bind to TNFR on the keratinocyte surface and to exert autocrine regulatory events including the induction of $PGE_2$ secretion [71, 76]. UV-induced, endogenous TNF-$\alpha$ may therefore mediate UV-induced ICAM-1 upregulation in human keratinocytes. In keeping with this hypothesis, we were able to demonstrate that supernatants derived from transformed keratinocytes 48 hours post-UV exposure were capable of inducing ICAM-1 surface expression in unirradiated cells, emphasizing the existence of a soluble ICAM-1–inducing activity, which was produced by UV-irradiated keratinocytes [70]. Surprisingly, biologically active anti-TNF-α antibodies, which effectively inhibited binding of endogenous TNF-α to TNFR on UV-irradiated keratinocytes as well as UV-induced, TNF-α–mediated $PGE_2$ release from these cells, did not even partially block this ICAM-1–inducing activity. Similarly, the same antibodies did not even partially decrease UV-induced keratinocyte ICAM-1 expression, if added to UV-irradiated cells [70]. However, UV-induced ICAM-1 expression in transformed human keratinocytes could be significantly inhibited, if irradiated cells were cultured in the continuous presence of anti-IL-1α antibodies [62] or if irradiated cells were transiently transfected with IL-1α anti-sense oligonucleotides (J. Krutmann, unpublished observation). Moreover, preincubation of conditioned medium derived from UV-irradiated, transformed human keratinocytes with antibodies directed against rhIL-1α completely blocked the ICAM-1–inducing activity present in these supernatants [62]. Finally, the capacity of IL-1α to induce ICAM-1 expression in UV-irradiated keratinocytes was associated with a markedly increased capacity of irradiated cells to bind rhIL-1α. These studies strongly suggest that IL-1α, but not TNF-α, is the principal mediator of UV-induced ICAM-1 upregulation in human keratinocytes [62].

In conclusion, UV radiation is capable of modulating human keratinocyte ICAM-1 expression in a biphasic manner. This modulatory activity was found to be due to UV radiation effects on keratinocyte cytokine production and secretion as well UV-induced alterations of keratinocyte responsiveness to ICAM-1–inducing cytokines.

## B. Cytokine Regulation of Keratinocyte-Derived Soluble ICAM-1 Molecules

Very recent studies from our laboratory indicate that supernatants derived from long-term cultured, normal as well as transformed human keratinocytes, upon appropriate stimulation, contain significant amounts of sICAM-1 molecules [19]. Interestingly, sICAM-1 molecules could not be detected in supernatants derived from unstimulated long-term cultured, normal human keratinocytes, but significant levels were present in supernatants of cells that had been stimulated with rhIFN-γ, rhTNF-α, or a combination of both cytokines. Moreover, supernatants of unstimulated transformed human keratinocytes contained low but significant amounts of sICAM-1, and the ICAM-1 content was again further enhanced after stimulation of cells with the above-mentioned cytokines. However, in marked contrast to the regulation of mICAM-1 expression, shedding of sICAM-1 molecules was not increased upon exposure of keratinocytes to UV light (A. Budnik and J. Krutmann, unpublished observation). These data clearly indicate that in addition to peripheral blood mononuclear cells and melanocytes, epithelial cells such as keratinocytes may be induced by selected cytokines to shed significant amounts of sICAM-1 molecules, and that ICAM-1 membrane expression and shedding of sICAM-1 molecules at least in this cell type may be differentially regulated.

## IV. CYTOKINE REGULATION OF MELANOCYTE/MELANOMA CELL ADHESION MOLECULE EXPRESSION

### A. Function and Regulation of Surface ICAM-1 Expression

In addition to keratinocytes, melanocytes recently were found to constitutively express low levels of ICAM-1 molecules on their surface [77–79]. Moreover, melanocyte ICAM-1 surface expression was markedly enhanced by cytokine stimulation [77, 79]. Specifically, in vitro exposure of human melanocytes to rhIFN-$\gamma$ and/or rhTNF-$\alpha$ was found to significantly upregulate melanocyte ICAM-1 surface expression, and the combination of both cytokines was found to act in an additive, but not in a synergistic manner. Moreover, melanocyte ICAM-1 surface expression could also be induced by stimulation of cells with rhIL-1$\alpha$, indicating that cytokine-induced ICAM-1 expression in melanocytes, as compared to keratinocytes, is differentially regulated [79]. This assumption is further supported by the notion that melanocytes are most sensitive to TNF-$\alpha$, whereas in keratinocytes, IFN-$\gamma$ is the strongest ICAM-1–inducing cytokine [44]. Moreover, preliminary data indicate that rhIL-6 as well as rhIL-7 may be capable of inducing melanocyte as well as melanoma cell mICAM-1 expression, although both cytokines did not affect ICAM-1 regulation in human keratinocytes [80, J. Krutmann, unpublished observation].

Although the exact function of melanocyte ICAM-1 surface expression remains to be determined, the role of ICAM-1 molecules in facilitating cytotoxicity mediated by lymphokine-activated killer cells, cytotoxic T cells, and antibody-dependent cellular cytotoxicity may indicate that binding of effector cells to melanocytes may be facilitated by melanocyte ICAM-1 surface expression [1, 4, 52]. Accordingly, melanocyte cytotoxicity appears to be a feature of certain forms of vitiligo characterized by vitiligo antigen expression as well as the presence of circulating antibodies against these antigens [80].

## B. Function and Regulation of ICAM-1 Shedding

In addition to melanocytes, melanoma cells were shown to express significant levels of mICAM-1 [78, 81]. Moreover, melanoma cell mICAM-1 expression appears to be positively correlated with melanoma progression [81, 82]. This finding is somewhat paradoxical if one assumes that melanoma cell ICAM-1 surface expression may be crucial for the generation of cell-mediated immune responses leading to melanoma cell injury. In this regard, it was of interest to learn that melanoma cells are capable of shedding functionally active ICAM-1 molecules [18]. Specifically, supernatants of unstimulated melanoma cells did not contain significant amounts of sICAM-1, but shedding of ICAM-1 molecules could be observed upon stimulation of cells with rhIFN-$\gamma$ and/or rhTNF-$\alpha$. Moreover, melanoma cell–derived supernatants containing sICAM-1 molecules significantly inhibited conjugate formation between lymphokine-activated killer cells and melanoma cells and markedly inhibited non–MHC-restricted cytotoxicity against melanoma cells mediated by lymphokine activated killer cells [18]. These in vitro data strongly indicate that shedding of ICAM-1 molecules may represent a mechanism by which melanoma cells may escape from non–MHC-restricted cytotoxicity. Selected cytokines may thus influence immunosurveillance against melanoma cells [82].

# V. FUNCTION AND CYTOKINE REGULATION OF LANGERHANS CELL ADHESION MOLECULES

ICAM-1 molecules on the surface of human antigen-presenting cells were shown to play an important role in helper T-cell activation. Accordingly, anti-ICAM-1 mAb markedly inhibited antigen-, mitogen-, and anti-CD3-antibody–induced T-cell responses [84–86]. Moreover, using DNA-mediated gene transfer, coexpression of ICAM-1 together with HLA-DR molecules by antigen-presenting cells was found to be critical for effective HLA-DR–restricted T-cell activation [87]. There is strong in vitro and in vivo evidence that human epidermal Langerhans cells are capable of functioning as accessory cells and antigen-presenting cells in responses of helper T cells [88, 89]. In addition, Langerhans cells were found to express a variety of adhesion molecules including ICAM-1, Mac-1, gp150.95, and LFA-3 [90–92]. Using antibody blocking experiments, Langerhans cell ICAM-1 expression was found to constitute an important costimulatory signal for allogeneic T-cell activation [93]. Similarly, anti-ICAM-1 mAb were found to significantly decrease the capacity of murine Langerhans cells to function as accessory cells for anti-CD3-antibody–induced T-cell activation [94]. The functional significance of mICAM-1 expression for Langerhans cell antigen-presenting cell function is further supported by the notion that UV radiation is capable of converting Langerhans cells from immunogenic to tolerogenic cells [95], and that this functional switch is most likely due to the inhibition of Langerhans cell ICAM-1 surface expression [86, 94, 96].

The mechanisms by which Langerhans cell ICAM-1 expression may be regulated are only poorly understood. It has been noticed, however, that freshly prepared Langerhans cells are ICAM-1 negative and that ICAM-1 molecules are reexpressed within a 72-hour culture period [90]. Moreover, this in vitro maturation, which was found to affect Langerhans cell antigen-presenting function, appears to be mediated by keratinocyte-derived cytokines [97]. Although the influence of epidermal cell–derived cytokines on Langerhans cell ICAM-1 expression is currently not known, it should be noted that cytokines are potent inducers of ICAM-1 expression in human antigen-presenting cells. Accordingly, human peripheral blood monocyte ICAM-1 surface and mRNA expression may be markedly induced by stimulation of cells with rhIFN-$\gamma$, rhIL-1$\alpha/\beta$, rhIL-6, and rhTNF-$\alpha$ [98].

## VI. ADHESION MOLECULES AS REGULATORY STRUCTURES FOR CYTOKINE SECRETION

Recent studies indicate that the interaction between adhesion molecules and cytokines may be bidirectional. Accordingly, cytokines, in addition to regulating adhesion molecule expression, may be regulated themselves via selected adhesion molecules including LFA-3, CD44, and ICAM-1. Stimulation of human thymocytes or peripheral blood monocytes with immobilized anti-LFA-3 or anti-CD44 antibodies was found to significantly induce the production and secretion of IL-1 and TNF-$\alpha$, indicating that binding of the physiological ligand to these molecules may represent a trigger for cytokine release [21, 22, 99]. Accordingly, induction of monocyte IL-1 secretion by anti-LFA-3 antibodies could be mimicked by stimulating monocytes with immobilized soluble CD2 molecules [22]. Whereas CD44 and LFA-3 molecules appear to mediate cytokine-inducing signals, there is one report indicating that the ICAM-1 molecule may serve in downregulation of cytokine production [23]. Accordingly, anti-ICAM-1 antibodies were found to significantly inhibit TNF-$\alpha$, IFN-$\gamma$, and IL-1 secretion in phytohemagglutinin-activated human peripheral blood mononuclear cells. In addition to ICAM-1, epidermal keratinocytes as well as Langerhans cells constitutively express LFA-3 molecules. Moreover, constitutive CD44 expression is a prominent feature of human keratinocytes in vitro as well as in vivo. It is therefore tempting to speculate that cytokine production in keratinocytes and/or Langerhans cells may be regulated by triggering these adhesion molecules.

## VII. CONCLUDING REMARKS

Recent research has provided new insights into the mechanisms by which adhesion of leukocytes to epidermal cells may be regulated. From these studies it appears that intraepidermal adhesion is regulated via an interacting network of cytokines, cytokine receptors, and adhesion molecules, in particular ICAM-1 molecules. Further studies are required to address the functional relevance of epidermal cell adhesion molecules distinct from ICAM-1, to clarify the role of adhesion molecules as regulatory structures for epidermal cell cytokine production, and to examine the functional and, in particular, the therapeutic role of soluble adhesion molecules for cytokine-mediated inflammatory/immunological reactions within the epidermis.

## ACKNOWLEDGMENT

This work was supported by a grant from the Deutsche Forschungsgemeinschaft DFG Kr 871/3-2.

## REFERENCES


1. D. A. Norris, *Immune Mechanisms in Cutaneous Disease*, Marcel Dekker, New York, 1989.
2. T. Kupper, *Arch. Dermatol. Res. 125*, 1406 (1989).
3. T. A. Springer, *Nature 346*, 425 (1990).
4. J. Krutmann, in *Pharmacology of the Skin* (H. Mukthar, ed.), CRC Press, Boca Raton, FL, 1992, p. 315.
5. Y. Shimizu, S. Shaw, N. Graber, T. V. Gopal, K. J. Horgan, G. A. Van Seventer, and W. Newmann, *Nature 349*, 799 (1991).
6. L. J. Picker, T. K. Kishimoto, C. W. Smith, R. A. Warnrock, and E. C. Butcher, *Nature 349*, 796 (1991).
7. J. B. Lowe, L. M. Stoolman, R. P. Nair, R. D. Larsen, T. L. Berhend, and R. M. Marks, *Cell 63*, 475 (1990).
8. M. L. Phillips, E. Nudelman, F. C. A. Gaeta, M. Perez, A. K. Singhal, S. Hakomori, and J. C. Paulson, *Science 250*, 1130 (1990).
9. G. Walz, A. Aruffo, W. Kolanus, M. P. Bevilaqua, and B. Seed, *Science 250*, 1132 (1990).
10. M. Tiemeyer, S. J. Swiedler, M. Ishihara, M. Moreland, H. Schweingruber, P. Hirtzer, and B. K. Brandley, *Proc. Natl. Acad. Sci. USA 88*, 1138 (1991).
11. S. E. Goelz, C. Hession, D. Goff, B. Griffiths, R. Tizard, B. Newman, G. Chi-Rosso, and R. Lobb, *Cell 63*, 1349 (1990).
12. T. M. Carlos, B. R. Schwartz, N. L. Kovach, E. Yee, M. Rosso, L. Osborn, G. Chi-Rosso, B. Newman, R. Lobb, and J. M. Harlan, *Blood 76*, 965 (1990).

13. L. Osborn, C. Hession, R. Tizard, C. Vassallo, S. Luhowskyi, G. Chi-Rosso, and L. Robb, *Cell 59*, 1203 (1989).
14. Y. Shimizu, W. Newman, T. V. Gopal, K. J. Horgan, N. Graber, L. D. Beall, G. A. Van Seventer, and S. A. Shaw, *J. Exp. Med. 113*, 1203 (1991).
15. M. L. Dustin and T. A. Springer, *J. Cell. Biol. 107*, 321 (1988).
16. J. Krutmann, in *Immunodermatology* (C. Hauser, ed.), Springer Seminars in Immunopathology, Berlin, 13, 333 (1992).
17. R. Rothlein, E. A. Mainolfi, M. Czajkowski, and S. D. Marlin, *J. Immunol. 147*, 3788 (1991).
18. J. C. Becker, R. Dummer, A. A. Hartmann, G. Burg, and R. E. Schmidt, *J. Immunol. 147*, 4398 (1991).
19. A. Budnik, U. Trefzer, F. Parlow, A. Kapp, E. Schöpf, and J. Krutmann, *Exp. Dermatol. 1*, 27 (1992).
20. U. Konter, I. Kellner, E. Klein, R. Kaufmann, V. Mielke, and W. Sterry, *Arch. Dermatol. Res. 281*, 454 (1989).
21. P. T. Le, L. W. Vollger, B. F. Haynes, and K. H. Singer, *J. Immunol. 15*, 4541 (1990).
22. D. S. A. Webb, Y. Shimizu, G. A. Van Seventer, S. Shaw, and T. L. Gerrard, *Science 249*, 1295 (1990).
23. D. Geissler, S. Gaggl, J. Möst, R. Greil, M. Herold, and M. Dierich, *Eur. J. Immunol. 20*, 2591 (1990).
24. M. L. Dustin, R. Rothlein, A. K. Bhan, C. A. Dinarello, and T. A. Springer, *J. Immunol. 137*, 245 (1986).
25. D. E. Staunton, S. D. Marlin, C. Stratowa, M. L. Dustin, and T. A. Springer, *Cell 52*, 925 (1988).
26. F. E. Katz, M. Parker, K. Stanley, L. J. Murray, E. A. Clark, and M. F. Greaves, *J. Immunol. 15*, 103 (1985).
27. R. Rothlein, M. L. Dustin, S. D. Marlin, and T. A. Springer, *J. Immunol. 137*, 1270 (1986).
28. D. E. Staunton, M. L. Dustin, and T. A. Springer, *Nature 339*, 61 (1989).
29. A. R. de Fougerolles, S. A. Stacker, R. Schwarting, and T. A. Springer, *J. Exp. Med. 174*, 252 (1991).
30. P. Nortamo, R. Li, R. Renkonen, T. Timonen, J. Prieto, M. Patarroyo, and C. A. Gahmberg, *Eur. J. Immunol. 21*, 2629 (1991).
31. M. S. Diamond, D. E. Staunton, S. D. Marlin, and T. A. Springer, *Cell 65*, 961 (1991).
32. Y. Rosenstein, J. K. Park, W. C. Hahn, F. S. Rosen, B. E. Bierer, and S. J. Burakoff, *Nature 354*, 233 (1991).
33. D. E. Staunton, V. J. Merluzzi, R. Rothlein, R. Barton, S. D. Marlin, and T. A. Springer, *Cell 56*, 849 (1989).
34. J. M. Greve, G. Favis, A. M. Meyer, C. P. Forte, S. C. Yost, C. W. Marlow, M. E. Kamarck, and A. McClelland, *Cell 56*, 839 (1989).
35. S. D. Marlin, D. E. Staunton, T. A. Springer, C. Stratowa, W. Sommergruber, and V. I. Merluzzi, *Nature 340*, 70 (1990).
36. H. C. Selinka, A. Zibert, and E. Wimmer, *Proc. Natl. Acad. Sci. USA 88*, 3598 (1991).

37. A. R. Behrendt, D. L. Simmons, J. Tansey, C. I. Newboldt, and K. Marsh, *Nature 341*, 57 (1989).
38. A. R. Berendt, A. McDowall, A. G. Craig, P. A. Bates, M. J. E. Sternberg, K. Marsh, C. I. Newbold, and N. Hogg, *Cell 68*, 71 (1992).
39. C. F. Ockenhaouse, R. Betageri, T. A. Springer, and D. E. Staunton, *Cell 68*, 63 (1992).
40. C. H. June, J. A. Ledbetter, P. S. Linsley, and C. B. Thompson, *Immunol. Today 11*, 211 (1990).
41. M. Augustin, P. Lindley, J. Ledbetter, C. Prinz, A. Kapp, E. Schöpf, J. Krutmann, and J. C. Simon, *J. Invest. Dermatol. 98*, 577 (1992).
42. T. A. Springer, M. L. Dustin, T. K. Kishimoto, and S. D. Marlin, *Annu. Rev. Immunol. 5*, 223 (1987).
43. B. F. Haynes, M. J. Telen, L. P. Hale, and S. M. Denning, *Immunol. Today 10*, 423 (1989).
44. M. L. Dustin, K. H. Singer, D. T. Tuck, and T. A. Springer, *J. Exp. Med. 167*, 1323 (1988).
45. F. W. Symington and E. B. Santos, *J. Immunol. 146*, 2169 (1991).
46. R. A. Kalish, *J. Immunol. 142*, 74 (1989).
47. J. C. Simon, P. D. Druz Jr., P. R. Bergstresser, L. S. Davis, and R. S. Tigelaar, *J. Immunol. 146*, 476 (1991).
48. G. L. Vejlsgaard, E. Ralfkiaer, C. Avnstrorp, M. Czajkowski, S. D. Marlin, and R. Rothlein, *J. Am. Acad. Dermatol. 20*, 782 (1989).
49. K. H. Singer, D. T. Tuck, H. A. Sampson, and R. P. Hall, *J. Invest. Dermatol. 92*, 746 (1989).
50. S. Lisby, E. Ralfkiaer, R. Rothlein, and G. L. Veljsgaard, *Br. J. Dermatol. 120*, 479 (1989).
51. B. J. Nickoloff, C. Griffiths, O. Baadsgard, J. J. Voorhes, C. A. Hanson, and K. D. Cooper, *JAMA 261*, 2217 (1989).
52. D. A. Norris, *J. Invest. Dermatol. 95*, 111S (1990).
53. D. A. Norris, M. B. Lyons, M. H. Middleton, J. J. Yohn, and M. Kashihara-Sawami, *J. Invest. Dermatol. 95*, 186 (1990).
54. J. Krutmann, A. Köck, E. Schauer, F. Parlow, A. Möller, A. Kapp, E. Förster, E. Schöpf, and T. A. Luger, *J. Invest. Dermatol. 95*, 178 (1990).
55. S. W. Caughman, L. Lian-Jie, and K. Degitz, *J. Invest. Dermatol. 94*, 22S (1990).
56. J. N. W. N. Barker, V. Sarma, R. S. Mitra, V. M. Dixit, and B. J. Nickoloff, *J. Clin. Invest. 85*, 605 (1990).
57. U. Trefzer, M. Brockhaus, F. Parlow, H. Lötscher, A. Kapp, E. Schöpf, and J. Krutmann, *J. Invest. Dermatol. 97*, 911 (1991).
58. B. B. Aggarwal, T. E. Eesalu, and P. E. Hass, *Nature 318*, 665 (1985).
59. B. M. Curtis, B. Gallis, R. O. Overell, J. C. McMahan, P. Deross, R. Oteland, J. Eisenman, S. Dower, and J. Sims, *Proc. Natl. Acad. Sci. USA 86*, 3045 (1989).
60. T. Kupper, *J. Clin. Invest. 86*, 1783 (1990).
61. T. Kupper, N. Birchall, B. Blanton, and S. Dower, *Clin. Res. 36*, 550A (1988).
62. J. Krutman, U. Trefzer, A. Kapp, E. Schöpf, and T. A. Luger, *J. Invest. Dermatol. 98*, 578 (1992).

63. J. N. W. N. Barker, M. H. Allen, and D. M. MacDonald, *J. Invest. Dermatol. 93*, 439 (1989).
64. A. Köck, T. Schwarz, R. Kirnbauer, A. Urbanski, P. Perry, J. C. Ansel, and T. A. Luger, *J. Exp. Med. 172*, 1609 (1990).
65. B. G. Stade, G. Messer, G. Riethmüller, and J. P. Johnson, *Immunobiology 182*, 79 (1990).
66. S. O. Wawryk, P. N. Cockerill, I. P. Wicks, and A. W. Boyd, *International Immunol. 3*, 83 (1991).
67. K. Degitz, L. Lian-Jie, and S. W. Caughman, *J. Biol. Chem. 266*, 14024 (1991).
68. G. Vorarberger, R. Schäfer, and C. Stratowa, *J. Immunol. 147*, 2777 (1991).
69. H. P. Hohmann, M. Brockhaus, P. A. Baeurle, R. Remy, R. Kolbeck, and A. P. G. M. van Loon, *J. Biol. Chem. 265*, 22409 (1990).
70. J. Krutmann, W. Czech, F. Parlow, U. Trefzer, A. Kapp, E. Schöpf, and T. A. Luger, *J. Invest. Dermatol. 98*, 923 (1992).
71. U. Trefzer, M. Grewe, M. Brockhaus, H. Lötscher, F. Parlow, A. Budnik, A. Kapp, E. Schöpf, T. A. Luger, and J. Krutmann, *J. Clin. Invest.* (in press).
72. L. Polla, R. Margolis, C. Goulston, J. A. Parrish, and R. D. Granstein, *J. Invest. Dermatol. 86*, 13 (1986).
73. K. Cooper, F. Fox, G. Neises, and S. Katz, *J. Immunol. 134*, 129 (1984).
74. D. A. Norris, S. D. Bennion, and M. H. Middleton, *J. Invest. Dermatol. 94*, 560A (1990).
75. P. Norris, R. N. Poston, S. D. Thomas, M. Thornhill, J. Hawk, and D. O. Haskard, *J. Invest. Dermatol. 96*, 763 (1991).
76. M. Grewe, U. Trefzer, M. Brockhaus, A. Kapp, E. Schöpf, and J. Krutmann, *Arch. Dermatol. Res. 284*, 40 (1992).
77. M. Tsujisaki, K. Igarashi, M. Eisinger, M. Herlyn, and S. Ferrone, *J. Immunol. 138*, 1310 (1987).
78. M. Temponi, G. Romano, C. M. D'Urso, Z. Wang, U. Kekish, and S. Ferrone, *Sem. Oncol. 15*, 595 (1988).
79. J. J. Yohn, M. Critelli, M. B. Lyons, and D. A. Norris, *J. Invest. Dermatol. 90*, 233 (1990).
80. R. Kirnbauer, E. Schauer, B. Charvat, A. Urbanski, E. Förster, P. Neuner, T. Schwarz, and T. A. Luger, *Arch. Dermatol. Res. 283*, 64A (1991).
81. J. C. Bystryn, in *Immune Mechanisms in Cutaneous Disease* (D. A. Norris, ed.), Marcel Dekker, New York, 1989, p. 447.
82. J. P. Johnson, B. G. Stade, B. Holzmann, W. Schwäble, and G. Riethmüller, *Proc. Natl. Acad. Sci. USA 86*, 641 (1989).
83. D. R. Welch, J. E. Bisi, B. E. Miller, D. Conaway, E. A. Seftor, K. H. Hohem, L. B. Gilmore, R. E. B. Seftor, M. Nakajima, and M. J. C. Hendrix, *Int. J. Cancer 47*, 227 (1991).
84. T. A. Fischer, A. Durandy, G. Sterkers, and C. Griscelli, *J. Immunol. 136*, 3198 (1986).
85. G. J. Dougherty, S. Murdoch, and N. Hogg, *Eur. J. Immunol. 18*, 35 (1988).
86. J. Krutmann, I. U. Khan, R. S. Wallis, F. Zhang, E. A. Rich, J. J. Ellner, and C. A. Elmets, *J. Clin. Invest. 85*, 1529 (1990).

87. D. M. Altmann, N. Hogg, J. Trowsdale, and D. Wilkinson, *Nature 338*, 512 (1989).
88. G. Stingl, S. I. Katz, L. Clement, I. Green, and E. M. Shevach, *J. Immunol. 121*, 2005 (1978).
89. K. Inaba, G. Schuler, M. D. Witmer, J. Valinsky, B. Atassi, and R. M. Steinman, *J. Exp. Med. 164*, 605 (1986).
90. N. Romani, A. Lenz, H. Glassel, H. Stössel, H. Stanzl, O. Majdic, P. Fritsch, and G. Schuler, *J. Invest. Dermatol. 93*, 600 (1989).
91. G. De Panfilis, D. Soligo, G. C. Manara, C. Ferrari, C. Torresani, *J. Invest. Dermatol. 93*, 60 (1989).
92. G. De Panfilis, G. C. Manara, C. Ferrari, and C. Torresani, *J. Invest. Dermatol. 94*, 317 (1990).
93. J. C. Simon, P. D. Cruz Jr., R. E. Tigelaar, R. D. Sontheimer, and P. R. Bergstresser, *J. Invest. Dermatol. 96*, 148 (1991).
94. A. Tang and M. C. Udey, *J. Immunol. 146*, 3347 (1991).
95. J. C. Simon, J. Krutmann, C. A. Elmets, P. R. Bergstresser, and P. D. Cruz, *J. Invest. Dermatol. 98*, 665 (1992).
96. J. Krutmann, F. Parlow, E. Schöpf, and C. A. Elmets, *Clin. Res. 39*, 194A (1991).
97. M. D. Wittmer-Pack, W. Olivier, J. Valinsky, G. Schuler, and R. M. Steinman, *J. Exp. Med. 167*, 1484 (1987).
98. J. Krutmann, U. Jonas, F. Parlow, U. Trefzer, M. Berger, E. Schöpf, and J. Bauer, *J. Invest. Dermatol. 98*, 539 (1992).
99. S. M. Denning, P. T. Le, K. H. Singer, and B. F. Haynes, *J. Immunol. 144*, 7 (1990).

# 21
# Melanocytic Cell Cytokines

**Cheryl A. Armstrong and John C. Ansel**
*Veterans Affairs Medical Center*
*and Oregon Health Sciences University*
*Portland, Oregon*

**Thomas A. Luger**
*Ludwig Boltzmann Institute for Cell Biology and Immunobiology of the Skin*
*University of Münster*
*Münster, Germany*

## I. INTRODUCTION

Melanocytes are neural crest–derived cells located in the epidermis, which historically have been evaluated primarily in terms of their ability to produce melanin and as precursor cells for malignant melanoma. During the last decade it has become possible to example melanocytic cells directly in vitro as a result of the successful cultivation of normal melanocytes and nevus cells in specialized tissue culture media [1, 2]. It is now clear that both epidermal melanocytes and nevus cells are capable of producing and responding to a number of distinct cytokines which have unique growth and immunomodulating properties. Although the biological relevance of these melanocytic cell–derived cytokines is not yet defined, they may play an important role in the growth and development of these cells. Malignant melanoma cells, the malignant counterpart of epidermal melanocytes, also produce a number of distinct cytokines. Recent evidence indicates that these melanoma-derived soluble mediators may influence the growth and progression of this neoplasm in vivo. This review will present current information regarding the ability of normal melanocytes, nevus cells, and melanoma cells to produce and respond to various growth factors, cytokines, and inflammatory mediators. The potential role of these factors in the biology of melanocytic cells will be discussed.

## II. MELANOCYTES

### A. Culture of Normal Melanocytes

Melanocytes are neural crest–derived cells that migrate to embryonic human skin at 7 weeks estimated gestational age (EGA) and become established in the epidermis at age 16–18 weeks EGA [3, 4]. One of the primary functions of epidermal melanocytes is to protect the host from the detrimental effects of ultraviolet (UV) irradiation by the production and transfer of melanin to keratinocytes. Melanin serves a protective function in the skin by filtering and reflecting UV radiation as well as acting as a scavenger of UV-induced reactive oxygen species (ROS) [5]. In adult human skin, there is a ratio of approximately 36 keratinocytes to every melanocyte [6]. Physical contact between these two cell types has long been recognized as essential for the transfer of melanosomes from melanocytes to keratinocytes. It has been proposed that keratinocytes may regulate the number of melanocytes in human fetal and neonatal skin by the production of growth factors and/or the expression of cell surface molecules [7].

In the last decade melanocytes were successfully cultured using newly described tissue culture methods [1]. With the advent of these techniques, melanocyte functions such as melanogenesis could be evaluated at a molecular level. Likewise, the response of normal melanocytes to peptide growth factors and inflammatory mediators as well as the capacity of melanocytes to produce cytokines could now be studied. In one of the first successful protocols for culturing human melanocytes, cells were grown in tissue culture media supplemented with serum, TPA (12-O-tetradecanoyl-phorbal-13-acetate), and cholera toxin [1]. Under these conditions melanocyte proliferation rates were similar to those of cultured melanoma cells [1]. Variations in this approach demonstrate that proliferation in vitro can also be induced by other tumor-promoting phorbal esters and by agents that increase intracellular cAMP levels [2, 8]. Other investigators developed serum-free melanocyte growth media supplemented with basic fibroblast growth factor (bFGF), which also functioned as a mitogen for melanocytes in vitro [9–11]. bFGF is a member of the small family of heparin-binding growth factors that is mitogenic for a variety of cell types of mesodermal and neuroectodermal origin [12].

It was recently observed that keratinocytes co-cultured with melanocytes supported the proliferation of melanocytes in vitro without TPA-supplemented media [13, 14]. This led to the proposal that keratinocytes may produce melanocyte growth-promoting factors. This concept was further supported by the demonstration that human keratinocyte–derived bFGF acted as a natural mitogen for cultured melanocytes [15]. In this study, antiserum to bFGF or synthetic mutant bFGF fragments neutralized the melanocyte proliferation induced by keratinocyte-conditioned media. Other studies suggested that keratinocyte-derived growth factors other than bFGF may also function as melanocyte mitogens [16]. Additionally, bFGF secreted by dermal fibroblasts was postulated to have a similar mitogenic effect on melanocytes in vitro [10]. These studies support the concept that an interactive relationship between melanocytes, keratinocytes, and fibroblasts in the skin could be mediated by soluble factors secreted by these cells.

Another cytokine termed melanoma growth stimulatory activity (MGSA/GRO) was reported to act as a weak mitogen when added as a single agent to cultured melanocytes [17]. However, in combination with TPA and insulin, MGSA stimulated the proliferation of melanocytes as effectively as bFGF [17]. The MGSA gene is identical to the GRO gene and belongs to the $\alpha$-thromboglobulin supergene family along with platelet factor-4, macrophage-derived growth factor, $\alpha$-thromboglobulin, interleukin 8 (IL-8), and monocyte chemotactic factor [18, 19]. Keratinocytes are also a source of MGSA and therefore may modulate the growth of epidermal melanocytes by the secretion of this cytokine [20, 21].

Mediators other than bFGF and MGSA are mitogenic for normal human melanocytes. Other members of the FGF family including acidic FGF, K-FGF-*hst*, FGF-5, and FGF-6 stimulated the proliferation of melanocytes [22–24]. Hepatocyte growth factor and mast cell growth factor were reported to act as melanocyte mitogens [25]. All of these factors required the addition of dibutyryl AMP (dbcAMP) or isobutylmethyl xanthine (IBMX) to mediate melanocyte proliferation [22–25]. Melanocytes also proliferated in vitro in response to melanocyte-stimulating hormone alpha (MSH-$\alpha$) when this peptide was added to TPA-supplemented tissue culture media [11]. Although the mechanism of this response is not yet clear, it may be due to the induction of intracellular cyclic AMP levels, which is associated with the proliferation of melanocytes [26]. MSH-$\alpha$ is a melanotropin secreted predominately by the pituitary. Diverse nonpituitary tissues such as lymphoid cells and malignant tumors also secrete active MSH-$\alpha$ [27, 28]. Recently, keratinocytes stimulated with phorbol-12-myristate-13-acetate (PMA), interleukin 1 (IL-1), or UV light were also found to express mRNA specific for proopiomelanocortin, the precursor for MSH [29]. Moreover, keratinocytes also released biologically active MSH-$\alpha$ [29]. Therefore, a potential paracrine effect of keratinocyte-derived MSH-$\alpha$ on the proliferation of melanocytes could occur in the epidermis. In contrast to these results, several other investigators failed to demonstrate a significant mitogenic effect of MSH on melanocyte growth [30–32].

When the ability of leukotrienes to stimulate melanocyte proliferation was addressed, it was found that leukotriene $C_4$ ($LTC_4$) and leukotriene $D_4$ ($LTD_4$) were both capable of stimulating melanocyte proliferation [33].

Moreover, it was noted that $LTC_4$ as well as transforming growth factor alpha (TGF-$\alpha$) were potent inducers of melanocyte movement [34].

Some cytokines may block the proliferation of normal human melanocytes. Exogenous transforming growth factor beta (TGF-$\beta$) inhibited the growth of melanocytes in culture [35]. Likewise, IL-1$\alpha$, interleukin 6 (IL-6), and tumor necrosis factor alpha (TNF-$\alpha$) suppressed the proliferation of cultured neonatal human melanocytes [36]. These cytokines also suppressed the activity of melanocyte tyrosinase, which resulted in decreased melanin synthesis [36]. In another study, interferon beta (IFN-$\beta$) also inhibited the proliferation of melanocytes cultured in serum free media, while interferon alpha (IFN-$\alpha$) and interferon gamma (IFN-$\gamma$) had no effect on proliferation [37].

The expression of cellular adhesion molecules such as intercellular adhesion molecule 1 (ICAM-1) is necessary for cell-cell interactions. The increased expression of ICAM-1 in melanoma was found to correlate with increased risk of metastasis [38, 39]. The regulation of ICAM-1 expression on normal human melanocytes and melanoma cells by cytokines was recently investigated. Melanocytes, which may lack constitutive ICAM-1 expression, were stimulated to express this adhesion molecule by IFN-$\gamma$, TNF-$\alpha$, TNF-$\beta$, IL-1, IL-6, and interleukin 7 (IL-7), depending on the culture conditions [40, 41]. Most interestingly, the cytokine IL-6, which does not influence adhesion molecule expression on other cells, significantly upregulated melanocyte and melanoma cell ICAM-1 expression [40]. Since IL-6 does not affect keratinocyte ICAM-1 expression, there may exist differences in IL-6 receptor structure and function or signal transduction mechanisms regulating ICAM-1 expression in a cell- and tissue-specific manner.

The biological effects of UV light are multiple and include the suppression of the immune response, which could contribute to carcinogenesis and the development of malignant melanoma [42, 43]. The effects of UV light on ICAM-1 expression on both human melanocytes and melanoma cells appeared to be biphasic; inhibiting cytokine-induced ICAM-1 expression within the first 16 hours, but inducing ICAM-1 expression between 48 and 96 hours [40]. This late induction may be due to the autocrine stimulation of the melanocytic cells by cytokines such as TNF-$\alpha$ and IL-1, as reported in another study when keratinocytes were treated with UV light [44].

## B. Cytokine Production by Normal Melanocytes

In addition to responding to particular cytokines and inflammatory mediators, melanocytes also produce a number of growth factors and immunomodulating cytokines. Cultured normal human melanocytes expressed IL-1$\alpha$ mRNA and IL-1$\beta$ mRNA and secreted IL-1$\alpha$ and IL-1$\beta$ peptides [45–47]. IL-1 is a pleotropic cytokine which is capable of mediating a wide range of immunological, inflammatory, endocrinological, and hematopoietic activities [48]. IL-1$\alpha$ and IL-1$\beta$ share the same spectrum of biological activity although they have only 30% amino acid homology [49]. Likewise, there are two discrete IL-1 receptors with preferential expression on different cell types [49]. Although IL-1$\alpha$ and IL-1$\beta$ bind to either IL-1 receptor, IL-1$\alpha$ has higher affinity for type I receptors and IL-1$\beta$ binds with higher affinity to type II receptors. IL-1$\alpha$ and IL-1$\beta$ are first synthesized as 33 kd precursor peptides that are cleaved by specific proteases (IL-1$\alpha$ and IL-1$\beta$ convertases) to biologically active 17 kd products. Although both the 33 and 17 kd forms of IL-1$\alpha$ are biologically active, only the 17 kd form of IL-1$\beta$ has bioactivity. Melanocyte lysates contained an IL-1$\beta$ convertase necessary to convert the precursor IL-1$\beta$ peptide (33 kd) to its biologically active processed (17 kd) form [45]. It is postulated that melanocytic IL-1$\beta$ convertase may act in vivo on the 33 kd keratinocyte IL-1$\beta$ precursor, which results in the biologically active 17 kd form [45]. In addition, it was reported that cultured human melanocytes constitutively produced IL-1 [46] and that the neuropeptides MSH-$\alpha$, MSH-$\beta$, MSH-$\gamma$, NLE-MSH-$\alpha$, substance P (SP), and neurotensin increased melanocyte IL-1 production. IL-1$\alpha$ added to cultured melanocytes inhibited melanocyte proliferation suggesting a possible autocrine inhibitory role for this cytokine in melanocyte growth [36].

Normal cultured melanocytes are also capable of the constitutive expression of TGF-$\beta$ mRNA [50]. TGF-$\beta$1 is a multifunctional polypeptide growth factor that belongs to a family of regulatory proteins with a wide range of biological activities [51]. Most mammalian cell types express specific receptors for TGF-$\beta$. This cytokine is capable of either stimulating or inhibiting cellular proliferation and differentiation depending on the cell type and the cell culture conditions. TGF-$\beta$ also inhibited the proliferation of melanocytes and could thus modulate the growth of these cells [35].

Recently, it was reported that normal human melanocytes produce IL-8 and monocyte chemotactic and activating factor (MCAF) following stimulation by rIL-1$\alpha$ and TNF-$\alpha$ [52]. IL-8 is a potent neutrophil chemoattractant originally isolated from activated monocytes. This cytokine has a wide range of proinflammatory effects such as neutrophil chemotaxis/degranulation, increased expression of cellular adhesion molecules, and chemotactic activity for basophils and subsets of human peripheral T lymphocytes [53, 54]. Subcutaneous injection of IL-8 results in neutrophil infiltration at the site of injection [55, 56]. MCAF is capable of attracting and activating monocytes, which results in increased cytostatic capacity [57]. The ability of melanocytes to produce IL-8 and MCAF further supports the potential role of melanocytes in mediating inflammatory processes in the skin [52].

Cultured melanocytes were also reported to constitutively produce IL-6 and TNF-$\alpha$ [46]. Melanocyte IL-6 and TNF-$\alpha$ production were also significantly induced by MSH-$\alpha$, MSH-$\beta$, MSH-$\gamma$, NLE-MSH-$\alpha$, SP, and neurotensin [46]. Neuropeptide-activated melanocytes were reported to secrete significantly more TNF-$\alpha$ than similarly treated keratinocytes [46]. Cultured human melanocytes were also found to produce interleukin 3 (IL-3) and granulocyte-macrophage colony-stimulating factor (GM-CSF) [58]. Melanocytes have not been found to produce bFGF, platelet-derived growth factor (PDGF), TGF-$\alpha$, or MGSA [17, 22, 50, 59].

## III. NEVUS CELLS

Melanocytic nevi are benign neuroectodermal neoplasms of the skin composed of proliferations of melanocytic cells. Nevi are classified as junctional, compound, or intradermal depending on the location of the nevus cells in the skin. Although most people have nevi, there are few reports regarding the biology of nevus cells. Melanocytic nevus cell cultures have been successfully established by a number of investigators [2, 60–62]. Removal of the epidermal portion of nevus biopsy specimens led to the unambiguous isolation of nevus cells from compound-acquired nevus explants in culture [60]. Nevus cells from congenital and dysplastic nevi were reported to proliferate in serum-supplemented media containing a mixture of TPA, IBMX, and/or cholera toxin [2]. Primary nevus cells cultures can be established in serum-free media supplemented with bFGF, insulinlike growth factor-1 (IGF-1) or insulin, TPA for protein kinase C activation, and MSH-$\alpha$ [61]. These cells were maintained in culture for over 6 months with doubling times between 7 and 14 days [61]. Nevus cells required fewer exogenous growth factors in chemically defined media than melanocytes [61]. While MSH-$\alpha$ appeared to remain an essential component for long-term growth of nevus cells, bFGF and TPA could be greatly reduced or even omitted from the culture media [61]. Nevus cells can be isolated selectively from the epidermis, the basal layer, or from the dermis of benign pigmented lesions [62]. Nevus cells isolated from the dermal component of compound nevi exhibited the most rapid growth in culture suggesting that they are the most biologically active melanocytic cells in this type of nevus [62].

Nevus cells share growth characteristics of both normal melanocytes and melanoma cells. They were reported to have a finite life span in culture similar to melanocytes with a capacity of approximately 50 doublings [61, 63]. In addition, like melanocytes, cultured nevus cells were reported to require supplemental mitogenic agents [2, 60–63]. This is in contrast to late vertical growth phase primary melanoma cells and metastatic melanoma cells, which are able to grow continuously in culture without exogenous growth factors [61]. Also like melanocytes, nevus cells were nontumorigenic when inoculated in nude mice [62]. However, in contrast to melanocytes and like melanoma cells, nevus cells were reported to grow in an anchorage-independent manner in soft agar and to express a large number of melanoma-associated antigens [62, 64]. It has been postulated that the malignant transformation of benign melanocytes to melanoma cells is associated with the loss of normal growth control mechanisms present in normal melanocytes. Nevus cells and dysplastic nevus cells may represent an intermediate step in this process.

Few studies have evaluated cytokine production by nevus cells. It was reported that monolayers of cultured nevus cells secrete a mitogenic factor that stimulates the proliferation of a melanoma cell line [65]. Another group of investigators detected bFGF mRNA in nevus cells by in situ hybridization of biopsy specimens [66]. In this study, nevus cells in dysplastic nevi expressed higher levels of bFGF mRNA than in nevi without atypical features. Nevus cells were also reported to produce MGSA [20]. Recently, nevus biopsy specimens were reported to demonstrate bFGF, TGF-$\alpha$, PDGF, and IL-1 by immunohistochemistry [67]. It is clear that more work is needed to adequately characterize the role that specific cytokines may play in the biology of nevus cells.

## IV. MELANOMA CELLS

### A. Growth and Development

Melanomas are malignant neoplasms that originate from melanocytic cells within the epidermis. While the majority of melanomas appear to arise de novo, some appear to arise from preexisting nevi [68]. Congenital nevi and nevi with atypical changes (dysplastic nevi) have been identified as precursor lesions in many malignant melanomas [69, 70]. The multistep process of malignant melanoma development from epidermal melanocytes has been well delineated [71]. The progression of malignant melanoma from benign melanocytic cells has been divided into six lesional steps: (a) common acquired melanocytic nevus, (b) melanocytic nevus with persistent architectural atypia, (c) dysplastic nevus with persistent architectural and cytologic atypia, (d) radial growth phase of primary melanoma, (e) vertical growth phase of primary melanoma, and (f) metastatic melanoma [71]. This classification, based on clinical and histological criteria, has facilitated the investigation of biological, immunological, and genetic features of these pigmented lesions.

Cultured melanoma cells from primary and metastatic human melanomas produce a number of cytokines including bFGF, MGSA, IL-8, TGF-$\alpha$, epidermal growth factor (EGF), TGF-$\beta$, PDGF, IL-1, IL-6, IL-3, and GM-CSF [29]. There is a distinct heterogeneity in the cytokine production profile of different human melanoma cell lines. As in other neoplasms, it is postulated that some of these cytokines could contribute to the progression of benign melanocytic cells to malignant melanoma cells by acting as transforming autocrine growth factors. Melanoma-derived cytokines may also have paracrine or endocrine effects on the host immune response to these developing tumors [29]. The identity, characterization, and potential role of melanoma-derived cytokines in the growth and development of this neoplasm will be discussed.

## B. Growth Factors and Cytokines

Supernatants of cultured melanoma cells contain a number of discrete cytokines which are mitogenic for melanomas [29, 30, 72]. More specifically, melanoma-derived bFGF, MGSA, IL-1, IL-8, and PDGF have been reported to stimulate in vitro growth of melanoma cells [21, 73–76]. This suggests that these factors may function as autocrine growth factors in certain melanoma cell lines. The role of bFGF and MGSA as melanoma autocrine growth factors has been most convincingly established [22, 74].

*Basic Fibroblast Growth Factor*

The ability of bFGF to promote the in vitro growth of human malignant melanoma cells has been recognized for some time [71, 73]. Recently, it was demonstrated that certain melanoma cell lines are capable of producing bFGF and that bFGF functioned as an autocrine growth factor for the cultured melanoma cells [22, 50]. However, the production of bFGF by melanocytes was not sufficient for transformation of these cells as demonstrated in transfection studies of bFGF into a murine melanocyte cell line [77].

*Melanoma Growth Stimulatory Activity/Interleukin 8*

MGSA can function as an autocrine growth factor for melanoma cells. MGSA secreted by the Hs294T human melanoma cell line stimulated the proliferation of melanoma cells in vitro [74, 78]. In another study, the transfection of a murine melanocyte line with the MGSA gene resulted in a transformed cellular phenotype, as demonstrated by the ability of these cells to form colonies in soft agar and tumors in nude mice [79]. Thus, overexpression of MGSA is associated with transformation of melanocytes to melanoma and may potentially play a role in melanoma tumor progression in vivo.

Melanoma cell lines have recently been reported to produce IL-8 [21, 52]. The major biological activity of IL-8 is the attraction and activation of neutrophils. IL-8 belongs to the same cytokine family as MGSA, sharing 44% sequence homology at the amino acid level, and binds to the same receptor on neutrophils [80, 81]. Certain human melanoma cell lines expressed IL-8 mRNA and secreted IL-8 following stimulation with IL-1$\alpha$ or TNF-$\alpha$ [52]. There is also evidence that IL-8 functioned as an autocrine growth factor like MGSA in some melanoma cell lines [21, 74, 78]. Exogenous IL-8 was also reported to induce in vitro migration of melanoma cells [82]. The production of IL-8 by melanoma cells may therefore augment the proliferation and migration of certain melanomas. The secretion of IL-8 by melanoma cells could also initiate a significant local host cellular inflammatory response. Further in vivo studies are necessary to determine if IL-8 production by melanomas mediates the inflammatory cell infiltrate that is observed in histological examination of certain human melanomas.

### *Transforming Growth Factor Alpha, Epidermal Growth Factor, and Transforming Growth Factor Beta*

It has been recognized for some time that certain human melanomas can produce TGF-$\alpha$ and EGF [83, 84]. TGF-$\alpha$ is a polypeptide growth factor that was initially identified as a product of a human melanoma cell line and in a number of virally transformed rat cell lines [83]. A wide variety of human tumor cell lines including cells transformed by oncogenes, retroviruses, or tumor promoters produce TGF-$\alpha$, suggesting that TGF-$\alpha$ may play an important role in cell growth and neoplastic development [85]. Normal cells such as keratinocytes, macrophages, and pituitary cells also produce TGF-$\alpha$ [85]. EGF is a peptide growth factor also produced by a wide variety of cells, which mediates normal cell growth and repair processes [86]. TGF-$\alpha$ and EGF bind to the same receptor, and thus share biological activities such as the stimulation of fibroblasts and angiogenesis. Human keratinocytes express high affinity receptors for EGF/TGF-$\alpha$. Clinical studies suggest that TGF-$\alpha$/EGF are important in wound healing and tissue repair in the skin [87, 88]. Although certain melanoma cell lines produce TGF-$\alpha$ and EGF and express receptors for these factors, the biological role of TGF-$\alpha$ and EGF in melanoma cells remains unclear. One group of investigators reported that benign melanocytes expressed fewer EGF receptors than primary and metastatic melanomas [71]. Other researchers reported no difference in the high level of EGF receptors on benign nevi compared to melanomas in situ and metastatic melanomas [89]. Recently, constitutive TGF-$\alpha$ secretion was demonstrated in three of four melanoma cell lines tested [50]. No change in the proliferation of these melanoma cells in vitro was observed with either the addition of TGF-$\alpha$ or neutralizing antibody to TGF-$\alpha$ [50]. These results suggest that the proliferation of these melanomas was not dependent on the autocrine stimulation of TGF-$\alpha$ acting through external receptors.

TGF-$\beta$ is another transforming growth factor produced by melanoma cells [50, 84, 90]. This multifunctional polypeptide growth factor can either stimulate or inhibit cellular proliferation and differentiation depending on the cell type and the cell culture conditions [51]. TGF-$\beta$ inhibited the growth of melanoma cells in soft agar (anchorage-independent growth) in several independent studies [50, 84, 91]. Additionally, TGF-$\beta$1 inhibited the growth of several melanoma cell lines in tissue culture (anchorage-dependent growth)

[50]. Since TGF-$\beta$ has also been reported to be produced by melanocytes and to inhibit their in vitro proliferation, this cytokine may function generally as a negative autocrine growth factor for melanocytic cell growth [35, 50].

### *Platelet-Derived Growth Factor*

Melanoma cell lines are also capable of producing PDGF [50, 59, 92]. This cytokine is a potent mitogen for cells of mesenchymal origin and is chemotactic for monocytes, neutrophils, and endothelial cells [93, 94]. A wide number of cell types produce PDGF, including platelets, monocytes, macrophages, endothelial cells, keratinocytes, and some human tumor cell lines [95, 96]. PDGF produced by platelets consists primarily of a heterodimer of A and B polypeptide chains linked by disulfide bonds, while other tissues may express homodimeric forms of PDGF designated A-A and B-B [97, 98]. The PDGF-B chain gene is transforming when transfected into murine fibroblasts [99]. PDGF-A was also reported to be an autocrine growth factor for a human osteosarcoma cell lines in vitro [100]. Several different human melanoma cell lines have been found to produce a PDGF-like growth factor and express mRNA for PDGF [59]. PDGF-producing cell lines were established from one primary and two individual lymph node metastatic lesions from the same patient. All of these melanoma cell lines expressed PDGF-A chain mRNA, but only the primary melanoma cells expressed PDGF-B mRNA. In another study, PDGF-AA was detected in the supernatants of melanoma cell lines as determined by ELISA using PDGF isotype-specific antibodies [91]. PDGF-A chain appeared to be the predominate PDGF gene expressed in melanoma cells [50, 59, 92].

The biological role of melanoma-derived PDGF is unknown. Moreover, exogenous PDGF did not appear to affect the in vitro proliferation of melanoma cell lines [50]. The addition of a neutralizing PDGF antiserum did not inhibit the growth of cultured melanoma cells [50]. These results indicate that secreted PDGF does not appear to function as an autocrine growth factor for these melanoma cells. Melanoma-derived PDGF, however, may modulate the surrounding stroma, thus influencing tumor growth and development.

### *Interleukin 1*

It is well established that certain melanomas produce IL-1 [92, 101, 102]. IL-1 activity was detected in supernatants from human melanoma cells derived from one primary nodular melanoma and five metastatic melanoma cell lines [101]. These cell lines expressed only IL-1$\alpha$ mRNA by Northern blot analysis, however, biochemical characterization of the cell supernatants by HPLC gel filtration identified a major peak corresponding to IL-1$\alpha$ and a minor peak corresponding to IL-1$\beta$ [101]. In another study, a widely used melanoma cell line obtained from the American Type Culture Collection (ATCC) constitutively expressed both IL-1$\alpha$ mRNA and IL-1$\beta$ mRNA, whereas a second ATCC melanoma cell line did not express IL-1 mRNA [92]. In another investigation, it was also reported that 4 of 7 primary and 5 of 20 metastatic melanoma cell lines secreted IL-1 activity [102]. Three of four IL-1–secreting lines in this study expressed both IL-1$\alpha$ and IL-1$\beta$ mRNA, however, again most of the secreted IL-1 activity was IL-1$\alpha$. Therefore, the major form of IL-1 produced by melanoma cells appears to be IL-1$\alpha$ [92, 101, 102].

The biological implications of IL-1 production by malignant melanoma cells are unclear. Because of the pleotropic biological properties of this cytokine, melanoma-derived IL-1 could either facilitate or inhibit the growth and development of these neoplasms. In one study, IL-1 was reported to be mitogenic for a melanoma cell line, but it was not clearly established as an autocrine growth factor [75]. Another potential mechanism by which melanoma-derived IL-1 could support tumor growth and dissemination is by local or systemic immune modulation of host defense mechanisms. The injection of recombinant IL-1 induced systemic immune suppression in mice [103]. IL-1 could also augment the adherence of melanoma cells to endothelial cells by the induction of adhesion molecule expression such as ICAM-1 on endothelial cells [104]. The adherence of tumor cells to specific binding sites on endothelial cells appears to be an early critical step in the metastasis of neoplasms [105]. IL-1 secretion by melanoma cells may also upregulate adhesion molecule expression on melanoma cells, which could influence the metastatic process. The IL-1–secreting A375 melanoma cell line expressed surface ICAM-1 after the addition of IFN-$\gamma$, TNF-$\alpha$, and IL-1 to the cultured cells [106]. It has been recently reported that ICAM-1 expression on melanoma surgical specimens occurs at a higher frequency on metastatic lesions than in primary melanomas [38, 39]. It was postulated that the expression of melanoma ICAM-1 may contribute to the metastatic process in these tumors [38, 39]. In an animal model of metastatic melanoma, the simultaneous injection of recombinant IL-1 and human melanoma cells in nude mice resulted in a significantly higher number of pulmonary metastases than when tumor cells were injected alone [107].

The release of IL-1 by melanoma cells could inhibit melanoma growth by the mobilization of host immune defenses against the IL-1–secreting tumor. IL-1 is capable of contributing to the activation of a number of lymphoid cells including T cells, B cells, and monocytes [48]. These activated immune cells could then secrete a number of other cytokines such as TNF-$\alpha$, interleukin 2 (IL-2), IL-6, and IL-1 itself, which have direct and indirect antitumor effects [48, 108–110]. Moreover, IL-1 was reported to be directly cytostatic and/or cytotoxic for melanoma cells in vitro [111, 112]. The quantitative differences in the production of IL-1 by different melanomas may also contribute to the heterogeneity of the host response to these pigmented neoplasms. Thus IL-1 production by melanoma cells appears to play a complex role in the biology and the progression of this neoplasm.

### *Interleukin 6*

It was recently reported that some human melanoma cell lines secrete IL-6 [92, 113]. Like IL-1, IL-6 is a pleotropic cytokine secreted by a number of different cell types [114, 115]. This cytokine shares many activities with IL-1 and TNF-$\alpha$ including the induction of acute phase proteins and activation of leukocytes such as B cells, T cells, and natural killer cells [110, 114, 115]. IL-6 has both stimulatory and inhibitory properties for different neoplasms. IL-6 can function as an autocrine growth factor for plasmacytoma cells and AIDS–Kaposi sarcoma cells [116, 117]. In contrast, it was reported that mice with established lung and liver micrometastases from sarcomas or adenocarcinomas have a significant regression in their neoplasms after intraperitoneal IL-6 injeciton [118]. Recently it was reported that there are distinct differences in the IL-6 production between different human metastatic melanoma cell lines [92]. One melanoma cell line constitutively expressed IL-6 mRNA and secreted IL-6 activity, whereas the other cell line produced little or no IL-6. Likewise, in another study, one of two human melanoma cell lines only produced IL-6 after induction with rIL-1$\alpha$ [113]. Using an in vitro cell culture system, these investigators demonstrated that exogenous IL-6 inhibited the proliferation of an IL-6–producing melanoma cell line [113]. This suggested that IL-6 may have growth inhibitory properties for certain melanomas. Melanoma-derived IL-6 may have a potent antitumor effect in vivo [119]. A B16-derived murine melanoma cell line was transfected with a murine IL-6 plasmid expression vector to generate a melanoma cell line that constitutively secreted high levels of IL-6. Syngeneic mice injected with the IL-6–transfected melanoma cells developed subcutaneous melanomas that were significantly smaller than the tumors that grew in animals injected with either the parental melanoma cells or with melanoma cells transfected with the IL-6 gene in the nonfunctional 3′-5′ orientation [119].

### *Colony-Stimulating Factors*

Human melanoma cell lines are also capable of producing the colony-stimulating factors GM-CSF and IL-3 [29, 58, 92, 120]. GM-CSF has multiple biological activities including the induction of the maturation of undifferentiated bone marrow hematopoietic cells into mature granulocytes and macrophages [121, 122]. It is produced by activated T cells, macrophages, bone marrow stem cells, and by nonhematopoietic cells including endothelial cells and keratinocytes [121–123]. It was recently reported that conditioned media from a human melanoma cell line contained significant amounts of GM-CSF activity [120]. This melanoma cell line also expressed mRNA for GM-CSF and secreted GM-CSF as determined by ELISA [92]. The melanoma-derived GM-CSF stimulated human monocytes and a human monocytoid cell line to produce TNF in vitro [120]. GM-CSF produced by melanoma cells could activate immature or mature granulocytes and macrophages to limit the growth and development of this tumor. In other tumor studies, however, GM-CSF production by the tumor cell lines was immunosuppressive and actually accelerated tumor metastases [124]. GM-CSF functioned as an autocrine growth factor for certain malignant cells such as myeloblastic leukemia cells [125]. The ability of GM-CSF to directly affect melanoma cell growth has not been evaluated.

A melanoma cell line was also recently reported to express IL-3 mRNA and secrete IL-3 activity [58]. IL-3 functions as a potent growth factor for basophils and mast cells in addition to stimulating primitive progenitor bone marrow cells [126]. This cytokine is produced predominently by T lymphocytes. The biological role of melanoma-derived IL-3 in the pathogenesis of the tumor has not been established.

## V. CONCLUSION

Melanocytes, nevus cells, and melanoma cells can secrete and respond to a variety of growth factors and cytokines. These secreted factors have a wide range of inflammatory and mitogenic activities. In some cases these factors have a demonstrated autocrine effect on the secreting melanocytic cells. Some melanocytic cell–derived factors may modulate the surrounding epidermal cells, dermal connective tissue and matrix, and immune cells, which could have a critical effect (positive or negative) on the biology of these cells. We are just beginning to appreciate the important role that these melanocytic cell–derived cytokines may play in the biology of both normal and transformed melanocytic cells.

## REFERENCES

1. M. Eisinger and O. Marko, *Proc. Natl. Acad. Sci. USA 79*, 1028 (1982).
2. R. Halaban, S. Ghosh, P. Duray, J. M. Kirkwood, and A. B. Lerner, *J. Invest. Dermatol. 87*, 95 (1986).
3. M. E. Rawles, *Physiol. Rev. 28*, 383 (1948).
4. K. A. Holbrook, A. M. Vogel, R. A. Underwood, and C. A. Foster, *Pigment Cell Res. 1* (Suppl.), 6 (1988).
5. M. A. Pathak, *Ann. N.Y. Acad. Sci. 453*, 328 (1985).

6. T. B. Fitzpatrick, M. Miyamoto, and K. Ishikawa, *Arch. Dermatol. 96*, 305 (1967).
7. G. A. Scott and A. R. Haake, *J. Invest. Dermatol. 97*, 776 (1991).
8. B. A. Gilchrest, M. A. Vrabel, E. Flynn, and G. Szabo, *J. Invest. Dermatol. 83*, 370 (1984).
9. R. Halaban, S. Ghosh, and A. Baird, *In Vitro Cell. Develop. Biol. 23*, 47 (1987).
10. G. P. Shipley and M. R. Pittelkow, *Pigment Cell Res. 1*, 27 (1988).
11. M. Herlyn, M. L. Mancianti, J. Jambrosic, J. B. Bolen, and H. Koprowski, *Exp. Cell. Res. 179*, 322 (1988).
12. Burgess, *Ann. Rev. Biochem. 58*, 575 (1989).
13. M. de Luca, F. D'Anna, S. Bondanza, A. T. Franzi, and R. Cancedda, *J. Cell. Biol. 107*, 1919 (1988).
14. I. T. Valyi-Nagy, G. F. Murphy, M.-L. Mancianti, D. Whitaker, and M. Herlyn, *Lab. Invest. 62*, 314 (1990).
15. R. Halaban, R. Langdon, N. Birchall, C. Cuono, A. Baird, G. Scott, G. Moellmann, and J. McGuire, *J. Cell. Biol. 107*, 1611 (1988).
16. P. R. Gordon, C. P. Mansur, and B. A. Gilchrest, *J. Invest. Dermatol. 92*, 565 (1989).
17. R. Bordoni, R. M. Fine, D. Murray, and A. Richmond, *J. Cell. Biochem. 44*, 207 (1990).
18. A. Anisowicz, L. Bardwell, and R. Sager, *Proc. Natl. Acad. Sci. USA 84*, 7188 (1987).
19. J. Westwick, S. W. Li, and R. D. Camp, *Immunol. Today 10*, 146 (1989).
20. A. Richmond and H. G. Thomas, *J. Cell. Biochem. 36*, 185 (1988).
21. E. Föster, R. Kirnbauer, A. Urbanski, A. Köck, T. A. Luger, and T. Schwarz, *J. Invest. Dermatol. 96*, 608 (1991).
22. R. Halaban, B. S. Kwon, S. Ghosh, P. Delli Bovi, and A. Baird, *Oncogene Res. 3*, 177 (1988).
23. R. Halaban, in *Human Melanoma* (S. Ferrone, ed.), Springer-Verlag, Berlin, 1990, p. 3.
24. R. Halaban, in *Cancer Treatment and Research Series* (L. Nathanson, ed.), Kluwer Acad. Publ., Norwell, MA, 1991, p. 19.
25. R. Halaban, Y. Funasaka, J. Rubin, Y. Yarden, D. Williams, S. Lyman, and D. Birnbaum, *J. Invest. Dermatol. 96*, 560 (1991).
26. M. Ranson, S. Posen, and R. S. Mason, *J. Invest. Dermatol. 91*, 593 (1988).
27. A. I. Smith and J. W. Funder, *Endocr. Rev. 9*, 159 (1988).
28. C. R. DeBold, J. K. Menefee, W. E. Nicholson, and D. N. Orth, *Mol. Endocrinol. 88*, 862 (1989).
29. A. Köck, T. Schwarz, M. Micksche, and T. A. Luger, in *Cancer Treatment and Research*, Vol. 5 (L. Nathanson, ed.), Kluwer Acad. Publ., Norwell, MA, 1991, p. 41.
30. M. Eisinger, O. Marko, S. Ogata, and L. J. Old, *Science 229*, 984 (1985).
31. L. M. Wilkins, G. Szabo, L. Connell, B. A. Gilchrest, and T. Maciag, in *Cold Spring Harbor Conferences on Cell Proliferation, Growth of Cells in Hormonally Defined Media*, Vol. 9 (G. Sato, A. Pardee, D. Sirbasku, eds.), Cold Spring Harbor, New York, 1982, p. 929.

32. R. Halaban, S. H. Pomerantz, S. Marshall, D. T. Lambert, and A. B. Lerner, *J. Cell. Biol. 97*, 480 (1983).
33. J. G. Morelli, J. J. Yohn, M. B. Lyons, R. C. Murphy, and D. A. Norris, *J. Invest. Dermatol. 93*, 719 (1989).
34. J. G. Morelli, J. Kincannon, J. J. Yohn, T. Zekman, W. L. Weston, and D. A. Norris, *J. Invest. Dermatol. 98*, 290 (1992).
35. M. R. Pittelkow and G. D. Shipley, *J. Cell. Physiol. 140*, 565 (1989).
36. V. Swope, Z. Abdel-Malek, and J. Nordlund, *J. Invest. Dermatol. 96*, 180 (1991).
37. K. Krasagakis, C. Garbe, S. Kruger, and C. E. Orfanos, *J. Invest. Dermatol. 97*, 364 (1991).
38. J. P. Johnson, B. G. Stade, B. Holzmann, W. Schwable, and B. G. Riethmuller, *Proc. Natl. Acad. Sci. USA 86*, 641 (1989).
39. P. Natali, M. R. Nicotra, R. Cavaliere, A. Bigotti, G. Romano, M. Temponi, and S. Ferrone, *Cancer Res. 50*, 1271 (1990).
40. R. Kirnbauer, B. Charvat, E. Schauer, A. Köck, A. Urbanski, E. Förster, P. Neuner, T. A. Luger, and T. Schwarz, *J. Invest. Dermatol. 98*, 320 (1992).
41. J. J. Yohn, M, Critelli, M. B. Lyons, and D. A. Norris, *J. Invest. Dermatol. 90*, 233 (1990).
42. M. L. Kripke, *J. Am. Acad. Dermatol. 14*, 149 (1986).
43. H. K. Koh, B. E. Kliger, and R. A. Lew, *Photochem. Photobiol. 5*, 765 (1990).
44. J. Krutmann, W. Czech, F. Parlow, U. Trefzer, A. Kapp, E. Schöpf, and T. A. Luger, *J. Invest. Dermatol. 98*, 923 (1992).
45. H. Mizutani, N. Miwa, T. Mizutani, and T. S. Kupper, *J. Invest. Dermatol. 94*, 556 (1990).
46. A. Köck, E. Schauer, A. Urbanski, T. Schwarz, and T. A. Luger, *J. Invest. Dermatol. 96*, 630 (1991).
47. V. B. Swope, Z. A. Abdel-Malek, G. F. Babcock, R. M. Skramkoski, and J. J. Nordlund, *J. Invest. Dermatol. 96*, 549 (1991).
48. C. A. Dinarello, *Adv. Immunol. 44*, 153 (1989).
49. T. A. Luger and T. Schwarz, in *Langerhans Cell System* (G. Schuler, ed.), CRC Press, Boca Raton, FL, 1991, p. 217.
50. U. Rodeck, K. Melber, R. Kath, H.-D. Menssen, M. Varello, B. Atkinson, and M. Herlyn, *J. Invest. Dermatol. 97*, 20 (1991).
51. A. B. Roberts and M. B. Sporn, in *Peptide Growth Factors and Their Receptors* (M. B. Sporn and A. B. Roberts, eds.), Springer-Verlag, Berlin, 1990, p. 419.
52. C. O. C. Zachariae, K. Thestrup-Pedersen, and K. Matsushima, *J. Invest. Dermatol. 97*, 593 (1991).
53. T. Yoshimura, K. Matsushima, S. Tanaka, E. A. Robinson, E. Appella, J. J. Oppenheim, and E. J. Leonard, *Proc. Natl. Acad. Sci. USA 84*, 9233 (1987).
54. C. G. Larsen, A. O. Anderson, E. Appella, J. J. Oppenheim, and K. Matsushima, *Science 243*, 1464 (1989).
55. M. Rampart, J. Van Damme, L. Zonnekeyn, and A. G. Herman, *Am. J. Path. 135*, 21 (1989).
56. S. J. Foster, D. M. Aked, J.-M. Schröder, and E. Christophers, *Immunology 67*, 181 (1989).

57. C. O. C. Zachariae, A. O. Anderson, H. L. Thompson, E. Appella, A. Manto, J. J. Oppenheim, and K. Matsushima, *J. Exp. Med. 171*, 2177 (1990).
58. A. Köck, A. Möiler, R. Van Lambaigen, A. Urbanski, T. Schwarz, M. Micksche, and T. A. Luger, *Clin. Res. 38*, 412A (1990).
59. B. Westermark, A. Johnsson, Y. Paulsson, C. Betsholtz, C.-H. Heldin, M. Herlyn, U. Rodeck, and H. Koproswki, *Proc. Natl. Acad. Sci. USA 83*, 7197 (1986).
60. B. A. Gilchrest, V. Treloar, A. M. Grassi, M. Yaar, G. Szabo, and E. Flynn, *J. Invest. Dermatol. 87*, 102 (1986).
61. R. Kath, U. Rodeck, H. D. Menssen, M. L. Mancianti, A. J. Linnenbach, D. E. Elder, and M. Herlyn, *Anticancer Res. 9*, 865 (1989).
62. M. L. Mancianti, M. Herlyn, D. Weil, J. Jambrosic, U. Rodeck, D. Becker, L. Diamond, W. H. Clark, and H. Koprowski, *J. Invest. Dermatol. 90*, 134 (1988).
63. M. L. Mancianti and M. Herlyn, in *Skin Tumors: Experimental and Clinical Aspects* (C. J. Conti et al., eds.), Raven Press, New York, 1989, p. 369.
64. M. Herlyn, D. Herlyn, D. E. Elder, E. Bondi, D. LaRossa, R. Hamilton, H. F. Sears, G. Balaban, D. Guerry, W. K. Clark, and H. Koprowski, *Cancer Res. 43*, 5502 (1983).
65. A. Richmond, R. Fine, D. Murray, D. H. Lawson, and J. H. Priest, *J. Invest. Dermatol. 86*, 295 (1986).
66. G. Scott, M. Stoler, S. Sarkar, and R. Halaban, *J. Invest. Dermatol. 96*, 318 (1991).
67. M. G. Fleming, S. F. Howe, and A. G. Candel, *J. Invest. Dermatol. 98*, 608 (1992).
68. V. J. McGovern, *Pathology 2*, 85 (1970).
69. W. H. Clark, D. E. Elder, D. Guerry, M. N. Epstein, M. H. Greene, and M. Van Horn, *Hum. Pathol. 15*, 1147 (1984).
70. H. M. Greene, W. H. Clark, M. A. Tucker, D. E. Elder, K. H. Kraemer, D. Guerry, W. K. Witmer, J. Thompson, I. Matozzo, and M. C. Fraser, *N. Engl. J. Med. 312*, 91 (1985).
71. M. Herlyn, W. H. Clark, U. Rodeck, M. L. Mancianti, J. Jambrosic, and H. Koprowski, *Lab. Invest. 56*, 461 (1987).
72. S. Sauvaigo, R. E. Fretts, R. J. Riopelle, and A. E. Lagarde, *Int. J. Cancer 37*, 123 (1986).
73. A. Richmond, D. H. Lawson, D. W. Nixon, J. S. Stevens, and R. K. Chawla, *Cancer Res. 42*, 3175 (1982).
74. A. Richmond and H. G. Thomas, *J. Cell. Physiol. 129*, 375 (1986).
75. J. A. Schmidt, S. B. Mizel, D. Cohen, and I. Green, *J. Immunol. 128*, 2177 (1982).
76. R. Bordoni, H. G. Thomas, and A. Richmond, *J. Cell. Biochem. 39*, 421 (1989).
77. G. P. Dotto, G. Moellmann, S. Ghosh, M. Edwards, and R. Halaban, *J. Cell. Biol. 109*, 3115 (1989).
78. A. Richmond, D. H. Lawson, D. W. Nixon, J. S. Stevens, and R. K. Chawla, *Cancer Res. 43*, 2106 (1983).
79. A. Richmond, *Semin. Dermatol. 10*, 246 (1991).
80. K. Matsushima and J. J. Oppenheim, *Cytokine 1*, 2 (1989).

81. N. Mukaida, A. Hishinuma, C. O. C. Zacharaie, J. J. Oppenheim, and K. Matsushima, *Adv. Exp. Med. Biol. 305*, 31 (1991).
82. J. M. Wang, G. Taraboletti, K. Matsushima, J. Van Damme, and A. Mantovani, *Biochem. Biophys. Res. Comm. 169*, 165 (1990).
83. H. Marquardt and G. J. Todaro, *J. Biol. Chem. 257*, 5220 (1982).
84. J. E. DeLarco, D. A. Pigott, and J. A. Lazarus, *Proc. Natl. Acad. Sci. USA 82*, 5015 (1985).
85. J. Massague, *J. Biol. Chem. 265*, 21393 (1990).
86. M. D. Waterfield, *Lancet 1*, 1243 (1989).
87. G. L. Brown, L. B. Namey, J. Griffen, A. B. Cramer, J. M. Gancey, L. J. Curtsinger, L. Holtzin, G. S. Schultz, M. Jurkiewicz, and J. B. Lynch, *N. Engl. J. Med. 321*, 76 (1989).
88. S. E. Lynch, R. B. Colvin, and H. N. Antoniades, *J. Clin. Invest. 84*, 640 (1989).
89. D. L. Ellis, L. B. Nanney, and L. E. King, Jr., *J. Invest. Dermatol. 94*, 521 (1990).
90. S. Bodmer, K. Strommer, K. Frei, C. Siepl, N. DeTribolet, I. Heid, and A. Fontana, *J. Immunol. 143*, 3222 (1989).
91. A. B. Roberts, M. A. Anzano, L. M. Wakefield, N. S. Roche, D. F. Stern, and M. B. Sporn, *Proc. Natl. Acad. Sci. USA 82*, 119 (1985).
92. C. A. Armstrong, D. C. Tara, C. E. Hart, A. Köck, T. A. Luger, and J. C. Ansel, *Exp. Dermatol. 1*, 37 (1992).
93. C. H. Heldin and B. Westermark, *Cell 37*, 9 (1984).
94. R. Ross, *Ann. Rev. Med. 38*, 71 (1987).
95. L. T. Williams, *Clin. Res. 36*, 5 (1988).
96. D. Damm, G. Shipley, C. Hart, and J. Ansel, in *Molecular and Cellular Biology of Cytokines* (J. Oppenheim, M. C. Powanda, M. J. Kluger, C. Dinarello, eds.), Wiley-Liss, New York, 1990, p. 111.
97. A. Hammacher, U. Hellman, A. Johnsson, A. Ostman, K. Gunnarsson, B. Westmark, A. Wasteson, and C.-A. Heldin, *Biol. Chem. 263*, 16493 (1988).
98. C. Betsholtz, A. Johnsson, C.-H. Heldin, B. Westermark, P. Lind, M. S. Urdea, R. Eddy, T. B. Shows, K. Philpott, A. L. Mellor, T. J. Knott, and J. Scott, *Nature 320*, 695 (1986).
99. M. P. Beckmann, C. Betsholtz, C.-H. Heldin, B. Westermark, E. DiMarco, P. P. Di Fiore, K. C. Robbins, and S. A. Aaronson, *Science 241*, 1346 (1988).
100. C. Betsholtz, B. Westermark, B. Ek, and C.-H. Heldin, *Cell 39*, 447 (1984).
101. A. Köck, T. Schwarz, A. Urbanski, Z. Peng, M. Vetterlein, M. Micksche, J. C. Ansel, H. F. Kung, and T. A. Luger, *J. Natl. Cancer Inst. 81*, 36 (1989).
102. J. L. Bennicelli, J. Elias, J. Kern, and D. Guerry, *Cancer Res. 49*, 930 (1989).
103. B. Robertson, L. Gahring, R. Newton, and R. Daynes, *J. Invest. Dermatol. 88*, 380 (1987).
104. M. L. Austin, R. Rothlein, A. K. Bhan, C. A. Dinarello, and T. A. Springer, *J. Immunol. 137*, 245 (1986).
105. L. Alby and R. Auerbach, *Proc. Natl. Acad. Sci. USA 81*, 5739 (1984).
106. M. Temponi, R. Romano, C. M. D'Urso, Z. Want, U. Kekish, and S. Ferrone, *Semin. Oncol. 15*, 595 (1988).

107. R. Giavazzi, A. Garofalo, M. R. Bani, M. Abbate, P. Ghezzi, D. Boraschi, A. Mantovani, and E. Dejana, *Cancer Res. 50*, 4771 (1990).
108. B. J. Sugerman, B. B. Aggarwal, P. E. Hass, I. S. Figari, M. A. Palladino, and H. Shepard, *Science 230*, 943 (1985).
109. A. S. Rosenberg, M. T. Lotze, L. M. Mull, S. Leitman, A. E. Chang, S. E. Ettinghausen, Y. L. Matory, J. M. Skibber, E. Shiloni, J. T. Vetto, C. A. Seipp, C. Simpson, and C. M. Reichert, *N. Engl. J. Med. 313*, 1485 (1985).
110. T. A. Luger, J. Krutmann, R. Kirnbauer, A. Urbanski, T. Schwarz, G. Klappacher, A. Köck, M. Micksche, J. Malejczyk, E. Schauer, L. T. May, and P. B. Sehgal, *J. Immunol. 143*, 1206 (1989).
111. L. B. Lachman, C. A. Dinarello, N. D. Llansa, and I. J. Fidler, *J. Immunol. 136*, 3098 (1986).
112. K. Onozaki, K. Matsushima, B. B. Aggarwal, and J. J. Oppenheim, *J. Immunol. 1353*, 3962 (1985).
113. Y. Morinaga, H. Suzuki, F. Takatsuki, Y. Akiyama, T. Taniyam, K. Matsushima, and K. Onozaki, *J. Immunol. 143*, 3538 (1989).
114. P. B. Sehgal and L. T. May, *J. Interferon Res. 7*, 521 (1987).
115. K. Yasukawa, T. Hirano, Y. Watanabe, K. Muratani, T. Matsuda, S. Nakai, and T. Kishimoto, *EMBO J. 6*, 2939 (1987).
116. N. Tohyama, H. Karasuyama, and T. Tada, *J. Exp. Med. 171*, 389 (1990).
117. S. A. Miles, A. R. Rezai, J. F. Salazar-Gonzelez, M. V. Meyden, R. Stevens, D. M. Logan, R. T. Mitsuyasu, T. Taga, R. Hirano, R. Kishimoto, and O. Martinez-Maza, *Proc. Natl. Acad. Sci. USA 87*, 4068 (1990).
118. J. J. Mule, J. K. McIntosh, D. M. Jablons, and S. A. Rosenberg, *J. Exp. Med. 171*, 629 (1990).
119. C. A. Armstrong, S. V. Koppula, D. C. Tara, and J. C. Ansel, *J. Invest. Dermatol. 98*, 565 (1992).
120. M. Sabatini, J. Chavez, G. R. Mundy, and L. F. Bonewald, *Cancer Res. 50*, 2673 (1990).
121. D. C. Metcalf, C. G. Begley, G. R. Johnson, N. A. Nicola, M. A. Vadas, A. F. Lopez, D. J. Williamson, G. G. Wong, S. C. Clark, and E. A. Wang, *Blood 67*, 37 (1986).
122. C. A. Sieff, S. G. Emerson, R. E. Conahue, D. G. Nathan, E. A. Wang, G. G. Wong, and S. C. Clark, *Science 230*, 1171 (1985).
123. T. S. Kupper, F. Lee, D. Coleman, J. Chodakewitz, P. Flood, and M. Horowitz, *J. Invest. Dermatol. 91*, 185 (1988).
124. Y. Tsuchiya, M. Igarashi, R. Suzuki, and K. Kumagai, *J. Immunol. 141*, 699 (1988).
125. D. C. Yound and J. D. Griffin, *Blood 68*, 1178 (1986).
126. J. E. Groopman, J. M. Molina, and D. T. Scadden, *N. Engl. J. Med. 321*, 1449 (1989).

# IV
# CYTOKINE THERAPY

# 22
# Cytokines—Therapeutic Aspects for Skin Diseases

**Thomas A. Luger, Franz Trautinger,* and Thomas Schwarz**
*Ludwig Boltzmann Institute for Cell Biology and Immunobiology of the Skin*
*University of Münster*
*Münster, Germany*

## I. INTRODUCTION

Cytokines represent a heterogeneous group of mediators regulating cell activation, differentiation, and proliferation. They are produced by a variety of cells and exert their biological activities in an autocrine, paracrine, and endocrine way via binding to specific cell surface receptors. Increasing information about the functional properties of cytokines provided insight into a complex network of interacting mediators [1, 2]. The crucial role of cytokines in the mediation of inflammatory and immunological reactions as well as in cell differentiation and tumor growth suggested a therapeutic potential for these mediators. With the elucidation of their molecular structure and the availability of recombinant factors, cytokines recently have been introduced in the treatment of various skin diseases. Although cytokines and growth factors have been used therapeutically in a variety of disorders, this chapter will include only dermatological aspects. In addition, a huge number of clinical studies is going on, thus the following can be only a selection of trials showing major trends. Moreover, clinicians should refer carefully to the original articles before attempting any new or even controversial therapy.

---

**Current affiliation*: University of Vienna, Vienna, Austria.

## II. INTERLEUKINS

Malignancies were the first diseases in which cytokines were applied therapeutically; clinical trials have been performed with interleukin (IL)-2 and IL-4 so far. Little experience exists concerning the clinical use of other interleukins due to the fact that many of these factors were identified quite recently and became available in recombinant form quickly.

IL-2 has been shown to be of benefit in the treatment of patients with melanoma, either as monotherapy or in conjunction with adoptive immunotherapy using concurrent transfer of either lymphokine activated killer cells (LAK) or tumor-infiltrating lymphocytes (TIL) [3–6]. Either circulating leukocytes (LAK) or lymphocytes derived from the peritumoral area (TIL) are expanded in vitro in the presence of IL-2 and subsequently reinfused with IL-2 [7, 8]. In general, the administration of LAK cells increases the incidence of transient complete remission, but not the overall response [9]. Upon infusion of TIL, 23% of melanoma patients responded [6]. Clinical trials are in progress in which IL-2 is used in combination with other lymphokines (IL-4, tumor necrosis factor [TNF-$\alpha$], interferons [IFN], or colony-stimulating factors [CSF]) and antitumor monoclonal antibodies or chemotherapy [9, 10]. Recent protocols include application of low-dose subcutaneous ($1.8–18 \times 10^6$ U/m$^2$/day) IL-2 and IFN-$\alpha$ ($3–6 \times 10^6$ U/m$^2$ 3x/week). Preliminary data indicate that this outpatient regimen can induce objective tumor regressions with low systemic toxicity (WHO grade I and II) in renal cancer and melanoma [11]. There is also recent evidence that IL-2 may be effective in the treatment of hemangioendothelioma. Intralesional administration resulted in a disappearance of the tumor, and no recurrence within 1 year was seen [12].

Recently, IL-2 has been demonstrated to inhibit the IL-4–induced human IgE and $IgG_4$ secretion in vivo [13], suggesting that IL-2 may be useful for treatment of patients with atopic dermatitis. Accordingly, IL-2 ($1–2 \times 10^4$ U/kg 3x/day for 9–12 days) was given to 6 patients suffering from severe atopic dermatitis. Although IL-2 therapy resulted in a significant improvement of clinical symptoms in all patients, the disease relapsed 4–6 weeks after stopping treatment [14]. Laboratory findings revealed a decrease in circulating $CD4^+$ T cells, but no change in serum IgE levels.

Due to the high doses of IL-2 usually administered, toxicity is severe and mainly related to the vascular leak syndrome [4, 6]. Therefore, IL-2 therapy appears to be restricted to experienced personnel in intensive care units. In addition, diffuse erythema, pruritis, and desquamation have been observed. Moreover, erythrodermic exacerbations of psoriasis in patients who are receiving IL-2 and LAK have been reported [15].

## III. TUMOR NECROSIS FACTORS

Based on its biological activities observed in animal studies and in in vitro assays, tumor necrosis factor alpha (TNF-$\alpha$) appeared to exhibit therapeutic potential [16]. However, TNF-$\alpha$ seems to be one of the primary mediators of septic syndrome and shock, thus its application is limited by severe systemic and local adverse reactions. Upon subcutaneous injection exceeding 150 $\mu g/m^2$/day, side effects include severe hypotension, fever, chills, headache, nausea, vomiting, diarrhea, and anorexia [17, 18]. Therefore, in most cases the concentrations applicable may be too low to provide therapeutic benefit. Accordingly, disappointing results were obtained by systemic and intratumoral application of TNF-$\alpha$ in various cancers including melanoma [18, 19]. Recently, however, regionally advanced melanoma has been treated with a combination of TNF-$\alpha$ (2–4 mg), IFN-$\gamma$ (200 $\mu$g), and melphalan (38–120 mg) by isolated limb perfusion. Using this technique, high levels of TNF-$\alpha$ in the affected area without significant systemic toxicity are achieved. Twenty-one complete responses and 2 partial responses have been observed in 23 patients [20]. Because of severe toxicity, the described regimen is only suitable for local treatment and not available for widespread disease. Intraperitoneal injection of TNF-$\alpha$ has been shown to induce resorption of malignant ascites caused by ovarian, breast, gastrointestinal, and other cancers. This treatment caused an improvement of subjective symptoms without affecting the course of the underlying disease [21].

Promising but preliminary results have been obtained by the systemic application of TNF-$\alpha$ in severe psoriasis. These studies were based on experimental data showing an absence of TNF-$\alpha$ and decreased levels of IL-1 in psoriatic skin. Of 5 patients treated with TNF-$\alpha$ ($2–5 \times 10^5$/U/$m^2$ 3–5x/week for 1–3 months), complete clearing of the lesions was observed in three patients and partial clearing in one patient [22, 23]. Tolerable and fully reversible side effects were observed including fever, chills, leukocytosis, and antistreptolysin elevation. However, long-term results are not available yet. In addition, placebo-controlled trials are necessary in order to appreciate the value of this therapy. There are also reports about the intralesional application of TNF-$\alpha$ for treatment of cutaneous tumors. Accordingly, one case of Merkel cell carcinoma was treated successfully with intratumoral administration of TNF-$\alpha$ [24]. Furthermore, in one patient with primary cutaneous plasmacytoma without systemic involvement, intralesional TNF-$\alpha$ resulted in a marked reduction of tumor size [25].

## IV. COLONY-STIMULATING FACTORS

Animal studies and clinical phase I trials with hematopoietic growth factors indicated their potential use in myelodysplasia, neutropenia, chemotherapy-induced bone marrow toxicity, and bone marrow transplantation [26, 27]. Meanwhile CSF can be regarded as an essential therapeutic tool in various hematological disorders.

## A. AIDS

In order to improve the immune function and to overcome chemotherapy-related side effects, CSF have been applied in human immunodeficiency virus (HIV-1)–infected patients. GM-CSF treatment resulted in a rapid dose-dependent increase of neutrophils and eosinophils as well as in an improvement of neutrophil function [28, 29]. Furthermore, in preliminary trials GM-CSF and G-CSF overcame the myelotoxicity of azidothymidine therapy [30, 31]. However, a beneficial effect on the overall clinical outcome of these patients has not been demonstrated so far. Neutropenia usually limits the use of ganciclovir, which in some patients with AIDS-related cytomegalovirus retinitis has to be given for lifetime [32]. The combination of GM-CSF and ganciclovir reversed ganciclovir-induced neutropenia in these patients. However, in some AIDS patients treated with GM-CSF, increased levels of p24 HIV antigen have been observed. Therefore, it may be speculated that GM-CSF induces HIV-1 replication via activation of virus harboring macrophages [33–35]. Thus GM-CSF should be administered only concurrently with antiretroviral drugs. On the other hand, in vitro studies have demonstrated that the antiviral effect of azidothymidine may be potentiated by GM-CSF, which suggests a therapeutic benefit of this combination [36, 37]. In contrast, neither in vivo nor in vitro does G-CSF appear to have any effect on HIV replication [30, 34].

## B. Cutaneous Tumors

Bone marrow toxicity with subsequent susceptibility to infection and hemorrhage is a dose-limiting side effect of most chemotherapeutic agents. Because of the ability of CSFs to counteract these complications, many patients undergoing chemotherapy including those with melanoma seem to be potential candidates for the application of hematopoietic growth factors. In phase I studies different routes of administration have been used to define the optimal biological dose, toxicity, and pharmacokinetics of GM-CSF, G-CSF, M-CSF, and IL-3 [27]. Application of these factors has been demonstrated to result in reduced episodes of infection and in fewer chemotherapy delays [38, 39]. In addition, because of the immunomodulating effects of CSF, neutrophils and monocytes, respectively, may become more efficient in attacking cancer cells, especially when used in combination with monoclonal antibodies directed against melanoma surface antigens [40].

## C. Other Dermatoses

GM-CSF is known to stimulate myeloid cells to activate monocytes and to potentiate Langerhans cell functions. In a recent study rhGM-CSF was administered subcutaneously to 35 patients with borderline and polar lepromatous forms of leprosy (7.5–45 μg/day for 10 days). There was no evidence of an enhanced cell-mediated response to *Mycobacterium leprae*, and bacillary numbers remained unchanged. However, an enhanced wound healing in 22 out of 26 4-mm punch biopsy sites of patients receiving GM-CSF was observed, when compared to the healing time of untreated patients. In addition to enhancing keratinocyte proliferation, the selective recruitment of Langerhans cells into the dermis was observed at the GM-CSF–treated site [41].

## D. Side Effects

In contrast to most other biological response modifiers, CSFs are quite well tolerated. At therapeutic doses, side effects of GM-CSF include malaise, mild elevation in transaminase levels, bone pain, and a cutaneous eruptions, all being rather mild to moderate and fully reversible [38, 39, 42–44]. Serious toxic effects, such as capillary leak syndrome with pleural and pericardial effusions, ascites, and large vessel thrombocytosis, have been observed only when the GM-CSF dose exceeded 30 μg/kg/day [42, 43]. These severe effects may not be related only to GM-CSF directly, but may also result from an increased endogenous production of IL-1 and TNF-α after GM-CSF administration [46]. Recently, the development of a cutaneous maculopapulous eruption was reported in patients receiving GM-CSF [47, 48].

G-CSF is well tolerated, and except bone pain no significant side effects have been reported. However, one case of neutrophilic organ infiltration that resembled acute febrile neutrophilic syndrome (Sweet's syndrome) has been described. So far no data describing the toxicity of other hematopoietic growth factors are available [42–44, 49, 50]. The important question whether CSF therapy in some cases could lead to development of leukemia needs to be clarified because GM-CSF produced leukemic transformation of retrovirus-infected cells in vitro [51]. Although exposure to GM-CSF and G-CSF leads to enhanced proliferation of various solid tumor cell lines in vitro, no enhancement of in vivo growth of solid or lymphoid tumors has been reported in the patients treated so far [52]. The therapeutic use of CSFs could be further limited by the development of circulating antibodies, which have recently been observed [53].

# V. INTERFERONS

Because of their potent in vitro effects on immune and inflammatory responses as well as cell growth, IFNs were one of the first cytokines applied in humans [54]. Accordingly, quite a number of clinical trials have been performed using interferons in several skin diseases.

## A. Viral Diseases

Based on their antiviral effect, IFNs have been widely used for the treatment of viral diseases mainly caused by herpes- and papillomaviruses [55]. In patients with frequent recurrences of herpes simplex virus (HSV) infection, different schedules of subcutaneous administration of recombinant IFN-$\alpha$ resulted in suppression and decreased duration of the infection. A high dose regimen ($5 \times 10^5$ U/kg/day for 2 weeks) as well as moderate doses ($6 \times 10^6$ U for 3 days) showed similar beneficial effects [56, 57]. The response of first-episode herpes genitalis was similar [58]. Furthermore, in labial and genital herpes the topical application of either IFN-$\beta$ or IFN-$\alpha$ preparations proved to be effective in reducing the number of recurrences and the duration of the eruption [59–61]. When the efficacy of IFN-$\alpha$ ($9 \times 10^6$ U/day) for the treatment of first-episode herpes genitalis was compared with topical acyclovir, it proved not to be superior in reducing the frequency or severity of relapses [62]. Placebo-controlled studies showed a beneficial effect of IFN-$\alpha$ (1.7–5.1 $\times 10^5$ U/kg/day) on the clinical course of herpes zoster in immunocompromised patients [63–65]. Similarly, intravenous IFN-$\beta$ ($2 \times 10^6$ U/day) in immunocompromised patients was found to be of clinical benefit [66]. When compared with acyclovir ($3 \times 5$ mg/kg/day), IFN-$\alpha$ ($1 \times 10^7$ U/day) turned out to be equally effective in herpes zoster. Side effects, however, were observed more frequently in IFN-treated patients than in those given acyclovir [67].

Early studies addressing the effect of IFN in the treatment of condylomata acuminata demonstrated that high-dose regimens of IFN-$\alpha$ ($1.8 \times 10^7$ U/day) are similarly effective as low-dose regimens ($1.5 \times 10^6$ U/day) [68]. Because of the side effects in association with high-dose IFN therapy in the following studies, IFN-$\alpha$ mostly was used at a dosage of $1 \times 10^6$ U 3x/week for 3 weeks either intralesionally or subcutaneously [69–71]. Complete remission usually was observed in 30–50% of IFN-treated lesions versus a 15–30% response to placebo therapy [55,68]. Although the in vitro antiviral effect of IFN-$\gamma$ is weaker compared to IFN-$\alpha$ in some studies, IFN-$\gamma$ also was used for treatment of condylomata acuminata. A "cyclic" therapy regimen consisted of subcutaneous injection of either IFN—$\alpha$ ($1.5 \times 10^6$ U) or IFN-$\gamma$ (50 $\mu$g) daily for 7 days followed by 4 weeks without therapy. After three to four cycles, a 60% response rate could be observed [72]. Considering the published data the beneficial effects of IFN-$\gamma$ in the treatment of condylomata acuminata are controversial [73]. Although monotherapy for condylomata acuminata with IFN-$\alpha$ did not prove to be significantly superior

In vitro, IFN-$\alpha$ inhibits collagen and glycosaminoglycan production, normalizes collagenase activity, and inhibits fibroblast proliferation [146]. These data suggested IFN-$\alpha$ to be a promising candidate for treatment of fibrotic disorders such as keloids or scleroderma. Two intralesional injections of IFN-$\alpha$ ($1.5 \times 10^6$ U/injection) into progressively enlarging keloids resulted in more than 40% reduction in size [146]. Similar results were obtained with IFN-$\gamma$ [147]. Clinical trials for treatment of systemic sclerosis have also been performed with IFN-$\beta$ ($1 \times 10^6$ U/day for 3 weeks 4x/year) or IFN-$\gamma$ (50 $\mu$g 3x/week for 12 months) [148, 149]. Treatment of systemic sclerosis with IFN-$\gamma$ resulted in an improvement in the total skin score, whereas dysphagia, Raynaud's phenomenon, and cardiac involvement was not affected [149].

It has been reported that IFN-$\alpha$ blocks the migration of endothelial cells in vitro and inhibits angiogenesis in mice [150, 151]. These findings prompted the investigation of the efficacy of subcutaneous injections of IFN-$\alpha$ (up to $3 \times 10^6$ U/m$^2$ daily) for treatment of infants with hemangiomas that failed to respond to corticosteroid treatment. In 18 out of 20 patients the hemangiomas regressed by 50% or more after an average 7.8 months of treatment [152]. No short-term side effects have been noticed so far, and the children's growth and development seems to be normal.

A remarkable response to IFN-$\alpha$ ($5 \times 10^6$ U 3x/week) was observed in one patient with systemic mastocytosis. As in the case with hematological disorders, the time until remission was quite long (2 months) [153]. Immunomodulatory agents were used with moderate success for treatment of alopecia areata, suggesting a potential therapeutic value of IFN. However, intralesional IFN-$\alpha$ had no significant effect on alopecia areata [154]. Systemic therapy with either IFN-$\alpha$ or IFN-$\gamma$ appears to be effective in patients with severe Behçet's disease, as most patients showed rapid clearing of cutaneous and mucosal lesions [155–158].

Cytokines also play an important role in infectious diseases characterized by granuloma formation, i.e., visceral and cutaneous leishmaniasis and lepromatous leprosy [159–161]. Based on in vitro investigations and animal studies, a stimulation of macrophages and an enhancement of the specific T-cell response in experimental leishmaniasis could be demonstrated [161, 162]. In a placebo-controlled study, intralesional IFN-$\gamma$ (25 $\mu$g 4x/week) injections resulted in complete clearance of 4 out of 13 lesions caused by *L. braziliensis* and 9 out of 13 lesions caused by *L. tropica* [161]. In addition, systemic IFN-$\gamma$ (50 $\mu$g/m$^2$/day for 4 weeks) proved to be useful in treating cutaneous leishmaniasis [162]. Systemic treatment with IFN-$\gamma$ in combination with pentavalent antimony has been shown to be effective in antimony-refractory visceral leishmaniasis as well as in unpretreated patients [160].

total tumor burden may be an important factor because tumors in an advanced stage rarely respond to IFN. Recent studies indicate that intralesional injection of IFN-$\alpha$ and IFN-$\beta$, respectively, may be effective in cutaneous metastases [100–103]. However, the overall survival is not significantly affected. The initially reported beneficial effect of cimetidine in combination with IFN-$\alpha$ could not be confirmed [104]. Recently, encouraging results (30% response) were obtained with a combination of IFN-$\alpha$ and DTIC [10, 101, 104–108]. Preliminary observations indicate a beneficial effect of IFN-$\alpha$ in an adjuvant setting in patients with high-risk melanoma [109]. Despite the low efficacy of IFN monotherapy in metastatic disease, several randomized prospective studies are now being performed with IFNs as an adjuvant or in combination with chemotherapy [104].

Treatment of patients with disseminated AIDS-associated Kaposi's sarcoma with IFN-$\alpha$ revealed that high doses resulted in regression in 20–50% of the patients [110, 111]. However, high-dose IFN therapy (up to $4 \times 10^7$ U/day) is limited due to the occurrence of severe side effects, and IFN-$\alpha$ in doses less than $2 \times 10^6$ U/m$^2$ did not prove to be useful [112]. In addition, a correlation between the immune profile and the response rate was observed. Patients with more than 400 CD4$^+$ cells responded best, whereas patients with fewer than 150 CD4$^+$ cells did not [113]. In advanced stages of disseminated Kaposi's sarcoma IFN-$\alpha$ therapy seems to be ineffective [114]. Although extracutaneous lesions of Kaposi's sarcoma do not respond to IFN-$\alpha$ therapy, single cutaneous tumors can be treated effectively with intralesional injection [115]. In contrast to the epidemic form, few data are available dealing with the response of classical Kaposi's sarcoma to IFN (objective regression of cutaneous lesions of more than 50% in 7 out of 10 patients) [116].

Recently, IFN-$\alpha$ applied intralesionally ($1.5 \times 10^6$ U 3x/week for 3 weeks) was introduced into the treatment of actinic keratoses, basal cell carcinomas, and squamous cell carcinomas [117]. In most cases the response has been evaluated during a 12-week posttreatment period, and in some cases the clearance has been confirmed by excisional biopsy specimens. The overall response rate in most trials has been between 80 and 100% [118-121]. In contrast, topically applied IFN-$\alpha$ ($3 \times 10^7$ U 4x/day for 4 weeks) was less effective [118]. According to a recent study, the number of applications can be reduced significantly by injecting a sustained-release formulation of IFN-$\alpha$ into basal cell carcinomas (3 injections of $1 \times 10^6$ U) [123]. Similarly, intralesional IFN-$\gamma$ seems to be effective in treating basal cell carcinomas [124], however, the results of controlled studies have not yet been reported [125]. Side effects are minimal except for moderate pain during injection, which has to be given in the base of the lesion and not directly into the neoplasm. Therefore, in certain subgroups of patients in whom to conventional therapy, adjuvant therapy with IFN-$\alpha$ or IFN-$\beta$ either topically or systemically after surgery, cryotherapy, or laser treatment alone or in combination with retinoids appears to be promising [74–76]. With regard to bowenoid papulosis preliminary data indicate that continuous treatment with IFN-$\gamma$ ($4 \times 10^6$ U 3x/week for 13 weeks) appears to be effective, showing a complete response in 3 of 4 patients [77].

Several studies focus on IFN treatment for common warts, but its value is still uncertain. Whereas in some trials no effect in comparison to a placebo group was reported, response rates up to 80% were observed in others [69, 78, 79]. Further controlled studies are needed to evaluate the efficacy of IFNs in the treatment of common warts. At present because of their questionable efficacy and the pain of intralesional injection, IFNs cannot be recommended as the first therapy of choice. In contrast, epidermodysplasia verruciformis can be treated successfully with systemic IFN-$\alpha$, however, discontinuation of treatment results in a rapid relapse [80].

## B. Cutaneous Neoplasms

Recombinant IFN-$\alpha$ either alone or in combination with other therapy regimens has been demonstrated to be effective to treat cutaneous T-cell lymphomas (CTLL). In initial studies high-dose IFN-$\alpha$ (up to $5 \times 10^7$ U/m$^2$) revealed a response rate of more than 50% [81]. In another randomized trial low-dose IFN-$\alpha$ ($3 \times 10^6$ U/m$^2$) was compared to an escalating dose regimen (up to $3.6 \times 10^7$ U/m$^2$) resulting in an overall response of 68% (optimal dose > $3 \times 10^6$ U/m$^2$) [82]. Intralesional application of low-dose IFN-$\alpha$ ($1 \times 10^6$ U/week for 4 weeks) into the plaques resulted in regression of most lesions, whereas systemic low-dose IFN-$\alpha$ ($5 \times 10^6$ U 3x/week for 4 weeks) was not effective in five patients [83, 84]. Promising data recently were reported by several groups with the use of a combination of IFN-$\alpha$ ($18 \times 10^6$ U 3x/week) and retinoids (0.7 mg/kg/day) yielding a response rate of about 50% (85–87]. Concurrent treatment of IFN-$\alpha$ ($6–30 \times 10^6$ U 3x/week) with PUVA in 15 patients gave an overall response rate of 93% [88]. A beneficial effect of low-dose IFN-$\alpha$ and extracorporal photopheresis recently was observed in a patient with Sézary syndrome [89]. Combinations of IFN-$\alpha$ with chemotherapeutic agents (e.g., deoxycoformicin) in the treatment of low-grade lymphoproliferative malignancies are under current investigation [90].

Because of their antiproliferative and immunomodulating effects in vitro, IFNs have been used in the treatment of melanoma [91, 92]. Response rates achieved with systemic IFN-$\alpha$ either high or low dose in metastatic melanoma were in the range of 5–30% [93–96]. IFN-$\gamma$ did not appear to be superior to IFN-$\alpha$ [97, 98]. Soft tissue metastases are more likely to respond, whereas bone or liver metastases seem to be resistant [91, 99]. In addition, excisions of cancer carries significant functional and surgical risks, intralesional IFN may offer a valuable alternative.

## C. Other Dermatoses

Mononuclear cells of patients with atopic dermatitis were found to produce increased levels of IL-4, but decreased levels of IFN-$\gamma$. Moreover, IL-4 levels correlated positively and IFN-$\gamma$ levels negatively with the patients' serum IgE levels [126–128]. In preliminary studies, subcutaneous injections of IFN-$\gamma$ (100 $\mu$g 5x/week followed by 100 $\mu$g 3x/week for 3 weeks) resulted in remarkable improvement of skin lesions associated with a decrease in serum IgE levels [129]. Another study revealed similar results when using three successive dose levels each for 5 days (100 $\mu$g, 50 $\mu$g, and 20 $\mu$g) or 50 $\mu$g/day for 6 weeks [130]. A recently completed multicenter randomized double-blind placebo-controlled trial applying IFN-$\gamma$ in atopic dermatitis (50 $\mu$g/m$^2$ daily for 12 weeks) revealed an overall response rate of 50% versus 21% in the placebo group. Patients less than 20 years old responded with a significant improvement of the skin lesions in 67%. In contrast to other studies, serum IgE levels did not change during therapy [131]. Although IFN-$\alpha$ treatment inhibited IgE synthesis and improved the cutaneous eruptions in a patient with hyper-IgE syndrome, patients with severe atopic dermatitis do not seem to benefit from IFN-$\alpha$ (3 $\times$ 10$^6$ U 3x/week) treatment [132, 133].

The efficacy of IFN-$\alpha$ or IFN-$\gamma$ in psoriasis is controversial. Favorable results have been observed in the treatment of psoriatic arthropathy with IFN-$\gamma$ [134]. However, IFN-$\gamma$ (100–250 $\mu$g/m$^2$/day for 4 weeks) only had minor effects on chronic plaque psoriasis [135, 136], while IFN-$\alpha$ appears to be of limited benefit or to cause even exacerbation in some cases [137, 138]. There is clinical evidence that IFN therapy is improving the clinical course of certain autoimmune diseases inducing rheumatoid arthritis, multiple sclerosis, and thrombocytopenic purpura [139–141]. Accordingly, clinical trials have been performed to evaluate the efficacy of IFN-$\alpha$ (40–120 U/week for 4–13 weeks) for treatment of discoid lupus erythematosus and subacute cutaneous lupus erythematosus [142]. A marked improvement was observed in 8 out of 10 patients. However, most patients relapsed after discontinuation of therapy.

Treatment of chronic hepatitis with IFN-$\alpha$ has been proven to be effective [143]. Recently, two patients with hepatitis B and concomitant lichen planus were treated with IFN-$\alpha$ (3 $\times$ 10$^6$ U 3x/week for 6 months). A total and prolonged disappearance of the lichen planus lesions was observed in both patients, who did not receive any other local or systemic therapies [144]. However it should be noted that in one case the appearance of lichen planus was observed during IFN-$\alpha$ therapy for a myeloma [145].

IFNs have also been used to treat chronic granulomatous disease in children and granuloma annulare [163–165]. Although some effectiveness was noticed, further studies are required.

## D. Side Effects

Most patients who receive systemic IFN therapy experience flulike symptoms such as fever, chills, headache, myalgia, and nausea that respond well to acetaminophen. Hematological changes include leukopenia and thrombopenia. Side effects usually do not exceed WHO grade II, and severe changes have been observed only at high doses. Usually the side effects are rapidly reversible, and no cumulative toxicity has been noticed. However, recently the occurrence of skin necrosis at the site of injection has been observed in a patient receiving IFN-$\alpha$ subcutaneously for treatment of AIDS-related Kaposi's sarcoma [166]. In some cases, IFN therapy has led to the formation of antinuclear antibodies and to the exacerbation of an underlying autoimmune disease [167]. Another worrisome observation during IFN therapy is the development of neutralizing antibodies [168, 169]. This is of importance because the resistance to IFN treatment in hairy cell leukemia correlates quite well with the development of neutralizing antibodies. However, patients who develop antibodies against recombinant IFN-$\alpha$ still respond well to natural IFN-$\alpha$.

# VI. GROWTH FACTORS

Growth factors originally have been regarded as a heterogeneous group of mediators regulating primarily cell proliferation. This family includes epidermal growth factor (EGF), transforming growth factor alpha (TGF-$\alpha$), fibroblast growth factors (FGF), nerve growth factor (NGF), insulin-like growth factors (IGF), and platelet-derived growth factor (PDGF). They control the growth of normal and malignant cells as well as the formation of matrix proteins. Furthermore, growth factors turned out to be important mediators of immunity and cell surface alteration [170–174].

Enhancement of wound healing and reepithelialization is a central problem in the treatment of poorly healing wounds and extensive burn injuries, particularly when autologous donor sites are limited. In vitro and in vivo studies have demonstrated that keratinocyte-derived cytokines and growth factors are involved in pathophysiological mechanisms of wound healing such as local inflammation, reepithelialization, and synthesis of matrix proteins [174–177]. The potential benefit of keratinocyte-derived mediators is further based on the observation that after transplantation of allogeneic-cultured keratinocytes, healing of chronic ulcers was observed in spite of rejection of the grafted cells [178]. Accordingly, donor-derived epidermal cells may produce growth factors such as bFGF, TGF-$\alpha$, TGF-$\beta$, IL-1, and IL-6, which may be responsible for accelerated wound healing [179].

Several studies have been performed to address the usefulness of in vivo application of these factors in animals as well as in humans. Recent observations showed a beneficial effect when either IL-1, EGF, TGF-$\alpha$, FGF, or PDGF was applied topically either in ointment or in buffered solution [180–185]. When experimental skin graft donor sites of patients who required skin transplantation were treated with silver sulfadiazine cream with or without EGF (10 $\mu$g/ml), EGF-containing cream significantly decreased the average duration of healing time [184]. Recently, in a randomized phase I/II double-blind placebo-controlled study, PDGF (100 $\mu$g/ml for 28 days) significantly improved the healing of chronic pressure ulcers [185]. Although these results appear promising, further studies are needed to clarify whether a single growth factor or, more likely, a combination of several mediators will be useful therapeutically to improve wound healing. In addition, TGF-$\beta$ seems to be essential for hypertrophic scar formation since anti-TGF-$\beta$ recently has been reported to be effective in controlling scar formation [186].

## VII. CONCLUSION

The availability of recombinant cytokines in sufficient amounts allowed the use of these potent regulatory mediators in clinical trials for a variety of diseases. In some instances they already can be regarded as useful therapeutic alternatives. Future aspects include application of cytokines in combination with standard regimens such as chemo- or radiation therapy. Another promising field is cytokine gene therapy. Accordingly, first clinical trials are being performed using TILs transfected with the TNF-$\alpha$ genes for treatment of patients with melanoma [187, 188]. However, much needs to be elucidated with regard to the knowledge of the complex cytokine interactions in order to get a better insight into the role of these mediators in the pathogenesis of diseases as well as to use them more efficiently in therapy.

## ACKNOWLEDGMENT

We wish to thank M. Orschel for her expert secretarial assistance.

## NOTE ADDED IN PROOF

### Interleukins

The occurrence of cutaneous side effects has been reported in 72% of patients receiving rhIL-2 for metastatic melanoma. In most cases they were mild, presenting as burning pruriginous erythema, but in some cases blister formation and necrotic lesions were observed. These non-treatment-limiting cutaneous side effects disappeared without sequelae upon discontinuation of rhIL-2 [189]. Treatment of a refractory B-cell lymphocytic lymphoma with IL-2 was reported to cause a reversible increase of peripheral monoclonal B-cell lymphocytes [190].

## Colony Stimulating Factors

Treatment induced mylosuppression in AIDS patients recently was reported to be successfully treated with G-CSF. Since G-CSF in contrast to GM-CSF does not stimulate HIV infected monocytes this cytokine preferentially should be used in HIV infected patients. However, one patient with HIV-associated Kaposi sarcoma developed a tumor-like infiltration resembling Burkitt's lymphoma during G-CSF therapy. Following discontinuation of G-CSF the tumor regressed spontaneously [191, 192]. Recently, it was reported that psoriasis in one patient with aplastic anemia completely cleared after treatment with GM-CSF (3 $\mu$g/kg/3 months) [193].

## Interferons

Intralesional rhIFN/$\beta$ ($1 \times 10^6$ U 3x/week/3 weeks) was shown to be effective in treating basal cell carcinoma [194]. An overall complete response rate of 88.2% was obtained when small sun-induced squamous cell carcinomas were treated intralesionally with rhIFN$\alpha$ ($1.5 \times 10^6$ U 3x/week/3 weeks) [195]. In one case the successful therapy of metastatic eccrine poroma using perilesional IFN$\alpha$ and IL-2 was reported [196]. IFN$\alpha$ also appears to be useful in treating Ofuji's papuloerythoderma [197]. In addition to IFN$\alpha$ IFN$\gamma$ (50 mg 3x/weeks/12 weeks) was also demonstrated to be very effective for the treatment of extensive lichen planus [198]. Treatment of systemic sclerosis with IFN$\gamma$ (0.5 mg/m$^2$ or 0.1 mg/m$^2$ 3x/week/18 weeks) therapy revealed a beneficial effect on the skin involvement [199]. Local or systemic application of IFN$\gamma$ seems to be useful in treating granuloma anulare [201]. Subcutaneous administration of IFN$\alpha$ ($5 \times 10^6$ U 5x/week/9 months) resulted in a marked relief of the clinical symptoms of urticaria pigmentosa [202]. Recently reported side effects of IFN$\alpha$ therapy include Telogen effluvium and [203] bullous eruptions with pemphigus-like antibodies [204].

## REFERENCES

1. F. R. Balkwill and F. Burke, *Immunol. Today 10*, 299 (1989).
2. A. R. Green, *Lancet i*, 705 (1989).
3. S. A. Rosenberg, *Immunol. Today 9*, 58 (1988).

4. M. T. Lotze, A. E. Chang, C. A. Seipp C. Simpson, J. T. Vetto, and S. A. Rosenberg, *JAMA 256*, 3117 (1986).
5. S. A. Rosenberg, B. S. Packard, P. M. Aebersold, D. Solomon, S. L. Topalian, S. T. Toy, P. Simon, M. T. Lotze, J. C. Yang, C. A. Seipp, C. Simpson, C. Carter, S. Bock, D. Schwartzentruber, J. P. Wei, and D. E. White, *N. Engl. J. Med. 319*, 1676 (1988).
6. R. L. Kradin, D. S. Lazarus, S. M. Dubinett, J. Gifford, B. Grove, J. T. Kurnick, F. I. Preffer, C. E. Pinto, E. Davidson, R. J. Callahan, and H. W. Strauss, *Lancet i*, 577 (1989).
7. S. Rosenberg, *J. Natl. Cancer Inst. 75*, 595 (1985).
8. S. A. Rosenberg, P. Spiess, and R. Lafreniere, *Science 223*, 1318 (1986).
9. M. T. Lotze and S. A. Rosenberg, in *Progress in Allergy and Clinical Immunology* (W. J. Pichler, ed.), Hogrefe & Huber Publishers, Toronto, 1989, p. 529.
10. S. A. Rosenberg, M. T. Lotze, J. C. Yang, W. M. Linehan, C. Seipp, S. Calabro, S. E. Karp, R. M. Sherry, S. Steinberg, and D. E. White, *J. Clin. Oncol. 7*, 1863 (1989).
11. J. Atzpodien, H. Kirchner, C. R. Franks, A. Körfer, P. A. Palmer, P. Evers, and H. Poliwoda, *Insights Immunother. 1*, 47 (1990).
12. M. Masuzawa, T. Asai, K. Nishioka, and S. Nishiyama, *J. Invest. Dermatol. 93*, 563A (1989).
13. H. Spiegelberg, R. J. Falkoff, R. D. O'Connor, and L. Beck, *Clin. Exp. Immunol. 84*, 400 (1991).
14. K. M. Hsieh, C. C. Chou, and S. F. Huang, *J. Clin. Immunol. 11*, 22 (1991).
15. R. E. Lee, A. A. Gaspari, M. T. Lotze, A. E. Chang, and S. A. Rosenberg, *Arch. Dermatol. 124*, 1811 (1988).
16. B. Beutler and A. Cerami, in *Immunophysiology* (J. J. Oppenheim and E. M. Shevach, ed.), Oxford University Press, New York, 1990, p. 226.
17. A. A. Jakubowski, E. S. Caspar, J. L. Gabrilove, M. A. Templeton, S. A. Sherwin, and H. F. Oettgen, *J. Clin. Oncol. 7*, 289 (1989).
18. K. W. Zamkoff, N. B. Newman, A. R. Rudolph, J. Young, and B. J. Poiesz, *J. Biol. Response Mod. 8*, 539 (1989).
19. S. Retsas, M. Leslie, and D. Bottomley, *Br. Med. J. 298*, 1290 (1989).
20. D. Lienard, P. Ewalenko, J. J. Delmotte, N. Renard, and F. J. Lejeune, *J. Clin. Oncol. 10*, 52 (1992).
21. H. Schmidt, M. Kaufmann, G. v. Minckwitz, E. M. Grischke, G. Basterty, J. Kempini, and V. Raeth, *Eur. Cytokine Network 3*, 246 (1992).
22. H. Takematsu, H. Ozawa, T. Yoshimura, M. Hara, A. Sakakibara, J. Oyama, and H. Tagami, *Br. J. Dermatol. 124*, 209 (1991).
23. P. J. Creaven and H. L. Stoll Jr., *J. Am. Acad. Dermatol. 24*, 735 (1991).
24. Y. Ito, K. Kawamura, T. Miura, U. Kowichi, H. Onodera, H. Takahashi, S. Sugiyama, and M. Takahashi, *Arch. Dermatol. 125*, 1093 (1989).
25. R. Tsuboi, R. Morioka, H. Yaguchi, R. Shimokawa, M. Inaba, and H. Ogawa, *Br. J. Dermatol. 126*, 395 (1992).
26. D. Metcalf, *Lancet i*, 885 (1989).

27. J. Laver and M. A. S. Moore, *J. Natl. Cancer Inst. 81*, 1370 (1989).
28. G. C. Baldwin, J. C. Gasson, S. G. Quan, J. Fleischmann, R. Weisbart, D. Oette, R. T. Mitsuyasu, and D. W. Golde, *Proc. Natl. Acad. Sci. USA 85*, 2763 (1988).
29. J. E. Groopman, R. T. Mitsuyasu, M. J. DeLeo, D. H. Oette, and D. W. Golde, *N. Engl. J. Med. 317*, 593 (1987).
30. S. Miles, R. T. Mitsuyasu, J. Moreno, G. Baldwin, N. K. Alton, L. Souza, and J. Glaspy, *Blood 77*, 2109 (1991).
31. J. D. Levine, J. D. Allan, J. H. Tessitore, N. Falcone, F. Galasso, R. J. Israel, and J. E. Groopman, *Blood 78*, 2148 (1991).
32. H. S. Grossberg, E. M. Bonnem, and W. Buhlers, *N. Engl. J. Med. 320*, 1560 (1989).
33. T. M. Folks, J. Justement, A. Kinter, C. A. Dinarello, and A. S. Fauci, *Science 238*, 800 (1987).
34. Y. Koyanagi, W. A. O'Brien, J. Q. Zhao, D. W. Golde, J. C. Gasson, and I. S. Chen, *Science 241*, 1673 (1988).
35. J. M. Pluda, Y. Yarchoan, P. D. Smith, N. McAtee, L. E. Shay, D. Oette, M. Maha, S. M. Wahl, C. E. Myers, and S. Broder, *Blood 76*, 463 (1990).
36. C. F. Perno, R. Yarchoan, D. A. Cooney, N. R. Hartman, D. S. Webb, Z. Hao, H. Mitsuya, D. G. Johns, and S. Broder, *J. Exp. Med. 169*, 933 (1989).
37. S. M. Hammer and J. M. Gillis, *Antimicrob. Agents Chemother. 31*, 1046 (1987).
38. G. J. Lieschke and A. W. Burgess, *New Engl. J. Med. 327*, 99 (1992).
39. W. P. Steward, D. J. Dunlop, and J. Cassidy, *Behring Inst. Mitt. 90*, 44 (1991).
40. R. H. Weisbart, J. C. Gassons, and D. W. Golde, *Ann. Int. Med. 110*, 297 (1989).
41. G. Kaplan, G. Walsh, L. S. Guido, P. Meyn, R. A. Burkhardt, R. M. Abalos, J. Barker, P. A. Frindt, T. T. Fajardo, R. Celona, and Z. A. Cohn, *J. Exp. Med. 175*, 1717 (1992).
42. J. A. Neidhart, *Cancer 70*, 913 (1992).
43. K. Welte, C. Zeidler, A. Reiter, W. Müller, E. Odenwald, L. Souza, and H. Riehm, *Blood 75*, 1056 (1990).
44. S. D. Nimer, *Cancer 70*, 921 (1992).
45. S. J. Brandt, W. P. Peters, S. K. Atwater, J. Kurtzberg, M. J. Borowitz, R. B. Jones, E. J. Shpall, R. C. Bast, C. J. Gilbert, and D. H. Oette, *N. Engl. J. Med. 318*, 869 (1988).
46. E. J. Wing, D. M. Magee, T. L. Whiteside, S. S. Kaplan, and R. K. Shadduck, *Blood 73*, 643 (1989).
47. T. D. Horn, P. J. Burke, J. E. Karp, and A. F. Hood, *Arch. Dermatol. 127*, 49 (1991).
48. D. R. Mehregan, A. F. Fransway, J. H. Edmonson, and K. M. Leiferman, *Arch. Dermatol. 128*, 1055 (1992).
49. J. A. Glaspy, G. C. Baldwin, P. A. Robertson, L. Souza, M. Vincent, J. Ambersley, and D. W. Golde, *Ann. Intern. Med. 109*, 789 (1988).

50. W. E. Berdel, S. Danhauser-Riedl, G. Steinhauser, and E. F. Winton, *Blood 73*, 80 (1989).
51. D. Metcalf, *Cancer 65*, 2185 (1990).
52. S. Dedhar, L. Gaboury, P. Galloway, and C. Eaves, *Proc. Natl. Acad. Sci. 85*, 9253 (1988).
53. J. G. Gribben, S. Devereux, N. S. B. Thomas, M. Keim, A. H. Goldstone, and D. C. Linch, *Lancet 335*, 434 (1990).
54. R. M. Friedmann, in *Immunophysiology* (J. J. Oppenheim and E. M. Shevach, ed.), Oxford University Press, New York, 1990, p. 194.
55. R. Stadler, A. Mayer-da-Silva, B. Bratzke, C. Garbe, and C. Orfanos, *J. Am. Acad. Dermatol. 20*, 650 (1989).
56. G. J. Pazin, J. H. Harger, J. A. Armstrong, M. K. Breinig, J. R. Caplan, K. Cantell, and M. Ho, *J. Infect. Dis. 156*, 891 (1987).
57. A. Lassus, I. Bergelin, A. Paloranta, E. Rinne, A. Eskelinen, and K. Saeilae, *Sex. Transm. Dis. 14*, 185 (1987).
58. M. Ho, *J. Invest. Dermatol. 92*, 556 (1989).
59. A. E. Friedman-Kien, R. J. Klein, R. D. Glaser, and S. M. Czelusniak, *J. Am. Acad. Dermatol. 15*, 989 (1986).
60. M. Glezerman, E. Lunenfeld, V. Cohen, I. Sarov, M. Movshovitz, T. Doerner, J. Shomam, and M. Revel, *Lancet 1*, 8578 (1988).
61. J. Shupack, M. Stiller, I. Davis, C. Kenny, and L. Jondreau, *Dermatology 184*, 40 (1992).
62. M. J. Levin, F. N. Judson, L. Eron, Y. J. Bryson, L. Corey, M. Murray, and R. R. Scheer, *Antimicrob. Agents Chemother. 33*, 649 (1989).
63. T. C. Merigan, K. H. Rand, R. B. Pollard, P. S. Abdallah, G. W. Jordan, and R. P. Fried, *N. Engl. J. Med. 298*, 981 (1978).
64. G. W. Jordan, R. P. Fried, and T. C. Merigan, *J. Infect. Dis. 130*, 56 (1974).
65. T. C. Merigan, J. C. Gallagher, R. B. Pollard, and A. M. Arvin, *Antimicrob. Agents Chemother. 19*, 193 (1981).
66. K. Uyeno, H. Yasuno, and M. Niimura, *J. Invest. Dermatol. 93*, 583 (1989).
67. P. Duschet, T. Schwarz, P. Soyer, A. Henk, H. Hausmaninger, and F. Gschnait, *Int. J. Dermatol. 27*, 4 (1988).
68. G. Gross, H. Ikenberg, A. Roussaki, N. Drees, and E. Schöpf, *Chemotherapy 32*, 537 (1986).
69. J. C. Vance, B. J. Bart, R. C. Hansen, R. C. Reichman, C. McEwen, K. D. Hatch, B. Berman, and D. T. Tanner, *Arch. Dermatol. 122*, 272 (1986).
70. L. J. Eron, F. Judson, S. Tucker, S. Prawer, J. Mills, K. Murphy, M. Hickey, M. Rogers, S. Flannigan, and N. Hien, *N. Engl. J. Med. 315*, 1069 (1986).
71. R. C. Reichman, D. Oakes, W. Bonnez, C. Greisberger, S. Tyring, L. Miller, R. Whitley, H. Carveth, M. Weidner, G. Krueger, L. Yorkey, N. J. Roberts, and R. Dolin, *Ann. Intern. Med. 108*, 675 (1988).
72. G. Gross, W. Degen, M. Hilgarth, L. Kowalzick, A. Roussaki, Th. Rufli, H. Schöfer, and J. Brzoska, *J. Invest. Dermatol. 93*, 553 (1989).
73. C. C. Zouboulis, R. Stadler, and H. Ikenberg, *J. Invest. Dermatol. 93*, 586 (1989).

74. G. Gross, H. Pfister, M. Hagedorn, and R. Stahn, *Dermatologica 166*, 48 (1983).
75. G. Gross, A. Roussaki, and H. Pfister, *Curr. Probl. Dermatol. 18*, 178 (1989).
76. E. A. Olsen, F. F. Kelly, R. T. Vollmer, D. A. Buddin, and P. K. Weck, *J. Am. Acad. Dermatol. 20*, 1023 (1989).
77. G. Gross, A. Roussaki, and I. Papendick, *J. Invest. Dermatol. 95*, 152S (1990).
78. J. R. Gibson, S. G. Harvey, D. Kemmett, J. Salisbury, and P. Marks, *Br. J. Dermatol. 115*, 76 (1986).
79. M. Niimura, *J. Dermatol.* (Tokyo) *10*, 217 (1983).
80. E. J. Androphy, I. Dvoretzky, A. E. Maluish, H. J. Wallace, and D. R. Lowy, *J. Am. Acad. Dermatol. 11*, 197 (1984).
81. P. A. Bunn, D. C. Ihde, and K. A. Foon, *Int. J. Cancer 1*, 9 (1987).
82. E. A. Olsen, S. T. Rosen, R. T. Vollmer, D. Variakojis, H. H. Roenigk, N. Diab, and J. Zefren, *J. Am. Acad. Dermatol. 20*, 395 (1989).
83. E. C. Vonderheid, R. Thompson, K. A. Smiles, and A. Lattanand, *Arch. Dermatol. 123*, 757 (1987).
84. J. M. Wolff, J. A. Zitelli, B. S. Rabin, K. A. Smiles, and E. Abell, *J. Am. Acad. Dermatol. 13*, 604 (1985).
85. L. R. Braathen and N. McFadden, *J. Dermatol. Treatm. 1*, 29 (1989).
86. K. Thestrup-Pedersen, R. Hammer, K. Kaltoft, H. Sogaard, and H. Zachariae, *Br. J. Dermatol. 118*, 811 (1988).
87. R. Knobler, F. Trautinger, E. M. Kokoschka, Th. Radaszkiewicz, and M. Micksche, *J. Invest. Dermatol. 93*, 559 (1989).
88. H. H. Roenigk Jr., T. M. Kunzel, A. P. Skoutelis, E. Springer, G. Yu, W. Caro, K. Gilyon, D. Variakojs, K. Kaul, P. A. Bunn Jr, L. Evans, and S. T. Rosen, *J. Invest. Dermatol. 95*, 198S (1990).
89. A. H. Rook, B. Prystowski, M. Cassis, M. Boufal, and S. R. Lessin, *Arch. Dermatol. 127*, 1535 (1991).
90. P. A. Bunn, Jr. and D. A. Norris, *J. Invest. Dermatol. 95*, 209 (1990).
91. S. S. Legha, *Cancer 57*, 1675 (1986).
92. J. M. Kirkwood and M. S. Erstoff, *J. Invest. Dermatol. 95*, 180S (1990).
93. J. H. Schiller, J. K. V. Willson, G. Bittner, W. H. Wollberg, M. J. Hawkins, and E. C. Borden, *J. Interferon Res. 6*, 615 (1986).
94. E. T. Creagan, D. L. Ahmann, S. Frytak, H. J. Long, M. N. Chang, and L. M. Itri, *Cancer 59*, 638 (1987).
95. T. Dorval, T. Palangie, M. Jouve, E. Garcia-Giralt, L. Israel, E. Falcoff, D. Schwab, and P. Pouillart, *Cancer 58*, 215 (1986).
96. J. M. Kirkwood and M. Ernstoff, *Semin. Oncol. 12*, 7 (1985).
97. E. T. Creagan, D. L. Ahmann, H. J. Long, S. Frytak, S. A. Sherwin, and M. N. Chang, *Cancer Treat. Rep. 71*, 843 (1987).
98. M. Landthaler and O. Braun-Falco, *J. Am. Acad. Dermatol. 20*, 687 (1989).
99. J. M. Kirkwood and M. Ernstoff, *Semin. Incol. 18*, 48 (1986).
100. P. Von Wussow, F. Hartmann, M. Freund, H. Poliwoda, and H. Deicher, *Cancer 61*, 1701 (1988).
101. R. Stadler and C. Garbe, *Zschr. Hautkrkh. 65*, 504 (1990).

102. R. Rosso, M. T. Nobile, M. R. Sertoli, A. Giannitelli, P. L. Santi, R. Volpe, and G. Nicolo, *Oncology 42*, 86 (1985).
103. G. Fierlbeck, B. d'Hoedt, W. Stroebel, H. Stutte, O. Bogenschütz, and G. Rassner, *Hautarzt 43*, 16 (1992).
104. G. R. McLeod, D. B. Thomson, and P. Hersey, *J. Invest. Dermatol. 95*, 185S (1990).
105. V. C. Ho and A. J. Sober, *J. Am. Acad. Dermatol. 22*, 159 (1990).
106. G. R. C. McLeod, D. B. Thomson, and P. Hersey, *Int. J. Cancer 1*, 31 (1987).
107. S. Wadler and E. L. Schwartz, *Cancer Res. 50*, 3473 (1990).
108. C. Garbe, C. Zouboulis, S. Krüger, M. Waibel, E. D. Kreuser, R. Stadler, and C. O. Orfanos, *Hautarzt 43*, 4 (1992).
109. E. M. Kokoschka, F. Trautinger, R. M. Knobler, H. Pohl-Markl, and M. Micksche, *J. Invest. Dermatol. 95*, 193S (1990).
110. S. E. Krown, F. X. Real, S. Cunningham-Rundles, P. L. Myskowski, B. Koziner, S. Fein, A. Mittelman, H. F. Oettgen, and B. Safai, *N. Engl. J. Med. 308*, 1071 (1983).
111. J. E. Groopman, M. S. Gottlieb, J. Goodman, R. T. Mitsuyasu, M. A. Conant, H. Prince, J. L. Fahey, M. Derezin, W. M. Weinstein, and C. Casavante, *An. Intern. Med. 100*, 671 (1984).
112. F. X. Real, H. F. Oettgen, and S. E. Krown, *J. Clin. Oncol. 4*, 544 (1986).
113. H. C. Lane, J. Feinberg, V. Davey, L. Deyton, M. Baseler, J. Manischewitz, H. Masur, J. A. Kovacs, B. Herpin, R. Walker, J. A. Metcalf, N. Salzman, G. Quinnan, and A. S. Fauci, *Lancet ii*, 1218 (1988).
114. W. Rozenbaum, S. Gharakhanian, B. Cardon, M. S. Navarette, and R. De Sahb, *J. Invest. Dermatol.* 93, 574 (1989).
115. M. Alecu, G. Ghyka, F. Halalau, A. Calugaru, and G. Coman, *Med. Intern. 28*, 61 (1991).
116. M. Ribojad, L. Burradori, O. Verola, J. Zeller, A. Puissant, and P. Morel, *J. Invest. Dermatol. 95*, 176S (1990).
117. L. Wickramashinghe, T. C. Hindson, and H. Wacks, *J. Am. Acad. Dermatol. 20*, 71 (1989).
118. H. T. Greenway, R. C. Cornell, D. J. Tanner, E. Peets, G. M. Bordin, and C. Nagi, *J. Am. Acad. Dermatol. 15*, 437 (1986).
119. L. Edwards, N. Levine, M. Weidner, M. Piepkorn, and K. Smiles, *Arch. Dermatol. 122*, 779 (1986).
120. J. J. Grob, A. M. Collet, M. H. Munoz, and J. J. Bonerandi, *Lancet i*, 232 (1988).
121. R. C. Cornell, H. T. Greenway, S. B. Tucker, L. Edwards, S. Ashworth, J. C. Vance, D. J. Tanner, E. L. Taylor, K. A. Smiles, and E. A. Peets, *J. Am. Acad. Dermatol. 23*, 694 (1990).
122. L. Edwards, N. Levine, and K. A. Smiles, *J. Dermatol. Surg. Oncol. 16*, 446 (1990).
123. L. Edwards, S. B. Tucker, D. Perednia, K. A. Smiles, E. L. Taylor, D. J. Tanner, and E. Peets, *Arch. Dermatol. 126*, 1029 (1990).
124. L. Edwards, D. Whiting, D. Rogers, K. Luck, and K. A. Smiles, *J. Am. Acad. Dermatol. 22*, 496 (1990).

125. D. E. Gormley, *J. Am. Acad. Dermatol. 16*, 885 (1987).
126. B. M. Stadler, D. Gauchat, C. Vasello, N. Kazunori, G. Qui, and J. F. Gauchat, in *Cytokines Regulating the Allergic Response* (C. Sorg, ed.), Karger, Basel, 1989, p. 37.
127. U. Reinhold, W. Wehrmann, S. Kukel, and H.-W. Kreysel, *Clin. Exp. Immunol. 79*, 374 (1990).
128. J. Pene, F. Rousset, F. Briere, I. Chretien, X. Paliard, J. Banchereau, H. Spits, and J. E. De Vries, *J. Immunol. 141*, 1218 (1988).
129. U. Reinhold, W. Wehrmann, S. Kukel, and H.-W. Kreysel, *Lancet i*. 1282 (1990).
130. M. Boguniewicz, M. S. Jaffe, A. Izu, M. Sullivan, D. York, R. S. Geha, and D. Y. De Leung, *Am. J. Med. 88*, 365 (1990).
131. J. M. Hanafin, L. C. Schneider, D. Y. M. Leung, C. N. Ellis, H. S. Jaffe, A. E. Izu, L. R. Bucalo, S. E. Hirabayashi, S. J. Tofte, G. Cantu-Gonzales, H. Milgrom, M. Boguniewicz, and K. D. Cooper, *J. Am. Acad. Dermatol. 28*, 189 (1993).
132. G. Souillet, F. Rousset, and J. E. de Vries, *Lancet ii*, 1384 (1990).
133. R. M. MacKie, *Lancet i*, 1282 (1990).
134. G. Fierlbeck and G. Rassner, *Dtsch. Med. Wschr. 111*, 1313 (1986).
135. V. B. Morhenn, K. Pregerson-Rodan, R. Henzl Mullen, G. S. Wood, B. J. Nickoloff, S. A. Sherwin, and E. M. Farber, *Arch. Dermatol. 123*, 1633 (1987).
136. J. Schulze and G. Mahrle, *Lancet ii*, 926 (1986).
137. R. Neumann, H. Pohl-Markl, and E. Aberer, *Dermatologica 175*, 28 (1987).
138. J. R. Quesado and J. H. Gutterman, *Lancet ii*, 1466 (1986).
139. R. A. Knobler, *Neurology 38*, 58 (1988).
140. M. K. Peddiani, F. Savery, and L. M. Hang, *Clin. Ther. 9*, 39 (1986).
141. A. M. L. Lever, M. G. Brook, I. Yaps, and H. C. Thomas, *Br. Med. J. 295*, 1519 81987).
142. J. F. Nicolas, J. Thivolet, J. Kanitakis, and S. Lyonnet, *J. Invest. Derm. 95*, 1425 (1990).
143. G. L. Davis, L. A. Balart, E. R. Schiff, *N. Engl. J. Med.* 321, 1501 (1989).
144. M. S. Doutre, C. Beylot, P. Couzigou, P. Long, P. Royer, and P. Beylot, *Dermatology* 184, 229 (1992).
145. B. Rodrigues, M. Oliveira, A. Inock, *Nouv. Dermatol.* 8, 29 (1989).
146. B. Berman and M. R. Duncan, *J. Am. Acad. Dermatol. 21*, 694 (1989).
147. R. D. Granstein, T. J. Flotte, and E. P. Amento, *J. Invest. Dermatol. 95*, 75S (1990).
148. A. Tulli, G. Capizzi, G. Petitti, and M. Biele, *J. Invest. Dermatol. 93*, 582A (1989).
149. R. Hein, J. Behr, M. Hündgen, N. Hunzelmann, M. Meurer, O. Braun-Falco, A. Urbanski, and T. Krieg, *Br. J. Dermatol. 126*, 496 (1992).
150. D. Brouty-Boyé and B. R. Zetter, *Science 208*, 516 (1980).
151. Y. A. Sidky and E. C. Borden, *Cancer Res. 47*, 5155 (1987).
152. R. A. B. Ezekowitz, J. B. Mulliken, and J. Folkman, *N. Engl. J. Med. 326*, 1456 (1992).

153. H. Klun-Nelemans, J. H. Jansen, B. G. Wolthers, P. M. Kluin, H. M. Kroon, and R. Willemze, *N. Engl. J. Med. 326*, 619 (1992).
154. K. L. Magee, S. M. Hsu, and S. B. Tucker, *Arch. Dermatol. 126*, 760 (1990).
155. R. Stadler, B. Bratzke, and I. Baumann, *Hautarzt 38*, 97 (1987).
156. D. Tsambaos, D. Eichelberg, and M. Goos, *Arch. Dermatol. Res. 278*: 335 (1986).
157. G. Mahrle and H. J. Schulze, *J. Invest. Dermatol. 95*, 132S (1990).
158. G. Fierlbeck and G. Rassner, *J. Invest. Dermatol. 93*, 549A (1989).
159. C. F. Nathan, G. Kaplan, W. R. Lewis, A. Nusrat, M. D. Witmer, S. A. Sherwin, C. K. Job, C. R. Horowitz, R. M. Steinman, and Z. A. Cohn, *N. Engl. J. Med. 315*, 6 (1986).
160. R. Badaro, E. Falcoff, F. S. Badaro, E. M. Carvalho, D. Pedral-Sampaio, A. Barral, J. S. Carvalho, M. Barral-Netto, M. Brandely, and L. Silva, *N. Engl. J. Med.* 322, 16 (1990).
161. G. Harms, K. Zwingenberger, A. K. Chehade, S. Talhari, P. RAcz, A. Mouakeh, M. Douba, L. Nakel, R. D. Naiff, and P. G. Kremsner, *Lancet ii*, 1287 (1989).
162. G. Kolde and T. Luger, *Arch. Dermatol. Res. 284*, 20A (1991).
163. J. M. Sechler, H. L. Malech, C. J. White, and J. I. Gallin, *Proc. Natl. Acad. Sci. USA 85*, 4874 (1988).
164. T. Baba, M. Hoshino, and K. Uyeno, *Arch. Dermatol. 124*, 1015 (1988).
165. J. I. Gallin, *Clin. Immunol. Immunopathol. 61*, S100 (1991).
166. F. Cnudde, S. Gharakhanian, J. Luboinski, J. Dry, and W. Rozenbaum, *Int. J. Dermatol. 30*, 147A (1991).
167. K. C. Conlon, W. J. Urba, J. W. Smith, II, R. G. Steis, D. L. Longo, and J. W. Clark, *Cancer 65*, 2237 (1990).
168. R. G. Steis, J. W. Smith, and W. J. Urba, *N. Engl. J. Med. 318*, 1409 (1988).
169. P. Von Wussow, *J. Invest. Dermatol. 93*, 583A (1989).
170. M. D. Waterfield, *Lancet i*, 1243 (1989).
171. S. M. Wahl, M. McCartney-Francis, and M. Mergenhagen, *Immunol. Today 10*, 258 (1989).
172. K. A. Thomas, *FASEB J* 1, 4334 (1987).
173. R. Ross, *Lancet ii*, 1179 (1989).
174. M. B. Sporn and A. B. Roberts, *J. Clin. Invest. 78*, 329 (1986).
175. T. K. Hunt and F. B. LaVan, *N. Engl. J. Med. 321*, 111 (1989).
176. V. B. Morhenn, *Immunol. Today 9*, 104 (1988).
177. M. Rothe and V. Falanga, *Arch. Dermatol. 125*, 1390 (1989).
178. P. J. Phillips, O. Kehinde, H. Green, and B. A. Gilchrest, *J. Am. Acad. Dermatol. 21*, 191 (1989).
179. T. Schwarz and T. Luger, in *Pharmacology of the Skin* (H. Mukhtar, ed.), CRC Press, Boca Raton, FL, 1992, p. 283.
180. G. L. Brown, L. B. Nanney, J. Griffen, A. B. Cramer, J. M. Yancey, L. J. Curtsinger III, L. Holtzin, G. S. Schultz, M. J. Jurkiewicz, and J. B. Lynch, *N. Engl. J. Med. 321*, 76 (1989).
181. D. N. Sauder, P. L. Killian, and J. A. McLane, *Cytokine 1*, 151A (1989).

182. G. F. Pierce, T. A. Mustoe, R. M. Senior, J. Reed, G. L. Griffin, A. Thomason, and T. F. Deuel, *J. Exp. Med. 167*, 974 (1988).
183. T. A. Mustoe, G. F. Pierce, A. Thomason, P. Gramates, M. B. Sporn, and T. F. Deuel, *Science 237*, 1333 (1987).
184. G. S. McGee, J. M. Davidson, A. Buckley, A. Sommer, S. C. Woodward, A. M. Aquino, R. Barbour, and A. A. Demetriou, *J. Surg. Res. 45*, 145 (1988).
185. M. C. Robson, L. G. Phillips, J. P. Heggers, M. A. McPherson, and L. S. Heiner, *Proc. Clin. Biol. Res. 365*, 95 (1991).
186. M. Shah, D. M. Foreman, and M. W. J. Ferguson, *Lancet 339*, 213, (1992).
187. W. F. Anderson, *Science 256*, 808 (1992).
188. A. Dusty Miller, *Nature 357*, 455 (1992).
189. P. Wolkenstein, O. Chosidow, J. Wechsler, J. C. Guillaume, M. C. Lescs, M. Brandely, M. F. Avril, and J. Revuz, *J. Am. Acad. Dermatol. 28*, 66 (1993).
190. P. Tiberghien, E. Racadot, M. Deschaseaux, M. Delain, L. Voillat, M. Billot, M. Flesch, A. Rozenbaum, M. Brandely, J-Y. Cahn, and P. Herve, *Cancer 69*, 2583 (1992).
191. K. Schröder, C. Garbe, M. Waibel, H. Reupke, M. Detmar, F. Dallenbach, and C. E. Orfanos, *Hautarzt 43*, 700 (1992).
192. U. R. Hengge, N. H. Brockmeyer, and M. Goos, *Clin. Invest. 70*, 922 (1992).
193. S. P. Raychaudhuri and M. M. Fiore, *J. Am. Acad. Dermatol. 27*, 451 (1992).
194. L. Kowalzick, G. Fierlbeck, S. Jablonska, H. Mensing, W. Remy, T. Rogozinski, C. Schober, C. Stetter, and J. Brzoska, *Arch. Derm. Res. 285*, 51 (1993).
195. L. Edwards, B. Berman, R. P. Rapini, D. A. Whiting, S. Tyring, H. T. Greenway, Jr., S. P. Eyre, D. J. Tanner, E. L. Taylor, and K. A. Smiles, *Arch. Dermatol. 128*, 1486 (1992).
196. R. Dummer, J. C. Becker, B. Boser, A. A. Hartmann, and G. Burg, *Arch. Dermatol. 128*, 1127 (1992).
197. P. Plantin, P. Milochau, J. P. Leroy, C. Berthou, L. Sensebe, J. F. Abgrall, and G. Guillet, *Ann. Dermatol. Venerol. 119*, 643 (1992).
198. L. Engelmann and J. Kunze, *Arch. Derm. Res. 284*, 20 (1992).
199. B. Freundlich, S. A. Jimeney, V. D. Steen, T. A. Medsger, Jr., M. Szkolnicki, and H. S. Jaffe, *Arthrit. Rheumat. 35*, 1134 (1992).
200. J. C. Simon, R. Niedner, and E. Schöpf, *Arch. Derm. Res. 285*, 51 (1993).
201. C. Müller, D. Abeck, H. Bildau, and H. Mensing, *Arch. Derm. Res. 285*, 51 (1993).
202. G. Kolde, C. Sunderkötter, and T. A. Luger, *J. Amer. Acad. Dermatol.* in press (1993).
203. A. Tosti, C. Misciali, F. Bardazzi, P. A. Fanti, and C. Varotti, *Dermatol. 184*, 124 (1992).
204. A. Parodi, M. Semino, and R. Gallo, *Dermatol. 186*, 155 (1993).

# Index

# About the Editors

THOMAS A. LUGER is Director and Chairman of the Department of Dermatology at the Ludwig Boltzmann Institute for Cell Biology and Immunobiology of the Skin, University of Münster, Germany. The author or coauthor of over 190 book chapters and professional papers, he is a member of the Society for Investigative Dermatology, the American Academy of Dermatology, and the American Federation for Clinical Research, among other organizations, and serves as Editor of the journal *Experimental Dermatology*, and on the editorial boards of eight other journals. Dr. Luger received the M.D. degree (1975) from the University of Vienna, Austria.

THOMAS SCHWARZ is Professor of Dermatology and Head of the Division of Photobiology and Phototherapy in the Department of Dermatology at the Ludwig Boltzmann Institute for Cell Biology and Immunobiology of the Skin, University of Münster, Germany. A member of the American Academy of Dermatology, the Society for Investigative Dermatology, and the American Association of Immunologists, among other organizations, and an Associate Editor of the journal *Experimental Dermatology*, he is the author or coauthor of more than 90 professional papers and book chapters. Dr. Schwarz received the M.D. degree (1980) from the University of Vienna, Austria.